Recent Progress in HIV Research

Recent Progress in HIV Research

Editor: Anabella Frost

hayle medical
New York

Hayle Medical,
750 Third Avenue, 9th Floor,
New York, NY 10017, USA

Visit us on the World Wide Web at:
www.haylemedical.com

ISBN 978-1-64647-569-8 (Hardback)

Cataloging-in-Publication Data

Recent progress in HIV research / edited by Anabella Frost.
p. cm.
Includes bibliographical references and index.
ISBN 978-1-64647-569-8
1. HIV infections. 2. AIDS (Disease). 3. HIV infections--Research.
4. AIDS (Disease)--Research. I. Frost, Anabella.
RC606.6 .R43 2023
616.979 2--dc23

Contents

Preface

HIV is a virus that severely affects the immune system resulting in acquired immunodeficiency syndrome (AIDS). The treatment of HIV involves combination antiretroviral therapy (cART). This therapy suppresses HIV-1 replication, blocks transmission, and improves immune responses. cART is a lifelong treatment, and does not eliminate the virus while also having side effects. The focus in the treatment of HIV is the reactivation of HIV reservoirs for subsequent termination by viral cytopathic effects or host immunity. The most researched HIV reservoir is resting memory CD4+ T cells in peripheral blood and lymphoid tissues. The antiretroviral therapies have expanded significantly in the recent times and comprise five categories of antiretrovirals, including nucleoside reverse transcriptase inhibitors (NRTIs), protease inhibitors, non-nucleoside reverse transcriptase inhibitors (NNRTIs), integrase strand transfer inhibitors (INSTIs) and entry inhibitors. This book unfolds the innovative aspects of HIV research which will be crucial for the progress of this field in the future. For someone with an interest and eye for detail, this book covers the most significant topics on HIV-AIDS and its treatment.

The information shared in this book is based on empirical researches made by veterans in this field of study. The elaborative information provided in this book will help the readers further their scope of knowledge leading to advancements in this field.

Finally, I would like to thank my fellow researchers who gave constructive feedback and my family members who supported me at every step of my research.

Editor

1

Current Status of Latency Reversing Agents Facing the Heterogeneity of HIV-1 Cellular and Tissue Reservoirs

Amina Ait-Ammar[1†], Anna Kula[2†], Gilles Darcis[3], Roxane Verdikt[1], Stephane De Wit[4], Virginie Gautier[5], Patrick W. G. Mallon[5], Alessandro Marcello[6], Olivier Rohr[7] and Carine Van Lint[1]*

[1] *Service of Molecular Virology, Department of Molecular Virology (DBM), Université Libre de Bruxelles (ULB), Gosselies, Belgium,* [2] *Malopolska Centre of Biotechnology, Laboratory of Virology, Jagiellonian University, Krakow, Poland,* [3] *Infectious Diseases Department, Liège University Hospital, Liège, Belgium,* [4] *Service des Maladies Infectieuses, CHU Saint-Pierre, Université Libre de Bruxelles, Bruxelles, Belgium,* [5] *UCD Centre for Experimental Pathogen Host Research (CEPHR), School of Medicine, University College Dublin, Dublin, Ireland,* [6] *Laboratory of Molecular Virology, International Centre for Genetic Engineering and Biotechnology (ICGEB), Trieste, Italy,* [7] *Université de Strasbourg, EA7292, FMTS, IUT Louis Pasteur, Schiltigheim, France*

***Correspondence:**
Carine Van Lint
cvlint@ulb.ac.be

† These authors have contributed equally to this work

One of the most explored therapeutic approaches aimed at eradicating HIV-1 reservoirs is the "shock and kill" strategy which is based on HIV-1 reactivation in latently-infected cells ("shock" phase) while maintaining antiretroviral therapy (ART) in order to prevent spreading of the infection by the neosynthesized virus. This kind of strategy allows for the "kill" phase, during which latently-infected cells die from viral cytopathic effects or from host cytolytic effector mechanisms following viral reactivation. Several latency reversing agents (LRAs) with distinct mechanistic classes have been characterized to reactivate HIV-1 viral gene expression. Some LRAs have been tested in terms of their potential to purge latent HIV-1 *in vivo* in clinical trials, showing that reversing HIV-1 latency is possible. However, LRAs alone have failed to reduce the size of the viral reservoirs. Together with the inability of the immune system to clear the LRA-activated reservoirs and the lack of specificity of these LRAs, the heterogeneity of the reservoirs largely contributes to the limited success of clinical trials using LRAs. Indeed, HIV-1 latency is established in numerous cell types that are characterized by distinct phenotypes and metabolic properties, and these are influenced by patient history. Hence, the silencing mechanisms of HIV-1 gene expression in these cellular and tissue reservoirs need to be better understood to rationally improve this cure strategy and hopefully reach clinical success.

Keywords: HIV-1, latency reversing agents, cure, latency, reservoirs, heterogeneity

INTRODUCTION

Approximately, 36.9 million people in the world are living with HIV, while there were 33.3 million in 2010, showing that HIV is still a global public health problem (UNAIDS 2018).

The development of ART has allowed the suppression of virus replication to undetectable levels. Thus, ART reduces HIV-associated morbidity, prolongs survival, prevents transmission, and results in a partial reconstitution of the immune system, as measured by an increase in circulating CD4$^+$ T cells. However, ART can cause cumulative toxic effects with the emergence of HIV-1 drug-resistant variants (Hu and Kuritzkes, 2014). Moreover, ART is unable to achieve complete virus eradication since it targets only actively replicating virus, and as such, treatment needs to be taken life-long. The main barrier to an HIV cure is the formation of stable reservoirs of latent HIV-1 that are defined as a cell type or an anatomical site in which integrated proviruses persist (Eisele and Siliciano, 2012). The latent reservoirs are highly heterogeneous and composed of multiple cell types, such as macrophages, but the best-characterized ones are a small population of HIV-1-infected memory CD4$^+$ T cells. In addition to cellular reservoirs, GALT, CNS, genital tract, and lymph nodes are the main anatomical reservoirs of HIV-1 (Coombs et al., 2003; Gras and Kaul, 2010; Yukl et al., 2013). The role of the respiratory tract (Cribbs et al., 2015), liver (Penton and Blackard, 2014), kidney (Winston et al., 2001), and adipose tissue (Couturier et al., 2015) as HIV-1 reservoirs is also gaining importance. Moreover, an anatomical site in which ART penetration is limited (called a sanctuary) or a site which is immune-privileged (such as B cell follicular centers within lymph nodes, testis, and the brain) may allow for residual replication contributing to viral persistence (Connick et al., 2007; Chomont et al., 2009; Buzón et al., 2011; Eisele and Siliciano, 2012; Fletcher et al., 2014). Together, these reservoirs can be induced to actively produce viruses by various cellular stimuli and therefore represent one potential source of rebound of viremia after ART interruption (Chun et al., 1997; Davey et al., 1999; Beliakova-Bethell et al., 2017; Ganor et al., 2019).

Viruses have developed different mechanisms to escape the host immune system. In addition to the rapid evolution of viral variants, the establishment of viral latency in the infected cells is one of these mechanisms (Deng et al., 2015). Latently-infected cells contain stably-integrated, replication-competent proviruses repressed by a plethora of silencing mechanisms operating at the transcriptional and post-transcriptional levels. The number of latently-infected cells carrying replication-competent proviruses is extremely low with a majority of defective proviruses (Ho et al., 2013; Bruner et al., 2016, 2019). Significant progress has been made in the development of various therapeutic approaches that target HIV-1 and prevent disease progression. Currently, two strategies are under investigation in order to reach long-term control of viral replication in the absence of ART: the first strategy is aiming at achieving a sterilizing cure (i.e., a total elimination of the virus from the human body), whereas the second is a functional cure (i.e., a remission or long-term control of HIV-1 in the absence of ART, without loss of CD4$^+$ T cells, no clinical progression, lack of HIV-1 transmission, and a reduction of the size of the reservoirs). Given the difficulty of achieving a sterilizing cure, one specific approach for a functional cure, called the "shock and kill" strategy, has become one of the major focus of attention (Thorlund et al., 2017). However, it now appears that the main barrier to reaching success with this "shock and kill" strategy is the heterogeneity of the latent HIV-1 reservoirs that is reflected by the diversity of infected cell types residing in the blood and in the different tissues and by the complexity of the molecular mechanisms governing latency and most likely differing from one cell to the other.

The present review will discuss the heterogeneity of the HIV-1 reservoirs that has been highlighted by studies using LRAs. We will describe the determinants responsible for these heterogeneous responses to LRAs, including the diversity of cell types composing the reservoirs (their origin, their differentiation, and their activation state). We will briefly present the multiple molecular mechanisms governing latency, the HIV-1 diversity within the latent and reactivated reservoirs, the patient-to-patient and cellular variations in response to LRAs. Finally, we will discuss why a better understanding of these elements is crucial for reaching an HIV-cure.

Abbreviations: 5-AzaC, 5-azacytidine; 5-azadC, 5-aza-2′deoxycytidine; 5′LTR, 5′ Long Terminal Repeat; 7SK snRNP, 7SK small nuclear ribonucleoprotein; APOBEC3A, Apolipoprotein B mRNA editing enzyme, catalytic polypeptide-like 3 A; ART, Antiretroviral therapy; ASP, Antisense protein; BETis, Bromodomain and Extraterminal (BET) bromodomain inhibitors; B-HIVE, Barcoded HIV ensembles; CA-US, Cell associated unspliced; CCR5/6/7, CC chemokine receptor 6/7; CGi, CpG island; CSF, Cerebrospinal fluid; CTIP2, COUP-TF (Chicken Ovalbumin Upstream Promoter Transcription Factor)-Interacting Protein 2; CXCR3/5, C-X-C Chemokine Receptor3/5; CNS, central nervous system; DCs, dendritic cells; DNA, Deoxyribonucleic acid; DNMT, DNA methyl-transferase; DSIF, DRB (5,6-dichloro-1-beta-D-ribofuranosylbenzimidazole) Sensitivity Inducing Factor; EDITS, Envelope Detection by Induced Transcription-based Sequencing; ESE_{tat}, Exonic Splice Enhancer tat; ESR-1, Estrogen receptor-1; EZH2, Enhancer Of Zeste 2 Polycomb Repressive Complex 2 Subunit; fDCs, follicular dendritic cells; GALT, Gut-Associated Lymphoid Tissue; HDAC, histone deacetylase; HIV, human immunodeficiency virus; HLA-DR, Human Leukocyte Antigen – DR isotype; HMBA, Hexamethylene bisacetamide; HP1, heterochromatin Protein 1; HSCs, hematopoietic Stem Cells; IL-2/4/7/15, Interleukin 2/4/7/15; ITIM, Immunoreceptor Tyrosine-based Inhibitory Motif; KAP1, KRAB (Krüppel-Associated Box) domain-Associated Protein 1; LAG-3, Lymphocyte Activation Gene-3; LARA, latency and reversion assay; lncRNA, Long non-coding RNA; LRA, latency-reversing agents; MAPK, mitogen-activated protein kinase; MATR3, Matrin 3; mDCs, myeloid dendritic cells; miRNA, Micro ribonucleic acid; MMQO, 8-methoxy-6-methylquinolin-4-ol; Nef, negative regulatory factor; NELF, Negative Elongation Factor; NFAT, Nuclear Factor of Activated T-cells; NF-κB, Nuclear Factor-kB; PBMCs, peripheral blood mononuclear cells; PCAF, p300/CBP (CREB Binding Protein)-Associated Factor; PD-1, programmed cell death-1; PHA, phytohemagglutinin; PMA, phorbol myristate acetate; PML, promyelocytic leukemia protein; PRC2, polycomb repressive complex 2; PSF, polypyrimidine tract-binding protein associated splicing factor; PTB, Polypyrimidine Tract Binding protein; P-TEFb, Positive Transcription Elongation Factor b; qPCR, Quantitative polymerase chain reaction; QVOA, quantitative viral outgrowth assays; Rev, regulator of virion expression; RNA, ribonucleic acid; RNAPII, RNA polymerase II; RT-ddPCR, teverse transcription droplet digital PCR; SAHA, suberoylanilide hydroxamic acid; SIV, simian immunodeficiency virus; SMAC, second mitochondrial activator of caspases; SMYD2, SET (Suppressor of variegation, Enhancer of Zeste, Trithorax) and MYND (Myeloid-Nervy-DEAF1) domain-containing protein 2; Sp1, specificity protein 1; STAT5, signal transducer and activator of transcription 5; Suv39H1, Suppressor of variegation 3-9 homolog 1; TAR, transactivation response element; Tat, transactivator of transcription; T_{CM}, central memory CD4$^+$ T cells; TCR, T Cell Receptor; T_{EM}, effector memory CD4$^+$ T cells; T_{fh}, T follicular helper cells; Th17, T helper cells 17; TIGIT, T-cell immunoreceptor with Ig ITIM domains; Tim-3, T cell immunoglobulin and mucin 3; TILDA, Tat/rev-induced limiting dilution assay; T_N, Naïve CD4$^+$ T cells; TNFα, tumor necrosis factor alpha; T_{reg}, Regulatory CD4$^+$ T cells; TRIM19, Tripartite Motif 19/22; TSA, trichostatin A; T_{SCM}, stem cell-like memory CD4$^+$ T cells; TSS, transcription start site; T_{TD}, terminally differentiated CD4$^+$ T cells; T_{TM}, Transitional memory CD4$^+$ T cells; UNAIDS, United Nations Programme on HIV and AIDS; UPF-1, up-frameshift protein 1.

HETEROGENEOUS COMPOSITION OF HIV-1 RESERVOIRS

$CD4^+$ T Cell Reservoirs

HIV-1 infects subsets of $CD4^+$ T lymphocytes, leading either to productively-infected cells or, rarely, to latently-infected cells. HIV-1 infected $CD4^+$ T cells can be distinguished either by their state of differentiation, by their function, or by the markers they express on their surface.

$CD4^+$ T Cell Differentiation Subsets

$CD4^+$ T cells infected with HIV-1 can be grouped by their state of differentiation into naive T cells (T_N, $CD45RA^+$, $CD62L^+$, and $CD95^-$) and memory $CD4^+$ T cells, which can be further divided into four subpopulations: central memory T cells (T_{CM}, $CD45RA^-$, $CCR7^+$, and $CD27^+$), effector memory T cells (T_{EM}, $CD45RA^-$, $CCR7^-$, and $CD27^-$), transitional memory T cells (T_{TM}, $CD45RA^-$, $CCR7^-$, and $CD27^+$), and stem cell-like memory T cells (T_{SCM}, $CD45RA^+$, $CCR7^+$, $CD27^+$, and $CD95^+$). T_N cells that are more resistant to HIV-1 infection than memory $CD4^+$ T cells and as such contain lower levels of HIV-1 DNA (Venanzi Rullo et al., 2019), produce as many virions (Zerbato et al., 2019) or greater (Venanzi Rullo et al., 2019) amount of replication-competent HIV-1 than the memory $CD4^+$ T cells following latency reversal with LRAs, indicating that T_N cells are an important reservoir of latent HIV-1. Moreover, the total proportion of T_N increases under ART regimen compared to memory T cells (Wightman et al., 2010). However, clonal expansion is more frequently observed in memory than in T_N cells, thus contributing to HIV-1 persistence (von Stockenstrom et al., 2015). Indeed, homeostatic proliferation driving clonal expansion has been evidenced by pioneering work of Chomont et al. (2009) that identified T_{CM} and T_{TM} as the main reservoir for HIV-1 infection. These two major subgroups are a more stable reservoir for HIV-1 than T_{EM} which are short-lived and, unlike T_{CM} and T_{TM}, express markers of activation (HLA-DR) (Pardons et al., 2019) and might be more sensitive to programmed cell death (Riou et al., 2007; Chomont et al., 2009; Cockerham et al., 2014). It has been previously shown by the group of Sarah Palmer that T_{EM} which are in an activation state carry the highest number of intact proviruses compared to T_{CM}, T_{TM}, and T_N (Hiener et al., 2017). This finding suggests that the resting phenotype of $CD4^+$ T cells (i.e., characterized by no expression of activation markers) is not a prerequisite for latent infection. These differences could be explained by patient-specific variations related to the duration of infection before ART initiation or to the duration of ART. Moreover, some evidence supports the theory that HIV-1 can establish latent infection in actively replicating $CD4^+$ T cells, suggesting that HIV-1 infection of both resting and activated primary $CD4^+$ T cells could result in latency (Chavez et al., 2015). The T_{TD}, corresponding to aged T-cell populations that reflect HIV-1 disease progression (Cao et al., 2009) and in which integrated HIV-1 DNA is also detected, are a very small reservoir with a reduced frequency in HIV-1 individuals under suppressive ART and improved $CD4^+$ T cell counts (Chomont et al., 2009; Behrens et al., 2018). Finally, T_{SCM} are permissive to HIV-1 infection and contribute to its persistence by their capacity of self-renewal and prolonged survival rate. The proportion of viral DNA associated with these T_{SCM} cells is higher than in T_{CM}. Although T_{SCM} are latently-infected, they represent only a small fraction of the total reservoir (Gattinoni et al., 2011; Buzon et al., 2014).

$CD4^+$ T Cell Functional Subsets

Different $CD4^+$ T cell subsets that are generated from T_N were shown to be HIV-1 infected. For instance, resting $CD4^+CD25^+$ T_{reg} were found to be sensitive to HIV-1 infection acting as a viral reservoir in patients under long ART (Tran et al., 2008). These cells are characterized by a lesser response to T cell activation which limits virus expression and inhibits $CD8^+$ T-cell cytotoxic function (Tran et al., 2008; Pardons et al., 2019). Additionally, the gamma-delta T cells (γδ T) which represent approximately 2 to 10% of total circulating $CD3^+$ T lymphocytes and whose majority express TCR from Vδ2 variable regions (hereafter referred as Vδ2 cells), are classified as memory cells according to the expression of CD45RO and CD27 markers (Miyawaki et al., 1990). These Vδ2 cells have been documented to be productively infected and depleted upon HIV-1 infection (Li and Pauza, 2011). More recently, it has been demonstrated that Vδ2 cells in ART-treated patients with complete suppression of HIV-1 plasma viremia harbor latent HIV-1 that can replicate following *ex vivo* stimulation indicating that peripheral Vδ2 T cells are a potential HIV-1 reservoir (Soriano-Sarabia et al., 2015). Also, Th17 $CCR6^+$ memory $CD4^+$ T-cell subsets in the blood and colon are long-lived cells that act as HIV-1 reservoirs during ART (Gosselin et al., 2010, 2017; Pardons et al., 2019). In addition, T follicular helper cells (T_{fh}) from the germinal center and peripheral blood (pT_{fh}) are highly susceptible to HIV-1 infection holding replication-competent virus and serve as reservoirs during ART (Perreau et al., 2013; Pallikkuth et al., 2015; Kohler et al., 2016; Pardons et al., 2019). These cells are characterized by surface expression of CXCR5 and PD-1, reside in the lymph node follicles in immediate anatomical proximity to B cells, and support the germinal center reaction essential for the generation of effective humoral immunity. Notably, the group of Matthieu Perreau, by investigating lymph node T_{fh} (expressing CXCR5 and PD-1) and pT_{fh} (expressing CXCR3), has shown that these subpopulations are the major sources of infectious replication-competent HIV-1 (Banga et al., 2016b, 2018).

Very recently, resident memory $CD4^+$ T cells (T_{RM}), present in tissues such as the lower female genital tract has been described as a critical HIV-1 reservoir in cervical mucosa (Cantero-Pérez et al., 2019). Interestingly, cervical tissues from aviremic ART-treated HIV-1 infected woman contained higher viral DNA content compared to blood samples and showed that $CD4^+$ T_{RM} harboring viral DNA and viral RNA are the main contributors to this reservoir.

Markers of Latently-Infected $CD4^+$ T Cells

Studies investigating the role in latency of activation markers such as HLA-DR and immune checkpoint molecules (i.e., PD-1, LAG-3, TIGIT and Tim-3) have indicated that these markers are preferentially expressed at the surface of memory

CD4$^+$ T cells (T_{CM} and T_{TM}) harboring latent HIV-1 provirus (Fromentin et al., 2016; Evans et al., 2018; Pardons et al., 2019). Although several studies, including those carried on SIV-infected macaques, have demonstrated that cells expressing these markers carry latent, replication-competent integrated viral DNA (Chomont et al., 2009; Hurst et al., 2015; Banga et al., 2016b; Fromentin et al., 2016; McGary et al., 2017), the replication competence of the integrated proviruses and the contribution of the cells bearing these markers to the latent reservoir still need to be fully elucidated.

Recently, the expression of CD32a has been reported as a potential marker of memory CD4$^+$ T cells harboring a replication-competent latent virus in aviremic patients under ART (Descours et al., 2017; Darcis et al., 2019). The role of CD32a as a cellular marker of HIV-1 reservoirs has been the subject of several works (Abdel-Mohsen et al., 2018; Martin et al., 2018; Osuna et al., 2018; Thornhill et al., 2019). A complete study presented at CROI by Darcis et al. (CROI 2019, Poster 346 - CD32$^+$ CD4$^+$ T cells are enriched in HIV-1 DNA) showed that active CD4$^+$ T cells co-expressing HLA-DR and CD32a are highly enriched with HIV-1 DNA.

The integrin $\alpha4\beta7$ has been shown on a T cell subset that is highly susceptible to HIV-1 infection (Cicala et al., 2009; Sivro et al., 2018). Moreover, the integrin $\alpha4\beta1$ was shown to be expressed by more than 70% of infected cells both in untreated and ART-suppressed individuals (Pardons et al., 2019). Integrins mediate the adhesion and transendothelial migration of lymphocytes facilitating their homing to GALT (for $\alpha4\beta7$) and to the inflamed central nervous system/bone marrow (for $\alpha4\beta1$) suggesting a role in HIV-1 persistence by enhancing T cell expansion.

In addition, high levels of CD2 receptor expression on latently infected resting memory CD4$^+$ T cells in virally suppressed HIV-1-infected subjects has been also identified (Iglesias-Ussel et al., 2013). Moreover, CD30 receptor was identified on transcriptionally active CD4$^+$ lymphocytes in individuals on suppressive ART suggesting that it might be a marker of residual, transcriptionally active HIV-1 infected cells in the setting of suppressive ART (Hogan et al., 2018). Last but not least, very recently the B lymphocyte antigen CD20 has also been identified as a marker of transcriptionally-active HIV-infected cells (Serra-Peinado et al., 2019).

Non-T Cell Reservoirs

Even though memory CD4$^+$ T cells are a long-term cellular reservoir for HIV-1, they are not the only source of viral rebound during treatment interruption. Macrophages, DCs, and tissue macrophages, such as microglial cells, are part of the viral reservoir (Kumar et al., 2014; Kandathil et al., 2016; Honeycutt et al., 2017; Schwartz et al., 2019).

Indeed, overwhelming evidence supports the notion that tissues, such as the CNS (Canestri et al., 2010; Gras and Kaul, 2010), lymph nodes (Sewald et al., 2015), testes (Darcis et al., 2016; Jenabian et al., 2016), gut (Yukl et al., 2013), genital tract (Iversen et al., 2004; Marcelin et al., 2008; Sheth et al., 2009), and lungs (Costiniuk and Jenabian, 2014), serve as HIV-1 sanctuaries that counteract viral eradication. In this regard, the group of Morgane Bomsel has recently reported that urethral tissue macrophages expressing IL-1 receptor, CD206, and IL-4 receptor, but not CD163, constitute a replication-competent HIV-1 reservoir (Ganor et al., 2019). Importantly, lipopolysaccharides specifically reactivate the production of replication-competent infectious proviruses from these tissue macrophages (Ganor et al., 2019).

In the case of circulating monocytes, they are more resistant to HIV-1 infection and their contribution as a viral reservoir is controversial and remains debatable. Monocytes have been proposed as a vehicle of HIV-1 dissemination throughout the body upon their entry in tissues where they differentiate into macrophages. Especially, due to their ability to cross the blood-tissue barrier, monocytes consequently, spread the infection into sanctuaries such as the brain (Pulliam et al., 1997; Valcour et al., 2009, 2010, 2013; Williams et al., 2014). These characteristics indicated the monocytes as an important viral reservoir. However, even if several studies have reported persistent infection of monocytes in ART treated individuals (Lambotte et al., 2000; Sonza et al., 2001; Gibellini et al., 2008), others failed to detect HIV-1 in circulating monocytes (Almodóvar et al., 2007). A recent work from the group of Nicolas Chomont indicated that monocyte infection is infrequent, and they highlighted the importance of using flow cytometry cell-sorting to minimize contamination by CD4$^+$ T cells (Massanella et al., 2019).

Follicular dendritic cells (fDCs) in lymphoid tissues specialized in the trapping and retention of antigens in the form of immune complexes on their surface, including HIV-1 virions, can serve as a potential viral reservoir (Smith et al., 2001). Using specific and sensitive next-generation *in situ* hybridization approach, Deleage et al. (2016) documented the importance of B cell follicles in active, latent, and persistent infections by analyzing lymphoid tissues from macaques prior to and during ART. These fDCs could thus transfer the virus to T cells present in the follicles of secondary lymphoid organs (Heesters et al., 2015). In addition, myeloid dendritic cells (mDCs) located in the lymph nodes may support a very low level of viral replication and have a role in HIV-1 latency (Shen et al., 2014). However, the mechanism of viral persistence in these cells is not yet clearly understood [reviewed in Kandathil et al. (2016)].

Viral DNA has also been detected in hematopoietic stem cells (HSCs) from ART-treated patients, which could demonstrate their involvement in HIV-1 persistence (Sebastian et al., 2017; Zaikos et al., 2018). Despite the limited infection and detection of HSCs in a subset of patients (McNamara et al., 2013), their role as a viral reservoir may be crucial. Finally, HIV-1 can infect kidney allografts after transplantation despite undetectable viremia thereby suggesting that podocytes can serve as viral reservoirs and revealing once again the heterogeneous composition of the HIV-1 reservoir (Canaud et al., 2014).

In conclusion, multiple cell subsets being present at various cellular differentiation states, either resting or activated, can serve as HIV-1 reservoir. All these cells contribute to the complexity and heterogeneity of the reservoirs of latent HIV-1. It is very likely that different molecular mechanisms of latency establishment and persistence are involved in different latently-infected cell types and even may vary among cells of the same lineage.

COMPLEXITY OF MOLECULAR MECHANISMS REGULATING HIV-1 LATENCY

It is well established that repression of HIV-1 expression is mediated through a plethora of molecular mechanisms both for the establishment and for the maintenance of post-integration latency (summarized in **Figure 1**). In fact, HIV-1 latency is a multifactorial phenomenon, controlled by several interlinked mechanisms operating at the transcriptional and post-transcriptional levels [reviewed in Van Lint et al., 2013)] and influenced by the transcriptional program of the host cell (Bradley et al., 2018). For instance, some studies have suggested that HIV-1 viral latency is related to the integration site and orientation of the provirus (Greger et al., 1998; Han et al., 2008; Lenasi et al., 2008; Chen et al., 2017; Einkauf et al., 2019). HIV-1 integration seems random but favors the introns of transcriptionally-active genes located in gene dense regions in the outer shell of the nucleus close to the nuclear pores (Schröder et al., 2002; Han et al., 2004; Marini et al., 2015; Singh et al., 2015; Chen et al., 2017). The importance of transcriptional interference as a mechanism suppressing the expression of the integrated provirus (including steric hindrance, convergent transcription, and enhancer trapping) has also been proposed (Greger et al., 1998; Han et al., 2008; Lenasi et al., 2008) [reviewed in Colin and Van Lint (2009)].

Moreover, during latency, the HIV-1 promoter is heavily controlled by epigenetic mechanisms, including DNA methylation (Blazkova et al., 2009; Kauder et al., 2009; Chávez et al., 2011) and histone post-translational modifications, such as histone acetylation (Lusic et al., 2003; Jiang et al., 2007; Tyagi and Karn, 2007; Li et al., 2018), methylation (du Chéné et al., 2007; Marban et al., 2007; Imai et al., 2010; Friedman et al., 2011; Ding et al., 2013; Tchasovnikarova et al., 2015, 2017; Boehm et al., 2017; Nguyen et al., 2017; Zhang et al., 2017; Huang et al., 2019), and crotonylation (Jiang et al., 2018). The degree of DNA methylation on the HIV-1 promoter was long considered controversial due to conflicting observations in patients (Blazkova et al., 2009, 2012; Kauder et al., 2009; Ho et al., 2013; Weber et al., 2014). However, this heterogeneity in promoter methylation profile between patients has now been explained by the duration of the infection (Palacios et al., 2012) and/or the duration of ART therapy (Trejbalová et al., 2016) which impacts the accumulation of cytosine methylation on the 5′LTR. Still, the exact mechanisms of this DNA methylation accumulation in the latent reservoir of HIV-1-infected individuals remain unclear.

Additionally, an antisense transcript originating from the 3′LTR (named the *ASP* RNA) (Zapata et al., 2017) was recently shown to recruit the PRC2 repressor complex to the HIV-1 5′LTR, increasing the repressive epigenetic mark H3K27me3 while reducing RNAPII occupancy at the viral promoter and promoting the establishment and maintenance of HIV-1 latency at the epigenetic level (Zapata et al., 2017). An HIV-encoded antisense long non-coding RNA directs the same epigenetic silencing mechanisms by recruiting and guiding chromatin-remodeling complex consisting of proteins such as DNMT3a, EZH2, and HDAC-1 to the viral promoter leading to transcriptional HIV-1 latency (Saayman et al., 2014).

HIV-1 latency is also associated with poor availability of transcriptional activating factors including NF-κB, NFAT, and STAT5 due to their cytoplasmic sequestration (Williams et al., 2006; Della Chiara et al., 2011; Hakre et al., 2012; Bosque et al., 2017) and with a low expression level of the viral transactivator Tat (Burnett et al., 2009; Weinberger et al., 2005). The interaction of the cellular transcriptional cofactor CTIP2 with HP1α is involved in the relocation of Tat to transcriptionally inactive regions of the chromatin (Rohr et al., 2003). However, HIV-1 counteracts CTIP2 mediated-repression by promoting its degradation by the HIV-1 accessory protein Vpr (Forouzanfar et al., 2019). Another recent finding has revealed that APOBEC3A, the restriction factor that suppresses HIV-1 infection in macrophages, maintains HIV-1 latency by recruiting KAP1 and HP1 inducing repressive histone marks (Taura et al., 2019). In addition, the importance of TRIM22, known to inhibit the binding of Sp1 to the 5′LTR promoter (Turrini et al., 2015) and to colocalize with HIV-1 transcriptional repressors TRIM19/PML (Forlani et al., 2017), contributes to the maintenance of HIV-1 latency (Turrini et al., 2019).

During latency and even after transcription initiation, the RNAPII is paused during early elongation, constraining its processivity and resulting in repression of HIV-1 gene expression (Adams et al., 1994). RNAPII terminates prematurely and accumulates at specific positions of the HIV-1 promoter that overlap with the position of the repressive nucleosome nuc-1, positioned in the 5′LTR just after the TAR region, inducing a block of transcriptional elongation (Verdin et al., 1993). This inhibition of HIV-1 transcription elongation is regulated by the binding of negative factors such as NELF and DSIF to the RNAPII (Yamaguchi et al., 1999; Jadlowsky et al., 2014) and by the limited availability of the cellular transcription factor P-TEFb due to its sequestration by the 7SK snRNP complex (Nguyen et al., 2001; Yang et al., 2001; Cherrier et al., 2013; Eilebrecht et al., 2014). P-TEFb is composed of CyclinT1 and CDK9 and requires the CDK9 Thr-186 phosphorylation for its activity to mediate the phosphorylation of the C-terminal domain of the paused RNAPII antagonizing its negatives factors (Wei et al., 1998; Ramakrishnan et al., 2009). The level of CDK9 phosphorylation has been found to be lower in resting $CD4^+$ T cells harboring latent HIV-1 (Budhiraja et al., 2013; Ramakrishnan et al., 2015). Furthermore, CTIP2 binds to the 7SK snRNP complex to inhibit P-TEFb and HIV-1 transcription in microglial cells (Cherrier et al., 2013; Eilebrecht et al., 2014).

Abortive TAR transcripts have been reported even during transcriptional elongation block (Adams et al., 1994; Core and Lis, 2008; Kaiser et al., 2017). In a very elegant manner, the group of Steven Yukl has evidenced that multiple blocks to transcription and even to splicing and export exist in patient cells. They developed a panel of RT-ddPCR assays to measure at the same time different HIV-1 transcripts (Telwatte et al., 2018; Yukl et al., 2018) in patient-derived

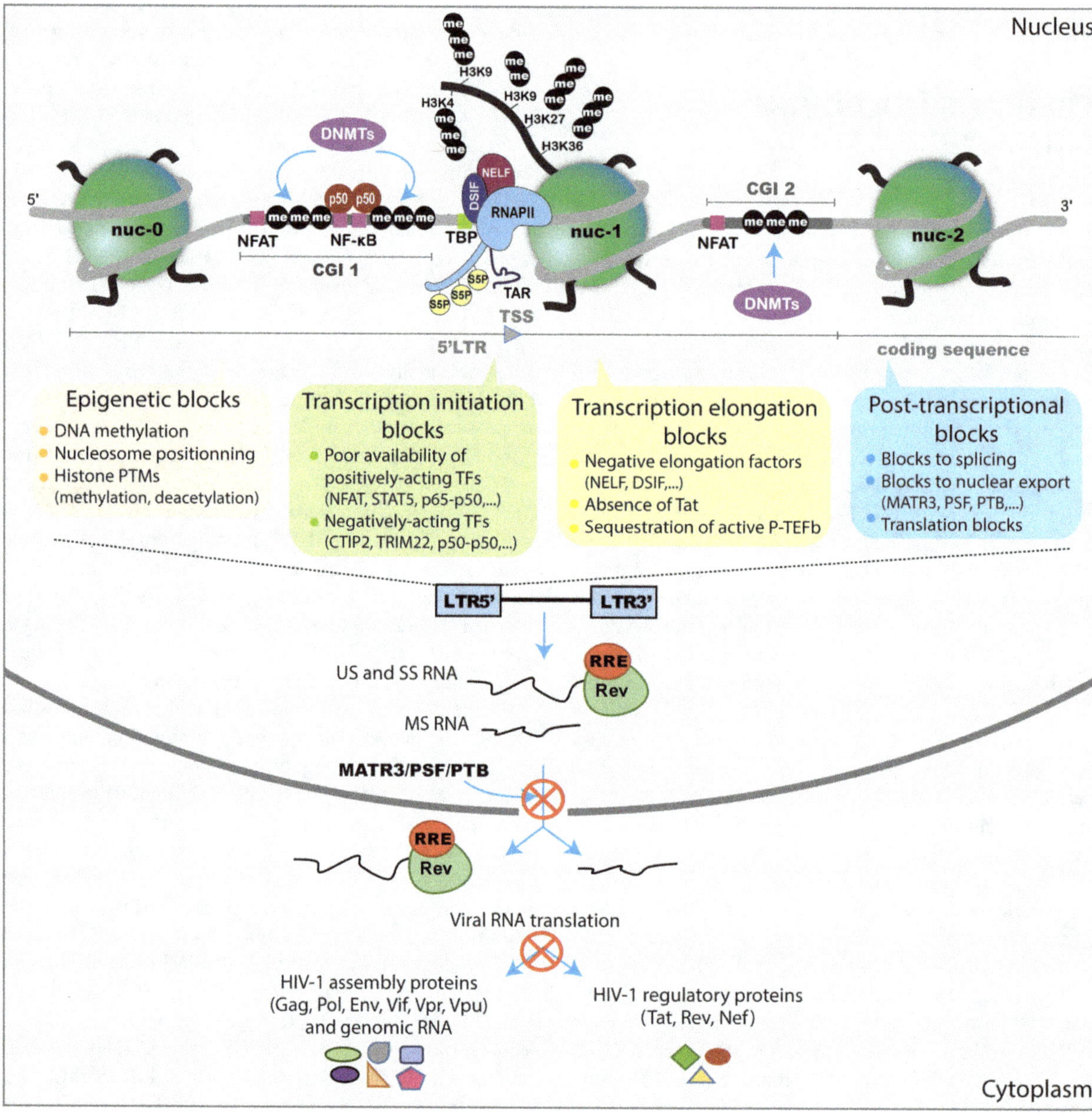

FIGURE 1 | Schematic representation of the different transcriptional and post-transcriptional blocks involved in HIV-1 latency. During HIV-1 latency, several blocks preventing viral production have been described. These are represented by the methylation of the two CGIs surrounding the HIV-1 TSS and the deposit of repressive epigenetic marks (histone deacetylation and methylation) maintaining the repressive nucleosome nuc-1 positioned in the HIV-1 5′LTR promoter just downstream the TSS. The transcription initiation is also blocked because of the cytoplasmic sequestration of the positive NF-κB heterodimer p50–p65 and the phosphorylated NFAT and STAT5. The presence of repressive factors (such as CTIP2, TRIM22 and the binding of the homodimer p50–p50 to the NF-κB binding sites in the HIV-1 promoter) acts negatively on HIV-1 transcription initiation. The RNAPII, with its phosphorylated serine 5 (S5P) residue in its C-terminal domain, pauses and accumulates at the promoter-proximal region due to the binding of the negative factors NELF and DSIF. The elongation is also blocked by the absence of the master regulator of viral transcription Tat and by the sequestration of the positive transcriptional elongation factor P-TEFb into the inactive complex named 7SK snRNP. The splicing and export of HIV-1 transcripts are inefficient during latency due to the low expression level of post-transcriptional factors such as PTB, MATR3, and PSF. Finally, translation of viral transcripts could be inhibited by mechanisms involving mRNA degradation and sequestration in cytoplasmic granules.

cells. They quantified the transcripts suggestive of transcriptional interference (U3-U5), initiation (TAR), 5′ elongation (R-U5-pre-Gag), distal transcription (Nef), completion (U3-polyA), and multiple splicing (Tat-Rev) (Yukl et al., 2018). Using blood $CD4^+$ T cells from HIV-1 individuals under ART, they showed a greater block to HIV-1 transcriptional elongation, distal HIV-1 transcription, completion, and multiple splicing than to transcriptional initiation (Yukl et al., 2018). This transcription profiling approach highlighted the blocks at distinct stages of HIV-1 transcription and splicing (which may be governed by different mechanisms), thereby underlying the heterogeneity of HIV-1 latency in $CD4^+$ T cells.

The work of Telwatte et al. (2018) and Yukl et al. (2018) and also of Pace et al. (2012) have highlighted the importance of post-transcriptional blocks in HIV-1 latency. Post-transcriptional blocks of the nuclear export of various viral transcripts including unspliced, partially spliced, multiply-spliced, and translation of HIV-1 RNA by miRNAs have also been reported (Pomerantz et al., 1990; Malim and Cullen, 1991; Lassen et al., 2006; Weng et al., 2014; Modai et al., 2019). Interestingly, a recent study from the group of Alessandro Marcello has demonstrated that the expression level of MATR3 and PSF, two known post-transcriptional cofactors of the HIV-1 protein Rev required for Rev-mediated export of RRE-containing HIV-1 RNAs (Kula et al., 2011, 2013), are poorly expressed in latently-infected patients cells (Sarracino et al., 2018), suggesting a novel post-transcriptional block linked to RNA export. This latter block was reversed by ectopic overexpression of MATR3 which boosted the action of the HDAC inhibitor SAHA in the J-Lat cell line model for HIV-1 latency (Sarracino et al., 2018). These results demonstrated the importance of post-transcriptional blocks, especially at the level of viral RNAs export, that need to be relieved to reach full viral reactivation by LRAs. Similarly, the work of Andrew Mouland and colleagues has demonstrated that UPF-1, a known RNA surveillance protein (Ajamian et al., 2015), acts as a positive post-transcriptional regulator of viral reactivation from latency (Rao et al., 2018).

Additional post-transcriptional mechanisms including the involvement of cellular miRNA and non-coding RNAs in latency have been described. More specifically, the regulation of viral expression and production by miRNAs targeting PCAF (Triboulet et al., 2007) and CyclinT1 (Sung and Rice, 2009; Budhiraja et al., 2013) have been related to latency (Huang et al., 2007). Many of these miRNAs involved in this process are expressed in resting cells but are downregulated during T-cell activation (Huang et al., 2007). For instance, the lower susceptibility to HIV-1 infection of monocytes in comparison to macrophages has been shown to be correlated with high and low expression of these miRNAs, respectively (Klase et al., 2007). Finally, lncRNA called NRON which is strongly expressed in resting $CD4^+$ T cells was shown to be involved in HIV-1 latency by inducing Tat degradation through the proteasome pathway (Li et al., 2016). The combination of SAHA with NRON knockdown significantly reactivates viral production from latently-infected primary $CD4^+$ T cells (Li et al., 2016).

Altogether, the complexity of the molecular mechanisms underlying HIV-1 latency marks the heterogeneous nature of the HIV-1 reservoirs.

SHOCK AND KILL STRATEGY TO ELIMINATE THE LATENT RESERVOIR

Mechanistic insights into HIV-1 transcriptional repression during latency have allowed to develop the "shock and kill" strategy. This approach is based on the use of small-size chemical compounds called LRAs which reactivate HIV-1 from latency (the "shock" phase) while maintaining ART in order to prevent new infection events (Sengupta and Siliciano, 2018). This kind of strategy would allow the "kill" phase during which latently-infected cells would then die from viral cytopathic effects or host cytolytic effector mechanisms following viral reactivation. Of note, this strategy does not discriminate between replication-competent and defective proviruses. Several classes of LRAs have been developed and studied (reviewed in Kim et al., 2018; Spivak and Planelles, 2018; Sadowski and Hashemi, 2019). These include: PKC agonists, MAPK agonists, CCR5 antagonist, Tat vaccine, SMAC mimetics, inducers of P-TEFb release, activators of Akt pathway, benzotriazole derivatives, epigenetic modifiers (including HDACis, HMTis, and DNMTis), and immunomodulatory LRAs (including TLR agonists, IL-15 agonist and immune checkpoint inhibitors) (summarized in **Table 1**).

It has been further demonstrated by several groups, including ours, that targeting a single mechanism might not be efficient enough to reactivate the majority of latent proviruses and that combinations of LRAs acting on several HIV-1 silencing molecular mechanisms are needed to obtain synergistic viral reactivations and achieve a more significant decrease in the size of the reservoirs (Reuse et al., 2009; Bouchat et al., 2012, 2016; Darcis et al., 2015; Jiang et al., 2015; Laird et al., 2015; Pache et al., 2015; Tripathy et al., 2015; Abdel-Mohsen et al., 2016; Chen et al., 2017; Rochat et al., 2017; Das et al., 2018). Moreover, when LRAs are used in combination, lower concentrations are effective, thereby reducing the toxicity of each LRA. However, even if these LRA combinations reverse latency, they could inhibit multiple $CD8^+$ T cell function [reviewed in Clutton and Jones (2018)]. Importantly, despite the potent effect of a single LRA and of LRA combinations *in vitro* and *ex vivo*, multiple clinical trials have failed to show a decrease in the size of the latent reservoir *in vivo*. A clear change in plasma HIV-1 RNA with a subsequent decrease in the reservoir size *in vivo* has been seen only for the immune check point inhibitor nivolumab (Guihot et al., 2018) and for romidepsin (combined with an immunovaccine) (Leth et al., 2016) but without prolonging time to viral rebound after ART interruption in this latter study (Leth et al., 2016). In the case of nivolumab, the study was conducted only on one patient who experienced a drastic and sustained decrease of the HIV-1 reservoir (Guihot et al., 2018). However, other controversial studies found no consistent changes in the size of the latent reservoir nor in HIV-specific $CD8^+$ T-cell responses in HIV-1-infected individuals treated with anti-PD1 antibodies (including nivolumab) (Le Garff et al., 2017; Evans et al., 2018; Lavolé et al., 2018; Scully et al., 2018). Success to completely eradicate latent viruses with LRAs is hampered by the heterogeneous nature of the latent reservoir and by the diversity of the silencing mechanisms governing latency that make the current "shock and kill" strategy inefficient.

LATENCY REVERSING AGENTS HIGHLIGHT THE HETEROGENEOUS NATURE OF THE LATENT RESERVOIR

All studies investigating LRAs have demonstrated the heterogeneous nature of the cellular and tissue reservoirs of

TABLE 1 | Classes of HIV-1 latency reversing agents.

LRA classes	Examples	Targets	References
PKC agonists	Prostratin Bryostatin-1 Ingenols: Ingenol-B, Ingenol 3,20-dibenzoate (Ingenol-db), ingenol-3-angelate (ingenol mebutate, PEP005)	NF-κB activation	Kulkosky et al., 2001; DeChristopher et al., 2012; Jiang et al., 2014; Darcis et al., 2015; Spivak et al., 2015
MAPK agonist	Procyanidin trimer C1	MAP Kinase activation	Cary and Peterlin, 2018
CCR5 antagonist	Maraviroc	NF-κB activation	López-Huertas et al., 2017; Madrid-Elena et al., 2018
Tat vaccine	Tat Oyi vaccine Tat-R5M4 protein	Activation of HIV-1 LTR	Geng et al., 2016
SMAC mimetics	SBI-0637142 Birinapant	Induction of non-canonical NF-κB pathways	Pache et al., 2015; Hattori et al., 2018
Inducers of P-TEFb release	BETis: JQ1, I-BET, I-BET151, OTX015, UMB-136, MMQO, CPI-203, RVX-208, PFI-1, BI-2536 and BI-6727 HMBA	Release of P-TEFb	Contreras et al., 2007; Bartholomeeusen et al., 2012; Darcis et al., 2015; Lu et al., 2016; Huang et al., 2017; Lu et al., 2017; Abner et al., 2018; Gohda et al., 2018; Liang et al., 2019
Activators of Akt pathway	Disulfiram	Upregulation of Akt signaling pathway	Xing et al., 2011; Doyon et al., 2013; Spivak et al., 2014
Benzotriazole derivatives	1-hydroxybenzotriazol (HOBt)	STAT5 activation	Bosque et al., 2017
Epigenetic modifiers	HDACis: TSA, trapoxin, SAHA, romidepsin, panobinostat, entinostat, givinostat, valproic acid, MRK-1/11, AR-42, fimepinostat, chidamide	HDAC inhibition	Van Lint et al., 1996; Quivy et al., 2002; Ylisastigui et al., 2004; Archin et al., 2009; Archin et al., 2012; Rasmussen et al., 2013, 2014; Wightman et al., 2013; Mates et al., 2015; Søgaard et al., 2015; Banga et al., 2016a; Kuai et al., 2018; Gunst et al., 2019; Yang et al., 2018
	HMTis: chaetocin, EPZ-6438, GSK-343, DZNEP, BIX-01294, UNC-0638	Suv39H1, G9a, SMYD2	Friedman et al., 2011; Bouchat et al., 2012; Nguyen et al., 2017
	DNMTis: 5-AzaC, 5-AzadC	DNMT1, 3a, 3b	Bouchat et al., 2016
Immunomodulatory LRAs	TLR agonists: TLR2 (Pam3CSK4), TLR7 (GS-9620), TLR8, TLR9 (MGN 1703) agonists IL-15 agonist (ALT-803) Immune checkpoint inhibitors: anti-PD-1 (nivolumab, pembrolizumab), anti-CTLA-4 (ipilimumab)		Schlaepfer and Speck, 2011; Novis et al., 2013; Wightman et al., 2015; Jones et al., 2016; Offersen et al., 2016; Tsai et al., 2017; Evans et al., 2018

latent HIV-1 and their diverse reactivation capacity, highlighting the different determinant responsible for the heterogeneous responses to LRAs. All these studies are summarized in **Table 2**.

HIV-1 Diversity Within the Latent and Reactivated Reservoirs

Few studies so far have focused on investigating the contribution of the viral diversity, the compartmentalization, the intact or defective nature of the viral reservoir, and the origin of the rebounding virus in latency reversal. A previous study in patients who initiated ART during acute infection showed that proviral sequences from PBMCs and GALT presented low level of genomic diversity and divergence and remained unchanged after treatment interruption (Lerner et al., 2011). Moreover, there was no phylogenetic link between the rebounded plasma viral sequences and those from the GALT proviral DNA, indicating that HIV-1 cellular reservoirs in the GALT may be different from those circulating in peripheral blood and might not contribute to the rebounded plasma viremia (Lerner et al., 2011). Other studies have supported the compartmentalization idea of the viral population in the gut with divergent opinions (van der Hoek et al., 1998; Lewis et al., 2013; Rozera et al., 2014). Depending on the stage of HIV-1 infection, the diversity of HIV-1 RNA appears lower in patients with early infection *versus* chronic infection, and thus, compartmentalization is lost during chronic infection (Rozera et al., 2014). However, other works have supported other conflicting ideas with findings showing absence of compartmentalization of HIV-1 between the gut and blood (Avettand-Fenoel et al., 2011; Imamichi et al., 2011; Evering et al., 2012), providing evidence for cross infection between these two compartments (Chun et al., 2008).

HIV-1 sequence diversity has been reported to be either higher (Klein et al., 2018) or similar (Piantadosi et al., 2019) to genital tract compared to blood. Viral compartmentalization between the blood and the male genital tract has been reported by multiple studies including SIV-infected macaques (Delwart et al., 1998; Paranjpe et al., 2002; Pillai et al., 2005; Coombs et al., 2006; Diem et al., 2008; Houzet et al., 2018). More recently, patients under suppressive ART exhibited a significant positive correlation between viral diversity and genetic compartmentalization in the blood and testes, but it was attributable to differential frequencies of identical HIV-1 sequences between the two sites (Miller et al., 2019). However, there was no evidence of compartmentalization when only unique sequences per sites are considered, suggesting that compartmentalization between blood and testes is linked to clonal expansion (Miller et al., 2019).

HIV-1 phylogenetic analysis of *post-mortem* CSF, brain, and spleen from HIV-1 patients under ART and presenting dementia symptoms showed that HIV-1 strains from the blood

TABLE 2 | The diverse responses of latently-infected cells to LRAs reflect the heterogeneity of the mechanisms driving HIV-1 latency.

Heterogeneity determinants	References	Cellular or tissue reservoir	Methodology	Heterogeneous responses to LRAs	
				LRAs	**Results illustrating heterogeneous responses to LRAs**
Virus genetic background	Norton et al., 2019	Jurkat cells infected with HIV-1 WT or mutated in ESE_{tat}.	Flow cytometry	PMA JQ1 Panobinostat	Mutations altering viral gene splicing (tat mRNA) lead to more silent phenotypes that are differently reactivated by diverse LRAs.
Cell model	Spina et al., 2013	J-Lat 6.3, 8.4, 11.1 and 5A8. Primary T-cell models of HIV-1 latency. *Ex vivo* T-cell cultures from HIV-1$^+$ individuals.	Flow cytometry QVOA	Anti-CD3 + anti-CD28, PHA, PMA, prostratin, bryostatin, PMA + ionomycin, TNFα, IL-7 + IL-2, SAHA, MRK-1, MRK-11, HMBA, ionomycin	None of the *in vitro* T cell model alone is able to capture accurately the *ex vivo* response characteristics of latently-infected T cells isolated from HIV$^+$ individuals.
Cell type	Grau-Expósito et al., 2019	Patient-derived diverse subsets of memory CD4$^+$ T cells.	Flow-based RNA FISH	Romidepsin Panobinostat JQ1 Ingenol-3-angelate Bryostain-1	Romidepsin acts on majority of the T-cell subsets (T_{CM}, T_{EM}, T_{TM}, and T_{NA}) except for T_{SCM}. Ingenol reactivates majority of T-cell subsets (T_{NA}, T_{SCM}, T_{CM}, and T_{TM}) except for T_{EM}. Panobinostat acts mainly on T_{CM} and slightly on T_{EM} and T_{NA}. Bryostatin-1 reactivates very modestly T_{NA}, T_{TD}, and T_{CM}. JQ1 acts very modestly on the majority of the subsets, except for T_{SCM}. Romidepsin + ingenol is the most potent combination generating p24 only in T_{CM}.
	Kulpa et al., 2019	*Ex vivo* T-cell cultures from HIV-1$^+$ individuals and *in vitro* model of HIV-1 latency LARA.	Flow cytometry Cell sorting TILDA	Bryostatin IL-15 PMA + ionomycin	T_{CM} cells differentiate into T_{EM} cells when exposed to LRAs. The increase of T_{EM} subset frequencies is predictive of higher prevalence of cells carrying an inducible reservoir.
	Baxter et al., 2016	Diverse subsets of patient-derived CD4$^+$ T cells.	Flow-based RNA FISH	Bryostatin-1 Ingenol-3-angelate	Bryostatin-1 mainly reactivates T_{EM}. Ingenol reactivates T_{CM}, T_{TM} and T_{EM}.
	Kula et al., 2019	U1, THP89, CHME5 and J-Lat 9.2, J-Lat A1 and A2.	Flow cytometry	Disulfiram	Disulfiram reactivates HIV-1 in 3 myeloid infected cell lines but not in the infected T-lymphoid cell lines.
Latency molecular mechanisms	Yukl et al., 2018	Patient-derived blood CD4$^+$ T cells.	RT-ddPCR	Panobinostat Romidepsin Ingenol mebutate	Panobinostat and romidepsin increase full-length and elongated transcripts, while ingenol mebutate increases polyadenylated and multiply spliced transcripts.
Tissue reservoir	Elliott et al., 2014	Patient-derived blood and rectal CD4$^+$ T cells.	Semi-nested RT-qPCR	SAHA	Fold change in CA-US HIV-1 RNA following SAHA is 5 times higher in CD4$^+$ T cells from blood compared to rectal tissue from HIV-1$^+$ individuals.
Integration site of the provirus and chromatin context	Chen et al., 2017	Jurkat cells infected with B-HIVE.	Sorting of the GFP$^+$ cells coupled with inverse PCR and provirus mapping	PHA SAHA	PHA and SAHA reactivate proviruses located at distinct integration sites but with an increased frequency in the proximity of enhancers for SAHA.

(Continued)

TABLE 2 | Continued

Heterogeneity determinants	References	Cellular or tissue reservoir	Methodology	Heterogeneous responses to LRAs	
				LRAs	Results illustrating heterogeneous responses to LRAs
	Abner et al., 2018	Jurkat cells infected with B-HIVE.	Sorting of the GFP^+ cells coupled with RT-qPCR and provirus mapping	MMQO JQ1 SAHA Prostratin	BETi (MMQO and JQ1) target viruses integrated at distinct sites as compared to those targeted by SAHA and prostratin.
	Battivelli et al., 2018	Primary $CD4^+$ T cells infected with dual-labeled HIV-1.	Cells sorting coupled with semi-nested ligation-mediated PCR and provirus sequencing	Panobinostat JQ1 Bryostatin-1 Anti-CD3 + anti-CD28	LRAs reactivate only 5% of latently-infected cells. The inducible and non-inducible populations exhibit distinct chromatin integration sites which were associated, respectively, with active chromatin and heterochromatin with non-accessible region.
Patient to patient and patient gender	Das et al., 2018	Patient-derived resting memory $CD4^+$ T cells.	EDITS	Anti-CD3 + anti-CD28 SAHA	Women have reduced inducible RNA reservoirs compared to men following treatment with anti-CD3 + anti-CD28. ESR-1 antagonists potentiate HIV-1 reactivation by SAHA, however, females show higher reactivation than males HIV-1^+ individuals.
	Darcis et al., 2017	Patient-derived $CD8^+$-depleted PBMCs and resting $CD4^+$ T cells.	Highly sensitive TaqMan based RT-qPCR	JQ1 + bryostatin JQ1 + ingenol-B 5-AzadC + panobinostat 5-AzadC + romidepsin	There is a positive correlation between the HIV-1 reservoir size and the *ex vivo* capacity of HIV-infected patient cell cultures to be reactivated by LRAs. However, some HIV-1^+ patients deviate from this linearity (for example, patients who, despite a low reservoir, are more easily reactivated than many other patients who have a larger reservoir).
	Yukl et al., 2018	Patient-derived $CD4^+$ T cells.	RT-ddPCR	JQ1, Disulfiram Chaetocin, Panobinostat Romidepsin, Ingenol mebutate, Ingenol 3,20-dibenzoate	All LRAs exhibit inter-patient variability to reverse the blocks to HIV-1 transcription with a very weak exception for romidepsin.

B-HIVE, barcoded HIV ensembles; CA-US RNA, cell-associated unspliced RNA; EDITS, envelope detection by induced transcription-based sequencing; LARA, latency and reversion assay; RNA FISH, RNA Fluorescence In Situ Hybridization; RT-ddPCR, reverse transcription droplet digital polymerase chain reaction; TILDA, Tat/rev-induced limiting dilution assay; QVOA, Quantitative Viral Outgrowth Assays.

and spleen are different from those in the brain and CSF (Caragounis et al., 2008). A more recent study of *env* and *nef* phylogeny on ART suppressed individuals confirmed the presence of considerable viral diversity in the spleen and lymph nodes (Nolan et al., 2018). However, there is no viral compartmentalization between spleen and PBMCs in SIV-infected and suppressed rhesus macaques (Siddiqui et al., 2019).

The comparison of latent HIV-1 from the blood and lymph node CD4$^+$ T cells from HIV-1 individuals undergoing ART interruption, after TLR9 coadministration with ART, suggests the same frequencies of intact proviruses in the blood and lymph nodes and the fact that CD4$^+$ T cells carrying latent viruses circulate between the blood and lymphoid tissues. However, there is no overlap between latent reservoirs and rebounded virus, thereby supporting the idea that recombinations may play a role in the emergence of the rebounded viremia (Vibholm et al., 2019).

Time to ART from estimated date of infection as an early ART initiation is associated with less molecular diversity in CSF without impacting HIV-1 DNA provirus compartmentalization in the CNS which occurs very early after infection (Schnell et al., 2010; Sturdevant et al., 2015; Oliveira et al., 2017). In the study of Oliveira et al. (2017), a higher diversity in PBMCs than in CSF is reported. The compartmentalized HIV-1 RNA in CNS is found to contribute to viral rebound within the CSF in patients undergoing treatment interruption but is phylogenetically distinct from those present in the paired blood plasma (Gianella et al., 2016).

Most of the previous studies estimated that blood memory CD4$^+$ T cells are the source of viral rebound after ART interruption or viral reactivation from latency. The first work of Timothy Schacker and colleagues examined HIV-1 variants by single-genome amplification and phylogenetic analyses in matched lymph nodes, GALT biopsies and blood from HIV-1 suppressed individuals under longstanding ART after treatment interruption (Rothenberger et al., 2015). The rebounded virus after treatment interruption was found to be detectable in latently-infected cells at multiple sites with a highly complex and genetically diverse population of virions which bring out the challenges facing the heterogeneity of HIV-1 reservoir (Rothenberger et al., 2015). Another study of the effect of a brief treatment interruption on the HIV-1 latent reservoir of individuals who initiated ART during chronic infection showed no alteration either in the size or in the diversity of the peripheral reservoir and highlighted the substantial variability and the prevalence of clonally-expanded viral populations (Salantes et al., 2018). Interestingly, the group of Sarah Palmer indicated that analytical treatment interruption (ATI) activated proviruses with similar sequence between plasma and intestinal lamina propria mononuclear cells (Barton et al., 2016), indicating that intestinal HIV-1 reservoir is contributing to viremia following ATI. A recent study by the group of Linos Vandekerckhove confirmed the heterogeneous source of viral rebound from distinct anatomical reservoirs in HIV-1 individuals undergoing treatment interruption, showing that genetically-identical viral expansions play a significant role in viral rebound (De Scheerder et al., 2019). In a study presented by Oliveira et al. (CROI 2019, Poster 327—Characterizing the HIV DNA reservoirs in whole-body tissues in the "Last Gift" cohort), HIV-1 DNA was detected in most body tissues with a nice distribution and compartmentalization of HIV-1 reservoir between tissues from the Last Gift cohort enrolling altruistic, terminally-ill persons living with HIV-1. They have successfully sequenced *env* from 10 different tissues with many identical HIV-*env* sequences sampled in multiple body tissues.

Some LRA interventions analyzed whether the increase of CA-US HIV-1 RNA is related to limited or to broad activation of HIV-1 proviruses. The single genome sequencing of viral RNA transcripts showed that panobinostat and vorinostat activate genetically diverse HIV-1 proviruses that are similar to that observed during ATI but with a high percentage of defective viral sequences (Barton et al., 2016). More precisely, T_{CM} contributed to the rebounded viremia, indicating once again the important role of this subset in the persistence of latent HIV-1 (Barton et al., 2016). Finally, romidepsin administration to HIV-1 individuals under suppressive ART activates transcription from blood CD4$^+$ T cells latent HIV-1 proviruses (Winckelmann et al., 2017). Importantly, the viremia induced by romidepsin contained few defective mutations and is characterized by low genetic diversity (Winckelmann et al., 2017, 2018).

Together, these studies illustrate that cure strategies should consider the complex and variable composition of the different viral reservoirs, the replication-competent capacity, the diversity and compartmentalization of HIV-1 reservoir, and the role of cellular clonal expansion and cellular proliferation in promoting HIV-1 persistence.

Weak Reactivation Potential of Latency Reversing Agents and Post-transcriptional Blocks

An important issue for the development of a more effective "shock and kill" approach is to determine how effective LRAs are in terms of full viral reactivation from all latently-infected cells composing the reservoirs. Indeed, most of the *in vivo* reactivation studies demonstrated a rather weak reactivation effect of LRAs, i.e., an effect only on HIV-1 transcription with much less or no effect on plasma HIV-1 RNA (Archin et al., 2012; Spivak et al., 2014; Elliott et al., 2015). For instance, a recent clinical trial using escalating doses of disulfiram demonstrated that even if all doses produced an increase in the level of intracellular HIV-1 RNA, only the highest dose increased plasma HIV-1 RNA level albeit with very low effect (Elliott et al., 2015). Similar observations have been reported for SAHA: i.e., weak effect at the level of viral particle production *in vivo* as assessed by measurement of plasma HIV-1 RNA (Archin et al., 2012). Mohammadi et al. (2014) have shown in their primary CD4$^+$ T cell models that disulfiram and SAHA treatments increased viral transcription, but failed to effectively enhance viral translation. In addition, the group of Maria Buzon has very recently demonstrated that a median of 16.28% of the whole HIV-reservoir exhibited HIV-1 transcripts induction after viral reactivation using various LRAs and their combinations, but only 10.10% of these HIV-1 RNA$^+$ cells produced viral p24 proteins (Grau-Expósito et al., 2019).

Recent work by the group of Andrew Lever (Norton et al., 2019) has demonstrated that inefficient splicing regulation may also influence the action of LRAs. They studied the polymorphisms occurring in a recently identified viral mRNA splicing regulatory element (ESE_{tat}) regulating *tat* mRNA splicing which results in more silent phenotypes of the virus. Indeed, higher doses of LRAs (PMA, JQ1, and panobinostat) were required to reactivate silent viruses bearing the polymorphisms in ESE_{tat}, reflecting their lower rate of inducibility as compared to wild-type HIV-1 (Norton et al., 2019). Therefore, different post-transcriptional mechanisms including blocks to export and alteration of mRNA splicing may be considered as druggable targets for a combined approach of more potent latency reversal (Sarracino et al., 2018; Norton et al., 2019).

Cell Model-Specific Effects of Latency Reversing Agents

Latency reversing agents were shown to be cell model-specific exhibiting diverse reactivation profiles across multiple HIV-1 latency model systems. A comprehensive study by Spina et al. (2013) tested the potency of a panel of thirteen LRAs for their ability to reactivate HIV-1 in several broadly used HIV-1 latency models (primary T-cell models, multiple J-Lat cell lines, and *ex vivo* T-cell cultures derived from the blood of HIV-1$^+$ individuals) (Spina et al., 2013). They showed that PHA was the only stimulus that uniformly reactivated latent HIV-1 in all these cell models, although other LRAs exerted largely heterogeneous responses among the various models (Spina et al., 2013). Importantly, following LRA treatment, none of the *in vitro* cell model systems could accurately capture the *ex vivo* response characteristics of latently-infected T cells from patients.

Cell Type-Specific Effects of Latency Reversing Agents

In addition to cell model-specific effects of LRAs, recent studies demonstrated the cell type-specific effects of LRAs. For instance, Baxter et al. (2016) highlighted heterogeneous responses of CD4$^+$ populations to bryostatin and ingenol. The authors showed that bryostatin induced HIV-1 expression in T_{EM} cells but had limited effect in T_{CM} and T_{TM} cells. While ingenol, on the other hand, exhibited more similar reactivation effects among the different memory T-cell subpopulations (Baxter et al., 2016). Similarly, the group of Maria Buzon has very recently demonstrated heterogeneous responses to LRAs of the latent reservoirs present in different CD4$^+$ T-cell subpopulations (Grau-Expósito et al., 2019). Romidepsin and ingenol and their combination were the most potent LRAs at reactivating HIV-1 in almost all the subsets of CD4$^+$ T cells by increasing, respectively, the proportion of T_{CM}, T_{EM}, T_{TM}, T_{NA}, and T_{NA}, T_{SCM}, T_{CM}, T_{TM} cells expressing HIV-1 RNA. Panobinostat successfully reactivated HIV-1 only in T_{CM} cells. Bryostatin-1 reactivated very modestly some T-cell subsets, including T_{NA}, T_{TD}, and T_{CM}. Therefore, T-cell differentiation status may impact the action of LRAs. Indeed, Kulpa et al. (2019) show in *ex vivo* and *in vitro* models that differentiated phenotype of T_{EM} cells from that of quiescent T_{CM} cells is associated with a potentiated response to LRAs and to a highest level of inducible HIV-1 reservoir. Additionally, the effects may also be cell type-specific. We have also recently demonstrated that disulfiram exhibited limited reactivation spectra, being active only in myeloid-derived HIV-1 latently infected cell lines (U1, THP89GFP monocytic, and CHME-5/HIV-1 microglial cells) but not in Jurkat-based T-cell lines (Kula et al., 2019). These heterogeneous cellular responses to LRAs indicate that distinct and cell-type dependent molecular mechanisms contribute to HIV-1 latency in diverse reservoirs.

Latency Molecular Mechanism-Specific and Tissue-Specific Effects of Latency Reversing Agent

It has recently been demonstrated by Yukl et al. (2018), using an elegant transcriptional profiling approach, that LRAs exhibit silencing mechanisms-specific effects. These authors found that HDACis (panobinostat and romidepsin) and PKC agonists (ingenol 3,20-dibenzoate and ingenol mebutate) exert differential effects on the latency blocks in the blood latently-infected CD4$^+$ T cells (Yukl et al., 2018). More specifically, HDACis increased total and elongated transcripts but had less or no effect on polyadenylated and multiply spliced transcripts, whereas ingenol mebutate strongly induced polyadenylated and multiply spliced transcripts but had lesser effects on transcription initiation and elongation (Yukl et al., 2018). These latter results are in agreement with another study showing that romidepsin administration after six doses of the therapeutic vaccine Vacc-4x, in HIV-1 individual under suppressive ART, increased early events in HIV-1 transcription (initiation and elongation) but had less effect on later stages (completion, multiple splicing) (Moron-Lopez et al., 2019). The differential effects of these LRAs suggest that the mechanisms underlying the blocks to completion and splicing may differ from those that mediate the blocks to initiation and elongation. The group of Yukl compared CD4$^+$ T cells from the blood and rectum tissue reservoirs using a similar transcriptional profiling approach and found a much greater block to HIV-1 transcription initiation in the rectum compared to blood (Telwatte et al., 2018). Indeed, the ratio of total to elongated transcripts was 6-fold lower in the rectum CD4$^+$ T cells, suggesting less of a block to HIV-1 transcriptional elongation in rectal CD4$^+$ T cells (Telwatte et al., 2018). In fact, a multi-dose trial of SAHA has evidenced that the cell-associated HIV-1 RNA in latently infected CD4$^+$ T cells from the blood was 5-fold higher compared to CD4$^+$ T cells from the rectal tissue (Elliott et al., 2014), suggesting that the LRA-driven effects may also be tissue-specific. Thus, further studies should investigate whether gut cells differ from blood cells in their response to LRAs in terms of HIV-1 transcript production and of cellular gene expression.

Integration Site-Specific Effects of Latency Reversing Agents

The group of Guillaume Fillion demonstrated that different LRAs reactivate different subsets of latent proviruses (Chen et al., 2018). Using a method called B-HIVE to map the chromosomal locations of individual proviruses, these authors revealed in Jurkat cells that responses to LRAs are also viral integration site-specific. They found that PHA and SAHA reactivated proviruses inserted at distinct genomic locations, suggesting that the insertion context of HIV-1 is a critical determinant of the viral response to LRAs (Chen et al., 2018). Using the same B-HIVE technology, the groups of Albert Jordan and Guillaume Fillion demonstrated that MMQO (an LRA which acts as an I-BET) and JQ1 reactivate latent HIV-1 proviruses integrated at distinct sites from those proviruses targeted by SAHA and prostratin (Abner et al., 2018). Interestingly, Battivelli et al. (2018) demonstrated that only less than 5% of latently-infected primary CD4$^+$ T cells are reactivated by LRAs. By further sequencing analysis, these authors showed the preference toward integration events in active chromatin sites for the reactivable cell population, while these regions were significantly disfavored in the non-reactivable group, highlighting that the role of chromatin environment is an important determinant of LRA effectiveness (Battivelli et al., 2018).

Patient-Specific and Sex-Specific Effects of Latency Reversing Agents

Many other determinants may also be responsible for the heterogeneous reactivation profile of LRAs. Patient-dependent effects of LRAs were reported. Indeed, viral productions evident in some patients but not in others were observed in all reactivation clinical trials (Spivak et al., 2014; Elliott et al., 2015; Leth et al., 2016; Tapia et al., 2017). Additionally, in our previous reactivation studies, we demonstrated patient-specific variations in terms of reactivation capacity of their *ex vivo* cell cultures following treatments with various LRAs (Darcis et al., 2015, 2017; Bouchat et al., 2016). Indeed, we established a positive correlation between the size of the HIV-1 reservoirs and the *ex vivo* capacity of HIV-1-infected patients' cell cultures to be reactivated by LRAs (Darcis et al., 2017), but we identified HIV-1$^+$ patients who deviated from this linearity relative to their corresponding HIV reservoir size (Darcis et al., 2017), indicating that the reservoirs size is one determinant of the cell capacity to produce virus but that this parameter alone is not sufficient. The patient-dependent heterogeneity in the responses to LRAs could be explained by patient characteristics such as genetic background, time to treatment initiation, duration and type of therapy and also by the gender-specificity, as recently proposed by the team of Jonathan Karn (Das et al., 2018). Sex-based differences in HIV-1 reservoir activity is characterized by a higher cell-associated HIV-1 RNA, higher plasma HIV-1 RNA, higher T-cell activation, and PD-1 expression in men compared to women (Scully et al., 2019). The group of Jonathan Karn has shown that the estrogen receptor-1 (ESR-1) is a key regulator of HIV-1 latency (Das et al., 2018). More specifically, antagonists of ESR-1 activate latent HIV-1 proviruses and potentiate HIV-1 reactivation by LRAs such as SAHA, TNFα, and IL-15, while ESR-1 agonists potently block HIV-1 reactivation. Despite a reduced inducible reservoir compared to men, women showed much higher levels of inhibition in response to TCR stimulation in the presence of ESR-1 agonists but exhibited a higher reactivation in response to ESR-1 antagonists when combined with SAHA than the group of male HIV$^+$ individuals (Das et al., 2018). The circadian rhythm is an additional biological process that can affect HIV-1 transcription and reactivation (Chang et al., 2018). The circadian rhythm has been first suggested in the clinical trial testing short term administration of disulfiram (Elliott et al., 2015) as a parameter influencing HIV-1 transcription. The authors find an unexpected large variation in pre-dosing CA-US HIV-1 RNA which was statistically significantly higher immediately prior to the first dose of disulfiram than at the two previous time points without changes in HIV-1 DNA or plasma HIV-1 RNA (Elliott et al., 2015). Indeed, Sharon Lewin and colleagues have subsequently demonstrated a significant time-dependent variation in CA-US HIV-1 RNA in CD4$^+$ T cells from HIV$^+$ individuals on suppressive ART, a variation which is modulated by circadian regulator factors driving transcription from the viral LTR (Chang et al., 2018). Thus, in *ex vivo* studies, the time of blood collection could affect LRA reactivation potency and should be considered to improve latency reversal.

The multiplicity of mechanisms that regulate HIV-1 latency and the diversity of factors responsible for the heterogeneity of the latent HIV-1 reservoir most likely vary from one patient to the other and even from one cell to the other in a single patient. Indeed, several single-cell studies reported cell-to-cell variability of the latent reservoir (Baxter et al., 2016; Yucha et al., 2017) and the heterogeneity of cellular response to LRAs (Passaes et al., 2017). A recent single-cell transcriptome profiling study from Angela Ciuffi laboratory has demonstrated that latently-infected cells are transcriptionally heterogeneous and can be separated into two different cell clusters based on their cellular states (Golumbeanu et al., 2018). These distinct states correlated with the susceptibility to cellular activation and HIV-1 reactivation, highlighting that the cellular environment could also contribute to the success of HIV-1 reactivation strategies (Golumbeanu et al., 2018).

CONCLUSION

In the frame of the "shock and kill" strategy, clinical trials using LRAs have so far produced unconvincing results. This strategy faces multiple barriers which prevent the complete eradication of replication competent viruses of the HIV-1 reservoir and must, therefore, be optimized. Targeting and reactivating latent cells is challenging due to the heterogeneous nature of the viral reservoirs. Recent studies demonstrating diverse responses of infected cells to LRAs point to their weak effect (Archin et al., 2012; Spivak et al., 2014; Elliott et al., 2015) and highlight the diversity of determinants responsible for the reservoirs' heterogeneity that were demonstrated so far to be virus genetic background-(Norton et al., 2019), cell model-(Spina et al., 2013), cell type-(Baxter et al., 2016; Grau-Expósito et al., 2019; Kula et al., 2019), silencing mechanism-(Elliott et al., 2014; Yukl et al., 2018), tissue reservoir-(Elliott et al., 2014; Telwatte et al., 2018; Yukl et al., 2018), integration site-(Chen et al., 2017; Abner et al., 2018; Battivelli et al., 2018), patient-(Darcis et al., 2017; Yukl et al., 2018), and gender-(Das et al., 2018) specific. In addition, some studies demonstrate a heterogeneous effect of LRAs on NK cells (Garrido et al., 2016) and cytotoxic T-cell lymphocyte (Walker-Sperling et al., 2016) activity with conflicting observations, suggesting either an immunosuppressive effect or a reduced impact of LRA activity on cells sensing HIV-1 reactivation (Archin et al., 2012; Jones et al., 2014; Clutton et al., 2016; Walker-Sperling et al., 2016; Desimio et al., 2017, 2018). Moreover, prolonged ART treatment is associated with a significant reduction in the frequency of HIV-1-specific $CD8^+$ T-cells (Gray et al., 1999; Casazza et al., 2001). Thus, as demonstrated by the group of Robert Siliciano, stimulating HIV-1-specific CTLs prior to reactivating latent HIV-1 should be considered for a successful eradication in future clinical trials (Shan et al., 2012). Another determinant of the effectiveness of a given LRA in reactivating and purging the viral reservoirs is its ability to efficiently induce latent HIV-1 by targeting not only transcriptional but also post-transcriptional mechanisms that need to be considered for a combined approach of more potent latency reversal. Additionally, an effective LRA needs to penetrate the multitude of HIV-1 tissue reservoirs and sanctuary sites. For instance, it has been shown that panobinostat did not sufficiently penetrate the central nervous system (Rasmussen et al., 2015) and romidepsin's concentration in CSF of non-human primate was only 2% of the level found in plasma (Berg et al., 2004). Consequently, ensuring a better tissue penetration of LRAs by enhancing the drug delivery system, and most importantly strengthening the killing of the LRA-reactivated cells by stimulating $CD8^+$ T responses are essential for the eradication strategy. Rational design of LRAs considering all these determinants is not possible at the moment, due to the lack of knowledge of all the cellular factors and pathways impacting HIV-1 gene expression and leading to productive viral replication. New approaches including single-cell technologies should be considered to understand why some cells respond to LRAs while others do not as this will be essential for improving the "shock and kill" strategy and hopefully reaching a cure. Moreover, due to the challenges that hinder the effectiveness of the "shock and kill" approach, some attention is also given to strategies aimed at completely suppressing HIV-1 transcription named the "block and lock." In this context, the Tat inhibitor didehydro-cortistatin A (dCA) has shown its ability to inhibit *ex vivo* residual viral replication under ART and to prolong the time to viral reactivation after treatment interruption (Kessing et al., 2017), but some *in vitro* resistance mutations to dCA were reported (Mousseau et al., 2019). Currently, several drugs are identified for their ability to be used as LPA (Latency Promoting Agents) to ensure a functional cure (Suzuki et al., 2013; Wan and Chen, 2014; Vranckx et al., 2016; Hayashi et al., 2017; Jean et al., 2017; Debyser et al., 2018). Undeniably several strategies must be exploited in order to reach a functional cure. Dealing with the residual viremia and the contribution of ongoing viral replication in the reservoir's replenishment is one of the major issues. If one of these strategies is promising its efficacy in clinic will be a long process and should, therefore, lead to the formation of a deep latency state preventing viral rebound after ART interruption.

AUTHOR CONTRIBUTIONS

AA-A, AK, GD, RV, and CV wrote the manuscript. SD, VG, PM, AM, and OR gave advice and suggestions for the writing of the manuscript.

REFERENCES

Abdel-Mohsen, M., Chavez, L., Tandon, R., Chew, G. M., Deng, X., Danesh, A., et al. (2016). Human galectin-9 is a potent mediator of HIV transcription and reactivation. *PLoS Pathog.* 12:e1005677. doi: 10.1371/journal.ppat.1005677

Abdel-Mohsen, M., Kuri-Cervantes, L., Grau-Exposito, J., Spivak, A. M., Nell, R. A., Tomescu, C., et al. (2018). CD32 is expressed on cells with transcriptionally active HIV but does not enrich for HIV DNA in resting T cells. *Sci. Transl. Med.* 10:eaar6759. doi: 10.1126/scitranslmed.aar6759

Abner, E., Stoszko, M., Zeng, L., Chen, H.-C., Izquierdo-Bouldstridge, A., and Konuma, T. (2018). A new quinoline BRD4 inhibitor targets a distinct latent HIV-1 reservoir for reactivation from other 'shock' drugs. *J. Virol.* 92:e02056-17. doi: 10.1128/JVI.02056-17

Adams, M., Sharmeen, L., Kimpton, J., Romeo, J. M., Garcia, J. V., Peterlin, B. M., et al. (1994). Cellular latency in human immunodeficiency virus-infected individuals with high CD4 levels can be detected by the presence of promoter-proximal transcripts. *Proc. Natl. Acad. Sci. U.S.A.* 91, 3862–3866. doi: 10.1073/pnas.91.9.3862

Ajamian, L., Abel, K., Rao, S., Vyboh, K., García-de-Gracia, F., Soto-Rifo, R., et al. (2015). HIV-1 recruits UPF1 but excludes UPF2 to promote nucleocytoplasmic export of the genomic RNA. *Biomolecules* 5, 2808–2839. doi: 10.3390/biom5042808

Almodóvar, S., Del, C., Colón, M., Maldonado, I. M., Villafañe, R., Abreu, S., et al. (2007). HIV-1 infection of monocytes is directly related to the success of HAART. *Virology* 369, 35–46. doi: 10.1016/j.virol.2007.07.010

Archin, N. M., Keedy, K. S., Espeseth, A., Dang, H., Hazuda, D. J., and Margolis, D. M. (2009). Expression of latent human immunodeficiency type 1 is induced by novel and selective histone deacetylase inhibitors. *AIDS* 23, 1799–1806. doi: 10.1097/QAD.0b013e32832ec1dc

Archin, N. M., Liberty, A. L., Kashuba, A. D., Choudhary, S. K., Kuruc, J. D., Crooks, A. M., et al. (2012). Administration of vorinostat disrupts HIV-1 latency in patients on antiretroviral therapy. *Nature* 487, 482–485. doi: 10.1038/nature11286

Avettand-Fenoel, V., Hocqueloux, L., Müller-Trutwin, M., Prazuck, T., and Melard, A. (2011). Greater diversity of HIV DNA variants in the rectum compared to variants in the blood in patients without HAART. *J. Med. Virol.* 83, 1499–1507. doi: 10.1002/jmv.22132

Banga, R., Procopio, F. A., Cavassini, M., and Perreau, M. (2016a). In vitro reactivation of replication-competent and infectious HIV-1 by histone deacetylase inhibitors. *J. Virol.* 90, 1858–1871. doi: 10.1128/JVI.02359-15

Banga, R., Procopio, F. A., Noto, A., Pollakis, G., Cavassini, M., and Ohmiti, K. (2016b). PD-1(+) and follicular helper T cells are responsible for persistent HIV-1 transcription in treated aviremic individuals. *Nat. Med.* 22, 754–761. doi: 10.1038/nm.4113

Banga, R., Procopio, F. A., Ruggiero, A., Noto, A., Ohmiti, K., Cavassini, M., et al. (2018). Blood CXCR3+ CD4 T cells are enriched in inducible replication competent HIV in aviremic antiretroviral therapy-treated individuals. *Front. Immunol.* 9:144. doi: 10.3389/fimmu.2018.00144

Bartholomeeusen, K., Xiang, Y., Fujinaga, K., and Peterlin, B. M. (2012). Bromodomain and extra-terminal (BET) bromodomain inhibition activate transcription via transient release of positive transcription elongation factor b (P-TEFb) from 7SK small nuclear ribonucleoprotein. *J. Biol. Chem.* 287, 36609–36616. doi: 10.1074/jbc.M112.410746

Barton, K., Hiener, B., Winckelmann, A., Rasmussen, T. A., Shao, W., and Byth, K. (2016). Broad activation of latent HIV-1 in vivo. *Nat. Commun.* 7:12731. doi: 10.1038/ncomms12731

Battivelli, E., Dahabieh, M. S., Abdel-Mohsen, M., Svensson, J. P., Tojal Da Silva, I., and Cohn, L. B. (2018). Distinct chromatin functional states correlate with HIV latency reactivation in infected primary CD4+ T cells. *eLife* 7:e34655. doi: 10.7554/eLife.34655

Baxter, A. E., Niessl, J., Fromentin, R., Richard, J., Porichis, F., and Charlebois, R. (2016). Single-cell characterization of viral translation-competent reservoirs in HIV-infected individuals. *Cell Host Microbe* 20, 368–380. doi: 10.1016/j.chom.2016.07.015

Behrens, N. E., Wertheimer, A., Klotz, S. A., and Ahmad, N. (2018). Reduction in terminally differentiated T cells in virologically controlled HIV-infected aging patients on long-term antiretroviral therapy. *PLoS One* 13:e0199101. doi: 10.1371/journal.pone.0199101

Beliakova-Bethell, N., Hezareh, M., Wong, J. K., Strain, M. C., Lewinski, M. K., and Richman, D. D. (2017). Relative efficacy of T cell stimuli as inducers of productive HIV-1 replication in latently infected CD4 lymphocytes from patients on suppressive cART. *Virology* 508, 127–133. doi: 10.1016/j.virol.2017.05.008

Berg, S. L., Stone, J., Xiao, J. J., Chan, K. K., Nuchtern, J., Dauser, R., et al. (2004). Plasma and cerebrospinal fluid pharmacokinetics of depsipeptide (FR901228) in nonhuman primates. *Cancer Chemother. Pharmacol.* 54, 85–88. doi: 10.1007/s00280-004-0766-5

Blazkova, J., Murray, D., Justement, J. S., Funk, E. K., Nelson, A. K., and Moir, S. (2012). Paucity of HIV DNA methylation in latently infected, resting CD4+ T cells from infected individuals receiving antiretroviral therapy. *J. Virol.* 86, 5390–5392. doi: 10.1128/JVI.00040-12

Blazkova, J., Trejbalova, K., Gondois-Rey, F., Halfon, P., Philibert, P., Guiguen, A., et al. (2009). CpG methylation controls reactivation of HIV from latency. *PLoS Pathog.* 5:e1000554. doi: 10.1371/journal.ppat.1000554

Boehm, D., Jeng, M., Camus, G., Gramatica, A., Schwarzer, R., Johnson, J. R., et al. (2017). SMYD2-mediated histone methylation contributes to HIV-1 latency. *Cell Host Microbe* 21, 569–579.e6. doi: 10.1016/j.chom.2017.04.011

Bosque, A., Nilson, K. A., Macedo, A. B., Spivak, A. M., Archin, N. M., Van Wagoner, R. M., et al. (2017). Benzotriazoles reactivate latent HIV-1 through inactivation of STAT5 SUMOylation. *Cell Rep.* 18, 1324–1334. doi: 10.1016/j.celrep.2017.01.022

Bouchat, S., Delacourt, N., Kula, A., Darcis, G., Van Driessche, B., Corazza, F., et al. (2016). Sequential treatment with 5-aza-2'-deoxycytidine and deacetylase inhibitors reactivates HIV-1. *EMBO Mol. Med.* 8, 117–138. doi: 10.15252/emmm.201505557

Bouchat, S., Gatot, J.-S., Kabeya, K., Cardona, C., Colin, L., Herbein, G., et al. (2012). Histone methyltransferase inhibitors induce HIV-1 recovery in resting CD4(+) T cells from HIV-1-infected HAART-treated patients. *AIDS* 26, 1473–1482. doi: 10.1097/QAD.0b013e32835535f5

Bradley, T., Ferrari, G., Haynes, B. F., Margolis, D. M., and Browne, E. P. (2018). Single-cell analysis of quiescent HIV infection reveals host transcriptional profiles that regulate proviral latency. *Cell Rep.* 25, 107–117.e3. doi: 10.1016/j.celrep.2018.09.020

Bruner, K. M., Murray, A. J., Pollack, R. A., Soliman, M. G., Laskey, S. B., and Capoferri, A. A. (2016). Defective proviruses rapidly accumulate during acute HIV-1 infection. *Nat. Med.* 22, 1043–1049. doi: 10.1038/nm.4156

Bruner, K. M., Wang, Z., Simonetti, F. R., Bender, A. M., Kwon, K. J., Sengupta, S., et al. (2019). A quantitative approach for measuring the reservoir of latent HIV-1 proviruses. *Nature* 566, 120–125. doi: 10.1038/s41586-019-0898-8

Budhiraja, S., Famiglietti, M., Bosque, A., Planelles, V., and Rice, A. P. (2013). Cyclin T1 and CDK9 T-loop phosphorylation are downregulated during establishment of HIV-1 latency in primary resting memory CD4+ T cells. *J. Virol.* 87, 1211–1220. doi: 10.1128/JVI.02413-12

Burnett, J. C., Miller-Jensen, K., Shah, P. S., Arkin, A. P., and Schaffer, D. V. (2009). Control of stochastic gene expression by host factors at the HIV promoter. *PLoS Pathog.* 5:e1000260. doi: 10.1371/journal.ppat.1000260

Buzón, M. J., Codoñer, F. M., Frost, S. D. W., Pou, C., Puertas, M. C., Massanella, M., et al. (2011). Deep molecular characterization of HIV-1 dynamics under suppressive HAART. *PLoS Pathog.* 7:e1002314. doi: 10.1371/journal.ppat.1002314

Buzon, M. J., Sun, H., Li, C., Shaw, A., Seiss, K., and Ouyang, Z. (2014). HIV-1 persistence in CD4+ T cells with stem cell-like properties. *Nat. Med.* 20, 139–142. doi: 10.1038/nm.3445

Canaud, G., Dejucq-Rainsford, N., Avettand-Fenoël, V., Viard, J.-P., Anglicheau, D., Bienaimé, F., et al. (2014). The kidney as a reservoir for HIV-1 after renal transplantation. *J. Am. Soc. Nephrol.* 25, 407–419. doi: 10.1681/ASN.2013050564

Canestri, A., Lescure, F.-X., Jaureguiberry, S., Moulignier, A., Amiel, C., and Marcelin, A. G. (2010). Discordance between cerebral spinal fluid and plasma HIV replication in patients with neurological symptoms who are receiving suppressive antiretroviral therapy. *Clin. Infect. Dis.* 50, 773–778. doi: 10.1086/650538

Cantero-Pérez, J., Grau-Expósito, J., Serra-Peinado, C., Rosero, D. A., Luque-Ballesteros, L., Astorga-Gamaza, A., et al. (2019). Resident memory T cells are a cellular reservoir for HIV in the cervical mucosa. *Nat. Commun.* 10:4739. doi: 10.1038/s41467-019-12732-2

Cao, W., Jamieson, B. D., Hultin, L. E., Hultin, P. M., Effros, R. B., and Detels, R. (2009). Premature aging of T cells is associated with faster HIV-1 disease progression. *J. Acquir. Immune Defic. Syndr.* 50, 137–147. doi: 10.1097/QAI.0b013e3181926c28

Caragounis, E.-C., Gisslén, M., Lindh, M., Nordborg, C., Westergren, S., Hagberg, L., et al. (2008). Comparison of HIV-1 pol and env sequences of blood, CSF, brain and spleen isolates collected ante-mortem and post-mortem. *Acta Neurol. Scand.* 117, 108–116. doi: 10.1111/j.1600-0404.2007.00914.x

Cary, D. C., and Peterlin, B. M. (2018). Procyanidin trimer C1 reactivates latent HIV as a triple combination therapy with kansui and JQ1. *PLoS One* 13:e0208055. doi: 10.1371/journal.pone.0208055

Casazza, J. P., Betts, M. R., Picker, L. J., and Koup, R. A. (2001). Decay kinetics of human immunodeficiency virus-specific CD8+ T cells in peripheral blood after initiation of highly active antiretroviral therapy. *J. Virol.* 75, 6508–6516. doi: 10.1128/jvi.75.14.6508-6516.2001

Chang, C. C., Naranbhai, V., Stern, J., Roche, M., Dantanarayana, A., and Ke, R. (2018). Variation in cell-associated unspliced HIV RNA on antiretroviral therapy is associated with the circadian regulator brain-and-muscle-ARNT-like-1. *AIDS* 32, 2119–2128. doi: 10.1097/QAD.0000000000001937

Chavez, L., Calvanese, V., and Verdin, E. (2015). HIV latency is established directly and early in both resting and activated primary CD4 T cells. *PLoS Pathog.* 11:e1004955. doi: 10.1371/journal.ppat.1004955

Chávez, L., Kauder, S., and Verdin, E. (2011). *In vivo*, *in vitro*, and *in silico* analysis of methylation of the HIV-1 provirus. *Methods* 53, 47–53. doi: 10.1016/j.ymeth.2010.05.009

Chen, H.-C., Martinez, J. P., Zorita, E., Meyerhans, A., and Filion, G. J. (2017). Position effects influence HIV latency reversal. *Nat. Struct. Mol. Biol.* 24, 47–54. doi: 10.1038/nsmb.3328

Chen, H.-C., Zorita, E., and Filion, G. J. (2018). Using barcoded HIV ensembles (B-HIVE) for single provirus transcriptomics. *Curr. Protoc. Mol. Biol.* 122:e56. doi: 10.1002/cpmb.56

Cherrier, T., Le Douce, V., Eilebrecht, S., Riclet, R., Marban, C., Dequiedt, F., et al. (2013). CTIP2 is a negative regulator of P-TEFb. *Proc. Natl. Acad. Sci. U.S.A.* 110, 12655–12660. doi: 10.1073/pnas.1220136110

Chomont, N., El-Far, M., Ancuta, P., Trautmann, L., Procopio, F. A., and Yassine-Diab, B. (2009). HIV reservoir size and persistence are driven by T cell survival and homeostatic proliferation. *Nat. Med.* 15, 893–900. doi: 10.1038/nm.1972

Chun, T.-W., Carruth, L., Finzi, D., Shen, X., DiGiuseppe, J. A., and Taylor, H. (1997). Quantification of latent tissue reservoirs and total body viral load in HIV-1 infection. *Nature* 387, 183–188. doi: 10.1038/387183a0

Chun, T.-W., Nickle, D. C., Justement, J. S., Meyers, J. H., Roby, G., Hallahan, C. W., et al. (2008). Persistence of HIV in gut-associated lymphoid tissue despite long-term antiretroviral therapy. *J. Infect. Dis.* 197, 714–720. doi: 10.1086/527324

Cicala, C., Martinelli, E., McNally, J. P., Goode, D. J., Gopaul, R., Hiatt, J., et al. (2009). The integrin alpha4beta7 forms a complex with cell-surface CD4 and defines a T-cell subset that is highly susceptible to infection by HIV-1. *Proc. Natl. Acad. Sci. U.S.A.* 106, 20877–20882. doi: 10.1073/pnas.0911796106

Clutton, G., Xu, Y., Baldoni, P. L., Mollan, K. R., Kirchherr, J., and Newhard, W. (2016). The differential short- and long-term effects of HIV-1 latency-reversing agents on T cell function. *Sci. Rep.* 6:30749.

Clutton, G. T., and Jones, R. B. (2018). Diverse impacts of HIV latency-reversing agents on CD8+ T-cell function: implications for HIV cure. *Front. Immunol.* 9:1452. doi: 10.3389/fimmu.2018.01452

Cockerham, L. R., Siliciano, J. D., Sinclair, E., O'Doherty, U., Palmer, S., Yukl, S. A., et al. (2014). CD4+ and CD8+ T cell activation are associated with HIV DNA in resting CD4+ T cells. *PLoS One* 9:e110731. doi: 10.1371/journal.pone.0110731

Colin, L., and Van Lint, C. (2009). Molecular control of HIV-1 postintegration latency: implications for the development of new therapeutic strategies. *Retrovirology* 6:111. doi: 10.1186/1742-4690-6-111

Connick, E., Mattila, T., Folkvord, J. M., Schlichtemeier, R., Meditz, A. L., Ray, M. G., et al. (2007). CTL fail to accumulate at sites of HIV-1 replication in lymphoid tissue. *J. Immunol.* 178, 6975–6983. doi: 10.4049/jimmunol.178.11.6975

Contreras, X., Barboric, M., Lenasi, T., and Peterlin, B. M. (2007). HMBA releases P-TEFb from HEXIM1 and 7SK snRNA via PI3K/Akt and activates HIV transcription. *PLoS Pathog.* 3:e146. doi: 10.1371/journal.ppat.0030146

Coombs, R. W., Lockhart, D., Ross, S. O., Deutsch, L., Dragavon, J., Diem, K., et al. (2006). Lower genitourinary tract sources of seminal HIV. *J. Acquir. Immune Defic. Syndr.* 41, 430–438. doi: 10.1097/01.qai.0000209895.82255.08

Coombs, R. W., Reichelderfer, P. S., and Landay, A. L. (2003). Recent observations on HIV type-1 infection in the genital tract of men and women. *AIDS* 17, 455–480. doi: 10.1097/00002030-200303070-00001

Core, L. J., and Lis, J. T. (2008). Transcription regulation through promoter-proximal pausing of RNA polymerase II. *Science* 319, 1791–1792. doi: 10.1126/science.1150843

Costiniuk, C. T., and Jenabian, M.-A. (2014). The lungs as anatomical reservoirs of HIV infection. *Rev. Med. Virol.* 24, 35–54. doi: 10.1002/rmv.1772

Couturier, J., Suliburk, J. W., Brown, J. M., Luke, D. J., Agarwal, N., Yu, X., et al. (2015). Human adipose tissue as a reservoir for memory CD4+ T cells and HIV. *AIDS* 29, 667–674. doi: 10.1097/QAD.0000000000000599

Cribbs, S. K., Lennox, J., Caliendo, A. M., Brown, L. A., and Guidot, D. M. (2015). Healthy HIV-1-infected individuals on highly active antiretroviral therapy harbor HIV-1 in their alveolar macrophages. *AIDS Res. Hum. Retroviruses* 31, 64–70. doi: 10.1089/AID.2014.0133

Darcis, G., Berkhout, B., and Pasternak, A. O. (2019). The quest for cellular markers of HIV reservoirs: any color you like. *Front. Immunol.* 10:2251. doi: 10.3389/fimmu.2019.02251

Darcis, G., Bouchat, S., Kula, A., Van Driessche, B., Delacourt, N., and Vanhulle, C. (2017). Reactivation capacity by latency-reversing agents ex vivo correlates with the size of the HIV-1 reservoir. *AIDS* 31, 181–189. doi: 10.1097/QAD.0000000000001290

Darcis, G., Coombs, R. W., and Van Lint, C. (2016). Exploring the anatomical HIV reservoirs: role of the testicular tissue. *AIDS* 30, 2891–2893. doi: 10.1097/qad.0000000000001281

Darcis, G., Kula, A., Bouchat, S., Fujinaga, K., Corazza, F., and Ait-Ammar, A. (2015). An in-depth comparison of latency-reversing agent combinations in various *in vitro* and *ex vivo* HIV-1 latency models identified bryostatin-1+JQ1 and ingenol-B+JQ1 to potently reactivate viral gene expression. *PLoS Pathog.* 11:e1005063. doi: 10.1371/journal.ppat.1005063

Das, B., Dobrowolski, C., Luttge, B., Valadkhan, S., Chomont, N., and Johnston, R. (2018). Estrogen receptor-1 is a key regulator of HIV-1 latency that imparts gender-specific restrictions on the latent reservoir. *Proc. Natl. Acad. Sci. U.S.A.* 115, E7795–E7804. doi: 10.1073/pnas.1803468115

Davey, R. T., Bhat, N., Yoder, C., Chun, T.-W., Metcalf, J. A., and Dewar, R. (1999). HIV-1 and T cell dynamics after interruption of highly active antiretroviral therapy (HAART) in patients with a history of sustained viral suppression. *Proc. Natl. Acad. Sci. U.S.A.* 96, 15109–15114. doi: 10.1073/pnas.96.26.15109

De Scheerder, M.-A., Vrancken, B., Dellicour, S., Schlub, T., Lee, E., and Shao, W. (2019). HIV rebound is predominantly fueled by genetically identical viral expansions from diverse reservoirs. *Cell Host Microbe* 26, 347–358.e7. doi: 10.1016/j.chom.2019.08.003

Debyser, Z., Vansant, G., Bruggemans, A., Janssens, J., and Christ, F. (2018). Insight in HIV integration site selection provides a block-and-lock strategy for a functional cure of HIV infection. *Viruses* 11:E12. doi: 10.3390/v11010012

DeChristopher, B. A., Loy, B. A., Marsden, M. D., Schrier, A. J., Zack, J. A., and Wender, P. A. (2012). Designed, synthetically accessible bryostatin analogues potently induce activation of latent HIV reservoirs in vitro. *Nat. Chem.* 4, 705–710. doi: 10.1038/nchem.1395

Deleage, C., Wietgrefe, S. W., Del Prete, G., Morcock, D. R., Hao, X. P., Piatak, M., et al. (2016). Defining HIV and SIV reservoirs in lymphoid tissues. *Pathog. Immun.* 1, 68–106.

Della Chiara, G., Crotti, A., Liboi, E., Giacca, M., Poli, G., and Lusic, M. (2011). Negative regulation of HIV-1 transcription by a heterodimeric NF-κB1/p50 and C-terminally truncated STAT5 complex. *J. Mol. Biol.* 410, 933–943. doi: 10.1016/j.jmb.2011.03.044

Delwart, E. L., Mullins, J. I., Gupta, P., Learn, G. H., Holodniy, M., Katzenstein, D., et al. (1998). Human immunodeficiency virus type 1 populations in blood and semen. *J. Virol.* 72, 617–623. doi: 10.1128/jvi.72.1.617-623.1998

Deng, K., Pertea, M., Rongvaux, A., Wang, L., Durand, C. M., Ghiaur, G., et al. (2015). Broad CTL response is required to clear latent HIV-1 due to dominance of escape mutations. *Nature* 517, 381–385. doi: 10.1038/nature14053

Descours, B., Petitjean, G., López-Zaragoza, J.-L., Bruel, T., Raffel, R., Psomas, C., et al. (2017). CD32a is a marker of a CD4 T-cell HIV reservoir harbouring replication-competent proviruses. *Nature* 543, 564–567. doi: 10.1038/nature21710

Desimio, M. G., Giuliani, E., and Doria, M. (2017). The histone deacetylase inhibitor SAHA simultaneously reactivates HIV-1 from latency and up-regulates NKG2D ligands sensitizing for natural killer cell cytotoxicity. *Virology* 510, 9–21. doi: 10.1016/j.virol.2017.06.033

Desimio, M. G., Giuliani, E., Ferraro, A. S., Adorno, G., and Doria, M. (2018). *In vitro* exposure to prostratin but not bryostatin-1 improves natural killer cell functions including killing of CD4+ T cells harboring reactivated human immunodeficiency virus. *Front. Immunol.* 9:1514. doi: 10.3389/fimmu.2018.01514

Diem, K., Nickle, D. C., Motoshige, A., Fox, A., Ross, S., Mullins, J. I., et al. (2008). Male genital tract compartmentalization of human immunodeficiency virus type 1 (HIV). *AIDS Res. Hum. Retroviruses* 24, 561–571. doi: 10.1089/aid.2007.0115

Ding, D., Qu, X., Li, L., Zhou, X., Liu, S., Lin, S., et al. (2013). Involvement of histone methyltransferase GLP in HIV-1 latency through catalysis of H3K9 dimethylation. *Virology* 440, 182–189. doi: 10.1016/j.virol.2013.02.022

Doyon, G., Zerbato, J., Mellors, J. W., and Sluis-Cremer, N. (2013). Disulfiram reactivates latent HIV-1 expression through depletion of the phosphatase and tensin homolog. *AIDS* 27, F7–F11. doi: 10.1097/QAD.0b013e3283570620

du Chéné, I., Basyuk, E., Lin, Y.-L., Triboulet, R., Knezevich, A., and Chable-Bessia, C. (2007). Suv39H1 and HP1gamma are responsible for chromatin-mediated HIV-1 transcriptional silencing and post-integration latency. *EMBO J.* 26, 424–435. doi: 10.1038/sj.emboj.7601517

Eilebrecht, S., Le Douce, V., Riclet, R., Targat, B., Hallay, H., Van Driessche, B., et al. (2014). HMGA1 recruits CTIP2-repressed P-TEFb to the HIV-1 and cellular target promoters. *Nucleic Acids Res.* 42, 4962–4971. doi: 10.1093/nar/gku168

Einkauf, K. B., Lee, G. Q., Gao, C., Sharaf, R., Sun, X., and Hua, S. (2019). Intact HIV-1 proviruses accumulate at distinct chromosomal positions during prolonged antiretroviral therapy. *J. Clin. Invest.* 129, 988–998. doi: 10.1172/JCI124291

Eisele, E., and Siliciano, R. F. (2012). Redefining the viral reservoirs that prevent HIV-1 eradication. *Immunity* 37, 377–388. doi: 10.1016/j.immuni.2012.08.010

Elliott, J. H., McMahon, J. H., Chang, C. C., Lee, S. A., Hartogensis, W., and Bumpus, N. (2015). Short-term administration of disulfiram for reversal of latent HIV infection: a phase 2 dose-escalation study. *Lancet HIV* 2, e520–e529. doi: 10.1016/S2352-3018(15)00226-X

Elliott, J. H., Wightman, F., Solomon, A., Ghneim, K., Ahlers, J., and Cameron, M. J. (2014). Activation of HIV transcription with short-course vorinostat in HIV-infected patients on suppressive antiretroviral therapy. *PLoS Pathog.* 10:e1004473. doi: 10.1371/journal.ppat.1004473

Evans, V. A., van der Sluis, R. M., Solomon, A., Dantanarayana, A., McNeil, C., Garsia, R., et al. (2018). Programmed cell death-1 contributes to the establishment and maintenance of HIV-1 latency. *AIDS* 32, 1491–1497. doi: 10.1097/QAD.0000000000001849

Evering, T. H., Mehandru, S., Racz, P., Tenner-Racz, K., Poles, M. A., Figueroa, A., et al. (2012). Absence of HIV-1 evolution in the gut-associated lymphoid tissue from patients on combination antiviral therapy initiated during primary infection. *PLoS Pathog.* 8:e1002506. doi: 10.1371/journal.ppat.1002506

Fletcher, C. V., Staskus, K., Wietgrefe, S. W., Rothenberger, M., Reilly, C., Chipman, J. G., et al. (2014). Persistent HIV-1 replication is associated with lower antiretroviral drug concentrations in lymphatic tissues. *Proc. Natl. Acad. Sci. U.S.A.* 111, 2307–2312. doi: 10.1073/pnas.1318249111

Forlani, G., Tosi, G., Turrini, F., Poli, G., Vicenzi, E., and Accolla, R. S. (2017). Tripartite motif-containing protein 22 interacts with class II transactivator and orchestrates its recruitment in nuclear bodies containing TRIM19/PML and cyclin T1. *Front. Immunol.* 8:564. doi: 10.3389/fimmu.2017.00564

Forouzanfar, F., Ali, S., Wallet, C., Rovere, M. D., Ducloy, C., Mekdad, H. E., et al. (2019). HIV-1 Vpr mediates the depletion of the cellular repressor CTIP2 to counteract viral gene silencing. *Sci. Rep.* 9:13154. doi: 10.1038/s41598-019-48689-x

Friedman, J., Cho, W.-K., Chu, C. K., Keedy, K. S., Archin, N. M., Margolis, D. M., et al. (2011). Epigenetic silencing of HIV-1 by the histone H3 lysine 27 methyltransferase enhancer of zeste 2∇. *J. Virol.* 85, 9078–9089. doi: 10.1128/JVI.00836-11

Fromentin, R., Bakeman, W., Lawani, M. B., Khoury, G., Hartogensis, W., DaFonseca, S., et al. (2016). CD4+ T cells expressing PD-1, TIGIT and LAG-3 contribute to HIV persistence during ART. *PLoS Pathog.* 12:e1005761. doi: 10.1371/journal.ppat.1005761

Ganor, Y., Real, F., Sennepin, A., Dutertre, C.-A., Prevedel, L., Xu, L., et al. (2019). HIV-1 reservoirs in urethral macrophages of patients under suppressive antiretroviral therapy. *Nat. Microbiol.* 4, 633–644. doi: 10.1038/s41564-018-0335-z

Garrido, C., Spivak, A. M., Soriano-Sarabia, N., Checkley, M. A., Barker, E., Karn, J., et al. (2016). HIV latency-reversing agents have diverse effects on natural killer cell function. *Front. Immunol.* 7:356. doi: 10.3389/fimmu.2016.00356

Gattinoni, L., Lugli, E., Ji, Y., Pos, Z., Paulos, C. M., and Quigley, M. F. (2011). A human memory T cell subset with stem cell-like properties. *Nat. Med.* 17, 1290–1297. doi: 10.1038/nm.2446

Geng, G., Liu, B., Chen, C., Wu, K., Liu, J., and Zhang, Y. (2016). Development of an attenuated tat protein as a highly-effective agent to specifically activate HIV-1 latency. *Mol. Ther.* 24, 1528–1537. doi: 10.1038/mt.2016.117

Gianella, S., Kosakovsky Pond, S. L., Oliveira, M. F., Scheffler, K., Strain, M. C., and De la Torre, A. (2016). Compartmentalized HIV rebound in the central nervous system after interruption of antiretroviral therapy. *Virus Evol.* 2:vew020. doi: 10.1093/ve/vew020

Gibellini, D., Borderi, M., De Crignis, E., Cicola, R., Cimatti, L., Vitone, F., et al. (2008). HIV-1 DNA load analysis in peripheral blood lymphocytes and monocytes from naïve and HAART-treated individuals. *J. Infect.* 56, 219–225. doi: 10.1016/j.jinf.2008.01.001

Gohda, J., Suzuki, K., Liu, K., Xie, X., Takeuchi, H., Inoue, J.-I., et al. (2018). BI-2536 and BI-6727, dual Polo-like kinase/bromodomain inhibitors, effectively reactivate latent HIV-1. *Sci. Rep.* 8:3521. doi: 10.1038/s41598-018-21942-5

Golumbeanu, M., Cristinelli, S., Rato, S., Munoz, M., Cavassini, M., Beerenwinkel, N., et al. (2018). Single-cell RNA-seq reveals transcriptional heterogeneity in latent and reactivated HIV-infected cells. *Cell Rep.* 23, 942–950. doi: 10.1016/j.celrep.2018.03.102

Gosselin, A., Monteiro, P., Chomont, N., Diaz-Griffero, F., Said, E. A., Fonseca, S., et al. (2010). Peripheral blood CCR4+CCR6+ and CXCR3+CCR6+CD4+ T cells are highly permissive to HIV-1 infection. *J. Immunol.* 184, 1604–1616. doi: 10.4049/jimmunol.0903058

Gosselin, A., Wiche Salinas, T. R., Planas, D., Wacleche, V. S., Zhang, Y., and Fromentin, R. (2017). HIV persists in CCR6+CD4+ T cells from colon and blood during antiretroviral therapy. *AIDS* 31, 35–48. doi: 10.1097/qad.0000000000001309

Gras, G., and Kaul, M. (2010). Molecular mechanisms of neuroinvasion by monocytes-macrophages in HIV-1 infection. *Retrovirology* 7:30. doi: 10.1186/1742-4690-7-30

Grau-Expósito, J., Luque-Ballesteros, L., Navarro, J., Curran, A., Burgos, J., and Ribera, E. (2019). Latency reversal agents affect differently the latent reservoir present in distinct CD4+ T subpopulations. *PLoS Pathog.* 15:e1007991. doi: 10.1371/journal.ppat.1007991

Gray, C. M., Lawrence, J., Schapiro, J. M., Altman, J. D., and Winters, M. A. (1999). Frequency of class I HLA-restricted anti-HIV CD8+ T cells in individuals receiving highly active antiretroviral therapy (HAART). *J. Immunol.* 162, 1780–1788.

Greger, I. H., Demarchi, F., Giacca, M., and Proudfoot, N. J. (1998). Transcriptional interference perturbs the binding of Sp1 to the HIV-1 promoter. *Nucleic Acids Res.* 26, 1294–1301. doi: 10.1093/nar/26.5.1294

Guihot, A., Marcelin, A.-G., Massiani, M.-A., Samri, A., Soulié, C., Autran, B., et al. (2018). Drastic decrease of the HIV reservoir in a patient treated with nivolumab for lung cancer. *Ann. Oncol.* 29, 517–518. doi: 10.1093/annonc/mdx696

Gunst, J. D., Kjær, K., Olesen, R., Rasmussen, T. A., Østergaard, L., Denton, P. W., et al. (2019). Fimepinostat, a novel dual inhibitor of HDAC and PI3K, effectively reverses HIV-1 latency *ex vivo* without T cell activation. *J. Virus Erad.* 5, 133–137.

Hakre, S., Chavez, L., Shirakawa, K., and Verdin, E. (2012). HIV latency: experimental systems and molecular models. *FEMS Microbiol. Rev.* 36, 706–716. doi: 10.1111/j.1574-6976.2012.00335.x

Han, Y., Lassen, K., Monie, D., Sedaghat, A. R., Shimoji, S., Liu, X., et al. (2004). Resting CD4+ T cells from human immunodeficiency virus type 1 (HIV-1)-infected individuals carry integrated HIV-1 genomes within actively transcribed host genes. *J. Virol.* 78, 6122–6133. doi: 10.1128/jvi.78.12.6122-6133.2004

Han, Y., Lin, Y. B., An, W., Xu, J., Yang, H.-C., O'Connell, K., et al. (2008). Orientation-dependent regulation of integrated HIV-1 expression by host gene transcriptional readthrough. *Cell Host Microbe* 4, 134–146. doi: 10.1016/j.chom.2008.06.008

Hattori, S., Matsuda, K., Tsuchiya, K., Gatanaga, H., Oka, S., and Yoshimura, K. (2018). Combination of a latency-reversing agent with a Smac mimetic minimizes secondary HIV-1 infection *in vitro*. *Front. Microbiol.* 9:2022. doi: 10.3389/fmicb.2018.02022

Hayashi, T., Jean, M., Huang, H., Simpson, S., Santoso, N. G., and Zhu, J. (2017). Screening of an FDA-approved compound library identifies levosimendan as a novel anti-HIV-1 agent that inhibits viral transcription. *Antiviral Res.* 146, 76–85. doi: 10.1016/j.antiviral.2017.08.013

Heesters, B. A., Lindqvist, M., Vagefi, P. A., Scully, E. P., Schildberg, F. A., and Altfeld, M. (2015). Follicular dendritic cells retain infectious HIV in cycling endosomes. *PLoS Pathog.* 11:e1005285. doi: 10.1371/journal.ppat.1005285

Hiener, B., Horsburgh, B. A., Eden, J.-S., Barton, K., Schlub, T. E., and Lee, E. (2017). Identification of genetically intact HIV-1 proviruses in specific CD4+ T cells from effectively treated participants. *Cell Rep.* 21, 813–822. doi: 10.1016/j.celrep.2017.09.081

Ho, Y.-C., Shan, L., Hosmane, N. N., Wang, J., Laskey, S. B., Rosenbloom, D. I. S., et al. (2013). Replication-competent noninduced proviruses in the latent reservoir increase barrier to HIV-1 cure. *Cell* 155, 540–551. doi: 10.1016/j.cell.2013.09.020

Hogan, L. E., Vasquez, J., Hobbs, K. S., Hanhauser, E., Aguilar-Rodriguez, B., and Hussien, R. (2018). Increased HIV-1 transcriptional activity and infectious burden in peripheral blood and gut-associated CD4+ T cells expressing CD30. *PLoS Pathog.* 14:e1006856. doi: 10.1371/journal.ppat.1006856

Honeycutt, J. B., Thayer, W. O., Baker, C. E., Ribeiro, R. M., Lada, S. M., Cao, Y., et al. (2017). HIV persistence in tissue macrophages of humanized myeloid-only mice during antiretroviral therapy. *Nat. Med.* 23, 638–643. doi: 10.1038/nm.4319

Houzet, L., Pérez-Losada, M., Matusali, G., Deleage, C., Dereuddre-Bosquet, N., Satie, A.-P., et al. (2018). Seminal simian immunodeficiency virus in chronically infected cynomolgus macaques is dominated by virus originating from multiple genital organs. *J. Virol.* 92:e00133-18. doi: 10.1128/JVI.00133-18

Hu, Z., and Kuritzkes, D. R. (2014). Altered viral fitness and drug susceptibility in HIV-1 carrying mutations that confer resistance to nonnucleoside reverse transcriptase and integrase strand transfer inhibitors. *J. Virol.* 88, 9268–9276. doi: 10.1128/JVI.00695-14

Huang, H., Kong, W., Jean, M., Fiches, G., Zhou, D., Hayashi, T., et al. (2019). A CRISPR/Cas9 screen identifies the histone demethylase MINA53 as a novel HIV-1 latency-promoting gene (LPG). *Nucleic Acids Res.* 47, 7333–7347. doi: 10.1093/nar/gkz493

Huang, H., Liu, S., Jean, M., Simpson, S., Huang, H., and Merkley, M. (2017). A novel bromodomain inhibitor reverses HIV-1 latency through specific binding with BRD4 to promote tat and P-TEFb association. *Front. Microbiol.* 8:1035. doi: 10.3389/fmicb.2017.01035

Huang, J., Wang, F., Argyris, E., Chen, K., Liang, Z., and Tian, H. (2007). Cellular microRNAs contribute to HIV-1 latency in resting primary CD4+ T lymphocytes. *Nat. Med.* 13, 1241–1247. doi: 10.1038/nm1639

Hurst, J., Hoffmann, M., Pace, M., Williams, J. P., Thornhill, J., Hamlyn, E., et al. (2015). Immunological biomarkers predict HIV-1 viral rebound after treatment interruption. *Nat. Commun.* 6:8495. doi: 10.1038/ncomms9495

Iglesias-Ussel, M., Vandergeeten, C., Marchionni, L., Chomont, N., and Romerio, F. (2013). High levels of CD2 expression identify HIV-1 latently infected resting memory CD4+ T cells in virally suppressed subjects. *J. Virol.* 87, 9148–9158. doi: 10.1128/JVI.01297-13

Imai, K., Togami, H., and Okamoto, T. (2010). Involvement of histone H3 lysine 9 (H3K9) methyltransferase G9a in the maintenance of HIV-1 latency and its reactivation by BIX01294. *J. Biol. Chem.* 285, 16538–16545. doi: 10.1074/jbc.M110.103531

Imamichi, H., Degray, G., Dewar, R. L., Mannon, P., Yao, M., Chairez, C., et al. (2011). Lack of compartmentalization of HIV-1 quasispecies between the gut and peripheral blood compartments. *J. Infect. Dis.* 204, 309–314. doi: 10.1093/infdis/jir259

Iversen, A. K. N., Attermann, J., Gerstoft, J., Fugger, L., Mullins, J. I., and Skinhøj, P. (2004). Longitudinal and cross-sectional studies of HIV-1 RNA and DNA loads in blood and the female genital tract. *Eur. J. Obstet. Gynecol. Reprod. Biol.* 117, 227–235. doi: 10.1016/j.ejogrb.2004.05.016

Jadlowsky, J. K., Wong, J. Y., Graham, A. C., Dobrowolski, C., Devor, R. L., Adams, M. D., et al. (2014). Negative elongation factor is required for the maintenance of proviral latency but does not induce promoter-proximal pausing of RNA polymerase II on the HIV long terminal repeat. *Mol. Cell Biol.* 34, 1911–1928. doi: 10.1128/MCB.01013-13

Jean, M. J., Hayashi, T., Huang, H., Brennan, J., Simpson, S., and Purmal, A. (2017). Curaxin CBL0100 blocks HIV-1 replication and reactivation through inhibition of viral transcriptional elongation. *Front. Microbiol.* 8:2007. doi: 10.3389/fmicb.2017.02007

Jenabian, M.-A., Costiniuk, C. T., Mehraj, V., Ghazawi, F. M., Fromentin, R., Brousseau, J., et al. (2016). Immune tolerance properties of the testicular tissue as a viral sanctuary site in ART-treated HIV-infected adults. *AIDS* 30, 2777–2786. doi: 10.1097/qad.0000000000001282

Jiang, G., Espeseth, A., Hazuda, D. J., and Margolis, D. M. (2007). c-Myc and Sp1 contribute to proviral latency by recruiting histone deacetylase 1 to the human immunodeficiency virus type 1 promoter. *J. Virol.* 81, 10914–10923. doi: 10.1128/jvi.01208-07

Jiang, G., Mendes, E. A., Kaiser, P., Sankaran-Walters, S., Tang, Y., and Weber, M. G. (2014). Reactivation of HIV latency by a newly modified Ingenol derivative via protein kinase Cδ-NF-κB signaling. *AIDS* 28, 1555–1566. doi: 10.1097/qad.0000000000000289

Jiang, G., Mendes, E. A., Kaiser, P., Wong, D. P., Tang, Y., Cai, I., et al. (2015). Synergistic reactivation of latent HIV expression by Ingenol-3-angelate, PEP005, targeted NF-kB signaling in combination with JQ1 induced p-TEFb activation. *PLoS Pathog.* 11:e1005066. doi: 10.1371/journal.ppat.1005066

Jiang, G., Nguyen, D., Archin, N. M., Yukl, S. A., Méndez-Lagares, G., Tang, Y., et al. (2018). HIV latency is reversed by ACSS2-driven histone crotonylation. *J. Clin. Invest.* 128, 1190–1198. doi: 10.1172/JCI98071

Jones, R. B., Mueller, S., O'Connor, R., Rimpel, K., Sloan, D. D., and Karel, D. (2016). A subset of latency-reversing agents expose HIV-infected resting CD4+ T-cells to recognition by cytotoxic T-lymphocytes. *PLoS Pathog.* 12:e1005545. doi: 10.1371/journal.ppat.1005545

Jones, R. B., O'Connor, R., Mueller, S., Foley, M., Szeto, G. L., and Karel, D. (2014). Histone deacetylase inhibitors impair the elimination of HIV-infected cells by cytotoxic T-lymphocytes. *PLoS Pathog.* 10:e1004287. doi: 10.1371/journal.ppat.1004287

Kaiser, P., Joshi, S. K., Kim, P., Li, P., Liu, H., and Rice, A. P. (2017). Assays for precise quantification of total (including short) and elongated HIV-1 transcripts. *J. Virol. Methods* 242, 1–8. doi: 10.1016/j.jviromet.2016.12.017

Kandathil, A. J., Sugawara, S., and Balagopal, A. (2016). Are T cells the only HIV-1 reservoir? *Retrovirology* 13:86.

Kauder, S. E., Bosque, A., Lindqvist, A., Planelles, V., and Verdin, E. (2009). Epigenetic regulation of HIV-1 latency by cytosine methylation. *PLoS Pathog.* 5:e1000495. doi: 10.1371/journal.ppat.1000495

Kessing, C. F., Nixon, C. C., Li, C., Tsai, P., Takata, H., and Mousseau, G. (2017). *In vivo* suppression of HIV rebound by didehydro-cortistatin A, a 'block-and-lock' strategy for HIV-1 treatment. *Cell Rep.* 21, 600–611. doi: 10.1016/j.celrep.2017.09.080

Kim, Y., Anderson, J. L., and Lewin, S. R. (2018). Getting the "kill" into "shock and kill": strategies to eliminate latent HIV. *Cell Host Microbe* 23, 14–26. doi: 10.1016/j.chom.2017.12.004

Klase, Z., Kale, P., Winograd, R., Gupta, M. V., Heydarian, M., Berro, R., et al. (2007). HIV-1 TAR element is processed by Dicer to yield a viral micro-RNA involved in chromatin remodeling of the viral LTR. *BMC Mol. Biol.* 8:63. doi: 10.1186/1471-2199-8-63

Klein, K., Nickel, G., Nankya, I., Kyeyune, F., Demers, K., Ndashimye, E., et al. (2018). Higher sequence diversity in the vaginal tract than in blood at early HIV-1 infection. *PLoS Pathog.* 14:e1006754. doi: 10.1371/journal.ppat.1006754

Kohler, S. L., Pham, M. N., Folkvord, J. M., Arends, T., Miller, S. M., Miles, B., et al. (2016). Germinal center T follicular helper cells are highly permissive to HIV-1 and alter their phenotype during virus replication. *J. Immunol.* 196, 2711–2722. doi: 10.4049/jimmunol.1502174

Kuai, Q., Lu, X., Qiao, Z., Wang, R., Wang, Y., and Ye, S. (2018). Histone deacetylase inhibitor chidamide promotes reactivation of latent human immunodeficiency virus by introducing histone acetylation. *J. Med. Virol.* 90, 1478–1485. doi: 10.1002/jmv.25207

Kula, A., Delacourt, N., Bouchat, S., Darcis, G., Avettand-Fenoel, V., and Verdikt, R. (2019). Heterogeneous HIV-1 reactivation patterns of disulfiram and combined disulfiram+romidepsin treatments. *J. Acquir. Immune Defic. Syndr.* 80, 605–613. doi: 10.1097/QAI.0000000000001958

Kula, A., Gharu, L., and Marcello, A. (2013). HIV-1 pre-mRNA commitment to Rev mediated export through PSF and matrin 3. *Virology* 435, 329–340. doi: 10.1016/j.virol.2012.10.032

Kula, A., Guerra, J., Knezevich, A., Kleva, D., Myers, M. P., and Marcello, A. (2011). Characterization of the HIV-1 RNA associated proteome identifies matrin 3 as a nuclear cofactor of Rev function. *Retrovirology* 8:60. doi: 10.1186/1742-4690-8-60

Kulkosky, J., Culnan, D. M., Roman, J., Dornadula, G., Schnell, M., Boyd, M. R., et al. (2001). Prostratin: activation of latent HIV-1 expression suggests a potential inductive adjuvant therapy for HAART. *Blood* 98, 3006–3015. doi: 10.1182/blood.v98.10.3006

Kulpa, D. A., Talla, A., Brehm, J. H., Ribeiro, S. P., Yuan, S., and Bebin-Blackwell, A.-G. (2019). Differentiation into an effector memory phenotype potentiates HIV-1 latency reversal in CD4+ T cells. *J. Virol.* 93:e00969-19. doi: 10.1128/JVI.00969-19

Kumar, A., Abbas, W., and Herbein, G. (2014). HIV-1 latency in monocytes/macrophages. *Viruses* 6, 1837–1860. doi: 10.3390/v6041837

Laird, G. M., Bullen, C. K., Rosenbloom, D. I. S., Martin, A. R., Hill, A. L., Durand, C. M., et al. (2015). Ex vivo analysis identifies effective HIV-1 latency-reversing drug combinations. *J. Clin. Invest.* 125, 1901–1912. doi: 10.1172/JCI80142

Lambotte, O., Taoufik, Y., de Goër, M. G., Wallon, C., Goujard, C., and Delfraissy, J. F. (2000). Detection of infectious HIV in circulating monocytes from patients on prolonged highly active antiretroviral therapy. *J. Acquir. Immune Defic. Syndr.* 23, 114–119. doi: 10.1097/00126334-200002010-00002

Lassen, K. G., Ramyar, K. X., Bailey, J. R., Zhou, Y., and Siliciano, R. F. (2006). Nuclear retention of multiply spliced HIV-1 RNA in resting CD4+ T cells. *PLoS Pathog.* 2:e68. doi: 10.1371/journal.ppat.0020068

Lavolé, A., Guihot, A., Veyri, M., Lambotte, O., Autran, B., Cloarec, N., et al. (2018). PD-1 blockade in HIV-infected patients with lung cancer: a new challenge or already a strategy? *Ann. Oncol.* 29, 1065–1066. doi: 10.1093/annonc/md x817

Le Garff, G., Samri, A., Lambert-Niclot, S., Even, S., Lavolé, A., and Cadranel, J. (2017). Transient HIV-specific T cells increase and inflammation in an HIV-infected patient treated with nivolumab. *AIDS* 31, 1048–1051. doi: 10.1097/ qad.0000000000001429

Lenasi, T., Contreras, X., and Peterlin, B. M. (2008). Transcriptional interference antagonizes proviral gene expression to promote HIV latency. *Cell Host Microbe* 4, 123–133. doi: 10.1016/j.chom.2008.05.016

Lerner, P., Guadalupe, M., Donovan, R., Hung, J., Flamm, J., Prindiville, T., et al. (2011). The gut mucosal viral reservoir in HIV-infected patients is not the major source of rebound plasma viremia following interruption of highly active antiretroviral therapy. *J. Virol.* 85, 4772–4782. doi: 10.1128/jvi.02409-10

Leth, S., Schleimann, M. H., Nissen, S. K., Højen, J. F., Olesen, R., and Graversen, M. E. (2016). Combined effect of Vacc-4x, recombinant human granulocyte macrophage colony-stimulating factor vaccination, and romidepsin on the HIV-1 reservoir (REDUC): a single-arm, phase 1B/2A trial. *Lancet HIV* 3, e463–e472. doi: 10.1016/S2352-3018(16)30055-8

Lewis, M. J., Frohnen, P., Ibarrondo, F. J., Reed, D., Iyer, V., Ng, H. L., et al. (2013). HIV-1 Nef sequence and functional compartmentalization in the gut is not due to differential cytotoxic T lymphocyte selective pressure. *PLoS One* 8:e75620. doi: 10.1371/journal.pone.0075620

Li, H., and Pauza, C. D. (2011). HIV envelope-mediated, CCR5/α4β7-dependent killing of CD4-negative γδ T cells which are lost during progression to AIDS. *Blood* 118, 5824–5831. doi: 10.1182/blood-2011-05-356535

Li, J., Chen, C., Ma, X., Geng, G., Liu, B., Zhang, Y., et al. (2016). Long noncoding RNA NRON contributes to HIV-1 latency by specifically inducing tat protein degradation. *Nat. Commun.* 7:11730. doi: 10.1038/ncomms11730

Li, Z., Mbonye, U., Feng, Z., Wang, X., Gao, X., Karn, J., et al. (2018). The KAT5-acetyl-histone4-Brd4 axis silences HIV-1 transcription and promotes viral latency. *PLoS Pathog.* 14:e1007012. doi: 10.1371/journal.ppat.1007012

Liang, T., Zhang, X., Lai, F., Lin, J., Zhou, C., and Xu, X. (2019). A novel bromodomain inhibitor, CPI-203, serves as an HIV-1 latency-reversing agent by activating positive transcription elongation factor b. *Biochem. Pharmacol.* 164, 237–251. doi: 10.1016/j.bcp.2019.04.005

López-Huertas, M. R., Jiménez-Tormo, L., Madrid-Elena, N., Gutiérrez, C., Rodríguez-Mora, S., and Coiras, M. (2017). The CCR5-antagonist maraviroc reverses HIV-1 latency in vitro alone or in combination with the PKC-agonist bryostatin-1. *Sci. Rep.* 7:2385. doi: 10.1038/s41598-017-02634-y

Lu, P., Qu, X., Shen, Y., Jiang, Z., Wang, P., and Zeng, H. (2016). The BET inhibitor OTX015 reactivates latent HIV-1 through P-TEFb. *Sci. Rep.* 6:24100. doi: 10.1038/srep24100

Lu, P., Shen, Y., Yang, H., Wang, Y., Jiang, Z., Yang, X., et al. (2017). BET inhibitors RVX-208 and PFI-1 reactivate HIV-1 from latency. *Sci. Rep.* 7:16646. doi: 10.1038/s41598-017-16816-1

Lusic, M., Marcello, A., Cereseto, A., and Giacca, M. (2003). Regulation of HIV-1 gene expression by histone acetylation and factor recruitment at the LTR promoter. *EMBO J.* 22, 6550–6561. doi: 10.1093/emboj/cdg631

Madrid-Elena, N., García-Bermejo, M. L., Serrano-Villar, S., Díaz-de Santiago, A., Sastre, B., and Gutiérrez, C. (2018). Maraviroc is associated with latent HIV-1 reactivation through NF-κB activation in resting CD4+ T cells from HIV-infected individuals on suppressive antiretroviral therapy. *J. Virol.* 92:e019 31-17.

Malim, M. H., and Cullen, B. R. (1991). HIV-1 structural gene expression requires the binding of multiple Rev monomers to the viral RRE: implications for HIV-1 latency. *Cell* 65, 241–248. doi: 10.1016/0092-8674(91)90158-u

Marban, C., Suzanne, S., Dequiedt, F., de Walque, S., Redel, L., Van Lint, C., et al. (2007). Recruitment of chromatin-modifying enzymes by CTIP2 promotes HIV-1 transcriptional silencing. *EMBO J.* 26, 412–423. doi: 10.1038/sj.emboj. 7601516

Marcelin, A.-G., Tubiana, R., Lambert-Niclot, S., Lefebvre, G., Dominguez, S., Bonmarchand, M., et al. (2008). Detection of HIV-1 RNA in seminal plasma samples from treated patients with undetectable HIV-1 RNA in blood plasma. *AIDS* 22, 1677–1679. doi: 10.1097/QAD.0b013e32830abdc8

Marini, B., Kertesz-Farkas, A., Ali, H., Lucic, B., Lisek, K., Manganaro, L., et al. (2015). Nuclear architecture dictates HIV-1 integration site selection. *Nature* 521, 227–231. doi: 10.1038/nature14226

Martin, G. E., Pace, M., Thornhill, J. P., Phetsouphanh, C., Meyerowitz, J., Gossez, M., et al. (2018). CD32-expressing CD4 T cells are phenotypically diverse and can contain proviral HIV DNA. *Front. Immunol.* 9:928. doi: 10.3389/fimmu. 2018.00928

Massanella, M., Bakeman, W., Sithinamsuwan, P., Fletcher, J. L. K., Chomchey, N., Tipsuk, S., et al. (2019). Infrequent HIV infection of circulating monocytes during antiretroviral therapy. *J. Virol.* 94:e01174-19. doi: 10.1128/JVI.01174-19

Mates, J. M., de Silva, S., Lustberg, M., Van Deusen, K., Baiocchi, R. A., Wu, L., et al. (2015). A novel histone deacetylase inhibitor, AR-42, reactivates HIV-1 from chronically and latently infected CD4+ T-cells. *Retrovirology* 7, 1–5.

McGary, C. S., Deleage, C., Harper, J., Micci, L., Ribeiro, S. P., Paganini, S., et al. (2017). CTLA-4+PD-1- memory CD4+ T cells critically contribute to viral persistence in antiretroviral therapy-suppressed, SIV-infected rhesus macaques. *Immunity* 47, 776–788.e5. doi: 10.1016/j.immuni.2017.09.018

McNamara, L. A., Onafuwa-Nuga, A., Sebastian, N. T., Riddell, J., Bixby, D., and Collins, K. L. (2013). CD133+ hematopoietic progenitor cells harbor HIV genomes in a subset of optimally treated people with long-term viral suppression. *J. Infect. Dis.* 207, 1807–1816. doi: 10.1093/infdis/jit118

Miller, R. L., Ponte, R., Jones, B. R., Kinloch, N. N., Omondi, F. H., and Jenabian, M.-A. (2019). HIV diversity and genetic compartmentalization in blood and testes during suppressive antiretroviral therapy. *J. Virol.* 93:e00755-19. doi: 10.1128/JVI.00755-19

Miyawaki, T., Kasahara, Y., Taga, K., Yachie, A., and Taniguchi, N. (1990). Differential expression of CD45RO (UCHL1) and its functional relevance in two subpopulations of circulating TCR-gamma/delta+ lymphocytes. *J. Exp. Med.* 171, 1833–1838. doi: 10.1084/jem.171.5.1833

Modai, S., Farberov, L., Herzig, E., Isakov, O., Hizi, A., and Shomron, N. (2019). HIV-1 infection increases microRNAs that inhibit Dicer1, HRB and HIV-EP2, thereby reducing viral replication. *PLoS One* 14:e0211111. doi: 10.1371/journal. pone.0211111

Mohammadi, P., di Iulio, J., Muñoz, M., Martinez, R., Bartha, I., and Cavassini, M. (2014). Dynamics of HIV latency and reactivation in a primary CD4+ T cell model. *PLoS Pathog.* 10:e1004156. doi: 10.1371/journal.ppat.1004156

Moron-Lopez, S., Kim, P., Søgaard, O. S., Tolstrup, M., Wong, J. K., and Yukl, S. A. (2019). Characterization of the HIV-1 transcription profile after romidepsin administration in ART-suppressed individuals. *AIDS* 33, 425–431. doi: 10.1097/ QAD.0000000000002083

Mousseau, G., Aneja, R., Clementz, M. A., Mediouni, S., Lima, N. S., Haregot, A., et al. (2019). Resistance to the tat inhibitor didehydro-cortistatin a is mediated by heightened basal HIV-1 transcription. *mBio* 10:e01750-18. doi: 10.1128/ mBio.01750-18

Nguyen, K., Das, B., Dobrowolski, C., and Karn, J. (2017). Multiple histone lysine methyltransferases are required for the establishment and maintenance of HIV-1 latency. *mBio* 8:e00133-17. doi: 10.1128/mBio.00133-17

Nguyen, V. T., Kiss, T., Michels, A. A., and Bensaude, O. (2001). 7SK small nuclear RNA binds to and inhibits the activity of CDK9/cyclin T complexes. *Nature* 414, 322–325. doi: 10.1038/35104581

Nolan, D. J., Rose, R., Rodriguez, P. H., Salemi, M., Singer, E. J., and Lamers, S. L. (2018). The spleen is an HIV-1 sanctuary during combined antiretroviral therapy. *AIDS Res. Hum. Retroviruses* 34, 123–125. doi: 10.1089/AID.2017.0254

Norton, N. J., Mok, H. P., Sharif, F., Hirst, J. C., and Lever, A. M. L. (2019). HIV silencing and inducibility are heterogeneous and are affected by factors intrinsic to the virus. *mBio* 10:e00188-19. doi: 10.1128/mBio.00188-19

Novis, C. L., Archin, N. M., Buzon, M. J., Verdin, E., Round, J. L., and Lichterfeld, M. (2013). Reactivation of latent HIV-1 in central memory CD4+ T cells through TLR-1/2 stimulation. *Retrovirology* 10:119. doi: 10.1186/1742-4690-10-119

Offersen, R., Nissen, S. K., Rasmussen, T. A., Østergaard, L., Denton, P. W., Søgaard, O. S., et al. (2016). A novel toll-like receptor 9 agonist, MGN1703, enhances HIV-1 transcription and NK cell-mediated inhibition of HIV-1-infected autologous CD4+ T cells. *J. Virol.* 90, 4441–4453. doi: 10.1128/JVI.00222-16

Oliveira, M. F., Chaillon, A., Nakazawa, M., Vargas, M., Letendre, S. L., and Strain, M. C. (2017). Early antiretroviral therapy is associated with lower HIV DNA molecular diversity and lower inflammation in cerebrospinal fluid but does not prevent the establishment of compartmentalized HIV DNA populations. *PLoS Pathog.* 13:e1006112. doi: 10.1371/journal.ppat.1006112

Osuna, C. E., Lim, S.-Y., Kublin, J. L., Apps, R., Chen, E., Mota, T. M., et al. (2018). Evidence that CD32a does not mark the HIV-1 latent reservoir. *Nature* 561, E20–E28.

Pace, M. J., Graf, E. H., Agosto, L. M., Mexas, A. M., Male, F., Brady, T., et al. (2012). Directly infected resting CD4+T cells can produce HIV Gag without spreading infection in a model of HIV latency. *PLoS Pathog.* 8:e1002818. doi: 10.1371/journal.ppat.1002818

Pache, L., Dutra, M. S., Spivak, A. M., Marlett, J. M., Murry, J. P., Hwang, Y., et al. (2015). BIRC2/cIAP1 is a negative regulator of HIV-1 transcription and can be targeted by Smac mimetics to promote reversal of viral latency. *Cell Host Microbe* 18, 345–353. doi: 10.1016/j.chom.2015.08.009

Palacios, J. A., Pérez-Piñar, T., Toro, C., Sanz-Minguela, B., Moreno, V., Valencia, E., et al. (2012). Long-term nonprogressor and elite controller patients who control viremia have a higher percentage of methylation in their HIV-1 proviral promoters than aviremic patients receiving highly active antiretroviral therapy. *J. Virol.* 86, 13081–13084. doi: 10.1128/JVI.01741-12

Pallikkuth, S., Sharkey, M., Babic, D. Z., Gupta, S., Stone, G. W., Fischl, M. A., et al. (2015). Peripheral T follicular helper cells are the major HIV reservoir within central memory CD4 T cells in peripheral blood from chronically HIV-infected individuals on combination antiretroviral therapy. *J. Virol.* 90, 2718–2728. doi: 10.1128/JVI.02883-15

Paranjpe, S., Craigo, J., Patterson, B., Ding, M., Barroso, P., Harrison, L., et al. (2002). Subcompartmentalization of HIV-1 quasispecies between seminal cells and seminal plasma indicates their origin in distinct genital tissues. *AIDS Res. Hum. Retroviruses* 18, 1271–1280. doi: 10.1089/088922202320886316

Pardons, M., Baxter, A. E., Massanella, M., Pagliuzza, A., Fromentin, R., and Dufour, C. (2019). Single-cell characterization and quantification of translation-competent viral reservoirs in treated and untreated HIV infection. *PLoS Pathog.* 15:e1007619. doi: 10.1371/journal.ppat.1007619

Passaes, C. P. B., Bruel, T., Decalf, J., David, A., Angin, M., and Monceaux, V. (2017). Ultrasensitive HIV-1 p24 assay detects single infected cells and differences in reservoir induction by latency reversal agents. *J. Virol.* 91:e02296-16. doi: 10.1128/JVI.02296-16

Penton, P. K., and Blackard, J. T. (2014). Analysis of HIV quasispecies suggests compartmentalization in the liver. *AIDS Res. Hum. Retroviruses* 30, 394–402. doi: 10.1089/AID.2013.0146

Perreau, M., Savoye, A.-L., De Crignis, E., Corpataux, J.-M., Cubas, R., and Haddad, E. K. (2013). Follicular helper T cells serve as the major CD4 T cell compartment for HIV-1 infection, replication, and production. *J. Exp. Med.* 210, 143–156. doi: 10.1084/jem.20121932

Piantadosi, A., Freije, C. A., Gosmann, C., Ye, S., Park, D., Schaffner, S. F., et al. (2019). Metagenomic sequencing of HIV-1 in the blood and female genital tract reveals little quasispecies diversity during acute infection. *J. Virol.* 93:e00804-18. doi: 10.1128/JVI.00804-18

Pillai, S. K., Good, B., Pond, S. K., Wong, J. K., Strain, M. C., Richman, D. D., et al. (2005). Semen-specific genetic characteristics of human immunodeficiency virus type 1 env. *J. Virol.* 79, 1734–1742. doi: 10.1128/jvi.79.3.1734-1742.2005

Pomerantz, R. J., Trono, D., Feinberg, M. B., and Baltimore, D. (1990). Cells nonproductively infected with HIV-1 exhibit an aberrant pattern of viral RNA expression: a molecular model for latency. *Cell* 61, 1271–1276. doi: 10.1016/0092-8674(90)90691-7

Pulliam, L., Gascon, R., Stubblebine, M., McGuire, D., and McGrath, M. S. (1997). Unique monocyte subset in patients with AIDS dementia. *Lancet* 349, 692–695. doi: 10.1016/s0140-6736(96)10178-1

Quivy, V., Adam, E., Collette, Y., Demonte, D., Chariot, A., Vanhulle, C., et al. (2002). Synergistic activation of human immunodeficiency virus type 1 promoter activity by NF-kappaB and inhibitors of deacetylases: potential perspectives for the development of therapeutic strategies. *J. Virol.* 76, 11091–11103. doi: 10.1128/jvi.76.21.11091-11103.2002

Ramakrishnan, R., Dow, E. C., and Rice, A. P. (2009). Characterization of Cdk9 T-loop phosphorylation in resting and activated CD4(+) T lymphocytes. *J. Leukoc. Biol.* 86, 1345–1350. doi: 10.1189/jlb.0509309

Ramakrishnan, R., Liu, H., and Rice, A. P. (2015). Short communication: SAHA (vorinostat) induces CDK9 Thr-186 (T-loop) phosphorylation in resting CD4+ T cells: implications for reactivation of latent HIV. *AIDS Res. Hum. Retroviruses* 31, 137–141. doi: 10.1089/AID.2013.0288

Rao, S., Amorim, R., Niu, M., Temzi, A., and Mouland, A. J. (2018). The RNA surveillance proteins UPF1, UPF2 and SMG6 affect HIV-1 reactivation at a post-transcriptional level. *Retrovirology* 15:42. doi: 10.1186/s12977-018-0425-2

Rasmussen, T. A., Schmeltz Søgaard, O., Brinkmann, C., Wightman, F., Lewin, S. R., and Melchjorsen, J. (2013). Comparison of HDAC inhibitors in clinical development: effect on HIV production in latently infected cells and T-cell activation. *Hum. Vaccin. Immunother.* 9, 993–1001. doi: 10.4161/hv.23800

Rasmussen, T. A., Tolstrup, M., Brinkmann, C. R., Olesen, R., Erikstrup, C., and Solomon, A. (2014). Panobinostat, a histone deacetylase inhibitor, for latent-virus reactivation in HIV-infected patients on suppressive antiretroviral therapy: a phase 1/2, single group, clinical trial. *Lancet HIV* 1, e13–e21. doi: 10.1016/S2352-3018(14)70014-1

Rasmussen, T. A., Tolstrup, M., Møller, H. J., Brinkmann, C. R., Olesen, R., and Erikstrup, C. (2015). Activation of latent human immunodeficiency virus by the histone deacetylase inhibitor panobinostat: a pilot study to assess effects on the central nervous system. *Open Forum Infect. Dis.* 2:ofv037. doi: 10.1093/ofid/ofv037

Reuse, S., Calao, M., Kabeya, K., Guiguen, A., Gatot, J.-S., Quivy, V., et al. (2009). Synergistic activation of HIV-1 expression by deacetylase inhibitors and prostratin: implications for treatment of latent infection. *PLoS One* 4:e6093. doi: 10.1371/journal.pone.0006093

Riou, C., Yassine-Diab, B., Van grevenynghe, J., Somogyi, R., Greller, L. D., and Gagnon, D. (2007). Convergence of TCR and cytokine signaling leads to FOXO3a phosphorylation and drives the survival of CD4+ central memory T cells. *J. Exp. Med.* 204, 79–91. doi: 10.1084/jem.20061681

Rochat, M. A., Schlaepfer, E., and Speck, R. F. (2017). Promising role of toll-like receptor 8 agonist in concert with prostratin for activation of silent HIV. *J. Virol.* 91:e02084-16. doi: 10.1128/JVI.02084-16

Rohr, O., Lecestre, D., Chasserot-Golaz, S., Marban, C., Avram, D., Aunis, D., et al. (2003). Recruitment of tat to heterochromatin protein HP1 via interaction with CTIP2 inhibits human immunodeficiency virus type 1 replication in microglial cells. *J. Virol.* 77, 5415–5427. doi: 10.1128/jvi.77.9.5415-5427.2003

Rothenberger, M. K., Keele, B. F., Wietgrefe, S. W., Fletcher, C. V., Beilman, G. J., and Chipman, J. G. (2015). Large number of rebounding/founder HIV variants emerge from multifocal infection in lymphatic tissues after treatment interruption. *Proc. Natl. Acad. Sci. U.S.A.* 112, E1126–E1134. doi: 10.1073/pnas.1414926112

Rozera, G., Abbate, I., Vlassi, C., Giombini, E., Lionetti, R., Selleri, M., et al. (2014). Quasispecies tropism and compartmentalization in gut and peripheral blood during early and chronic phases of HIV-1 infection: possible correlation with immune activation markers. *Clin. Microbiol. Infect.* 20, 157–166. doi: 10.1111/1469-0691.12367

Saayman, S., Ackley, A., Turner, A.-M. W., Famiglietti, M., Bosque, A., Clemson, M., et al. (2014). An HIV-encoded antisense long noncoding RNA epigenetically regulates viral transcription. *Mol. Ther.* 22, 1164–1175. doi: 10.1038/mt.2014.29

Sadowski, I., and Hashemi, F. B. (2019). Strategies to eradicate HIV from infected patients: elimination of latent provirus reservoirs. *Cell. Mol. Life Sci.* 76, 3583–3600. doi: 10.1007/s00018-019-03156-8

Salantes, D. B., Zheng, Y., Mampe, F., Srivastava, T., Beg, S., Lai, J., et al. (2018). HIV-1 latent reservoir size and diversity are stable following brief treatment interruption. *J. Clin. Invest.* 128, 3102–3115. doi: 10.1172/JCI120194

Sarracino, A., Gharu, L., Kula, A., Pasternak, A. O., Avettand-Fenoel, V., Rouzioux, C., et al. (2018). Posttranscriptional regulation of HIV-1 gene expression during replication and reactivation from latency by nuclear matrix protein MATR3. *mBio* 9:e02158-18. doi: 10.1128/mBio.02158-18

Schlaepfer, E., and Speck, R. F. (2011). TLR8 activates HIV from latently infected cells of myeloid-monocytic origin directly via the MAPK pathway and from latently infected CD4+ T cells indirectly via TNF-α. *J. Immunol.* 186, 4314–4324. doi: 10.4049/jimmunol.1003174

Schnell, G., Price, R. W., Swanstrom, R., and Spudich, S. (2010). Compartmentalization and clonal amplification of HIV-1 variants in the cerebrospinal fluid during primary infection. *J. Virol.* 84, 2395–2407. doi: 10.1128/JVI.01863-09

Schröder, A. R. W., Shinn, P., Chen, H., Berry, C., Ecker, J. R., and Bushman, F. (2002). HIV-1 integration in the human genome favors active genes and local hotspots. *Cell* 110, 521–529. doi: 10.1016/s0092-8674(02)00864-4

Schwartz, C., Wallet, C., De Rovere, M., Van Assche, J., Daoud, F., and Rohr, O. (2019). Microglial cells: the main HIV-1 reservoir in the brain. *Front. Cell. Infect. Microbiol.* 9:362. doi: 10.3389/fcimb.2019.00362

Scully, E. P., Gandhi, M., Johnston, R., Hoh, R., Lockhart, A., and Dobrowolski, C. (2019). Sex-based differences in human immunodeficiency virus type 1 reservoir activity and residual immune activation. *J. Infect. Dis.* 219, 1084–1094. doi: 10.1093/infdis/jiy617

Scully, E. P., Rutishauser, R. L., Simoneau, C. R., Delagrèverie, H., Euler, Z., Thanh, C., et al. (2018). Inconsistent HIV reservoir dynamics and immune responses following anti-PD-1 therapy in cancer patients with HIV infection. *Ann. Oncol.* 29, 2141–2142. doi: 10.1093/annonc/mdy259

Sebastian, N. T., Zaikos, T. D., Terry, V., Taschuk, F., McNamara, L. A., Onafuwa-Nuga, A., et al. (2017). CD4 is expressed on a heterogeneous subset of hematopoietic progenitors, which persistently harbor CXCR4 and CCR5-tropic HIV proviral genomes in vivo. *PLoS Pathog.* 13:e1006509. doi: 10.1371/journal.ppat.1006509

Sengupta, S., and Siliciano, R. F. (2018). Targeting the latent reservoir for HIV-1. *Immunity* 48, 872–895. doi: 10.1016/j.immuni.2018.04.030

Serra-Peinado, C., Grau-Expósito, J., Luque-Ballesteros, L., Astorga-Gamaza, A., Navarro, J., Gallego-Rodriguez, J., et al. (2019). Expression of CD20 after viral reactivation renders HIV-reservoir cells susceptible to rituximab. *Nat. Commun.* 10:3705. doi: 10.1038/s41467-019-11556-4

Sewald, X., Ladinsky, M. S., Uchil, P. D., Beloor, J., Pi, R., Herrmann, C., et al. (2015). Retroviruses use CD169-mediated trans-infection of permissive lymphocytes to establish infection. *Science* 350, 563–567. doi: 10.1126/science.aab2749

Shan, L., Deng, K., Shroff, N. S., Durand, C. M., Rabi, S. A., and Yang, H.-C. (2012). Stimulation of HIV-1-specific cytolytic T lymphocytes facilitates elimination of latent viral reservoir after virus reactivation. *Immunity* 36, 491–501. doi: 10.1016/j.immuni.2012.01.014

Shen, R., Kappes, J. C., Smythies, L. E., Richter, H. E., Novak, L., and Smith, P. D. (2014). Vaginal myeloid dendritic cells transmit founder HIV-1. *J. Virol.* 88, 7683–7688. doi: 10.1128/JVI.00766-14

Sheth, P. M., Kovacs, C., Kemal, K. S., Jones, R. B., Raboud, J. M., and Pilon, R. (2009). Persistent HIV RNA shedding in semen despite effective antiretroviral therapy. *AIDS* 23, 2050–2054. doi: 10.1097/QAD.0b013e3283303e04

Siddiqui, S., Perez, S., Gao, Y., Doyle-Meyers, L., Foley, B. T., Li, Q., et al. (2019). Persistent viral reservoirs in lymphoid tissues in SIV-infected rhesus macaques of Chinese-origin on suppressive antiretroviral therapy. *Viruses* 11:E105. doi: 10.3390/v11020105

Singh, P. K., Plumb, M. R., Ferris, A. L., Iben, J. R., and Wu, X. (2015). LEDGF/p75 interacts with mRNA splicing factors and targets HIV-1 integration to highly spliced genes. *Genes Dev.* 29, 2287–2297. doi: 10.1101/gad.267609.115

Sivro, A., Schuetz, A., Sheward, D., Joag, V., Yegorov, S., and Liebenberg, L. J. (2018). Integrin α4β7 expression on peripheral blood CD4+ T cells predicts HIV acquisition and disease progression outcomes. *Sci. Transl. Med.* 10:eaam6354. doi: 10.1126/scitranslmed.aam6354

Smith, B. A., Gartner, S., Liu, Y., Perelson, A. S., Stilianakis, N. I., Keele, B. F., et al. (2001). Persistence of infectious HIV on follicular dendritic cells. *J. Immunol.* 166, 690–696. doi: 10.4049/jimmunol.166.1.690

Søgaard, O. S., Graversen, M. E., Leth, S., Olesen, R., Brinkmann, C. R., and Nissen, S. K. (2015). The depsipeptide romidepsin reverses HIV-1 latency *in vivo*. *PLoS Pathog.* 11:e1005142. doi: 10.1371/journal.ppat.1005142

Sonza, S., Mutimer, H. P., Oelrichs, R., Jardine, D., Harvey, K., and Dunne, A. (2001). Monocytes harbour replication-competent, non-latent HIV-1 in patients on highly active antiretroviral therapy. *AIDS* 15, 17–22. doi: 10.1097/00002030-200101050-00005

Soriano-Sarabia, N., Archin, N. M., Bateson, R., Dahl, N. P., Crooks, A. M., Kuruc, J. D., et al. (2015). Peripheral Vγ9Vδ2 T cells are a novel reservoir of latent HIV infection. *PLoS Pathog.* 11:e1005201. doi: 10.1371/journal.ppat.1005201

Spina, C. A., Anderson, J., Archin, N. M., Bosque, A., Chan, J., and Famiglietti, M. (2013). An in-depth comparison of latent HIV-1 reactivation in multiple cell model systems and resting CD4+ T cells from aviremic patients. *PLoS Pathog.* 9:e1003834. doi: 10.1371/journal.ppat.1003834

Spivak, A. M., Andrade, A., Eisele, E., Hoh, R., Bacchetti, P., and Bumpus, N. N. (2014). A pilot study assessing the safety and latency-reversing activity of disulfiram in HIV-1-infected adults on antiretroviral therapy. *Clin. Infect. Dis.* 58, 883–890. doi: 10.1093/cid/cit813

Spivak, A. M., Bosque, A., Balch, A. H., Smyth, D., Martins, L., and Planelles, V. (2015). *Ex vivo* bioactivity and HIV-1 latency reversal by ingenol dibenzoate and panobinostat in resting CD4(+) T cells from aviremic patients. *Antimicrob. Agents Chemother.* 59, 5984–5991. doi: 10.1128/AAC.01077-15

Spivak, A. M., and Planelles, V. (2018). Novel latency reversal agents for HIV-1 cure. *Annu. Rev. Med.* 69, 421–436. doi: 10.1146/annurev-med-052716-031710

Sturdevant, C. B., Joseph, S. B., Schnell, G., Price, R. W., Swanstrom, R., and Spudich, S. (2015). Compartmentalized replication of R5 T cell-tropic HIV-1 in the central nervous system early in the course of infection. *PLoS Pathog.* 11:e1004720. doi: 10.1371/journal.ppat.1004720

Sung, T.-L., and Rice, A. P. (2009). miR-198 inhibits HIV-1 gene expression and replication in monocytes and its mechanism of action appears to involve repression of cyclin T1. *PLoS Pathog.* 5:e1000263. doi: 10.1371/journal.ppat.1000263

Suzuki, K., Hattori, S., Marks, K., Ahlenstiel, C., Maeda, Y., and Ishida, T. (2013). Promoter targeting shRNA suppresses HIV-1 infection *in vivo* through transcriptional gene silencing. *Mol. Ther. Nucleic Acids* 2:e137. doi: 10.1038/mtna.2013.64

Tapia, G., Højen, J. F., Ökvist, M., Olesen, R., Leth, S., and Nissen, S. K. (2017). Sequential Vacc-4x and romidepsin during combination antiretroviral therapy (cART): immune responses to Vacc-4x regions on p24 and changes in HIV reservoirs. *J. Infect.* 75, 555–571. doi: 10.1016/j.jinf.2017.09.004

Taura, M., Song, E., Ho, Y.-C., and Iwasaki, A. (2019). Apobec3A maintains HIV-1 latency through recruitment of epigenetic silencing machinery to the long terminal repeat. *Proc. Natl. Acad. Sci. U.S.A.* 116, 2282–2289. doi: 10.1073/pnas.1819386116

Tchasovnikarova, I. A., Timms, R. T., Douse, C. H., Roberts, R. C., Dougan, G., Kingston, R. E., et al. (2017). Hyperactivation of HUSH complex function by charcot-marie-tooth disease mutation in MORC2. *Nat. Genet.* 49, 1035–1044. doi: 10.1038/ng.3878

Tchasovnikarova, I. A., Timms, R. T., Matheson, N. J., Wals, K., Antrobus, R., and Göttgens, B. (2015). Epigenetic silencing by the HUSH complex mediates position-effect variegation in human cells. *Science* 348, 1481–1485. doi: 10.1126/science.aaa7227

Telwatte, S., Lee, S., Somsouk, M., Hatano, H., Baker, C., Kaiser, P., et al. (2018). Gut and blood differ in constitutive blocks to HIV transcription, suggesting tissue-specific differences in the mechanisms that govern HIV latency. *PLoS Pathog.* 14:e1007357. doi: 10.1371/journal.ppat.1007357

Thorlund, K., Horwitz, M. S., Fife, B. T., Lester, R., and Cameron, D. W. (2017). Landscape review of current HIV 'kick and kill' cure research - some kicking, not enough killing. *BMC Infect. Dis.* 17:595. doi: 10.1186/s12879-017-2683-3

Thornhill, J. P., Pace, M., Martin, G. E., Hoare, J., Peake, S., Herrera, C., et al. (2019). CD32 expressing doublets in HIV-infected gut-associated lymphoid tissue are associated with a T follicular helper cell phenotype. *Mucosal Immunol.* 12, 1212–1219. doi: 10.1038/s41385-019-0180-2

Tran, T.-A., de Goër de Herve, M.-G., Hendel-Chavez, H., Dembele, B., Le Névot, E., and Abbed, K. (2008). Resting regulatory CD4 T cells: a site of HIV persistence in patients on long-term effective antiretroviral therapy. *PLoS One* 3:e3305. doi: 10.1371/journal.pone.0003305

Trejbalová, K., Kováøová, D., Blažková, J., Machala, L., Jilich, D., and Weber, J. (2016). Development of 5′ LTR DNA methylation of latent HIV-1 provirus in cell line models and in long-term-infected individuals. *Clin. Epigenetics* 8:19. doi: 10.1186/s13148-016-0185-6

Triboulet, R., Mari, B., Lin, Y.-L., Chable-Bessia, C., Bennasser, Y., Lebrigand, K., et al. (2007). Suppression of microRNA-silencing pathway by HIV-1 during virus replication. *Science* 315, 1579–1582. doi: 10.1126/science.1136319

Tripathy, M. K., McManamy, M. E. M., Burch, B. D., Archin, N. M., and Margolis, D. M. (2015). H3K27 demethylation at the proviral promoter sensitizes latent HIV to the effects of vorinostat in *ex vivo* cultures of resting CD4+ T cells. *J. Virol.* 89, 8392–8405. doi: 10.1128/JVI.00572-15

Tsai, A., Irrinki, A., Kaur, J., Cihlar, T., Kukolj, G., Sloan, D. D., et al. (2017). Toll-like receptor 7 agonist GS-9620 induces HIV expression and HIV-specific immunity in cells from HIV-infected individuals on suppressive antiretroviral therapy. *J. Virol.* 91:e02166-16. doi: 10.1128/JVI.02166-16

Turrini, F., Marelli, S., Kajaste-Rudnitski, A., Lusic, M., Van Lint, C., Das, A. T., et al. (2015). HIV-1 transcriptional silencing caused by TRIM22 inhibition of Sp1 binding to the viral promoter. *Retrovirology* 12:104. doi: 10.1186/s12977-015-0230-0

Turrini, F., Saliu, F., Forlani, G., Das, A. T., Van Lint, C., Accolla, R. S., et al. (2019). Interferon-inducible TRIM22 contributes to maintenance of HIV-1 proviral latency in T cell lines. *Virus Res.* 269:197631. doi: 10.1016/j.virusres.2019.05.009

Tyagi, M., and Karn, J. (2007). CBF-1 promotes transcriptional silencing during the establishment of HIV-1 latency. *EMBO J.* 26, 4985–4995. doi: 10.1038/sj.emboj.7601928

Valcour, V. G., Ananworanich, J., Agsalda, M., Sailasuta, N., Chalermchai, T., Schuetz, A., et al. (2013). HIV DNA reservoir increases risk for cognitive disorders in cART-naïve patients. *PLoS One* 8:e70164. doi: 10.1371/journal.pone.0070164

Valcour, V. G., Shiramizu, B. T., and Shikuma, C. M. (2010). HIV DNA in circulating monocytes as a mechanism to dementia and other HIV complications. *J. Leukoc. Biol.* 87, 621–626. doi: 10.1189/jlb.0809571

Valcour, V. G., Shiramizu, B. T., Sithinamsuwan, P., Nidhinandana, S., Ratto-Kim, S., and Ananworanich, J. (2009). Asia research collaboration with the University of Hawaii 001 protocol team. HIV DNA and cognition in a thai longitudinal HAART initiation cohort: the SEARCH 001 cohort study. *Neurology* 72, 992–998. doi: 10.1212/01.wnl.0000344404.12759.83

van der Hoek, L., Sol, C. J., Maas, J., Lukashov, V. V., Kuiken, C. L., and Goudsmit, J. (1998). Genetic differences between human immunodeficiency virus type 1 subpopulations in faeces and serum. *J. Gen. Virol.* 79(Pt 2), 259–267. doi: 10.1099/0022-1317-79-2-259

Van Lint, C., Bouchat, S., and Marcello, A. (2013). HIV-1 transcription and latency: an update. *Retrovirology* 10:67. doi: 10.1186/1742-4690-10-67

Van Lint, C., Emiliani, S., Ott, M., and Verdin, E. (1996). Transcriptional activation and chromatin remodeling of the HIV-1 promoter in response to histone acetylation. *EMBO J.* 15, 1112–1120. doi: 10.1002/j.1460-2075.1996.tb00449.x

Venanzi Rullo, E., Cannon, L., Pinzone, M. R., Ceccarelli, M., Nunnari, G., and O'Doherty, U. (2019). Genetic evidence that Naïve T cells can contribute significantly to the HIV intact reservoir: time to re-evaluate their role. *Clin. Infect. Dis.* 69, 2236–2237. doi: 10.1093/cid/ciz378

Verdin, E., Paras, P., and Van Lint, C. (1993). Chromatin disruption in the promoter of human immunodeficiency virus type 1 during transcriptional activation. *EMBO J.* 12, 3249–3259. doi: 10.1002/j.1460-2075.1993.tb05994.x

Vibholm, L. K., Lorenzi, J. C. C., Pai, J. A., Cohen, Y. Z., Oliveira, T. Y., and Barton, J. P. (2019). Characterization of intact proviruses in blood and lymph node from HIV-infected individuals undergoing analytical treatment interruption. *J. Virol.* 93:e01920-18. doi: 10.1128/JVI.01920-18

von Stockenstrom, S., Odevall, L., Lee, E., Sinclair, E., Bacchetti, P., Killian, M., et al. (2015). Longitudinal genetic characterization reveals that cell proliferation maintains a persistent HIV type 1 DNA pool during effective HIV therapy. *J. Infect. Dis.* 212, 596–607. doi: 10.1093/infdis/jiv092

Vranckx, L. S., Demeulemeester, J., Saleh, S., Boll, A., Vansant, G., and Schrijvers, R. (2016). LEDGIN-mediated inhibition of integrase-LEDGF/p75 interaction reduces reactivation of residual latent HIV. *EBioMedicine* 8, 248–264. doi: 10.1016/j.ebiom.2016.04.039

Walker-Sperling, V. E., Pohlmeyer, C. W., Tarwater, P. M., and Blankson, J. N. (2016). The effect of latency reversal agents on primary CD8+ T cells: implications for shock and kill strategies for human immunodeficiency virus eradication. *EBioMedicine* 8, 217–229. doi: 10.1016/j.ebiom.2016.04.019

Wan, Z., and Chen, X. (2014). Triptolide inhibits human immunodeficiency virus type 1 replication by promoting proteasomal degradation of Tat protein. *Retrovirology* 11:88. doi: 10.1186/s12977-014-0088-6

Weber, S., Weiser, B., Kemal, K. S., Burger, H., Ramirez, C. M., and Korn, K. (2014). Epigenetic analysis of HIV-1 proviral genomes from infected individuals: predominance of unmethylated CpG's. *Virology* 449, 181–189. doi: 10.1016/j.virol.2013.11.013

Wei, P., Garber, M. E., Fang, S. M., Fischer, W. H., and Jones, K. A. (1998). A novel CDK9-associated C-type cyclin interacts directly with HIV-1 Tat and mediates its high-affinity, loop-specific binding to TAR RNA. *Cell* 92, 451–462. doi: 10.1016/s0092-8674(00)80939-3

Weinberger, L. S., Burnett, J. C., Toettcher, J. E., Arkin, A. P., and Schaffer, D. V. (2005). Stochastic gene expression in a lentiviral positive-feedback loop: HIV-1 Tat fluctuations drive phenotypic diversity. *Cell* 122, 169–182. doi: 10.1016/j.cell.2005.06.006

Weng, K.-F., Hung, C.-T., Hsieh, P.-T., Li, M.-L., Chen, G.-W., Kung, Y. A., et al. (2014). A cytoplasmic RNA virus generates functional viral small RNAs and regulates viral IRES activity in mammalian cells. *Nucleic Acids Res.* 42, 12789–12805. doi: 10.1093/nar/gku952

Wightman, F., Lu, H. K., Solomon, A. E., Saleh, S., Harman, A. N., and Cunningham, A. L. (2013). Entinostat is a histone deacetylase inhibitor selective for class 1 histone deacetylases and activates HIV production from latently infected primary T cells. *AIDS* 27, 2853–2862. doi: 10.1097/QAD.0000000000000067

Wightman, F., Solomon, A., Khoury, G., Green, J. A., Gray, L., and Gorry, P. R. (2010). Both CD31(+) and CD31- naive CD4(+) T cells are persistent HIV type 1-infected reservoirs in individuals receiving antiretroviral therapy. *J. Infect. Dis.* 202, 1738–1748. doi: 10.1086/656721

Wightman, F., Solomon, A., Kumar, S. S., Urriola, N., Gallagher, K., Hiener, B., et al. (2015). Effect of ipilimumab on the HIV reservoir in an HIV-infected individual with metastatic melanoma. *AIDS* 29, 504–506. doi: 10.1097/qad.0000000000000562

Williams, D. W., Veenstra, M., Gaskill, P. J., Morgello, S., Calderon, T. M., and Berman, J. W. (2014). Monocytes mediate HIV neuropathogenesis: mechanisms that contribute to HIV associated neurocognitive disorders. *Curr. HIV Res.* 12, 85–96. doi: 10.2174/1570162x12666140526114526

Williams, S. A., Chen, L.-F., Kwon, H., Ruiz-Jarabo, C. M., Verdin, E., and Greene, W. C. (2006). NF-kappaB p50 promotes HIV latency through HDAC recruitment and repression of transcriptional initiation. *EMBO J.* 25, 139–149. doi: 10.1038/sj.emboj.7600900

Winckelmann, A., Barton, K., Hiener, B., Schlub, T. E., Shao, W., and Rasmussen, T. A. (2017). Romidepsin-induced HIV-1 viremia during effective antiretroviral therapy contains identical viral sequences with few deleterious mutations. *AIDS* 31, 771–779. doi: 10.1097/QAD.0000000000001400

Winckelmann, A., Morcilla, V., Shao, W., Schleimann, M. H., Hojen, J. F., Schlub, T. E., et al. (2018). Genetic characterization of the HIV-1 reservoir after Vacc-4x and romidepsin therapy in HIV-1-infected individuals. *AIDS* 32, 1793–1802. doi: 10.1097/QAD.0000000000001861

Winston, J. A., Bruggeman, L. A., Ross, M. D., Jacobson, J., Ross, L., D'Agati, V. D., et al. (2001). Nephropathy and establishment of a renal reservoir of HIV type 1 during primary infection. *N. Engl. J. Med.* 344, 1979–1984. doi: 10.1056/nejm200106283442604

Xing, S., Bullen, C. K., Shroff, N. S., Shan, L., Yang, H.-C., and Manucci, J. L. (2011). Disulfiram reactivates latent HIV-1 in a Bcl-2-transduced primary CD4+ T cell model without inducing global T cell activation. *J. Virol.* 85, 6060–6064. doi: 10.1128/JVI.02033-10

Yamaguchi, Y., Takagi, T., Wada, T., Yano, K., Furuya, A., Sugimoto, S., et al. (1999). NELF, a multisubunit complex containing RD, cooperates with DSIF to repress RNA polymerase II elongation. *Cell* 97, 41–51. doi: 10.1016/s0092-8674(00)80713-8

Yang, W., Sun, Z., Hua, C., Wang, Q., Xu, W., Deng, Q., et al. (2018). Chidamide, a histone deacetylase inhibitor-based anticancer drug, effectively reactivates latent HIV-1 provirus. *Microbes Infect.* 20, 626–634. doi: 10.1016/j.micinf.2017.10.003

Yang, Z., Zhu, Q., Luo, K., and Zhou, Q. (2001). The 7SK small nuclear RNA inhibits the CDK9/cyclin T1 kinase to control transcription. *Nature* 414, 317–322. doi: 10.1038/35104575

Ylisastigui, L., Archin, N. M., Lehrman, G., Bosch, R. J., and Margolis, D. M. (2004). Coaxing HIV-1 from resting CD4 T cells: histone deacetylase inhibition allows latent viral expression. *AIDS* 18, 1101–1108. doi: 10.1097/00002030-200405210-00003

Yucha, R. W., Hobbs, K. S., Hanhauser, E., Hogan, L. E., Nieves, W., and Ozen, M. O. (2017). High-throughput characterization of HIV-1 reservoir reactivation using a single-cell-in-droplet PCR assay. *EBioMedicine* 20, 217–229. doi: 10.1016/j.ebiom.2017.05.006

Yukl, S. A., Kaiser, P., Kim, P., Telwatte, S., Joshi, S. K., Vu, M., et al. (2018). HIV latency in isolated patient CD4+ T cells may be due to blocks in HIV transcriptional elongation, completion, and splicing. *Sci. Transl. Med.* 10:eaa9927. doi: 10.1126/scitranslmed.aap9927

Yukl, S. A., Shergill, A. K., Ho, T., Killian, M., Girling, V., Epling, L., et al. (2013). The distribution of HIV DNA and RNA in cell subsets differs in gut and blood of HIV-positive patients on ART: implications for viral persistence. *J. Infect. Dis.* 208, 1212–1220. doi: 10.1093/infdis/jit308

Zaikos, T. D., Terry, V. H., Sebastian Kettinger, N. T., Lubow, J., Painter, M. M., and Virgilio, M. C. (2018). Hematopoietic stem and progenitor cells are a distinct HIV reservoir that contributes to persistent viremia in suppressed patients. *Cell Rep.* 25, 3759–3773.e9. doi: 10.1016/j.celrep.2018.11.104

Zapata, J. C., Campilongo, F., Barclay, R. A., DeMarino, C., Iglesias-Ussel, M. D., Kashanchi, F., et al. (2017). The human immunodeficiency virus 1 ASP RNA promotes viral latency by recruiting the polycomb repressor complex 2 and promoting nucleosome assembly. *Virology* 506, 34–44. doi: 10.1016/j.virol.2017.03.002

Zerbato, J. M., McMahon, D. K., Sobolewski, M. D., Mellors, J. W., and Sluis-Cremer, N. (2019). Naïve CD4+ T cells harbor a large inducible reservoir of latent, replication-competent HIV-1. *Clin. Infect. Dis.* 69, 1919–1925. doi: 10.1093/cid/ciz108

Zhang, Z., Nikolai, B. C., Gates, L. A., Jung, S. Y., Siwak, E. B., and He, B. (2017). Crosstalk between histone modifications indicates that inhibition of arginine methyltransferase CARM1 activity reverses HIV latency. *Nucleic Acids Res.* 45, 9348–9360. doi: 10.1093/nar/gkx550

2

Memory CD4+ T-Cells Expressing HLA-DR Contribute to HIV Persistence During Prolonged Antiretroviral Therapy

Eunok Lee[1,2], Peter Bacchetti[3], Jeffery Milush[4], Wei Shao[5], Eli Boritz[6], Daniel Douek[6], Remi Fromentin[7], Teri Liegler[4], Rebecca Hoh[4], Steve G. Deeks[4], Frederick M. Hecht[4], Nicolas Chomont[7] and Sarah Palmer[1,2]*

[1] Centre for Virus Research, The Westmead Institute for Medical Research, Sydney, NSW, Australia, [2] Sydney Medical School, The University of Sydney, Sydney, NSW, Australia, [3] Department of Epidemiology and Biostatistics, University of California, San Francisco, San Francisco, CA, United States, [4] Department of Medicine, University of California, San Francisco, San Francisco, CA, United States, [5] Leidos Biomedical Research, Inc., Frederick National Laboratory for Cancer Research, Frederick, MD, United States, [6] Human Immunology Section, Vaccine Research Center, National Institutes of Allergy and Infectious Diseases, National Institute of Health, Bethesda, MD, United States, [7] Centre de Recherche du CHUM et Département de Microbiologie, Infectiologie et Immunologie, Université de Montreal, Montreal, QC, Canada

***Correspondence:**
Eunok Lee
eunok.lee@sydney.edu.au

To date, most assays for measuring the human immunodeficiency virus (HIV-1) reservoir do not include memory CD4+ T-cells expressing the activation marker, human leukocyte antigen-antigen D related (HLA-DR). However, little is known concerning the role these cells play in maintaining persistent HIV-1 during effective antiretroviral therapy (ART). To address this issue, we examined, cellular activation/exhaustion markers (Ki67, CCR5, PD-1, Lag-3 and Tim-3) and viral gag-pol DNA sequences within HLA-DR− and HLA-DR+ memory CD4+ T-cell subsets longitudinally from the peripheral blood of six participants over 3 to ≥15 years of effective therapy. HLA-DR expression was readily detected during the study period in all participants. The average expression levels of CCR5, PD-1 and Tim-3 were higher on the HLA-DR+ T-cell subset whereas the average of LAG-3 expression was higher on their HLA-DR− counterpart. The proportion of HIV-infected cells increased within the HLA-DR+ subset by an average of 18% per year of ART whereas the frequency of infected HLA-DR− T-cells slightly decreased over time (5% per year). We observed that 20–33% of HIV-DNA sequences from the early time points were genetically identical to viral sequences from the last time point within the same cell subset during ART. This indicates that a fraction of proviruses persists within HLA-DR+ and HLA-DR− T-cell subsets during prolonged ART. Our HIV-DNA sequence analyses also revealed that cells transitioned between the HLA-DR+ and HLA-DR− phenotypes. The Ki67 expression, a marker for cellular proliferation, and the combined markers of Ki67/PD-1 averaged 19-fold and 22-fold higher on the HLA-DR+ T-cell subset compared to their HLA-DR− counterpart. Moreover, cellular proliferation, as reflected by the proportion of genetically identical HIV-DNA sequences, increased within both T-cell subsets over the study period; however, this increase was greater within the HLA-DR+ T-cells. Our research revealed that cellular transition and proliferation contribute to the persistence of HIV in HLA-DR+ and HLA-DR− T-cell subsets during prolonged therapy. As such, the HIV reservoir expands during effective ART when both the HLA-DR+ and HLA-DR− cell subsets are included, and therapeutic interventions aimed at reducing the HIV-1 reservoir should target HLA-DR+ and HLA-DR− T-cells.

Keywords: HLA-DR, CD4+ T-cells, prolonged ART, HIV persistence, cell activation/exhaustion markers, cellular proliferation, single-proviral sequencing

INTRODUCTION

Since 1996, antiretroviral therapy (ART) has dramatically reduced the mortality and morbidity caused by HIV infection (Palella et al., 1998). However, ART alone does not eradicate HIV. HIV-DNA persists as an integrated genome in long-lived or slowly dividing cells throughout therapy (Finzi et al., 1997; Siliciano and Siliciano, 2004); and viral replication resumes within a few weeks after the termination of ART (Chun et al., 2010; Hocqueloux et al., 2010).

Studies have shown that persistent HIV cellular reservoirs are established when an activated CD4+ T-cell becomes infected by HIV but transitions to a long-lived and quiescent memory T-cells instead of undergoing lytic infection (Finzi et al., 1997; Siliciano et al., 2003, 2007; Chomont et al., 2009; Shan et al., 2017). In addition, resting memory T cells can be infected directly by HIV (Swiggard et al., 2005; Agosto et al., 2007; Saleh et al., 2007; Dai et al., 2009). Many studies that investigate HIV persistence use CD4+ T-cells depleted for Human Leukocyte Antigen-antigen D Related (HLA-DR) as those cells that express HLA-DR are thought to be productively infected and short-lived (Chun et al., 1995). However, the degree to which the HLA-DR+ T-cells contribute to HIV persistence during effective therapy is unknown.

In treatment naïve HIV-infected individuals, the expression of HLA-DR on CD4+ memory T-cells is associated with HIV disease progression (Kestens et al., 1994). Recent studies have linked T-cell activation to HIV persistence including a study by Murray et al. (2014) which revealed that HIV-DNA persists in activated memory CD4+ T-cells (HLA-DR+) up to 1 year after therapy initiation (Chun et al., 2005). In addition, Cockerham et al. (2014) found that the most consistent association was between the frequencies of CD4+ or CD8+ T-cells expressing HLA-DR and HIV-DNA copy number as measured by digital droplet PCR in resting CD4+ T-cells. These observations suggest that HIV-DNA persists in memory CD4+ T-cells displaying an activated phenotype long after active viral replication is dramatically reduced by ART.

In order to fully define the role of CD4+ memory T-cells expressing HLA-DR in maintaining HIV persistence, we measured the levels of cellular activation and exhaustion markers over time in HIV-infected individuals who have been on ART for more than 15 years. By using single-proviral sequencing targeting the *gag-pol* region (p6 through nucleotides 1–900 of the gene encoding reverse transcriptase, p6-RT), we determined how these immunological markers are related to the frequency of HIV-infected T-cells. In addition, we investigated how these cellular markers are related to the genetic composition of HIV-DNA within HLA-DR− and HLA-DR+ CD4+ memory T-cell subsets during prolonged ART. Furthermore, we examined the persistence of HIV-infected HLA-DR+ memory T-cells and cellular transition between the HLA-DR+ and HLA-DR− cellular phenotypes by following HIV-DNA levels and viral DNA sequences longitudinally over 3 to ≥15 years of therapy.

Our study revealed that CD4+ memory T-cells that express HLA-DR are readily detected in both acute/early and chronic participants on prolonged therapy. Also, we found the proportion of HIV-infected HLA-DR+ T cells increases after prolonged therapy (≥15 years). Sequencing the HIV-1 genome revealed the same HIV viral sequences persisted over years of therapy in both the HLA-DR+ and HLA-DR− T-cell subsets. In addition, this sequence analysis showed some evidence that CD4+ memory T-cells have a capacity to change their cellular phenotypes between HLA-DR+ and HLA-DR− during ART. We observed that HLA-DR+ T-cells expressed higher levels of cellular activation/exhaustion and proliferation markers compared to their HLA-DR− counterpart. Therefore, our findings suggest that HIV persists in both HLA-DR+ and HLA-DR− CD4+ memory T-cell subsets and inclusion of both cell types should be considered when quantifying the viral reservoir and during the development of immune based treatment strategies.

MATERIALS AND METHODS

Study Approval

This study was carried out in accordance with the recommendations of the institutional review board at the Western Sydney Health Department for the Westmead Institute for Medical Research (AU RED LNR/13/WMEAD/315), and the ethics review committees at the University of California San Francisco (UCSF) (10-01330/068192, 10-02631/083640) and Vaccine Gene Therapy Institute-Florida (VGTI-FL) (FWA 00004139). The protocol was approved by these committees. All study participants provided written informed consent in accordance with the Declaration of Helsinki.

Participant and Clinical Samples

We included six HIV-1 subtype-B positive individuals on prolonged ART (> 15 years) from the SCOPE cohort in the study; 2 who initiated therapy during acute/early HIV infection (<6 months of infection before initiation of ART, AHI group) and 4 who initiated therapy during chronic HIV infection (>1 year of infection before initiation of ART, CHI group) (**Supplementary Table 1**). For five of these participants, peripheral blood was collected at 4 visits (Visit ID 1-4; after approximately 3, 5, 10, and 15 years of therapy) for this study. Participant 2518 provided peripheral blood during two visits (Visit ID 4 and 5, after approximately 15 and 17 years of therapy) (**Supplementary Table 1**). The viral load around the time of these visits was <40–75 copies (HIV-RNA) per ml. The CD4 counts were 462 cells/μL or greater during the study period.

Sample Processing and Cell Sorting

The CD4+ T-cell subsets were sorted from frozen aliquots of peripheral blood mononuclear cells (PBMCs) stored for 4–16 years which contained 50–100 × 10^6 cells that were collected from 5 of the participants at approximately years 3, 5, 10 on ART (Visit ID 1–3). At approximately 15 years of therapy, CD4+ T-cells were isolated from a leukapheresis for all 6 participants (Visit ID 4). Participant 2518 had a second leukapheresis sample collected for this study 2 years later at approximately 17 years on therapy (Visit ID 5). The cells were sorted using the following antibodies: CD3-Brilliant Violet 711 (clone OKT3, BioLegend), CD4-APC-eFluor 780 (clone OKT4, Thermo Fisher), CD14-V500 (clone M5E2, BD# 561391), LIVE/DEAD Aqua marker (Invitrogen# L34957), CD45RA-PECF594 (clone HI100, BD Biosciences), and HLA-DR− Brilliant Violet 421 (clone L243, BioLegend). CD3+CD4+ T-cells were gated on memory cells defined as CD45RA negative. HLA-DR± cells were then sorted on a BD FACS ARIA-II (**Supplementary Figure 1**). The HLD-DR± populations were sorted to >99% purity. Following sorting, the cell subsets were processed at 4°C and stored as a dry cell pellet at −80°C until analysis.

Quantification of Immune Activation and Exhaustion Markers

Cryopreserved PBMC samples were thawed at 37°C and washed with Roswell Park Memorial Institute (RPMI) medium containing 10% heat inactivated fetal bovine serum, 1% L-glutamine, 1% sterile penicillin-streptomycin and 2 μg/mL DNase I (Sigma-Aldrich, St. Louis, MO, United States). PBMC were counted using Guava ViaCount Reagent on an BD Accuri flow cytometer (BD Bioscience). PBMC were plated in a 96-well v-bottom plate and stained for 15 min at 4°C, then washed twice with FACS buffer (phosphate-buffered saline containing 0.5% bovine serum albumin and 1 mM Ethylenediaminetetraacetic Acid). Finally, cells were fixed in 0.5% formaldehyde and data was acquired on a customized 4-laser BD LSR II Flow cytometer (BD Biosciences), with ≥200,000 lymphocytes collected for each sample. CPT beads (BD Bioscience) were used for instrument set up and target values were established using single peak medium range Rainbow Fluorescent Particles (Spherotech). BD™ CompBead Plus Anti-Mouse Ig, ê beads or single stained PBMC were used for compensation controls. Data was compensated and analyzed in FlowJo V9 (TreeStar). A fluorescence minus one control was utilized to determine where to place the gate for PD-1-, CD38- and HLA-DR− cells. We analyzed results as total CD4+ T-cells, divided out as naïve and memory based CD45RA expression and as CD4+ T-cells plus double negative T-cells (CD4-CD8- T-cells) in the event that CD4 was downregulated on the cell surface due to infection. The antibodies, fluorochrome conjugates and clones used for this analysis are included in the **Supplementary Table 2**. The cell viability of the frozen and leukapheresis samples used to measure the cellular activation/exhaustion markers ranged from 69.7–88.2% and 68.8–87%, respectively.

Quantification of Intracellular HIV-DNA Levels

Intracellular HIV DNA levels within the sorted HLA-DR− and HLA-DR+ CD4+ memory T-cell subsets were measured using a previously described real-time RT-PCR method (Kumar et al., 2007). For this analysis, 96-12,186 HLA-DR− and HLA-DR+ memory T-cells per μL were used.

DNA Extraction for Sequence Analyses

DNA was extracted from CD4+ HLA-DR− and HLA-DR+ memory T-cell subsets. For this extraction, 400 μL RNAzolRT (MRC, Inc.) was added to 1.5 mL Eppendorf tube containing the cell pellet. Next, 160 μL of sterile nuclease free water (Invitrogen) was added and mixed by inversion for 15 s followed by incubation for 15 min. The mixture was centrifuged at 16000 *g* for 15 min at room temperature. The top phase was removed and the bottom phase was used for DNA extraction. Nine hundred μL of DNAzol (MRC, Inc.) followed by 10 μL of glycogen (20 μg/μL, Qiagen) was added to the bottom phase. DNA was precipitated by adding 500 μL of 200 proof ethanol (Sigma-Aldrich). The mixture was incubated for 10 min at room temperature and centrifuged at full speed for 30 min. The supernatant was removed and the DNA pellet was washed with 75% ethanol twice. The pellet was air dried until no ethanol was visible. The pellet was dissolved in 300 μL of 8 mM NaOH (Sigma-Aldrich) followed by neutralization by adding 24 μL of 0.1 M HEPES (Gibco).

Single-Proviral Sequencing (SPS)

Individual intracellular HIV-DNA sequences were obtained from the extracted DNA by single-proviral sequencing (SPS) that amplifies the *gag-pol* region of HIV genome (p6-RT) as previously described (Palmer et al., 2005; Kearney et al., 2008, 2009; Josefsson et al., 2012, 2013; von Stockenstrom et al., 2015). Briefly, the extracted DNA molecules were serially diluted (1:1-1:81) to endpoint dilution. Single HIV-DNA molecules were amplified using primers flanking the p6-RT region. We obtained single HIV-DNA molecules from approximately 206 to 200 × 10^3 and 740 to 1.6 × 10^6 HLA-DR+ and HLA-DR− memory T-cells, respectively (**Supplementary Tables 3, 4**). We obtained a total of 618 and 832 HIV-DNA sequences from the HLA-DR+ and HLA-DR− memory T-cell subsets, respectively. PCR amplification and sequencing of the HIV-DNA molecules at limiting dilution allowed us to determine the HIV infection frequency of the memory T-cells and also identify those HIV DNA sequences which were part of expansions of identical sequences (EIS) (Josefsson et al., 2013; von Stockenstrom et al., 2015).

HIV-DNA Genetic Analysis

Inter-Participant Contamination Assessment

HIV-DNA p6-RT sequences derived from HLA-DR+ and HLA-DR− memory T-cell subsets were assessed for inter-participant contamination using a program for Maximum Likelihood based inference of large phylogenetic trees (Randomized Axelerated Maximum Likelihood; RAxML version 7.2.8.) with general time reversible and gamma distribution for the nucleotide model and rapid hill-climbing for the tree building algorithm (Stamatakis, 2006). The HIV sequences from the T-cell subsets and positive control for SPS were aligned using MAFFT (Katoh and Standley, 2013). The phylogenetic tree was annotated by ggtree in R (Yu et al., 2017). From this maximum likelihood phylogenetic tree, we found no evidence of cross-contamination between participant samples (**Supplementary Figure 2**).

Expansions of Identical HIV-DNA Sequences (EIS)

The expansions of identical HIV-DNA p6-RT sequences within HLA-DR− and HLA-DR+ memory T-cell subsets were identified within the CHI group using ElimDupes from the Los Alamos HIV sequence database[1] with a pairwise genetic identity of 100%. HIV-DNA sequences from each participant were aligned using MAFFT (Katoh and Standley, 2013). For three participants from the CHI group, as the number of DNA sequences obtained from the frozen cell aliquots were at times limited, we analyzed the HIV-DNA sequences obtained from the 3 earlier visits together (Visit ID 1-3). The viral sequences from leukapheresis sample collected at the 4th visit were analyzed separately. For participant 2518, the viral sequences from visits 4 and 5 were independently analyzed for EIS. An EIS must contain at least two genetically identical HIV-DNA sequences derived from a specific CD4+ memory T-cell subset. However, if an HIV-DNA sequence from one of three earlier time points was genetically identical to a sequence from the later time point, these matching sequences were not considered a part of an EIS.

Identification of Genetically Defective HIV-DNA p6-RT Sequences

HIV-DNA p6-RT sequences containing G-A hypermutations were identified using Los Alamos Hypermut tool (Rose and Korber, 2000). The sequences containing premature stop codons, insertions/deletions causing a frameshift and/or internal deletions were identified by manual screening and the Los Alamos quality control tool (see footnote 1). All the defective sequences were included in the subsequent genetic analyses.

HIV-DNA Sequence Analysis

The longitudinal analysis of HIV genomic material allowed us to determine persistence of HIV within HLA-DR+ and HLA-DR− CD4+ memory T-cell subsets and investigate the amount of transition between these two cell types. For each participant, we constructed maximum likelihood phylogenetic trees using HIV-DNA sequences derived from the HLA-DR+ and HLA-DR− memory T-cell subsets during therapy using MEGA6 (1000 bootstrap replicates, general time reversible model with gamma distribution and proportion of invariant sites, gamma category 5) (Tamura et al., 2013). For 5 of the participants, we combined the HIV-DNA sequences obtained from 3 earlier time points (Visit ID 1–3) and compared these sequences to those obtained at the last time point (Visit ID 4). For the CHI participant, 2518, we compared the viral sequences obtained at 15.1 and 17.0 years on ART (Visit ID 4 and 5). To investigate whether the HIV genomes sequenced from the HLA-DR+ and HLA-DR− cells persist over time, we calculated the percentage of viral sequences from the earlier time points (visits 1–3 or for 2518, visit 4) that were genetically identical to at least one HIV-DNA sequence from the last time point (visit 4, or for 2518 visit 5) within the HLA-DR+ or HLA-DR− memory T-cell subsets. In addition, we investigated the transition between the HLA-DR+ and HLA-DR− cellular phenotypes using sequence analyses. In conducting these analyses we calculated the percentage of (HLA-DR+)-derived viral sequences from the earlier time points (visits 1–3 or for 2518, visit 4) that were genetically identical to at least one HIV-DNA sequence from the HLA-DR− T-cells at last time point (visit 4, or for 2518 visit 5). We also calculated the percentage of (HLA-DR−)-derived HIV-DNA sequences from earlier time points which were later found in the HLA-DR+ T-cell subset during ART. All the phylogenetic trees were annotated and visualized by R package, ggtree, and MEGA6 (Tamura et al., 2013; Yu et al., 2017, 2018).

Statistics

We used restricted maximum likelihood to fit linear random-intercept-random-slope models to expression levels of HLA-DR, CCR5, LAG-3 and Tim-3 within HLA-DR+ and HLA-DR− CD4+ memory T-cell subsets at different time points during ART (Stata 15, StataCorp. 2017. Stata Statistical Software: Release 15. College Station, TX: StataCorp LLC). This method allows expression levels and their rates of change to differ in different participants. For proportions of HIV-infected T-cells in the HLA-DR+ and HLA-DR− subsets at longitudinal time points during ART, we used maximum likelihood statistical analysis modified from methods described previously (Josefsson et al., 2012, 2013; von Stockenstrom et al., 2015). We used the estimated model coefficients to derive estimated fold-differences of the proportions of infected cells and the expression of cellular activation/exhaustion markers between the HLA-DR+ and HLA-DR− cell subsets at various time points during therapy (Stata lincom command).

We defined dichotomous dependent variables for each HIV-DNA sequence being a part of an EIS and those sequences which indicate cellular persistence and transition. For these viral sequences, we applied mixed effects logistic regression with random person effects to obtain odds ratios to compare the last time point with the early time points during therapy, and to compare the HLA-DR+ to HLA-DR− T-cells.

[1] https://www.hiv.lanl.gov/

RESULTS

Persistent Expression of HLA-DR Within CD4+ Memory T-Cells During ART

We measured the expression of HLA-DR on memory CD4+ T-cells derived from HIV-infected individuals who initiated ART during acute/early and chronic infection at multiple time points during prolonged ART. The frequency of HLA-DR+ memory CD4+ T-cells ranged from 3.4 to 12.2% during 2.9–17.7 years of ART and increased by an average of 0.22% per year of therapy (95% CI = 0.02–0.42%, *p*-value = 0.038) (**Figure 1**). Our findings indicate HLA-DR+ memory CD4+ T-cells persist and even increase at a slow rate during therapy.

Different Expression Profiles of Cellular Activation/Exhaustion Markers Within HLA-DR+ and HLA-DR− CD4+ Memory T-Cell Subsets During ART

Immune exhaustion during chronic HIV infection is a process that causes T-cell dysfunction which is associated with high expression levels of immune checkpoint molecules (Kim and Ahmed, 2010; Khaitan and Unutmaz, 2011; Cox et al., 2017). However, the expression profile of cellular activation/exhaustion markers on HLA-DR+ CD4+ memory T-cells when HIV is suppressed by ART has not been characterized. Also, it is not clear whether the HLA-DR+ cellular compartment in an HIV-infected individual is characterized by T-cell dysfunction during ART. Therefore, we measured the frequency of HLA-DR+ and HLA-DR− memory CD4+ T cells expressing PD-1, LAG-3 and Tim-3 (markers for immune exhaustion, Cox et al., 2017); and CCR5 (virus-mediated pathogenesis and T-cell co-stimulation; Contento et al., 2008; Portales et al., 2012; Yang et al., 2012) by flow cytometry in samples from the six participants. We performed a linear prediction using a mixed effects regression model after performing a log transformation of percent T-cells expressing each of the cellular markers. The relative change in the frequency of the CD4+ memory T-cells expressing each cellular marker per year on therapy was determined by $e^{(slope)}$ [exp(slope) in **Figure 2**], where the slope is estimated from the fitted linear line. For this calculation, an $e^{(slope)}$ of greater than 1 indicates an increasing rate of expression and less than 1 indicates a decreasing rate of expression.

For each cellular marker, we estimated the fold-difference in their expression levels on HLA-DR+ versus HLA-DR− memory T-cells at 3, 5, 10, and 15 years of ART (calculated using the predicted linear line for each marker; **Figure 2** and **Table 1**). HLA-DR+ cells had a higher level of expression of all the cellular markers except LAG-3 compared to HLA-DR− cells during ART. For CCR5 expression, the greatest difference between the HLA-DR+ and HLA-DR− cells was observed at 3 years of ART (Fold-difference = 6.36, 95% CI = 3.76–10.77, $p < 0.001$), but the difference was reduced to 3.43-fold at 15 years of therapy (95% CI = 2.26–5.21, $p < 0.001$). For PD-1 and Tim-3, HLA-DR+ cells had a 2-fold higher expression of these markers compared to HLA-DR− cells at all time points ($p < 0.001$–0.14). However, the HLA-DR− T-cells had approximately 3-fold higher expression of LAG-3 than the HLA-DR+ cells throughout ART ($p < 0.001$). Overall, most of the cellular activation/exhaustion markers were associated with the HLA-DR+ cells whereas LAG-3 was highly expressed on the HLA-DR− cells during ART.

We also investigated the rate of the cellular activation/exhaustion marker expression throughout the treatment period of 3 to ≥15 years. An average of 3% ($p = 0.17$) and 9% ($p < 0.001$) increase in CCR5 expression per year of therapy was observed for the HLA-DR+ and HLA-DR− T-cells, respectively (**Figure 2A**). The rate of increase over time in

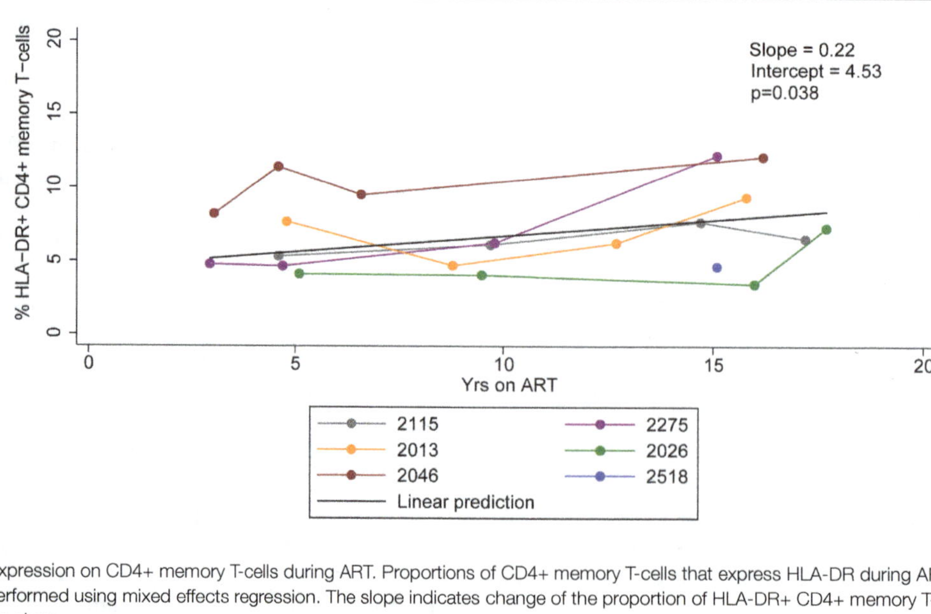

FIGURE 1 | HLA-DR expression on CD4+ memory T-cells during ART. Proportions of CD4+ memory T-cells that express HLA-DR during ART were quantified. The linear prediction was performed using mixed effects regression. The slope indicates change of the proportion of HLA-DR+ CD4+ memory T-cells per year on ART and *p*-value (p) is for the slope.

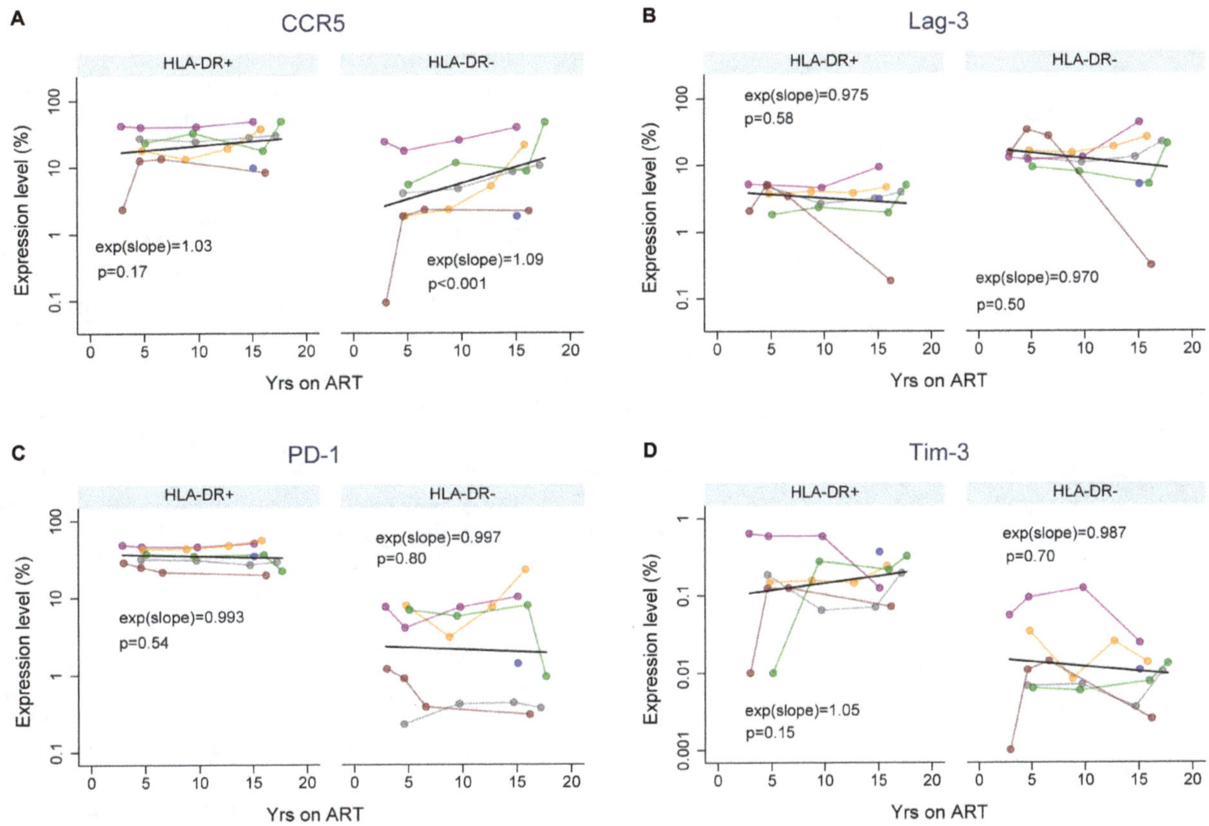

FIGURE 2 | Expression of cellular activation/exhaustion markers on HLA-DR+ and HLA-DR– CD4+ memory T-cells during ART. Proportions of HLA-DR+ and HLA-DR– CD4+ memory T-cells that express CCR5 **(A)**, LAG-3 **(B)**, PD-1 **(C)**, and Tim-3 **(D)**. The colors of data points and lines indicate different participants; 2115 (gray), 2275 (purple), 2013 (orange), 2026 (green), 2046 (maroon), and 2518 (blue). A linear prediction was performed on the log transformed values using mixed-effects linear regression (black line). The changes of expression levels per year on therapy are indicated by exp(slope) (or e^{slope}). An $e^{(slope)}$ greater than 1 indicates an increasing rate and less than 1 indicates a decreasing rate of expression. The *p*-values (p) are derived by comparing the slopes to the null hypothesis of slope = 0, or $e^{(slope)} = 1$.

CCR5 expression appeared to be greater in HLA-DR–, but the difference in rates between the HLA-DR+ and HLA-DR– T-cells had a *p*-value of 0.10. Both T-cell subsets revealed a slight decrease in the expression of LAG-3 and PD-1 (0.3–3%, $p = 0.50–0.80$, **Figures 2B,C**). The decrease in LAG-3 and PD-1 expression over time was similar between the T-cell subsets. Tim-3 expression increased by 5% on HLA-DR+ cells with each additional year of therapy ($p = 0.15$) whereas the HLA-DR– cells had a decreasing expression of Tim-3 of 1.3% per year (**Figure 2D**). However, the difference in the rates of change for Tim-3 expression during ART between the T-cell subsets was not statistically significant ($p = 0.19$). Overall, the changes in the expression of these cellular activation/exhaustion markers per year on ART were not found to be significant except for the expression of CCR5 on the HLA-DR– subset.

Persistence of HIV-Infected Cells Within HLA-DR+ and HLA-DR– CD4+ Memory T-Cell Subsets During ART

HIV persistence within HLA-DR+ CD4+ memory T-cells during prolonged ART is not clearly defined. We performed a previously described maximum likelihood method to estimate the number of cells infected within the HLA-DR+ and HLA-DR– CD4+ memory T-cell subsets in each participant at multiple time points during ART (Josefsson et al., 2012, 2013; Rosenbloom et al., 2015; von Stockenstrom et al., 2015). We employed multilevel mixed-effects negative binomial regression to estimate the change in the proportion of the infected T-cells per year on ART within the cell subsets. Using this model, we predicted the fold-difference of infection frequency between the HLA-DR+ and HLA-DR– subsets at 3, 5, 10, and 15 years of therapy. The change in the proportion of the infected T-cells is calculated by the $e^{(slope)}$ of the predicted line [exp(slope) in **Figure 3**], where a value of <1 indicates a decrease and a value of >1 indicates an increase.

We observed an average of 18% increase in the proportion of infected HLA-DR+ T-cells during each additional year of therapy when participants from both the AHI and CHI groups were included (fold-change = 1.18/year, 95%CI = 1.09–1.27, $p < 0.001$) (**Figure 3**). However, the proportion of HIV-infected HLA-DR– T-cells decreased at an average rate of 5.3% per year of ART (fold-change = 0.947/year, 95% CI = 0.877–1.023, $p = 0.17$). During 3–10 years of ART, the proportion of the HIV-infected HLA-DR+ cells remained about 30–84% lower than the HLA-DR–

TABLE 1 | Estimated fold-difference of expression levels of cellular activation/exhaustion markers between HLA-DR+ and HLA-DR− CD4+ memory T-cells.

Cellular marker	Years on ART	Fold-difference (HLA-DR+ vs. HLA-DR−)	95% CI		*p*-value
			Lower	Upper	
CCR5	3	6.36	3.76	10.77	<0.001
	5	5.74	3.72	8.87	<0.001
	10	4.44	3.27	6.02	<0.001
	15	3.43	2.26	5.21	<0.001
LAG-3	3	0.368	0.240	0.565	<0.001
	5	0.372	0.261	0.530	<0.001
	10	0.382	0.298	0.489	<0.001
	15	0.391	0.279	0.550	<0.001
PD-1	3	1.97	1.63	2.38	<0.001
	5	1.95	1.67	2.28	<0.001
	10	1.91	1.72	2.13	<0.001
	15	1.88	1.62	2.18	<0.001
Tim-3	3	1.80	0.82	3.95	0.143
	5	2.03	1.06	3.89	0.032
	10	2.76	1.75	4.35	<0.001
	15	3.74	2.01	6.97	<0.001

counterpart (**Table 2**). After 15 years of treatment, however, the frequency of HLA-DR+ infected cells was 2-fold greater than the HLA-DR− cells ($p = 0.013$).

In addition, we quantified intracellular HIV-DNA levels by qPCR targeting the long terminal repeat (LTR) region of the HIV genome during ART (Kumar et al., 2007). Many of these measurements were below the limit of the assay (1 copy of HIV-DNA) due to the low numbers of T-cells that were used in the assay (**Supplementary Table 5**).

Persistence of Viral p6-RT DNA Sequences Within HLA-DR+ and HLA-DR− CD4+ T-Cell Subsets During ART

Phylogenetic trees provide another way to visualize HIV persistence within the HLA-DR+ and HLA-DR− T-cell subsets. Therefore, we assessed the persistence of HIV-DNA p6-RT sequences within HLA-DR+ and HLA-DR− CD4+ memory T-cell subsets using phylogenetic analysis. The phylogenetic trees derived from the participants of the AHI group showed that HIV-DNA p6-RT sequences without stop codons within the HLA-DR+ and HLA-DR− T-cell subsets obtained during 2.9–17.2 years of therapy were genetically homogeneous (**Figure 4** and **Supplementary Figures 3–5**).

For the participants from the CHI group, the HIV sequences derived from the HLA-DR+ T-cell subset at different time points during ART intermingled (**Figure 5** and **Supplementary Figures 6–8**). For more accurate visualization of those HIV-DNA sequences that persisted over different time points during ART, we constructed phylogenetic trees using the

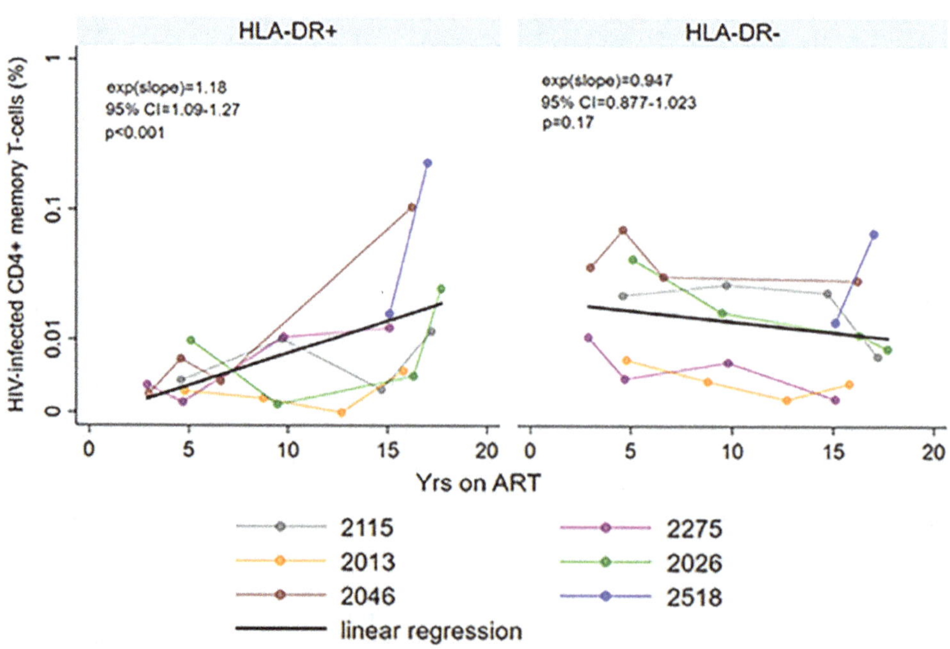

FIGURE 3 | Persistence of HIV-infected HLA-DR+ and HLA-DR− CD4+ memory T-cells during ART. The proportion of HIV-infected T-cells (%) was estimated using maximum likelihood model derived from single-proviral sequencing. The change in the frequency of HIV-infected T-cells per year on ART [exp(slope)] was derived from mixed-effects negative binominal regression (black line). The 95% confidence intervals (95% CI) and *p*-value of the exp(slope) are also shown. The colors of the data points and the lines indicate different participants as shown in the legend.

TABLE 2 | Estimated fold-differences of proportions of HIV-infected cells within HLA-DR+ and HLA-DR− CD4+ memory T-cell subsets during ART.

Years on ART	Fold-difference (HLA-DR+ vs. HLA-DR−)	95% CI		*p*-value
		Lower	Upper	
3	0.156	0.068	0.359	<0.001
5	0.240	0.120	0.483	<0.001
10	0.708	0.440	1.139	0.155
15	2.09	1.17	3.73	0.013

viral sequences derived from monophyletic clades (**Figure 6**). For two participants (2026 and 2518), we found a total of six sequences that persisted over two years in the HLA-DR+ T-cell subset (**Supplementary Table 6** and **Figure 6**). However, for all CHI participants, a total of 57 viral sequences derived from the HLA-DR− cell subset obtained at the earlier time points (3.0–10.0 years of ART; Visit ID 1-3) were genetically identical to sequences obtained at the last time point (15.8- years of ART; Visit ID 4; for 2518 this was compared from Visit ID 4 to Visit ID 5) (**Supplementary Table 6** and **Supplementary Figure 9**). For all of the participants combined, the odds that an HIV-DNA sequence derived from one of the three earlier time points was identical to at least one sequence from the last time point during ART was approximately 2-fold higher within HLA-DR+ cell subset compared to the HLA-DR− (p = 0.043) (**Figure 7**). Within the HLA-DR+ cell subset, 33% of the HIV-DNA sequences at the earlier time points were identical to at least one viral sequence from the last time point. For the HLA-DR− cell subset, we found 20% of HIV-DNA sequences derived from the earlier time points were genetically identical to at least one viral sequence derived from the last time point.

HIV-DNA Sequence Analysis Reveals a Fraction of CD4+ Memory T-Cells Change Between HLA-DR+ and HLA-DR− Phenotypes

Currently it is unclear as to the number of HIV-infected CD4+ memory T-cells transitioning between activated and resting cellular phenotypes. Therefore, we determined whether HLA-DR+ CD4+ memory T-cells containing HIV-DNA revert to the HLA-DR− phenotype during therapy. To do this, we calculated the number of HIV-DNA p6-RT sequences derived from the HLA-DR+ cell subset collected at the earlier time points that were genetically identical to the viral sequences derived from the HLA-DR− cell subset collected at the last time point from all of the participants (**Supplementary Table 6**). Also, we assessed whether the HLA-DR− memory T-cells transition to HLA-DR+ cellular phenotype by comparing the viral sequences from the HLA-DR− cell subset obtained at the earlier time points to those from the HLA-DR+ cell subset obtained at the last time point during ART (**Supplementary Table 6**).

For three participants (2026, 2046, and 2518), we found a total of eight phylogenetic clades which contained genetically identical HIV-DNA sequences derived from the HLA-DR+ cell subset obtained at the three earlier time points and the HLA-DR− cell subset obtained at last time point (**Figure 8**). In all CHI participants, we found a total of ten clades that contained HIV sequences derived from the HLA-DR− cell subset obtained at the 3 earlier time points being genetically identical to viral sequences obtained from HLA-DR+ cell subset sorted at last time points (**Figure 9**). For all of the participants combined, the proportion of HIV-DNA sequences that indicate cellular transition from HLA-DR+ to HLA-DR− (30%) or from HLA-DR− to HLA-DR+ CD4+ memory T-cells (21%) was not statistically significant (OR = 1.58, 95% CI = 0.86–2.89, p = 0.14) (**Figure 10**).

EIS Contribute to Proviral Persistence Within HLA-DR+ CD4+ Memory T-Cells During ART

Several studies have assessed the contribution of cellular proliferation to the persistence of HIV in different memory T cells by identifying and/or quantifying the number of genetically identical HIV-DNA sequences found in these cells at one time point or over time (Josefsson et al., 2013; Wagner et al., 2013; Imamichi et al., 2014; Kearney et al., 2015; von Stockenstrom et al., 2015; Simonetti et al., 2016; Hiener et al., 2017; Lee et al., 2017). However, many of these previous studies excluded HLA-DR expressing cells. We first determined the expression levels of the markers for cellular proliferation (Ki67 and the combined marker of Ki67/PD-1) on the HLA-DR+ and HLA-DR− CD4+ memory T-cells derived from the 4th visit during ART (Scholzen and Gerdes, 2000). We then compared these cellular expression levels with the genetically identical HIV-DNA p6-RT sequences obtained from the 4th visit during therapy. We also used a mixed effects logistic regression model to estimate changes in the frequency of genetically identical HIV-DNA p6-RT sequences during therapy within the HLA-DR+ and HLA-DR− CD4+ memory T-cell subsets derived from the CHI cohort, as these participants who initiated antiviral treatment during chronic infection contain genetically diverse intracellular viral DNA (Anderson et al., 2011; Josefsson et al., 2013; von Stockenstrom et al., 2015). In this study, we defined EIS as $\geq$2 genetically identical sequences which were derived from the same T-cell subset. For participants 2013, 2026, and 2046, we assessed the total number of sequences contributing to an EIS from the 3 earlier time points together (Visit ID 1-3) as these clinical samples were stored for 4–16 years and the number of cells sorted and the sequenced HIV genomes from these cells were at times quite low. We characterized the number of viral sequences contributing to an EIS from the samples obtained at the last time point separately, as the Visit ID 4 samples for all participants was a leukapheresis. For participant 2518, we characterized the number of sequences contributing to an EIS after 15.1 and 17.0 years of ART separately as the cells sorted at these time points (Visit ID 4 and 5) came from a leukapheresis.

To determine the proliferative nature of the HLA-DR+ and HLA-DR− CD4+ T-cells, we measured their expression

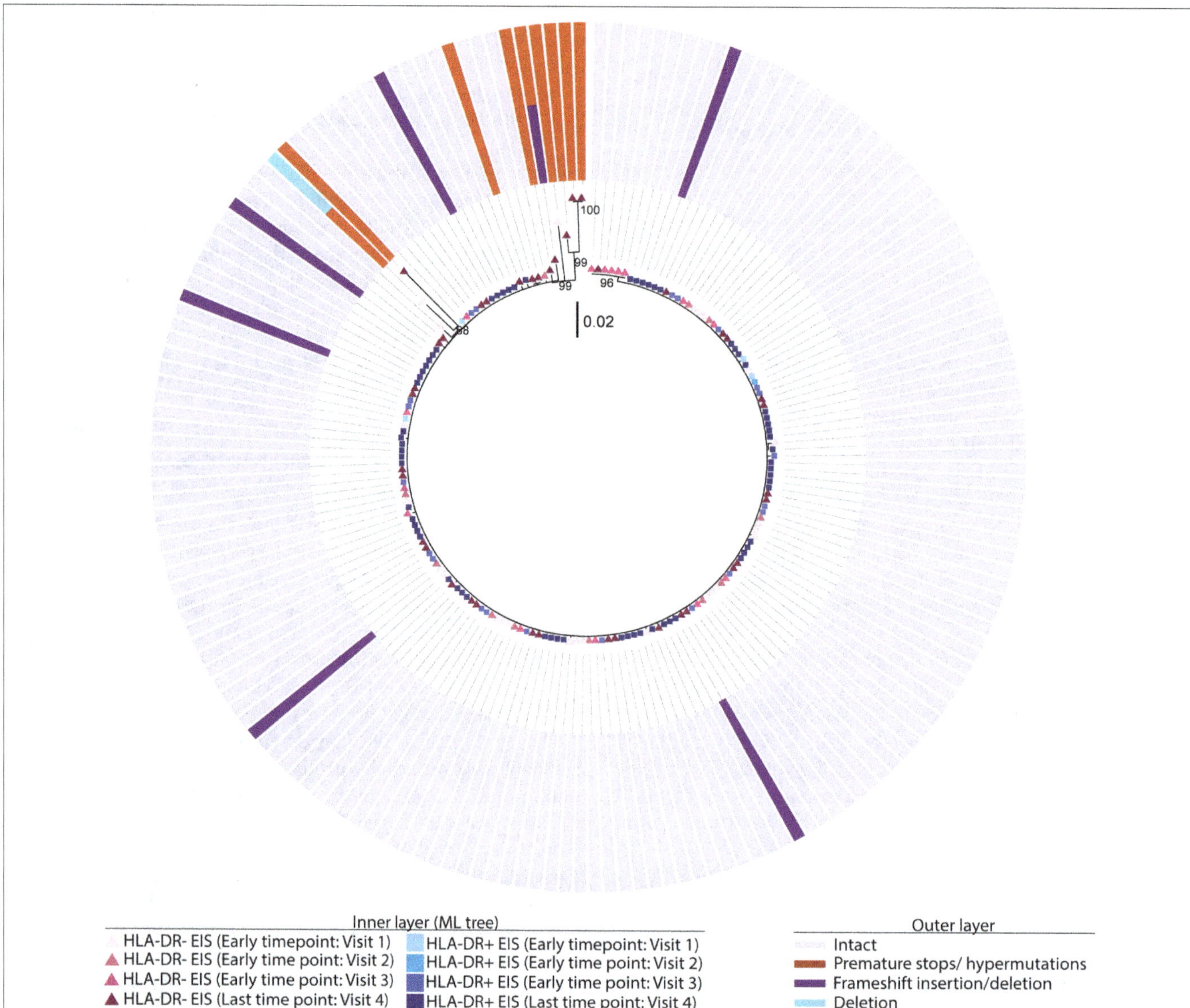

FIGURE 4 | Intact and defective HIV-DNA p6-RT sequences within HLA-DR+ and HLA-DR− CD4+ memory T-cell subsets derived from an acute/early participant. A representative phylogenetic tree of a participant from the AHI group (2275). The inner layer shows the phylogenetic tree constructed by all HIV-DNA p6-RT sequences derived from the HLA-DR+ and HLA-DR− T-cells obtained from participant 2275 during therapy (Visits 1–4; 2.9–15.1 years after ART initiation). The outer layer shows defective genetic features for individual HIV-DNA sequences as shown in the legend.

of the cellular proliferation marker Ki67 alone or Ki67/PD-1 co-expression (Scholzen and Gerdes, 2000). The expression of these markers was determined for all 6 participants at Visit ID 4 (after approximately 15 years of therapy). We found that Ki67 expression averaged 19-fold higher on the HLA-DR+ cells (range = 17.3–29.7%) compared to the HLA-DR− cells (range = 0.829–2.63%) (p = 0.0005) (**Supplementary Figure 10**). Also, we the found Ki67/PD-1 co-expression level averaged approximately 22-fold higher on the HLA-DR+ cells (range = 6.11–18.3%) compared to the HLA-DR− cells (0.246–0.824) (p = 0.0008) (**Supplementary Figure 10**). For the CHI group, we did not find a strong positive correlation between the proportion of identical HIV-DNA sequences within their HLA-DR+ and HLA-DR− CD4+ memory T-cells and the level of Ki67 or Ki67/PD-1 expression on these cells at Visit ID 4 (**Supplementary Table 7**).

When the HIV-DNA p6-RT sequences were visualized by phylogenetic trees, we found that these EIS contain both intact and defective viral sequences (**Figure 5** and **Supplementary Figures 6–8**). We also compared the number of HIV-DNA sequences from HLA-DR+ and HLA-DR− T-cell subsets contributing to an EIS at the earlier time points and the last time point during therapy. At the earlier time points during ART, the odds that an HIV-DNA sequence was part of an EIS within the HLA-DR+ or the HLA-DR− T-cell subset was similar (OR = 0.61–1.26, p = 0.20–0.82) (**Supplementary Table 8**).

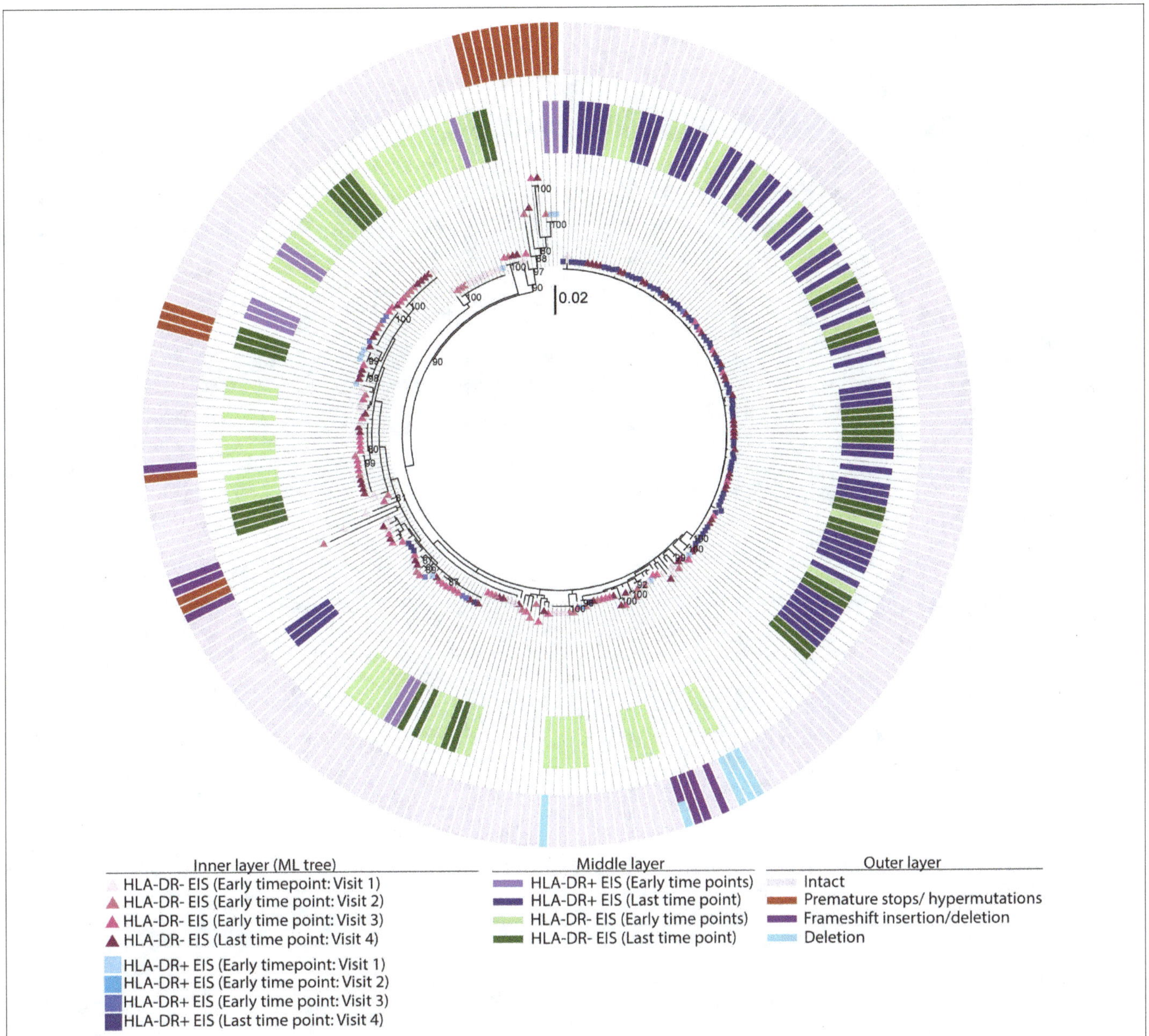

FIGURE 5 | EIS, intact and defective HIV-DNA p6-RT sequences within HLA-DR+ and HLA-DR– CD4+ memory T-cell subsets derived from a chronic participant. A representative phylogenetic tree of a participant from the CHI group (2026). The inner layer shows a maximum likelihood phylogenetic tree that includes all HIV-DNA p6-RT sequences derived from the HLA-DR+ and HLA-DR– T-cells obtained from participant 2026 during therapy (CHI group). The middle layer shows individual HIV-DNA sequences which are part of an EIS within the HLA-DR+ and HLA-DR– T-cells obtained at three earlier time points (Visits 1–3; 5.1–16.0 years after ART initiation) and last time point (Visit 4; 17.7 years after ART initiation), The outer layer shows defective genetic features for individual viral sequences as shown in the legend.

However, the odds that an HIV-DNA sequence contributes to an EIS in the HLA-DR+ T-cell subset was approximately 3 to 19-fold higher than their HLA-DR– counterpart at the last time point ($p < 0.001$). In addition, the proportion of HIV-DNA sequences derived from EIS was positively correlated with the proportion of HIV-infected CD4+ memory T-cells within the HLA-DR+ T-cell subset ($\rho = 1.00$, $p = 0.083$), whereas a negative correlation was observed within the HLA-DR– T-cells ($\rho = -0.800$, $p = 0.20$) (**Supplementary Table 7**).

For participants 2013, 2026, and 2046, the number of genetically identical HIV-DNA p6-RT sequences within the HLA-DR+ T-cell subset was 4-fold greater at last time point (Visit ID 4) compared to three earlier time points combined (Visit ID 1-3) (**Figure 11A**). Within this HLA-DR+ cell subset, the odds of a viral sequence being a part of an EIS was 12-fold greater at the last time point compared to the earlier time points (95% CI = 5.4–26.9, $p < 0.001$). For the HLA-DR– cell subset, we found that the proportion of genetically identical HIV DNA sequences was only

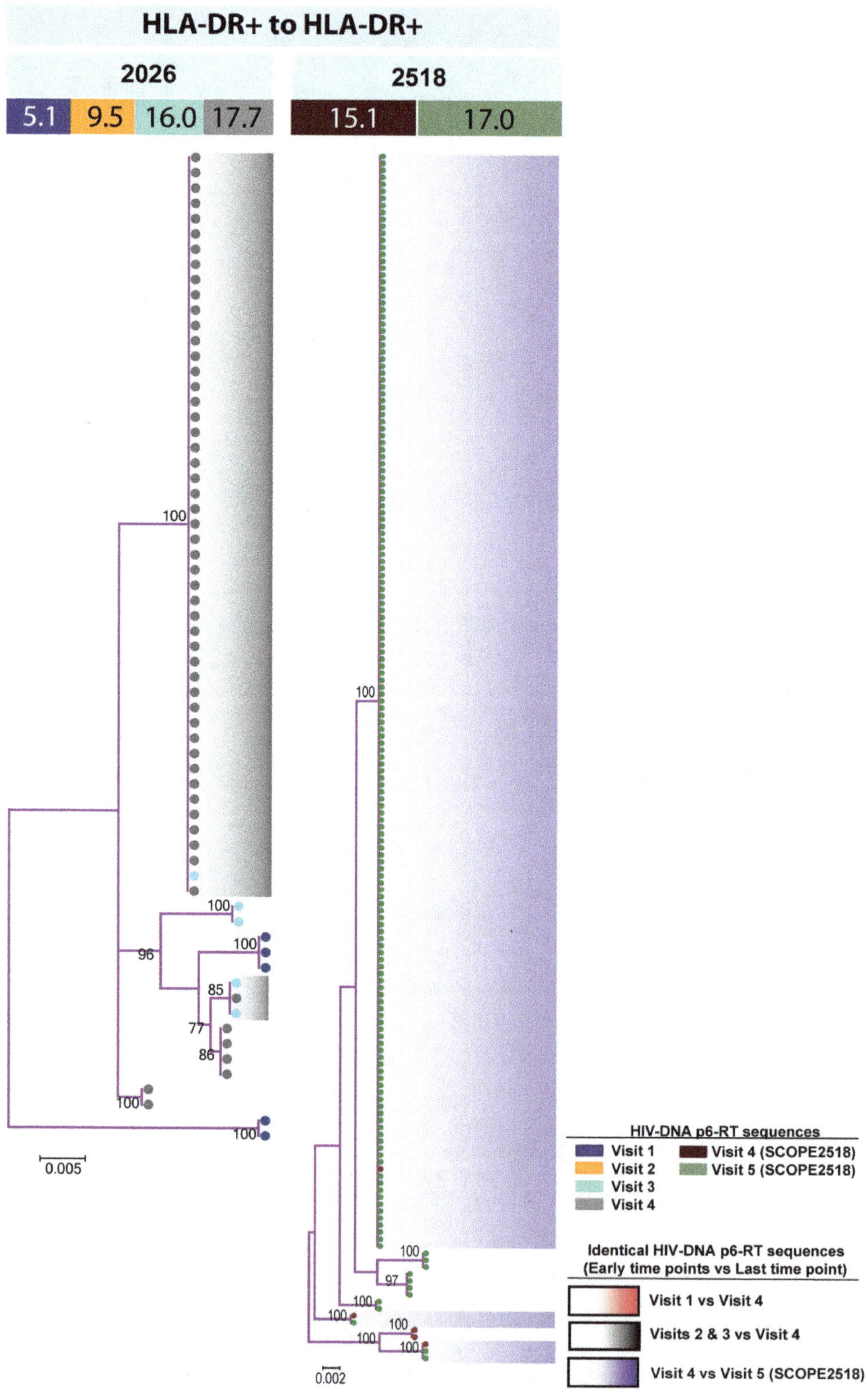

FIGURE 6 | HIV-DNA p6-RT sequences persist within HLA-DR+ CD4+ memory T-cell subset during ART. Maximum likelihood phylogenetic trees using HIV-DNA sequences derived from monophyletic clades within the HLA-DR+ T-cell subset (HLA-DR+ to HLA-DR+). The trees were constructed for participants 2026 and 2518. The sampling time points (years after ART initiation) for individual HIV-DNA sequences are indicated under the participant IDs. The viral sequences derived from different sampling time points are shown with different colors that correspond to the visit IDs as shown in the legend. The shades indicate phylogenetic clades that contain identical HIV-DNA sequences derived from the three earlier time points and the last time point.

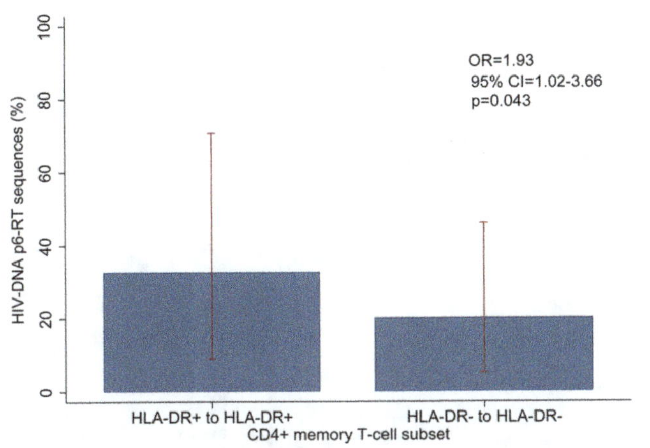

FIGURE 7 | Overall comparison of the HIV-DNA p6-RT sequences that persist within the HLA-DR+ and HLA-DR− CD4+ T-cell subsets during ART. The percent of HIV-DNA sequences that persist within the HLA-DR+ and HLA-DR− T-cells are indicated as "HLA-DR+ to HLA-DR+" and "HLA-DR− to HLA-DR−", respectively. The percent was estimated by fitting the mixed-effects logistic regression to all participants (blue bar). The 95% CIs of the percent values are shown as red capped lines. The odds ratio (OR) and its 95% CI and p-value compare "HLA-DR+ to HLA-DR+" to "HLA-DR− to HLA-DR−".

about 1.5-fold higher at the last time point compared to the earlier time points (OR = 2.32, 95% CI = 1.52–3.55, $p < 0.001$). For participant 2518, the proportion of the sequences derived from an EIS increased from 18 to 95% within the HLA-DR+ T-cells over two years of therapy (OR = 93.9, 95% CI = 17.4–508.3, $p < 0.001$) (**Figure 11B**). However, within the HLA-DR− T-cell subset, a smaller increase of genetically identical HIV sequences compared to the HLA-DR+ T-cell subset was observed (15–53%). Overall, for the CHI group, the number of viral sequences contributing to an EIS was 45.7 times greater within the HLA-DR+ T-cell subset obtained at the last time point compared to the earlier time points combined when the HIV-DNA sequences were normalized by the number of the HLA-DR+ cells we used in the sequencing ($p < 0.001$, **Figure 11C**). For the HLA-DR− T-cell subset, we found a 1.78-fold increase in the number of the viral sequences contributing to an EIS from the earlier time points compared to the last time point, however, this was not statistically significant.

DISCUSSION

HIV persists in resting memory CD4 T-cells during ART, but the contribution of CD4+ memory T cells expressing cellular markers of activation to the HIV reservoir is undefined. Understanding the contribution of CD4+ memory T-cells expressing HLA-DR to the persistent HIV reservoir is important for an accurate measurement of this HIV reservoir and would be crucial for the development of new immune based interventions. Here we performed a detailed longitudinal analysis of HIV persistence in HLA-DR+ and HLA-DR− memory T-cells sorted from peripheral blood of participants who initiated ART during acute/early and chronic infection. We also investigated the expression of cellular activation/exhaustion markers on these HLA-DR+ and HLA-DR− CD4+ memory T-cell subsets.

The assays currently used to detect inducible HIV proviruses commonly exclude CD4+ T-cells that express HLA-DR as these cells are believed to be actively transcribing HIV; thus, do not play an important role in HIV persistence during therapy (Chun et al., 1995; Siliciano and Siliciano, 2005). In our study, however, we found evidence for prolonged persistence of proviruses within HLA-DR+ CD4+ memory T-cell subset during therapy. First, the expression of HLA-DR+ on CD4+ memory T-cells and the proportion of HIV-infected HLA-DR+ T-cells increased with the duration of treatment. Second, for two participants treated during acute/early infection, the HIV-DNA p6-RT sequences derived from the HLA-DR+ T-cell subset over 2.9–17.2 years of ART were genetically homogeneous indicating stable infection of these cells from acute infection and throughout years of therapy. Lastly, we found two cases in the CHI group where HIV-DNA p6-RT sequences persisted within the HLA-DR+ T-cell subset over two years of therapy. Taken together our results suggest that we should consider including cells that express HLA-DR when measuring the HIV reservoir as HIV-infected HLA-DR+ T-cells do persist over years of therapy.

Studies have shown that HLA-DR expression correlates with the HIV-DNA level in CD4+ T-cells during 5.8–8.0 of therapy (Cockerham et al., 2014). In the current study, when participants were on therapy for 3 to ≥15 years, the proportion of HIV-infected HLA-DR+ T-cells increased at a rate of 18% per year. In the HLA-DR− memory T-cell subset, however, we found evidence for a decay in the proportion of the infected cells during ART at a rate of 5% per year, although it was not statistically significant. In addition, we measured HIV-DNA levels using qPCR targeting the LTR region, but many of these values were below the limit of the assay (1 HIV-DNA copy) due to the small numbers of cells assayed and therefore, were not informative. Nevertheless, our findings suggest a substantially slower decay rate of the HIV reservoir during therapy than previously reported ($t_{1/2}$ = 43.9–44.2 months) when both the HLA-DR+ and HLA-DR− cell subsets are included (Finzi et al., 1999; Siliciano et al., 2003). We found that the frequency of HIV-infected cells increased within the HLA-DR+ T-cell subset during therapy, and this increase could compensate for the slow decrease of HIV-infected HLA-DR− T-cells.

Our genetic analysis of the HIV-DNA p6-RT genomic region suggests that two cellular mechanisms contribute to HIV persistence during therapy. First, over years of therapy, our HIV-DNA sequence analysis indicated that a fraction of the HLA-DR+ T-cells contribute to the persistent HIV reservoir of the HLA-DR− T-cell subset. For example, 30% of the HIV-DNA sequences from HLA-DR+ T-cells from the three earlier time points on ART were genetically identical to viral sequences derived from the HLA-DR− subset obtained at the last time point on ART. This suggests that a fraction of the HLA-DR+ T-cells transitioned to the HLA-DR− phenotype, downregulating their HLA-DR expression during therapy. We also found 21% of HIV-DNA sequences within the HLA-DR− subset identified at the three earlier time points were only found in the HLA-DR+ T cells at the last time point, indicating a cellular transition from a resting

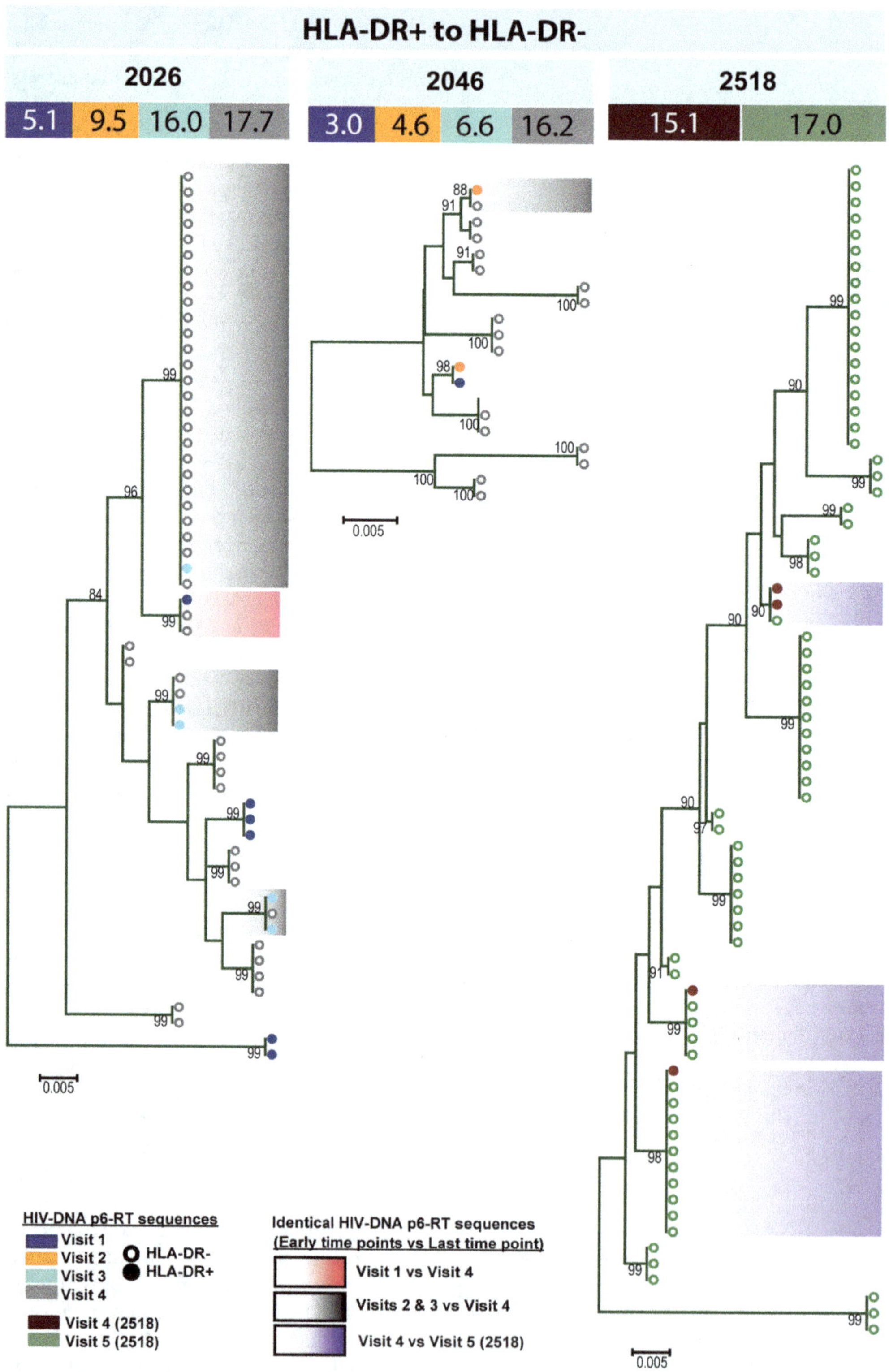

FIGURE 8 | HIV-DNA p6-RT sequences from HLA-DR+ T-cells that are identical to sequences from HLA-DR– T-cells during ART. Maximum likelihood phylogenetic trees using HIV-DNA sequences derived from monophyletic clades that show sequences from the first time points of HLA-DR+ T-cells being identical to sequences from HLA-DR– T-cells at the last time point (HLA-DR+ to HLA-DR–). The trees were constructed for participants 2026, 2046, and 2518. The sampling time points (years after ART initiation) for individual HIV-DNA sequences are indicated under the participant IDs. The viral sequences derived from different sampling time points are shown with different colors that correspond to the visit IDs as shown in the legend. The shades indicate phylogenetic clades that contain identical HIV-DNA sequences derived from the HLA-DR+ T-cells obtained from the three earlier time points and the HLA-DR– T-cells from the last time point.

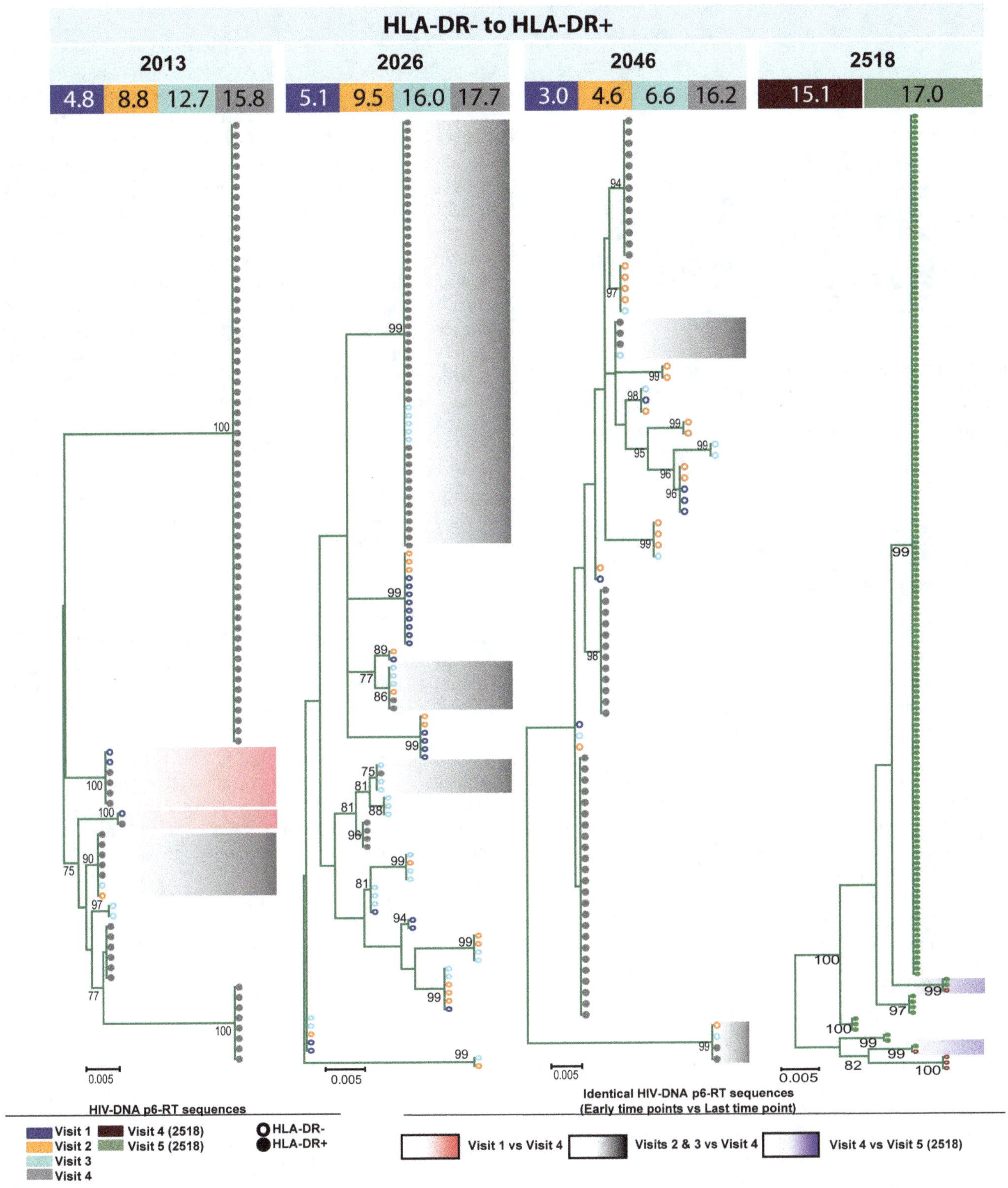

FIGURE 9 | HIV-DNA p6-RT sequences from HLA-DR– T-cells that are identical to sequences from the HLA-DR+ T-cells during ART. Maximum likelihood phylogenetic trees using HIV-DNA sequences derived from monophyletic clades that show sequences from the first time points of HLA-DR– T-cells being identical to sequences from HLA-DR+ T-cells at the last time point (HLA-DR– to HLA-DR+). The trees were constructed for all CHI participants. The sampling time points (years after ART initiation) for individual HIV-DNA sequences are indicated under the participant IDs. The viral sequences derived from different sampling time points are shown with different colors that correspond to the visit IDs as shown in the legend. The shades indicate phylogenetic clades that contain identical HIV-DNA sequences derived from the HLA-DR– T-cells obtained from the three earlier time points and the HLA-DR+ T-cells from the last time point.

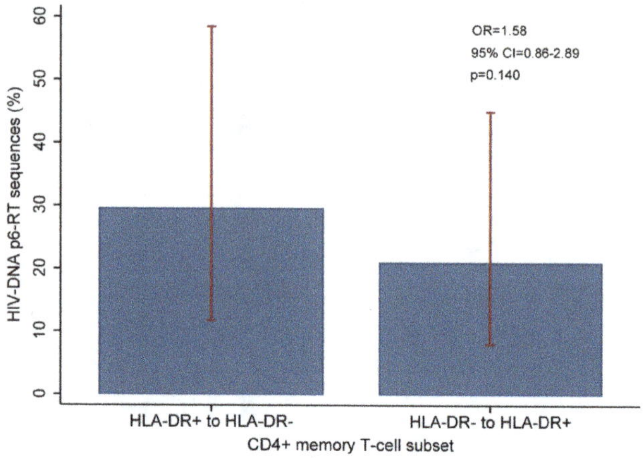

FIGURE 10 | Overall comparison of the HIV-DNA p6-RT sequences that switch between HLA-DR+ and HLA-DR– CD4+ T-cell subsets during ART. The percent of viral sequences derived from the HLA-DR+ T-cell subset from the three early time points which were identical to at least one (HLA-DR–)-derived viral sequence from the last time point is indicated as "HLA-DR+ to HLA-DR–". The percent of viral sequences derived from the HLA-DR– T-cell subset from the three early time points which were identical to at least one (HLA-DR+)-derived viral sequence from the last time point is indicated as "HLA-DR– to HLA-DR+". The percent was estimated from the mixed-effects logistic regression fitted to all participants (blue bar). The 95% CIs of the percent values are shown as red capped lines. The odds ratio (OR) and its 95% CI and p-value compare "HLA-DR+ to HLA-DR–" versus "HLA-DR– to HLA-DR+".

to activated (i.e., HLA-DR+) phenotype during therapy. Studies have shown that the HIV reservoir resides within an array of resting CD4+ memory T-cells with specific phenotypic markers during ART (Chomont et al., 2009; Perreau et al., 2013; Buzon et al., 2014). Also that effector and terminally differentiated effector CD4+ memory T-cell subsets commonly express HLA-DR (Corneau et al., 2017). Our genetic analysis suggests that a proportion of these differentiated CD4+ T-cell subsets cycle from HLA-DR– to HLA-DR+ phenotypes or vice versa during therapy and thus HLA-DR+ T-cells can contribute to the HIV reservoir in resting memory T-cells (Corneau et al., 2017).

In agreement with recent studies, we found cellular proliferation is the second cellular mechanism that contributes to HIV persistence during therapy (Josefsson et al., 2013; Wagner et al., 2013; Imamichi et al., 2014; Kearney et al., 2015; von Stockenstrom et al., 2015; Simonetti et al., 2016; Hiener et al., 2017; Lee et al., 2017). In our study, we found that genetically identical HIV-DNA p6-RT sequences increase during therapy within HLA-DR+ and HLA-DR– T-cells, indicating cellular proliferation continuously contributes to HIV persistence in both these cell subsets over years of ART. Also, we found a strong trend that the proportion of HIV-DNA sequences contributing to identical sequence clusters is positively correlated with the proportion of infected HLA-DR+ T-cells, but not within their HLA-DR– counterpart. We found that identical sequence expansions are comprised of either genetically intact or defective p6-RT HIV-DNA sequences. This indicates that cellular proliferation maintains the pool of HIV-infected cells containing genetically intact and defective p6-RT sequences, particularly within the HLA-DR+ T-cells.

Interestingly, we did not find a strong correlation between the proportion of HIV-DNA sequences belonging to a cluster of identical sequences and the markers for cellular proliferation (Ki67 and/or Ki67/PD-1 co-expression) within the HLA-DR+ and HLA-DR– T-cell subsets (Scholzen and Gerdes, 2000). This could be affected by the small number of CHI participants included in the correlation analysis. Also, this could be due to the fact that the expression of Ki67 and/or Ki67/PD-1 was determined within total CD4+ T-cells whereas identical sequence clusters were characterized within CD4+ memory T-cells. Cells expressing Ki67 are normally in the G_1 phase which is before the division of a cell (Combadere et al., 2000). Perhaps the lack of correlation between Ki67 expression and clusters of identical sequences indicates that these identical sequences represent cells which have already proliferated whereas Ki67 expression represents those cells which have the capacity to proliferate.

The integration of the HIV genome occurs during the acute phase of infection when HIV is mainly M-tropic or non-syncytium-inducing and utilizes CCR5 for viral entry (Bjorndal et al., 1997; Berger et al., 1999; Rambaut et al., 2004; Colby et al., 2018). This indicates that CCR5-tropic proviruses are present within the HIV reservoir and can release CCR5-tropic virions when ART is interrupted. We found the frequency of CCR5 expression was greater on the HLA-DR+ T-cell subset at all time points during ART. These findings could indicate that the HLA-DR+ T-cell subset would be a major target for HIV-infection when HIV-infected individuals on long-term ART undergo treatment interruption.

We found Tim-3 expression was extremely low on both the HLA-DR+ and HLA-DR– CD4+ memory T-cell subsets compared to other cellular activation/exhaustion markers; however, it was highly associated with the HLA-DR+ T-cell subset during ART. In agreement with an earlier study, our finding indicates that Tim-3 expression can be observed on both activated and resting CD4+ T-cells (Corneau et al., 2017). A recent study showed that the CD4+ T-cell count and Tim-3 expression level are inversely correlated (Rallon et al., 2018). The low expression of Tim-3 within the HLA-DR+ and HLA-DR– T-cell subsets could be related to CD4+ T-cell restoration during therapy, as the participants we studied had near normal CD4+ T-cell counts during ART (Rallon et al., 2018).

Among the cellular activation/exhaustion markers we studied, the expression profiles of PD-1 and LAG-3 were particularly interesting, as it has been shown that CD4+ memory T-cells expressing these immune checkpoint molecules are highly enriched with inducible HIV proviruses (Fromentin et al., 2016). We found PD-1 expression was higher on the HLA-DR+ memory T-cell subset compared to their HLA-DR– counterpart during therapy. Conversely, we found LAG-3 expression was higher on the HLA-DR– T-cell subset when compared to the HLA-DR+ during ART. Together, our results indicate that both HLA-DR+ and HLA-DR– T-cell subsets express cellular activation/exhaustion markers which indicate they could contain inducible HIV proviruses.

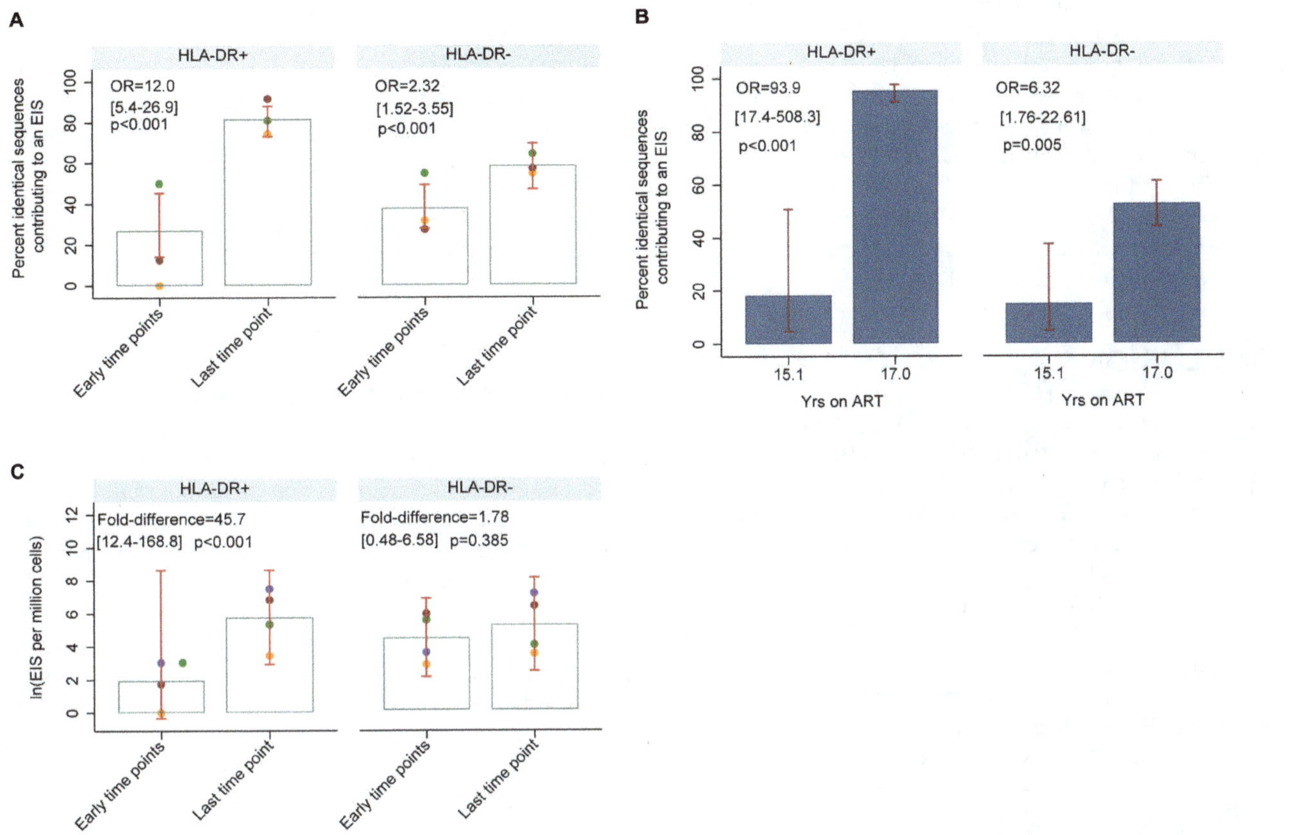

FIGURE 11 | HIV-DNA p6-RT sequences derived from EIS within HLA-DR+ and HLA-DR– CD4+ memory T-cells during therapy (CHI participants). **(A)** Percent of HIV-DNA p6-RT sequences derived from EIS (% EIS) for participants 2013 (orange data points), 2026 (green data points) and 2046 (maroon data points). EIS was characterized using HIV-DNA sequences derived from the three earlier time points combined ("Early time points") and the viral sequences derived from last time point ("Last time point"). The odds ratio (OR) compares "Last time point" to "Early time points." The 95% CI (in square brackets) and the *p*-value (p) of the OR are also shown. The open gray bars indicate mean % EIS and the 95% CI of the mean is shown as the red capped lines. **(B)** Percent of HIV-DNA p6-RT sequences derived from EIS (% EIS) for participant 2518. The OR compares 17.0 to 15.1 years of ART. The 95% CI (in square brackets) and the *p*-value (p) are also shown. The filled blue bars indicate % EIS and its 95% CI is shown as the red capped lines. **(C)** Quantity of HIV-DNA sequences derived from EIS per million cells analyzed within the HLA-DR+ and HLA-DR– T-cell subsets. The gray open bars indicate mean of log transformed EIS per million cells and red capped lines indicate 95% CI of this mean. The fold-difference compares EIS per million cells of "Last time point" to "Early time points." The 95% CI (in square brackets) and *p*-value (p) of the fold-difference are also shown. Different colors of the data points represent different participants; 2013 (orange), 2026 (green), 2046 (maroon), and 2518 (blue).

The expression profiles of cellular activation/exhaustion markers suggest several therapeutic strategies that could reduce the persistent viral reservoir in these memory T-cells. First, the high level of CCR5 receptors on HLA-DR+ T-cells suggest that CCR5-antagonists such as maraviroc would be effective in reducing the HIV infection in these T-cells (Fatkenheuer et al., 2008; Rusconi et al., 2013). Second, the high frequency of PD-1 expression on HLA-DR+ T-cells provides a rationale for the use of immune checkpoint blockers as anti-latency agents to target these infected cells during ART. The effect of these anti-PD-1 agents would be greater against the HLA-DR+ T-cell subset compared to their HLA-DR– counterpart (Day et al., 2006; Teigler et al., 2017). However, anti-LAG-3 checkpoint blockers would be more effective against HLA-DR– T-cells, as these cells more frequently expressed LAG-3 compared to HLA-DR+ T-cells (Gandhi et al., 2006; Brignone et al., 2007, 2009). Overall, our study indicates that the immune checkpoint blockers could target different CD4+ memory T-cell subsets.

There are several limitations to our study, first we sequenced the p6-RT region of HIV not the full-length HIV genome, which could cause an over estimation of the HIV infection frequency and the identification of identical HIV-DNA sequences in both T-cell subsets (Hiener et al., 2017). Second, the long-term storage of some of the clinical samples limited the number of cells we could sort and our ability to sequence many HIV-DNA molecules from these cells, and this was especially true for HLA-DR+ T-cells. A longitudinal study using full-length HIV sequencing and integration site analysis from leukapheresis samples would be ideal to reconfirm our findings, as no sub-genomic viral region can accurately predict cellular proliferation (Ho et al., 2013; Maldarelli et al., 2014; Wagner et al., 2014; Cohn et al., 2015; Laskey et al., 2016; Hiener et al., 2017; Lee et al., 2017). However, such longitudinal assays are time consuming, costly and would also be limited by cell numbers that can be sorted from long-term frozen cell aliquots. Nonetheless, it is worth noting that the region we used for our genetic analysis (p6-RT) has been shown to be the best predictor for the full-length HIV genome and the clonality of this genome (clonal prediction score of 95) (Laskey et al., 2016). In addition, our cell sorting strategy excludes terminally differentiated effector memory CD4+ memory T-cells (T_{EMRA}) which are a CD45RA positive cellular population as we focused on the memory T-cells which are CD45RA negative in this study. Due to the high expression of HLA-DR on T_{EMRA} cell subset, however, it is highly likely that this cellular subset can contribute to the persistence of CD4+ T-cells that express HLA-DR during prolonged ART (Corneau et al., 2017).

CONCLUSION

Our study showed that although CD4+ HLA-DR+ memory T-cells express a high frequency of activation and exhaustion markers, this memory T-cell subset contributes to the persistent viral reservoir by cellular proliferation. Our sequence analyses provided evidence that the same HIV-DNA sequence can persist in HLA-DR+ T-cells for over two years of ART, indicating this T-cell subset has the potential to continually contribute to the persistent viral reservoir. Our research revealed cellular proliferation contributes to the persistence of HIV in HLA-DR+ and HLA-DR− T-cell subsets during prolonged therapy. Moreover, HIV sequence comparisons between early and late time points of ART also suggest a fraction of CD4+ memory T-cells can undergo cellular transition between HLA-DR+ and HLA-DR− cellular phenotypes. Importantly, both HLA-DR+ and HLA-DR− CD4+ memory T-cells should be included in future studies of the HIV reservoir, as these cells express critical immune checkpoint molecules that could be used for therapeutic strategies.

ETHICS STATEMENT

The studies involving human participants were reviewed and approved by this study was approved by the institutional review board at the Western Sydney Health Department for the Westmead Institute for Medical Research (AU RED LNR/13/WMEAD/315), and the ethics review committees at the University of California San Francisco (UCSF) (10-01330/068192, 10-02631/083640) and Vaccine Gene Therapy Institute-Florida (VGTI-FL) (FWA 00004139). All participants provided written informed consent prior to inclusion in the study. The patients/participants provided their written informed consent to participate in this study.

AUTHOR CONTRIBUTIONS

EL conducted SPS on the participant samples, analyzed the resulting data, and wrote the original manuscript. RH, SD, FH, JM, NC, and RF enrolled the participants, collected the tissues and/or sorted the cell subsets from the participant samples. EL, TL, and JM prepared the participant samples. EB and DD developed and assisted with the HIV-DNA extraction from cells of the participants. JM measured the cell activation/exhaustion markers and contributed to methods. TL performed the qPCR. WS designed the sequence alignment workflows. PB conducted the statistical analysis and contributed to review and editing of the results and methods. SP designed the study and supervised the work performed. All authors read and edited the manuscript.

ACKNOWLEDGMENTS

We acknowledge with gratitude the participants who donated samples for this study. We thank Andrea Wright for reviewing the genetic analysis on a subset of the participants.

REFERENCES

Agosto, L. M., Yu, J. J., Dai, J., Kaletsky, R., Monie, D., and O'Doherty, U. (2007). HIV-1 integrates into resting CD4+ T cells even at low inoculums as demonstrated with an improved assay for HIV-1 integration. *Virology* 368, 60–72. doi: 10.1016/j.virol.2007.06.001

Anderson, J. A., Archin, N. M., Ince, W., Parker, D., Wiegand, A., Coffin, J. M., et al. (2011). Clonal sequences recovered from plasma from patients with residual HIV-1 viremia and on intensified antiretroviral therapy are identical to replicating viral RNAs recovered from circulating resting CD4+ T cells. *J. Virol.* 85, 5220–5223. doi: 10.1128/JVI.00284-11

Berger, E. A., Murphy, P. M., and Farber, J. M. (1999). Chemokine receptors as HIV-1 coreceptors: roles in viral entry, tropism, and disease. *Annu. Rev. Immunol.* 17, 657–700. doi: 10.1146/annurev.immunol.17.1.657

Bjorndal, A., Deng, H., Jansson, M., Fiore, J. R., Colognesi, C., Karlsson, A., et al. (1997). Coreceptor usage of primary human immunodeficiency virus type 1 isolates varies according to biological phenotype. *J. Virol.* 71, 7478–7487.

Brignone, C., Escudier, B., Grygar, C., Marcu, M., and Triebel, F. (2009). A phase I pharmacokinetic and biological correlative study of IMP321, a novel MHC class II agonist, in patients with advanced renal cell carcinoma. *Clin. Cancer Res.* 15, 6225–6231. doi: 10.1158/1078-0432.Ccr-09-0068

Brignone, C., Grygar, C., Marcu, M., Perrin, G., and Triebel, F. (2007). IMP321 (sLAG-3) safety and T cell response potentiation using an influenza vaccine as a model antigen: a single-blind phase I study. *Vaccine* 25, 4641–4650. doi: 10.1016/j.vaccine.2007.04.019

Buzon, M. J., Sun, H., Li, C., Shaw, A., Seiss, K., Ouyang, Z., et al. (2014). HIV-1 persistence in CD4+ T cells with stem cell-like properties. *Nat. Med.* 20, 139–142. doi: 10.1038/nm.3445

Chomont, N., El-Far, M., Ancuta, P., Trautmann, L., Procopio, F. A., Yassine-Diab, B., et al. (2009). HIV reservoir size and persistence are driven by T cell survival and homeostatic proliferation. *Nat. Med.* 15, 893–900. doi: 10.1038/nm.1972

Chun, T. W., Finzi, D., Margolick, J., Chadwick, K., Schwartz, D., and Siliciano, R. F. (1995). In vivo fate of HIV-1-infected T cells: quantitative analysis of the transition to stable latency. *Nat. Med.* 1, 1284–1290. doi: 10.1038/nm1295-1284

Chun, T. W., Justement, J. S., Murray, D., Hallahan, C. W., Maenza, J., Collier, A. C., et al. (2010). Rebound of plasma viremia following cessation of antiretroviral therapy despite profoundly low levels of HIV reservoir: implications for eradication. *AIDS* 24, 2803–2808. doi: 10.1097/QAD.0b013e328340a239

Chun, T. W., Nickle, D. C., Justement, J. S., Large, D., Semerjian, A., Curlin, M. E., et al. (2005). HIV-infected individuals receiving effective antiviral therapy for extended periods of time continually replenish their viral reservoir. *J. Clin. Invest.* 115, 3250–3255. doi: 10.1172/jci26197

Cockerham, L. R., Siliciano, J. D., Sinclair, E., O'Doherty, U., Palmer, S., Yukl, S. A., et al. (2014). CD4+ and CD8+ T cell activation are associated with HIV DNA in resting CD4+ T cells. *PLoS One* 9:e110731. doi: 10.1371/journal.pone.0110731

Cohn, L. B., Silva, I. T., Oliveira, T. Y., Rosales, R. A., Parrish, E. H., Learn, G. H., et al. (2015). HIV-1 integration landscape during latent and active infection. *Cell* 160, 420–432. doi: 10.1016/j.cell.2015.01.020

Colby, D. J., Trautmann, L., Pinyakorn, S., Leyre, L., Pagliuzza, A., Kroon, E., et al. (2018). Rapid HIV RNA rebound after antiretroviral treatment interruption in persons durably suppressed in Fiebig I acute HIV infection. *Nat. Med.* 24, 923–926. doi: 10.1038/s41591-018-0026-6

Combadere, B., Blanc, C., Li, T., Carcelain, G., Delaugerre, C., Calvez, V., et al. (2000). CD4+Ki67+ lymphocytes in HIV-infected patients are effector T cells accumulated in the G1 phase of the cell cycle. *Eur. J. Immunol.* 30, 3598–3603. doi: 10.1002/1521-4141(200012)30:12<3598::AID-IMMU3598<3.0.CO;2-E

Contento, R. L., Molon, B., Boularan, C., Pozzan, T., Manes, S., Marullo, S., et al. (2008). CXCR4-CCR5: a couple modulating T cell functions. *Proc. Natl. Acad. Sci. U.S.A.* 105, 10101–10106. doi: 10.1073/pnas.0804286105

Corneau, A., Cosma, A., Even, S., Katlama, C., Le Grand, R., Frachet, V., et al. (2017). Comprehensive mass cytometry analysis of cell cycle, activation, and coinhibitory receptors expression in CD4 T Cells from healthy and HIV-infected individuals. *Cytometry Part B Clin. Cytom.* 92, 21–32. doi: 10.1002/cyto.b.21502

Cox, M. A., Nechanitzky, R., and Mak, T. W. (2017). Check point inhibitors as therapies for infectious diseases. *Curr. Opin. Immunol.* 48, 61–67. doi: 10.1016/j.coi.2017.07.016

Dai, J., Agosto, L. M., Baytop, C., Yu, J. J., Pace, M. J., Liszewski, M. K., et al. (2009). Human immunodeficiency virus integrates directly into naive resting CD4+ T cells but enters naive cells less efficiently than memory cells. *J. Virol.* 83, 4528–4537. doi: 10.1128/jvi.01910-08

Day, C. L., Kaufmann, D. E., Kiepiela, P., Brown, J. A., Moodley, E. S., Reddy, S., et al. (2006). PD-1 expression on HIV-specific T cells is associated with T-cell exhaustion and disease progression. *Nature* 443, 350–354. doi: 10.1038/nature05115

Fatkenheuer, G., Nelson, M., Lazzarin, A., Konourina, I., Hoepelman, A. I., Lampiris, H., et al. (2008). Subgroup analyses of maraviroc in previously treated R5 HIV-1 infection. *N. Engl. J. Med.* 359, 1442–1455. doi: 10.1056/NEJMoa0803154

Finzi, D., Blankson, J., Siliciano, J. D., Margolick, J. B., Chadwick, K., Pierson, T., et al. (1999). Latent infection of CD4+ T cells provides a mechanism for lifelong persistence of HIV-1, even in patients on effective combination therapy. *Nat. Med.* 5, 512–517. doi: 10.1038/8394

Finzi, D., Hermankova, M., Pierson, T., Carruth, L. M., Buck, C., Chaisson, R. E., et al. (1997). Identification of a reservoir for HIV-1 in patients on highly active antiretroviral therapy. *Science* 278, 1295–1300. doi: 10.1126/science.278.5341.1295

Fromentin, R., Bakeman, W., Lawani, M. B., Khoury, G., Hartogensis, W., DaFonseca, S., et al. (2016). CD4+ T Cells expressing PD-1, TIGIT and LAG-3 contribute to HIV Persistence during ART. *PLoS Pathog.* 12:e1005761. doi: 10.1371/journal.ppat.1005761

Gandhi, M. K., Lambley, E., Duraiswamy, J., Dua, U., Smith, C., Elliott, S., et al. (2006). Expression of LAG-3 by tumor-infiltrating lymphocytes is coincident with the suppression of latent membrane antigen-specific CD8+ T-cell function in Hodgkin lymphoma patients. *Blood* 108, 2280–2289. doi: 10.1182/blood-2006-04-015164

Hiener, B., Horsburgh, B. A., Eden, J.-S., Barton, K., Schlub, T. E., Lee, E., et al. (2017). Identification of genetically Intact HIV-1 proviruses in Specific $CD4^+$ T Cells from Effectively Treated participants. *Cell Rep.* 21, 813–822. doi: 10.1016/j.celrep.2017.09.081

Ho, Y. C., Shan, L., Hosmane, N. N., Wang, J., Laskey, S. B., Rosenbloom, D. I., et al. (2013). Replication-competent noninduced proviruses in the latent reservoir increase barrier to HIV-1 cure. *Cell* 155, 540–551. doi: 10.1016/j.cell.2013.09.020

Hocqueloux, L., Prazuck, T., Avettand-Fenoel, V., Lafeuillade, A., Cardon, B., Viard, J.-P., et al. (2010). Long-term immunovirologic control following antiretroviral therapy interruption in patients treated at the time of primary HIV-1 infection. *AIDS* 24, 1598–1601. doi: 10.1097/QAD.0b013e32833b61ba

Imamichi, H., Natarajan, V., Adelsberger, J. W., Rehm, C. A., Lempicki, R. A., Das, B., et al. (2014). Lifespan of effector memory CD4+ T cells determined by replication-incompetent integrated HIV-1 provirus. *AIDS* 28, 1091–1099. doi: 10.1097/QAD.0000000000000223

Josefsson, L., Eriksson, S., Sinclair, E., Ho, T., Killian, M., Epling, L., et al. (2012). Hematopoietic precursor cells isolated from patients on long-term suppressive HIV therapy did not contain HIV-1 DNA. *J. Infect. Dis.* 206, 28–34. doi: 10.1093/infdis/jis301

Josefsson, L., von Stockenstrom, S., Faria, N. R., Sinclair, E., Bacchetti, P., Killian, M., et al. (2013). The HIV-1 reservoir in eight patients on long-term suppressive antiretroviral therapy is stable with few genetic changes over time. *Proc. Natl. Acad. Sci. U.S.A.* 110, E4987–E4996. doi: 10.1073/pnas.1308313110

Katoh, K., and Standley, D. M. (2013). MAFFT multiple sequence alignment software version 7: improvements in performance and usability. *Mol. Biol. Evol.* 30, 772–780. doi: 10.1093/molbev/mst010

Kearney, M., Maldarelli, F., Shao, W., Margolick, J. B., Daar, E. S., Mellors, J. W., et al. (2009). Human immunodeficiency virus type 1 population genetics and adaptation in newly infected individuals. *J. Virol.* 83, 2715–2727. doi: 10.1128/JVI.01960-08

Kearney, M., Palmer, S., Maldarelli, F., Shao, W., Polis, M. A., Mican, J., et al. (2008). Frequent polymorphism at drug resistance sites in HIV-1 protease and reverse transcriptase. *AIDS* 22, 497–501. doi: 10.1097/QAD.0b013e3282f29478

Kearney, M. F., Wiegand, A., Shao, W., Coffin, J. M., Mellors, J. W., Lederman, M., et al. (2015). Origin of rebound plasma HIV includes cells with identical proviruses that are transcriptionally active before stopping of antiretroviral therapy. *J. Virol.* 90, 1369–1376. doi: 10.1128/JVI.02139-15

Kestens, L., Vanham, G., Vereecken, C., Vandenbruaene, M., Vercauteren, G., Colebunders, R. L., et al. (1994). Selective increase of activation antigens HLA-DR and CD38 on CD4+ CD45RO+ T lymphocytes during HIV-1 infection. *Clin. Exp. Immunol.* 95, 436–441. doi: 10.1111/j.1365-2249.1994.tb07015.x

Khaitan, A., and Unutmaz, D. (2011). Revisiting immune exhaustion during HIV infection. *Curr. HIV/AIDS Rep.* 8, 4–11. doi: 10.1007/s11904-010-0066-0

Kim, P. S., and Ahmed, R. (2010). Features of responding T cells in cancer and chronic infection. *Curr. Opin. Immunol.* 22, 223–230. doi: 10.1016/j.coi.2010.02.005

Kumar, A. M., Borodowsky, I., Fernandez, B., Gonzalez, L., and Kumar, M. (2007). Human immunodeficiency virus type 1 RNA levels in different regions of human brain: quantification using real-time reverse transcriptase-polymerase chain reaction. *J. Neurovirol.* 13, 210–224. doi: 10.1080/13550280701327038

Laskey, S. B., Pohlmeyer, C. W., Bruner, K. M., and Siliciano, R. F. (2016). Evaluating clonal expansion of HIV-infected cells: optimization of PCR strategies to predict clonality. *PLoS Pathog.* 12:e1005689. doi: 10.1371/journal.ppat.1005689

Lee, G. Q., Orlova-Fink, N., Einkauf, K., Chowdhury, F. Z., Sun, X., Harrington, S., et al. (2017). Clonal expansion of genome-intact HIV-1 in functionally polarized Th1 CD4+ T cells. *J. Clin. Investig.* 127, 2689–2696. doi: 10.1172/JCI93289

Maldarelli, F., Wu, X., Su, L., Simonetti, F. R., Shao, W., Hill, S., et al. (2014). HIV latency. Specific HIV integration sites are linked to clonal expansion and persistence of infected cells. *Science* 345, 179–183. doi: 10.1126/science.1254194

Murray, J. M., Zaunders, J. J., McBride, K. L., Xu, Y., Bailey, M., Suzuki, K., et al. (2014). HIV DNA subspecies persist in both activated and resting memory CD4+ T cells during antiretroviral therapy. *J. Virol.* 88, 3516–3526. doi: 10.1128/JVI.03331-13

Palella, F. J. Jr., Delaney, K. M., Moorman, A. C., Loveless, M. O., Fuhrer, J., Satten, G. A., et al. (1998). Declining morbidity and mortality among patients with advanced human immunodeficiency virus infection. HIV Outpatient Study Investigators. *N. Engl. J. Med.* 338, 853–860. doi: 10.1056/nejm199803263381301

Palmer, S., Kearney, M., Maldarelli, F., Halvas, E. K., Bixby, C. J., Bazmi, H., et al. (2005). Multiple, linked human immunodeficiency virus type 1 drug resistance mutations in treatment-experienced patients are missed by standard genotype analysis. *J. Clin. Microbiol.* 43, 406–413. doi: 10.1128/JCM.43.1.406-413.2005

Perreau, M., Savoye, A. L., De Crignis, E., Corpataux, J. M., Cubas, R., Haddad, E. K., et al. (2013). Follicular helper T cells serve as the major CD4 T cell compartment for HIV-1 infection, replication, and production. *J. Exp. Med.* 210, 143–156. doi: 10.1084/jem.20121932

Portales, P., Psomas, K. C., Tuaillon, E., Mura, T., Vendrell, J. P., Eliaou, J. F., et al. (2012). The intensity of immune activation is linked to the level of CCR5 expression in human immunodeficiency virus type 1-infected persons. *Immunology* 137, 89–97. doi: 10.1111/j.1365-2567.2012.03609.x

Rallon, N., Garcia, M., Garcia-Samaniego, J., Cabello, A., Alvarez, B., Restrepo, C., et al. (2018). Expression of PD-1 and Tim-3 markers of T-cell exhaustion is associated with CD4 dynamics during the course of untreated and treated HIV infection. *PLoS One* 13:e0193829. doi: 10.1371/journal.pone.0193829

Rambaut, A., Posada, D., Crandall, K. A., and Holmes, E. C. (2004). The causes and consequences of HIV evolution. *Nat. Rev. Genet.* 5, 52–61. doi: 10.1038/nrg1246

Rose, P. P., and Korber, B. T. (2000). Detecting hypermutations in viral sequences with an emphasis on G -> A hypermutation. *Bioinformatics* 16, 400–401. doi: 10.1093/bioinformatics/16.4.400

Rosenbloom, D. I., Elliott, O., Hill, A. L., Henrich, T. J., Siliciano, J. M., and Siliciano, R. F. (2015). Designing and interpreting limiting dilution assays: general principles and applications to the latent reservoir for human immunodeficiency Virus-1. *Open Forum Infect. Dis.* 2:ofv123. doi: 10.1093/ofid/ofv123

Rusconi, S., Vitiello, P., Adorni, F., Colella, E., Foca, E., Capetti, A., et al. (2013). Maraviroc as intensification strategy in HIV-1 positive patients with deficient immunological response: an Italian randomized clinical trial. *PLoS One* 8:e80157. doi: 10.1371/journal.pone.0080157

Saleh, S., Solomon, A., Wightman, F., Xhilaga, M., Cameron, P. U., and Lewin, S. R. (2007). CCR7 ligands CCL19 and CCL21 increase permissiveness of resting memory CD4+ T cells to HIV-1 infection: a novel model of HIV-1 latency. *Blood* 110, 4161–4164. doi: 10.1182/blood-2007-06-097907

Scholzen, T., and Gerdes, J. (2000). The Ki-67 protein: from the known and the unknown. *J. Cell. Physiol.* 182, 311–322. doi: 10.1002/(sici)1097-4652(200003)182:3<311::Aid-jcp1<3.0.Co;2-9

Shan, L., Deng, K., Gao, H., Xing, S., Capoferri, A. A., Durand, C. M., et al. (2017). Transcriptional reprogramming during effector-to-memory transition renders CD4(+) T Cells permissive for latent HIV-1 infection. *Immunity* 47, 766.e3–775.e3. doi: 10.1016/j.immuni.2017.09.014

Siliciano, J. D., Kajdas, J., Finzi, D., Quinn, T. C., Chadwick, K., Margolick, J. B., et al. (2003). Long-term follow-up studies confirm the stability of the latent reservoir for HIV-1 in resting CD4+ T cells. *Nat. Med.* 9, 727–728. doi: 10.1038/nm880

Siliciano, J. D., Lai, J., Callender, M., Pitt, E., Zhang, H., Margolick, J. B., et al. (2007). Stability of the latent reservoir for HIV-1 in patients receiving valproic acid. *J. Infect. Dis.* 195, 833–836. doi: 10.1086/511823

Siliciano, J. D., and Siliciano, R. F. (2004). A long-term latent reservoir for HIV-1: discovery and clinical implications. *J. Antimicrob. Chemother.* 54, 6–9. doi: 10.1093/jac/dkh292dkh292

Siliciano, J. D., and Siliciano, R. F. (2005). Enhanced culture assay for detection and quantitation of latently infected, resting CD4+ T-cells carrying replication-competent virus in HIV-1-infected individuals. *Methods Mol. Biol.* 304, 3–15. doi: 10.1385/1-59259-907-9:003

Simonetti, F. R., Sobolewski, M. D., Fyne, E., Shao, W., Spindler, J., Hattori, J., et al. (2016). Clonally expanded CD4+ T cells can produce infectious HIV-1 in vivo. *Proc. Natl. Acad. Sci. U.S.A.* 113, 1883–1888. doi: 10.1073/pnas.1522675113

Stamatakis, A. (2006). RAxML-VI-HPC: maximum likelihood-based phylogenetic analyses with thousands of taxa and mixed models. *Bioinformatics* 22, 2688–2690. doi: 10.1093/bioinformatics/btl446

Swiggard, W. J., Baytop, C., Yu, J. J., Dai, J., Li, C., Schretzenmair, R., et al. (2005). Human immunodeficiency virus type 1 can establish latent infection in resting CD4+ T cells in the absence of activating stimuli. *J. Virol.* 79, 14179–14188. doi: 10.1128/jvi.79.22.14179-14188.2005

Tamura, K., Stecher, G., Peterson, D., Filipski, A., and Kumar, S. (2013). MEGA6: molecular evolutionary genetics analysis version 6.0. *Mol. Biol. Evol.* 30, 2725–2729. doi: 10.1093/molbev/mst197

Teigler, J. E., Zelinskyy, G., Eller, M. A., Bolton, D. L., Marovich, M., Gordon, A. D., et al. (2017). Differential inhibitory receptor expression on T Cells delineates functional capacities in chronic viral infection. *J. Virol.* 91:e0126317. doi: 10.1128/jvi.01263-17

von Stockenstrom, S., Odevall, L., Lee, E., Sinclair, E., Bacchetti, P., Killian, M., et al. (2015). Longitudinal genetic characterization reveals that cell proliferation maintains a persistent HIV Type 1 DNA pool during effective HIV therapy. *J. Infect. Dis.* 212, 596–607. doi: 10.1093/infdis/jiv092

Wagner, T. A., McKernan, J. L., Tobin, N. H., Tapia, K. A., Mullins, J. I., and Frenkel, L. M. (2013). An increasing proportion of monotypic HIV-1 DNA sequences during antiretroviral treatment suggests proliferation of HIV-infected cells. *J. Virol.* 87, 1770–1778. doi: 10.1128/JVI.01985-12

Wagner, T. A., McLaughlin, S., Garg, K., Cheung, C. Y., Larsen, B. B., Styrchak, S., et al. (2014). HIV latency. Proliferation of cells with HIV integrated into cancer genes contributes to persistent infection. *Science* 345, 570–573. doi: 10.1126/science.1256304

Yang, X., Jiao, Y.-M., Wang, R., Ji, Y.-X., Zhang, H.-W., Zhang, Y.-H., et al. (2012). High CCR5 density on central memory CD4+ T Cells in acute HIV-1 infection is mostly associated with rapid disease progression. *PLoS One* 7:e49526. doi: 10.1371/journal.pone.0049526

Yu, G., Lam, T. T.-Y., Zhu, H., and Guan, Y. (2018). Two methods for mapping and visualizing associated data on phylogeny using Ggtree. *Mol. Biol. Evol.* 35, 3041–3043. doi: 10.1093/molbev/msy194

Yu, G., Smith, D. K., Zhu, H., Guan, Y., and Lam, T. T.-Y. (2017). ggtree: an r package for visualization and annotation of phylogenetic trees with their covariates and other associated data. *Methods Ecol. Evol.* 8, 28–36. doi: 10.1111/2041-210x.12628 doi: 10.1111/2041-210x.12628

3

New Frontiers in Measuring and Characterizing the HIV Reservoir

*Shane D. Falcinelli[1,2], Cristina Ceriani[1,3], David M. Margolis[1,2,3] and Nancie M. Archin[1,3]**

[1] UNC HIV Cure Center, The University of North Carolina at Chapel Hill, Chapel Hill, NC, United States, [2] Department of Microbiology and Immunology, The University of North Carolina at Chapel Hill, Chapel Hill, NC, United States, [3] Department of Medicine, The University of North Carolina at Chapel Hill, Chapel Hill, NC, United States

***Correspondence:**
Nancie M. Archin
nancie_archin@med.unc.edu

A cure for HIV infection remains elusive due to the persistence of replication-competent HIV proviral DNA during suppressive antiretroviral therapy (ART). With the exception of rare elite or post-treatment controllers of viremia, withdrawal of ART invariably results in the rebound of viremia and progression of HIV disease. A thorough understanding of the reservoir is necessary to develop new strategies in order to reduce or eliminate the reservoir. However, there is significant heterogeneity in the sequence composition, genomic location, stability, and expression of the HIV reservoir both within and across individuals, and a majority of proviral sequences are replication-defective. These factors, and the low frequency of persistently infected cells in individuals on suppressive ART, make understanding the reservoir and its response to experimental reservoir reduction interventions challenging. Here, we review the characteristics of the HIV reservoir, state-of-the-art assays to measure and characterize the reservoir, and how these assays can be applied to accurately detect reductions in reservoir during efforts to develop a cure for HIV infection. In particular, we highlight recent advances in the development of direct measures of provirus, including intact proviral DNA assays and full-length HIV DNA sequencing with integration site analysis. We also focus on novel techniques to quantitate persistent and inducible HIV, including RNA sequencing and RNA/*gag* protein staining techniques, as well as modified viral outgrowth methods that seek to improve upon throughput, sensitivity and dynamic range.

Keywords: HIV, cure, reservoir, stability, replication-competent, defective provirus, QVOA, IPDA

INTRODUCTION

An estimated 40 million people are living with HIV, and over 30 million have died because of it. The incidence of new HIV infections globally is approximately 2 million each year (GBD 2015 HIV Collaborators, 2016; WHO, 2019). While antiretroviral therapy (ART) can control viremia and improve health outcomes, durably ART-suppressed HIV seropositive individuals are still at higher risk for diseases related to immune dysfunction and inflammation compared to uninfected individuals (Hunt et al., 2016). Moreover, lifelong adherence to ART is required for optimal health outcomes and is associated with financial burden, drug interactions, and unknown long-term effects of treatment (Deeks et al., 2017; Devanathan et al., 2019). Further, the stigma associated with HIV disease contributes to negative health outcomes (Rueda et al., 2016). Therefore, a cure for HIV is of substantial public health interest.

However, eliminating HIV infection remains an elusive goal due to the viral reservoir—HIV proviral DNA in the host genome of resting CD4+ T lymphocytes and possibly other cells (Bukrinsky et al., 1991; Chun et al., 1997, 1998; Finzi et al., 1997; Wong et al., 1997b; Finzi et al., 1999; Ganor et al., 2019). For the purposes of this review, we define the viral reservoir as a cell that encodes integrated, replication-competent virus that can fuel viral rebound after treatment interruption, even after years of suppressive ART (Eisele and Siliciano, 2012; Margolis et al., 2016). When referring broadly to HIV DNA that is integrated but includes both replication-competent and replication-incompetent HIV, we use the term persistent HIV (Wang et al., 2018b). On suppressive ART, transcription of proviral DNA from persistently infected cells during immune activation or other normal cellular processes can result in viral gene expression and viral particle release (Shen and Siliciano, 2008; Pasternak et al., 2013). Whether these particles are able to establish new infections under suppressive ART is a historical area of debate (Shen and Siliciano, 2008; Lorenzo-Redondo et al., 2016; Margolis et al., 2016; Martinez-Picado and Deeks, 2016); however, the overwhelming majority of evidence supports the notion that active viral replication does not occur during suppressive therapy. Rather, (1) long-lived cells infected prior to ART-initiation and (2) expansion of infected cells through cell division during suppressive therapy are responsible for persistence of the reservoir on long-term suppressive ART (Maldarelli, 2015; Bui et al., 2017; Kearney et al., 2017; Anderson and Maldarelli, 2018; Mok et al., 2018; Wang et al., 2018a; Bozzi et al., 2019). Nonetheless, upon cessation of suppressive ART, there is a rebound of viremia from the reservoir on the timescale of weeks and in general, progression of HIV disease if ART is not resumed (Chun et al., 1999; Hamlyn et al., 2012).

Research efforts over the past 30 years have sought to understand the reservoir in order to facilitate the development of interventions that could eradicate the reservoir (a cure) or enable HIV seropositive individuals to maintain suppressed viremia in the absence of ART (a functional cure) (Deeks et al., 2016). A central strategy for eradication (cure) is the use of latency reversal agents (LRAs) to induce proviral expression in conjunction with a vaccine, antibody, and/or cellular immunotherapy in order facilitate immune clearance of virally infected cells (Margolis et al., 2016). With regard to a functional cure, major strategies include the use of long-acting broadly neutralizing antibodies (passive immunotherapy), vaccination (active immunotherapy), modification of host cells to prevent viral replication (gene therapy), or permanent silencing of provirus ("block and lock") (Cillo and Mellors, 2016; Kessing et al., 2017; Elsheikh et al., 2019).

Common to all of these approaches for a cure or functional cure is a need for careful characterization and measurement of the viral reservoir. In recent years, advances in technology and the HIV cure field have resulted in the development of an arsenal of assays to characterize and measure the HIV reservoir. In this review, we first provide an overview of the characteristics of HIV reservoir—including the cell types thought to harbor the reservoir, the spectrum of viral expression within the reservoir, and the diversity of proviruses within the reservoir. Next, we review standard as well as emerging assays for measuring the reservoir. Throughout, we discuss ongoing and future applications of these assays to (1) improve understanding of the stability of the HIV reservoir and (2) accurately and reliably detect a reduction in the frequency of the HIV reservoir in cure research.

THE HIV RESERVOIR: CELL TYPES THAT HARBOR THE RESERVOIR

Here, we define the HIV reservoir as any cell that can produce replication-competent virus despite years of suppressive ART (Eisele and Siliciano, 2012; Margolis et al., 2016). To date, in humans, resting CD4+ T lymphocytes represent the largest and most well-characterized viral reservoir. However, there is mounting evidence from both animal models and human donors that other cell types may contribute to the total HIV reservoir. To provide context for our review of assays to measure the reservoir, we provide a brief overview of the cell types that may compose the reservoir.

CD4 T Cells

Resting CD4 T cells, defined as CD3+CD4+CD25-CD69-HLADR-, were the first cells to be identified as a reservoir for HIV (Chun et al., 1997, 1998; Finzi et al., 1997, 1999; Wong et al., 1997b). At the time, it was generally not believed that HIV exhibited a latent stage in its lifecycle, and so the use of this resting cell population allowed the demonstration of a definable pool of cells that lacked HIV expression when isolated, but could be induced (activated) *ex vivo* to express replication-competent HIV — hence a definitive proof of the presence of true virologic latency.

This reservoir in resting CD4 T cells is known to be very stable with a long half-life (~44.5 months) (Siliciano et al., 2003; Crooks et al., 2015). Therefore, to date, these cells represent the most formidable barrier to cure because of their frequency and slow decay rate. Within resting CD4 T cells, the HIV reservoir is most frequently detected in the central memory compartment (Finzi et al., 1997; Soriano-Sarabia et al., 2014). Of note, some studies using total CD4 T cells have detected higher frequencies of persistent HIV in the effector memory subset (Hiener et al., 2017), whereas others describe the highest frequency of persistent HIV in the central memory compartment (Chomont et al., 2009). In addition, replication-competent HIV has been recovered from naïve T cells and transitional memory T cells (Chomont et al., 2009; Soriano-Sarabia et al., 2014; Zerbato et al., 2019). HIV reservoirs have also been detected in gamma/delta T cells (Soriano-Sarabia et al., 2015) (**Figure 1**). The half-life of the reservoir in each of these cell compartments is little studied, and is complicated by the natural differentiation of these immune cells across compartments (i.e., central memory to effector memory). Furthermore, in the case of gamma/delta T cells, their low frequency and dual function as reservoirs and immune effectors complicates efforts to understand their contribution as a stable source of HIV under ART (Soriano-Sarabia et al., 2015; Garrido et al., 2018). Finally, long-lived CD4+

A Cell Types

CD4 T cells		Other Cell Types
Differentiation Status	Functional Polarization	
T_{NA}	**Tfh**	Macrophages:
T_{SCM}	Th1	• **Urethral**
T_{CM}	Th2	• Microglia
T_{TM}	Th9	• Lung
T_{EM}	Th17	• Skin
T_{TD}	**Treg**	• Gut
T_{MM}		• Others
T_{RM}		Mast cells
γδ		Renal epithelium
		Astrocytes
		Hematopoietic progenitors

B Anatomic Sites

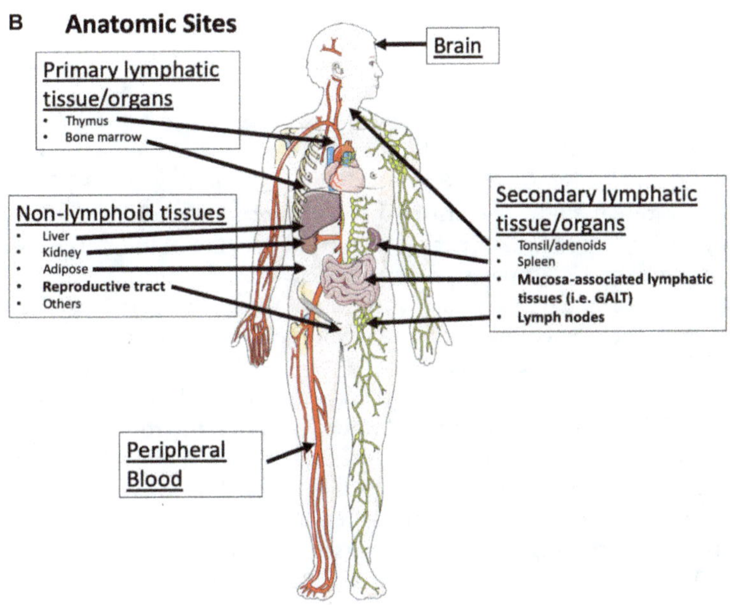

FIGURE 1 | Overview of cell types and anatomic sites reported to harbor the latent reservoir. **(A)** Cell types thought to harbor the HIV reservoir. Cell types with demonstrated recovery of replication-competent virus (defined as propagating virus in an outgrowth assay) in humans following years of suppressive ART are in bold. Cell types in regular font represent cells where HIV nucleic acid has been detected by PCR and/or sequencing either in humans or animal models but recovery of replication-competent virus in humans after years of suppressive ART has not been demonstrated. It is important to note that for many cell types, there has been very sparse sampling for replication-competent virus. NA, naïve; SCM, stem cell memory; CM, central memory; TM, transitional memory; EM, effector memory; TD, terminally differentiated; MM, migratory memory; RM, resident memory. **(B)** Anatomic sites with demonstrated recovery of replication-competent virus in humans following years of suppressive ART are highlighted in bold. Potential replication-competent anatomic reservoir sites are in regular font. These sites represent tissues/organs where HIV nucleic acid has been detected either in humans or animal models but recovery of replication-competent virus in humans after years of suppressive ART has not been demonstrated. It is important to note that for many tissue types, there has been very sparse sampling for replication-competent virus. Images were derived and modified from Servier Medical Arts under a Creative Commons Attribution 3.0 Unported License.

T memory stem cells may also contribute significantly to the viral reservoir in some individuals (Buzon et al., 2014).

Non-resting CD4 T cells that express one or more markers associated with activation (CD25, CD69, and/or HLA-DR) may also contain persistent, replication-competent HIV; however, the stability of persistent HIV within these cells remains to be proven. HIV DNA is enriched in non-resting CD4 T cells (Chun et al., 2005) and markers of immune activation and dysfunction are moderately correlated with DNA and RNA markers of viral persistence in some studies (Chomont et al., 2009; Hatano et al., 2013; Cockerham et al., 2014). A recent study demonstrated the recovery of identical *gag-pol* sequences from HLA-DR expressing-CD4 T cells over multiple time points in durably suppressed participants (Lee et al., 2019). This underscores the importance of interrogating non-resting CD4 T cells for HIV during suppressive therapy. Whether virus found in non-resting T cells originated from resting cells that acquired activation markers, or if some of these cells later return to the resting state is not well understood. As most activated T cells die in the contraction phase of the immune response (Alderson et al., 1995; Swain et al., 1996; Green et al., 2003; Marrack et al., 2010; McKinstry et al., 2010), activated T cells likely do not represent a stable reservoir. However, it is unclear if HLA-DR, CD25, and/or CD69 expression are always indicators of fully activated T cells that are destined to die via immune contraction. In addition, CD25 and/or HLA-DR expressing cells likely represent a heterogenous population of T regulatory cells and activated T cells (Simonetta and Bourgeois, 2013; Corneau et al., 2017). Thus, further evaluation of persistent HIV within these non-resting cells is warranted.

Functional polarization of CD4 T cells may also influence reservoir formation and stability. Within the B cell follicle and in the periphery, T follicular helper (T_{fh}) cells also represent an important cell type that harbors replication-competent HIV (Pallikkuth et al., 2015; Banga et al., 2016). Given the central role of T_{fh} cells in HIV replication during active infection, the reservoir may be highly enriched within tissue T_{fh} cells (Banga et al., 2016). In addition, HIV DNA is enriched in CD4 T cells with Th1/17 and Treg polarizations (Tran et al., 2008; Kulpa and Chomont, 2015; Sun et al., 2015; Dunay et al., 2017).

Studies of viremia in individuals on suppressive therapy (viral "blips" or residual viremia) demonstrate that the residual viremia is not always representative of the proviruses that compose the latent reservoir in CD4 T cells from peripheral blood (Bailey et al., 2006; Sahu et al., 2009; Anderson et al., 2011). However, this does not exclude the possibility that a small pool of peripheral blood CD4 T cells is responsible for residual viremia. Another possibility is that this residual viremia may be derived from CD4 T cells in tissues, or other cell types in tissues.

Other Cell Types

Until recently no study has demonstrated recovery, following years of suppressive therapy, of replication-competent virus from any other purified human cell type other than CD4+ T cells. However, a recent study demonstrated recovery of replication-competent HIV from macrophages harvested from urethral tissue of durably ART-suppressed donors (Ganor et al., 2019). In addition to urethral macrophages, there are several lines of reasoning and evidence that underscore the need to evaluate other cell types for HIV reservoir.

Cells from non-lymphoid lineages can be infected and produce HIV virions during active infection. However, the role and stability of these cells under suppressive ART is highly debated. Bone-marrow derived macrophages, as well as yolk-sac derived microglia and other tissue-resident macrophages may also represent potential HIV reservoirs (Gomez Perdiguero et al., 2015; Gama et al., 2018; Wong et al., 2019). Importantly, there is an increasing appreciation for the ability of tissue resident macrophages to self-renew and potentially serve as a long-lived reservoir of replication-competent virus (Gama et al., 2018; Roszer, 2018; Wong et al., 2019). In addition, neuroepithelial progenitor-derived astrocytes also harbor HIV provirus, though the replication competency and potential for reactivation of this virus *in vivo* is poorly understood (Al-Harti et al., 2018; Barat et al., 2018). HIV can infect multipotent hematopoietic CD34+ progenitor cells; however, in general during stable therapy detection of HIV DNA in this population is rare and no recovery of replication-competent virus has been demonstrated (Carter et al., 2010; Durand et al., 2012; Josefsson et al., 2012; Sebastian et al., 2017; Zaikos et al., 2018). Similarly, HIV DNA has been detected rarely in monocytes from durably suppressed individuals; however, monocytes have a half-life of days *in vivo* and do not represent a stable reservoir. Furthermore, purification of monocytes is complicated by their tendency to stick to CD4 T cells (Burel et al., 2019; Massanella et al., 2019). Infectious virus was recovered from placenta-associated mast cells from women on suppressive ART; however, the period of ART was on a timescale of months rather than years and suppression was defined as <400 copies HIV RNA/mL of plasma (Sundstrom et al., 2007). In all of these cases, however, no longitudinal study of the viral sequences that would appear to be replication-competent, or the recovery of virus from these populations over time, has been demonstrated in any of these cell types.

While there is a substantial body of evidence supporting the presence of HIV DNA or RNA in these cell populations, there has been no detection of replication-competent HIV that is directly attributable to a non-lymphoid lineage in ART-suppressed human donors, except for urethral macrophages (Ganor et al., 2019; Wong et al., 2019). Nevertheless, the finding of persistent HIV in urethral macrophages despite long-term ART, demonstration of rebound viremia in humanized myeloid-only mice, and recovery of replication-competent SIV from brain macrophages of ART-suppressed macaques underscores the need to further evaluate non-lymphoid lineage cells as potential long-lived reservoirs of replication-competent HIV in humans (Honeycutt et al., 2017; Gama et al., 2018; Ganor et al., 2019).

THE HIV RESERVOIR: ANATOMIC SITES OF THE RESERVOIR

The majority of studies of the HIV reservoir under suppressive ART have been in peripheral blood CD4 T cells. While these studies have yielded key insights into the HIV reservoir, it is critical to acknowledge that circulating CD4 T cells represent less than 2% of total body CD4 T cells (Westermann and Pabst, 1992; Di Mascio et al., 2009). There is an increasing appreciation for the microenvironment of tissue in the study of the reservoir of persistent HIV infection, and in the evaluation of cure or functional cure interventions (**Figure 1**) (Barton et al., 2016; Churchill et al., 2016; Wong and Yukl, 2016). This tissue context may include factors such as viral sequence compartmentalization, variation in viral expression levels, differential ART penetration, and availability of immune effector mechanisms to clear infected cells expressing viral RNA or protein (Fletcher et al., 2014; Deeks et al., 2016; Margolis et al., 2016; Baxter et al., 2018; van Zyl et al., 2018; Miller et al., 2019; Pardons et al., 2019).

Detailed HIV reservoir measurements of different tissues are reviewed elsewhere (Yukl and Wong, 2015; Barton et al., 2016; Churchill et al., 2016; Wong and Yukl, 2016). For the purposes of this review, we consider both defined and potential anatomic reservoir sites (**Figure 1**) in the context of current and emerging reservoir assays. Defined anatomic replication-competent HIV reservoir sites in humans who have been treated with long-term (years) of fully suppressive ART include CD4 T cells from peripheral blood and some secondary lymphoid tissues (Siliciano et al., 2003; Crooks et al., 2015; Sanyal et al., 2018), and recently the reproductive tract in the form of urethral macrophages (Ganor et al., 2019). It is critical to note that because of limited access to human tissue, there is sparse sampling of many tissue types (i.e., spleen) that undoubtedly harbor CD4 T cells with replication-competent HIV (**Figure 1**).

However, there are many long-lived cell types, such as other tissue resident macrophages in other sites (e.g., microglia), astrocytes, hematopoietic progenitor cells, among others, in which HIV DNA or RNA has been detected but replication-competent HIV has not (Carter et al., 2010; Canaud et al., 2014; Yukl and Wong, 2015; Al-Harti et al., 2018; Ko et al., 2019; Wong et al., 2019) (**Figure 1**). Therefore, we consider tissues with these cell types as potential reservoir sites. These cell types are found throughout the body in a variety of different tissues. Again, it is important to note that the absence of recovery of replication-competent virus in these tissues does not mean that reservoir does not exist in these locations. Limited access to human tissues, and the technical complexities associated with viral outgrowth assays in these samples limits the sensitivity of studies performed to date (Churchill et al., 2016; Deeks et al., 2016, 2017; Ganor et al., 2019). Understanding the composition and frequency of the replication-competent reservoir across different tissues is a critical issue for future cure research, as cure interventions must be assessed by their effect on the viral reservoir, wherever it is located.

THE HIV RESERVOIR: SPECTRUM OF VIRAL EXPRESSION, DIVERSITY, AND REPLICATION COMPETENCY

HIV proviral expression and diversity varies greatly across cells, tissues, and individuals. Cells with proviruses in their genomic DNA can increase in frequency (through homeostatic or antigen-driven proliferation) or decrease in frequency (through activation-induced cell death, viral cytolysis, or immune clearance) (Chomont et al., 2009; Wang et al., 2018a). Importantly, in HIV+ individuals on stable, suppressive ART, the net effect of the above processes universally result in a very slow decay of the replication-competent HIV reservoir in resting CD4 T cells (Siliciano et al., 2003; Crooks et al., 2015).

Critically, the exact threshold of viral expression sufficient for viral cytolysis or immune recognition and clearance is not well defined. CD4 T cells expressing HIV RNA and sometimes viral proteins are often detectable in ART-suppressed individuals, in the absence of any latency reversal intervention (Baxter et al., 2018). These cells, which represent a portion of provirus that is competent for viral transcription and translation, may reach a threshold of viral expression that renders them susceptible to either immune clearance or cell death. Alternatively these cells expressing HIV RNA or protein may return to a more quiescent state and contribute to the maintenance of the HIV reservoir (Barton et al., 2016; Margolis et al., 2016). Careful definition of how much viral RNA and/or protein antigen is necessary to render an infected cell amenable to immune clearance or apoptosis is needed to inform cure strategies.

In addition to the wide spectrum of viral expression, the HIV reservoir also contains a large diversity of proviral sequences, reviewed in van Zyl et al. (2018). This diversity is primarily attributed to the absence of a proofreading mechanism in the HIV reverse transcriptase enzyme, as well as high levels of viremia and recombination (van Zyl et al., 2018). Other factors that contribute to this diversity include: host immune response (APOBEC enzyme hypermutations) (Bruner et al., 2016), length of infection (accumulation of mutations and depletion of CD4 T cell targets) (Arrildt et al., 2015; Zhou et al., 2016), viral compartmentalization (Yukl and Wong, 2015; van Zyl et al., 2018; Miller et al., 2019), and selection for viral quasispecies that are able to evade killing by host immune mechanisms (Phillips et al., 1991; Wei et al., 2003; Kearney et al., 2009; van Zyl et al., 2018).

Associated with this diversity is a significant frequency of replication-defective proviruses, as well as clonally expanded sequences that may or may not be replication-competent (Bruner et al., 2016; Bui et al., 2017; Wiegand et al., 2017). Critically, most estimates posit that over 90% of proviruses are replication-defective. This, combined with the low frequency (0.01–100 per 1,000,000 CD4 T cells) of replication-competent proviruses (Siliciano et al., 2003; Crooks et al., 2015; Bruner et al., 2019) makes measurement of the replication-competent HIV reservoir extremely difficult. Given the diversity of persistent HIV and large number of defective proviruses, it is critical to consider what each reservoir assay measures in the context of the scientific or clinical question being asked, and whether it overestimates or underestimates the true frequency of the replication-competent HIV reservoir.

MEASURING THE HIV RESERVOIR

To provide a framework for our review of HIV reservoir assays, we have organized our discussion into assays that (1) directly measure proviral genomes (i.e., DNA PCR and DNA sequencing-based assays) and (2) assays that measure basal or experimentally inducible persistent HIV expression (i.e., RNA, viral proteins, or propagating viral infection). The best use of each assay is dependent on the aims of the scientific study and the type(s) of samples available (**Table 1**).

MEASURING THE HIV RESERVOIR: DIRECT MEASUREMENT OF VIRAL GENOMES

DNA PCR Assays

One of the first, and to date most widely used methods to estimate the frequency of persistent HIV is the detection of HIV DNA by quantitative PCR (qPCR). Of note, these assays all measure proviruses directly, but do not provide any information about their inducibility. An economical and rapid method, DNA PCR assays have been widely applied in different cell types and tissues (Malnati et al., 2008; Chomont et al., 2009; Yukl et al., 2013). However, it is often difficult to compare DNA PCR measurements across different assays (assay performance characteristics and cell normalization methods), individuals (proviral sequence heterogeneity) and tissues (differential extraction efficiencies and levels of PCR inhibitors across tissues) (Henrich et al., 2017). Specific DNA PCR assays are too numerous to discuss here, but primarily target conserved regions of *gag*, the LTR, or *pol*.

Digital droplet PCR (ddPCR) assays for HIV DNA have also been developed, and in general relative to qPCR have greater precision and tolerance for primer/probe mismatches, which are common because of the sequence heterogeneity of proviral DNA (Strain et al., 2013; Rutsaert et al., 2018). One limitation of HIV ddPCR assays, however, is the presence of false positives in no template control (NTC) wells and in DNA samples from HIV seronegative participants. This limitation, discussed in detail elsewhere (Strain et al., 2013; Kiselinova et al., 2014; Bosman et al., 2015; Rutsaert et al., 2018), is problematic for participants with very low reservoir frequencies. In contrast, false positives in qPCR assays occur much less frequently, and false positives can be excluded by sequencing, which is not possible on current ddPCR platforms (Strain et al., 2013; Bosman et al., 2015). Thus, for discriminating the absolute presence or absence of HIV DNA, qPCR-based approaches are preferred.

qPCR and ddPCR DNA assays overestimate the frequency of replication-competent reservoir primarily because there are many mutations with a replication-defective phenotype that

TABLE 1 | Overview of reservoir assays.

Assay target	Assay	Sensitivity for HIV	Specificity for HIV	Specificity for intact provirus	Specificity for integrated provirus	Cost	Cell number requirement	Assay time requirement	Over/under estimation of replication-competent reservoir	Examples
DNA	**qPCR/ddPCR (one region)**	Yes	Yes**	No	No	Low	Low	Low	Over	Malnati et al., 2008; Strain et al., 2013; Bosman et al., 2015
	Integrated DNA Assay	Yes	Yes	No	Yes	Medium	Low	Medium	Over	Reviewed in Liszewski et al., 2009
	IPDA	Yes	Yes**	Partial	No	Low	Low	Medium	Over	Bruner et al., 2019
	Q4PCR	Yes	Yes	Yes*	No	Medium	Low	High	Over	Gaebler et al., 2019
	SGS or NGS (one region)	Yes	Yes	No	No	Medium	Low	High	Over	Reviewed in Wang and Palmer, 2018
	Near-full length genome sequencing	Yes	Yes	Yes*	No	High	Medium	High	Over	Ho et al., 2013; Bruner et al., 2016; Hiener et al., 2017; Lee et al., 2017
	Integration site + full length genome sequencing	Yes	Yes	Yes*	Yes	High	Medium	High	Over	Einkauf et al., 2019; Patro et al., 2019
RNA	**Bulk cell PCR**	Yes	Yes	No	N/A	Low	Low	Low	Over	Archin et al., 2012; Shan et al., 2013
	Single cell PCR	Yes	Yes	No	N/A	Low	Low	High	Over	Procopio et al., 2015; Yucha et al., 2017
	Single copy assay (SCA)	Yes	Yes	No	N/A	Medium	N/A	Medium	Over	Reviewed in Wang and Palmer, 2018
	SGS or NGS	Yes	Yes	No	N/A	Medium	Medium	High	Over	Wiegand et al., 2017; Das et al., 2018
	***In situ* hybridization/RNA flow**	Yes	Yes	No	N/A	Medium	Medium	Medium	Over	Zhang et al., 2018; Porichis et al., 2014; Martrus et al., 2016; Baxter et al., 2017; Grau-Exposito et al., 2017
p24	**FAST/Digital Microscopy**	Yes	Partial***	Partial	N/A	High	Medium	High	Over	DeMaster et al., 2015
	Flow Cytometry	Yes	Partial***	Partial	N/A	Medium	Medium	Medium	Over	Baxter et al., 2016; Martrus et al., 2016; Baxter et al., 2017; Pardons et al., 2019
	ELISA (Digital and Standard)	Yes	Partial***	Partial	N/A	Medium	Medium	Medium	Over	Wu et al., 2017
	Mass Cytometry	Yes	Partial***	Partial	N/A	Medium	Medium	Medium	Over	Cavrois et al., 2017
Outgrowth	**QVOA**	Yes	Yes	Yes	N/A	High	High	High	Under	Siliciano and Siliciano, 2005; Archin et al., 2017

**Sequencing assays slightly overestimate the replication-competent reservoir. **ddPCR-based assays are associated with low false positive rates. ***p24-antibody based assays have false positive rates.*

occur outside of the viral region assayed, including APOBEC hypermutations, insertions, deletions, and packaging signal defects (Bruner et al., 2015, 2016). In addition, because most DNA PCR primers are designed inside the HIV genome region, these assays also detect linear unintegrated DNA and episomal forms of HIV DNA such 2-long terminal repeat (2-LTR) circles, though these unintegrated forms are significantly less frequent, and their stability in durably ART-suppressed individuals is debated (Eriksson et al., 2013; Bruner et al., 2015; Martinez-Picado et al., 2018). To overcome the problem of unintegrated forms of HIV DNA, assays for integrated HIV DNA were developed, taking advantage of the high frequency (~11%) of Alu short interspersed elements within the human genome as a host target to guarantee the exclusion of unintegrated forms of HIV (Deininger, 2011). One primer targets Alu elements while the other primer targets *gag*, followed by a nested PCR for the HIV LTR, enabling the detection of integrated provirus (O'Doherty et al., 2002; Liszewski et al., 2009). However, these assays are subject to variable efficiency depending on the proximity of human Alu sequence and the HIV genome that requires correction, and often require a high number of replicates for accurate frequency estimation (Liszewski et al., 2009; Graf and O'Doherty, 2013). Other methods to assay for integrated HIV DNA, including gel fractionation, inverse PCR, and linker ligation PCR, are reviewed in Liszewski et al. (2009).

In most PCR assays, the use of primers and probes targeting only one highly conserved proviral region detect HIV genomes that are defective or mutated in regions external of the assay amplicon (Eriksson et al., 2013; Bruner et al., 2016). Recent efforts have developed assays to simultaneously detect several conserved regions of the HIV genome. Bruner et al. (2019) developed the Intact Proviral DNA Assay (IPDA) that, based on ddPCR multiplex technology, simultaneously interrogate the presence of an intact packaging signal (PS) and the Rev-responsive element (RRE) within *env*. This innovative approach enables estimates of intact proviral DNA with as few as 5 million CD4 T cells. Moreover, the IPDA does not depend on long-distance PCR, the inefficiency of which might limit the ability of near full-length DNA sequencing approaches to accurately estimate the frequency of intact provirus. However, because the IPDA detects only a small sub-genomic region (2% of the HIV genome), there is still a risk of overestimation of intact proviral DNA. The IPDA may also quantify possible non-inducible provirus that may permanently remain latent for the lifetime of an individual. Bruner et al. (2019), in a bioinformatics analysis of several hundred proviral sequences, report that of the proviruses that would be amplified by the IPDA, approximately 70% are intact. To what extent this percentage varies from participant to participant, however, was not studied as it was not possible to perform sequencing following ddPCR in this study.

This knowledge gap was recently addressed by Gaebler et al. (2019), using a combined quadruplex qPCR and next-generation sequencing approach, termed Q4PCR. Q4PCR employs probes for PS, *env* (RRE), *pol* and *gag* that are highly conserved in intact proviruses. Q4PCR employs the same primer/probe set for *env* (RRE) as in the published version of the IPDA as well as the patent application (Siliciano, 2016; Bruner et al., 2019; Gaebler et al., 2019). Compared to the published version of the IPDA (Bruner et al., 2019), the primers for the PS region are different in Q4PCR (Gaebler et al., 2019); however, the probe is nearly identical. The PS primers and probe used in Q4PCR are identical to the sequences in the patent application for the IPDA (Siliciano, 2016).

Gaebler et al. (2019), in a separate bioinformatics analysis of >1000 near-full length sequences found that approximately 60% of proviruses detected by the PS and *env* primer/probe combination were intact. However, in sequence analysis of six individuals, they found that no amplification occurred for PS and *env* probes in 2/6 individuals. This variability was attributed to sequence polymorphisms in proviral genomes across individuals. While a potential issue, it appears to occur relatively infrequently (Bruner et al., 2019) and is readily corrected with alternative primers. In four individuals studied by Gaebler et al. (2019), the percentage of proviruses called intact by the IPDA probes that were truly intact by near-full-length sequencing varied from 9.1 to 96%. Gaebler et al. (2019) findings highlight a potential limitation of the IPDA: the percentage of proviruses that are correctly called intact by the IPDA may vary widely between individuals. This may be less troublesome if the assay is used to measure the effect of an intervention in an individual, but problematic if the assay is used to categorize different individuals. Further evaluation of more individuals with head-to-head comparisons of the Q4PCR method (modified to include the most current version of the IPDA PS primer sequences) and the IPDA is warranted. Moreover, development of intact proviral DNA assays that are optimized for all HIV subtypes will be necessary (Bruner et al., 2019). Nonetheless, the IPDA represents an attractive addition to the reservoir assay toolkit, as it is currently the most accurate high-throughput DNA assay for estimating the size of the replication-competent reservoir (Bruner et al., 2019).

HIV DNA Sequencing

Sequencing of HIV proviral genomes enables measurements of reservoir frequency, diversity, and evolution. While single genome/proviral sequencing (SGS/SPS) assays provide important information about proviral diversity, they overestimate the replication competent reservoir because they are based on sequencing of subgenomic regions and miss proviruses with deletions or mutations in the primer binding sites (Wang and Palmer, 2018). To reduce the former limitation, several near full-length HIV sequencing assays were developed (Ho et al., 2013; Bruner et al., 2016; Hiener et al., 2017; Lee et al., 2017) and are reviewed in Wang and Palmer (2018) and Wang et al. (2018b). Although laborious and expensive, they provide an assessment of persistent HIV diversity across different cell subsets and tissues, and with longitudinal sampling, could provide insight into the dynamics of reservoir frequency and diversity over time (Hiener et al., 2017; Lee et al., 2017). Limitations of these near-full-length sequencing assays include poor coverage of the viral LTRs and slight overestimation of replication-competent reservoir frequency (Wang and Palmer, 2018; Einkauf et al., 2019). In addition, application of these technologies to a higher number of individuals and time points is necessary to make generalizable findings about the sequence composition of the HIV reservoir (Wang et al., 2018b).

Sequencing of HIV integration sites has also provided critical insights into the HIV reservoir. Initial integration site mapping efforts underscored the importance of clonal expansion in HIV reservoir maintenance (Maldarelli et al., 2014; Wagner et al., 2014). Simultaneous detection of near-full length provirus as well as its integration site could improve knowledge of the reservoir and inform cure strategies. Two research groups are developing integrated full length HIV sequencing assays capable of linking HIV genome sequences and their integration site. Both the methods use a multiple displacement amplification (MDA) combined with SGS (Full length integrated proviral single genome sequencing, FLIP-SGS) (Patro et al., 2019) or followed by NGS (matched integration site and proviral sequencing, MIP-Seq) (Einkauf et al., 2019). These methods may yield important insights into reservoir dynamics and formation, as well as reservoir maintenance through clonal expansion. Early studies suggest that in participants on durable therapy, intact proviruses, relative to defective proviruses, are enriched in non-genic regions of the genome (Einkauf et al., 2019).

MEASURING THE HIV RESERVOIR: ASSESSMENT OF BASAL OR INDUCIBLE RESERVOIR EXPRESSION

Cell-associated HIV RNA is readily detectable at baseline, even in resting CD4 T cells (Archin et al., 2012; Archin et al., 2017). This suggests that at least in some cells, HIV is not completely quiescent. Thus, measurements of persistent HIV can be made on (1) unstimulated cells or (2) cells stimulated with T cell activating agents (the inducible reservoir). It is important to note for assays that measure the inducible reservoir, whether at the level of RNA, protein, or viral outgrowth, not all replication-competent proviruses are induced by a single round of T cell activation (Ho et al., 2013).

HIV RNA PCR

While proviruses that are transcription-competent are more likely to be replication-competent than any given sample of proviral DNA, there are still many defective proviruses that can be expressed at the RNA level (Bruner et al., 2016; Imamichi et al., 2016; Pollack et al., 2017; Wiegand et al., 2017). That said, baseline ca-RNA expression (and bulk HIV DNA) is predictive of time to viral rebound upon therapy cessation and may serve as a biomarker to guide future analytical treatment interruption studies (Pasternak and Berkhout, 2018).

Unlike proviral DNA where there is (generally) one integrated copy per infected cell, many copies of RNA can be present in a single cell, which makes reservoir frequency measurements using RNA more challenging. Bulk qPCR or ddPCR assays of HIV RNA can provide a sensitive and low cost estimation of HIV transcription. Of note, for one reported HIV-RNA assay, semi-nested qPCR appeared to have greater quantitative linearity, accuracy, and sensitivity relative to ddPCR (Kiselinova et al., 2014). However, these assays of bulk RNA cannot determine the frequency of HIV RNA positive cells, or the phenotype of the cell(s) expressing HIV RNA. Furthermore, similar issues discussed above in the DNA PCR section for comparisons across assays, individuals, and tissues apply to RNA as well. Targets of cell-associated RNA assays include assays for unspliced *gag* (Archin et al., 2012), polyadenylated transcripts (Shan et al., 2013), among others (Fischer et al., 2002; Pasternak et al., 2013; Pasternak and Berkhout, 2018). In addition, Yukl et al. (2018) recently published a ddPCR assay for multiple HIV transcripts (read-through, TAR, elongated, spliced, etc.) which may yield insights into the nature of blocks to HIV transcription from the reservoir at baseline or in response to latency reversal agents. Inducible HIV cell-free RNA from culture supernatants can also be measured (Spivak et al., 2015). Furthermore, measurements of residual viremia from individuals on suppressive ART using ultrasensitive single-copy HIV RNA assays (SCA) may serve as a measurement of inducible persistent HIV, as this residual viremia may reflect persistent HIV that is expressed following T cell activation due to normal immune physiology. SCA have limits of detection of 1 copy/mL of plasma (or lower, depending on the volume of plasma used), and have been used to study ART treatment intensification and latency reversal in clinical studies (reviewed in Wang and Palmer, 2018).

Other RNA PCR approaches have been developed to estimate the frequency of RNA expressing reservoir cells. Limiting dilution single cell RNA PCR assays estimate the frequency of HIV cell-associated RNA expressing cells (Pasternak and Berkhout, 2018). A major limiting dilution assay is the Tat/rev induced limiting dilution assay, or TILDA (Procopio et al., 2015). By assaying multiply spliced HIV RNA, TILDA assay reduces reservoir frequency overestimation because multiply spliced HIV RNA is less likely to (but still may) have replication defects than DNA measurements (Procopio et al., 2015; Imamichi et al., 2016; Pollack et al., 2017). Another innovative approach for estimating the frequency of RNA-expressing cells is single cell ddPCR (Yucha et al., 2017). Of note, all of these assays require further cross-sectional and longitudinal validation, to determine if they can categorize individuals in a useful way, or if they have appropriate discriminatory power to register the effect of a reservoir depletion strategy over time.

HIV RNA Sequencing

Limiting dilution sequencing assays have been developed, but are restricted by cost and sequence coverage. However, these assays are able to estimate the number of RNA copies per cell in addition to the frequency of RNA-expressing cells (Pasternak and Berkhout, 2018). Wiegand et al. (2017) developed the cell-associated HIV RNA and DNA single-genome sequencing (CARD-SGS) assay to estimate the frequency of HIV proviruses that express RNA at baseline. In addition, Das et al. (2018) recently reported a multi spliced RNA assay called EDITS (envelope detection by induced transcription-based sequencing) based on RT-nested PCR amplification of multiply spliced *env* RNA followed by NGS.

The sequencing of HIV RNA by SGS/NGS has been performed in several experimental contexts. SGS remains the gold standard even though it is expensive and time consuming. The use of

NGS, however, is limited. The frequency of PCR errors, PCR bias, recombination and rearrangement that occurs during NGS library construction need to be carefully considered. Methods such as primer ID (Jabara et al., 2011; Zhou et al., 2015) and alternative adaptor attachment strategies (Boltz et al., 2016) can mitigate the errors associated with NGS library preparation.

HIV RNA Staining Assays

In situ hybridization (ISH) of RNA at the single cell level was developed in the 1990s, and subsequently modified to simultaneously detect HIV RNA and host or virus RNA or protein (Wong et al., 1997a; Schacker et al., 2000; Baxter et al., 2018; Deleage et al., 2018). The development of these assays is reviewed elsewhere (Baxter et al., 2018). We highlight the recent development of next-generation HIV ISH assays, such as RNAscope and FISH-flow, that enable the detection of single HIV RNA positive cells with microscopy visualization (Estes et al., 2017; Zhang et al., 2018) or flow cytometry (Porichis et al., 2014; Martrus et al., 2016; Baxter et al., 2017; Grau-Exposito et al., 2017). Using these techniques, some inference about the levels (copies) of RNA per cell can be made based on staining intensities, in addition to the frequency of HIV RNA-expressing cells. A novel multiplex microscopy ISH approach allows for detections of viral DNA, RNA and protein. However, this has yet to be evaluated in cells from ART-suppressed participants (Puray-Chavez et al., 2017).

HIV *gag* p24 Assays

Recent efforts in the cure field have developed assays to quantify baseline or inducible expression of viral proteins, in particular the p24 capsid protein in whole cells. The rationale behind this effort is that quantification of inducible viral protein reduces overestimation of the frequency of the replication-competent reservoir, as proviruses that can progress through transcription and translation are less likely to have major defects (Bruner et al., 2016). All assays that employ antibodies to p24 are limited by a false positive rate from non-specific antibody binding. The use of two p24 antibodies may, at least partially, overcome this limitation.

Graf et al. (2013) demonstrated that in ART-suppressed participants, *gag* protein positive cells could be detected at a frequency of ~1 *gag*+ cell per million PBMCs. This finding supported the notion that at baseline, some persistent HIV is expressed at a protein level. However, this technique had a high false positive rate. To mitigate false positives, groups endeavored to detect *gag* positive cells in tandem with CD4 downregulation, suggestive of the presence of the Nef protein. O'Doherty and colleagues used a combination of Fiber-optic Array Scanning Technology (FAST) and automated digital microscopy to detect *gag* positive with concomitant CD4 downregulation, suggesting the presence of actively transcribed and translated viral proteins (DeMaster et al., 2015). While this technology improved the false positive rate, it is not yet widely used. Other groups focused on honing the specificity of p24 flow cytometry assays. The combination of *gag* staining with RNA flow (discussed above) proved useful in some trials but not others, likely due to RNA sequence heterogeneity (Baxter et al., 2016, 2017; Martrus et al., 2016; Grau-Exposito et al., 2017). Using a high number of RNA probes resulted in robust detection of *gag*+RNA+ cells, with the expected CD4 downregulation and enrichment in cell populations such as T_{fh} and PD1+ cells (Baxter et al., 2016, 2017, 2018).

More recent efforts have focused on using two *gag* protein probes in flow cytometry application to quantify inducible persistent HIV at the protein level. Chomont and colleagues recently published a flow cytometry protocol that utilizes two capsid antibodies for dual intracellular staining of p24 (Pardons et al., 2019). In ART-suppressed individuals, p24 double positive cells correlated with TILDA and QVOA measures. However, in this study, no p24 double positive cells were detected in ART-suppressed participants at baseline, in contrast to previous work using a single p24 antibody (Graf et al., 2013; Baxter et al., 2016). Notably, this novel technology might permit characterization of reservoir cells from ART-suppressed donors using standard flow cytometry surface markers and intracellular staining.

Another focus in quantification of viral reservoirs has utilized digital ELISA technology to quantify the very low levels of p24 produced from CD4 T cells after stimulation with a latency reversal agent or global T cell activator. This assay can be applied to cell lysates or culture supernatants and is able to detect sub-femtomolar levels of p24; however, the correlation of these measures with other assays of persistent HIV infection is not yet fully assessed (Wu et al., 2017).

Finally, high parameter mass cytometry techniques using heavy-metal tagged antibodies have been applied to *in vitro* studies of HIV infection to phenotype tonsillar CD4 T cells infected with a mass-cytometry compatible reporter virus (Cavrois et al., 2017). Assays to detect HIV p24 using mass cytometry are an area of active investigation and development.

OUTGROWTH ASSAYS

HIV Outgrowth Assays

Significant effort has been deployed recently to develop new or improved assays to measure clinical interventions aimed at depleting the HIV replication-competent reservoir. While assays based on PCR of HIV DNA offer a streamlined method to quantitate persistent HIV infection, a significant fraction of persistently infected cells harbor defective proviruses that cannot be distinguished from replication-competent provirus by amplification of one genomic region (Eriksson et al., 2013; Ho et al., 2013; Bruner et al., 2016). Thus, approaches to eradicate HIV infection will likely need to incorporate assays that reflect depletion of replication-competent viruses to measure the efficacy of anti-latency therapeutics. The quantitative viral outgrowth assay (QVOA or simply VOA) is probably the most well-known assay used to quantitate replication-competent HIV.

During the early days of the HIV epidemic, co-culture assays of PBMC from HIV-infected individuals with Phytohaemagglutinin (PHA)-stimulated PBMC from uninfected donors were used to confirm the presence of replicating virus and provide an estimation of the viral burden within infected people (Castro et al., 1988; Jackson et al., 1988; Ho et al., 1989;

Dimitrov et al., 1990). As it became evident that resting CD4 T cells were a major source of integrated proviral DNA during therapy (Chun et al., 1995), a derivative of these earlier co-culture assays was developed to quantify replication-competent HIV in purified CD4 T cells from HIV-infected individuals (Finzi et al., 1997; Wong et al., 1997b; Siliciano and Siliciano, 2005). Several detailed protocols for the traditional QVOA are available (Siliciano and Siliciano, 2005; Laird et al., 2016; Archin et al., 2017). Highly purified total or resting CD4+ T-cells are isolated from whole blood, leukapheresis product, or tissue-derived mononuclear cells for QVOA, and are stimulated with mitogen and co-cultured in a limiting dilution format with PHA-activated CD8-depleted PBMCs from HIV-seronegative individuals to exponentially expand the virus. Supernatant from co-culture assays are then assessed for the presence of p24 protein and Poisson statistics applied to estimate the frequency of resting cell infection that is reported as infectious unit per million CD4+ T cells (IUPM).

The QVOA is considered the gold standard for measuring replication-competent HIV and provides a definitive minimal estimate of reservoir size. However, the assay is costly and labor intensive, and given the low frequency of latently infected cells, often large numbers of cells are required to increase the limit of detection. The QVOA reports a minimal estimate of the frequency of latent but replication-competent proviruses, due to the presence of "non-induced" proviruses unresponsive to a single round of cell stimulation (Ho et al., 2013; Hosmane et al., 2017). Despite its limitations, the QVOA remains a reproducible and reliable method to measure the HIV latent reservoir and has been used to accurately assess the stability the reservoir over time. Using the QVOA, we measured resting CD4+ T-cell infection (RCI) in 37 HIV+ participants, on stable suppressive ART who donated resting CD4+ T cells via leukapheresis, over a period of 6 years and found that despite the long duration of ART, the half live of the reservoir in resting CD4+ T cells to be about 43 months, a value that is very close to that reported by Siliciano et al. (2003) a decade earlier, using an earlier version of the QVOA in a clinical cohort 10 years prior, on older ART (Crooks et al., 2015). This highlights (1) the stability of the replication-competent reservoir and (2) the reliability of the QVOA to probe reservoir dynamics.

Given the importance of the QVOA in assessing replication-competent HIV, many laboratories have introduced modifications to the original assay to streamline the assay and improve upon throughput, sensitivity and dynamic range (Avalos et al., 2016; Laird et al., 2016; Charlins et al., 2017; Fun et al., 2017; Metcalf Pate and Blankson, 2017; Sanyal et al., 2017; Massanella et al., 2018; Rosenbloom et al., 2019) (**Table 2**). Examples of modifications made to the standard QVOA to streamline and improve sensitivity involved replacing the uninfected donor PHA-blasts normally used in the co-culture to expand virus, with cell lines permissive for HIV infection such as the MOLT-4/CCR5, or using RT-PCR with primers specific for polyadenylated HIV-1 or *gag* RNA to detect virus released into culture supernatant (Laird et al., 2013; Massanella et al., 2018). In their mQVOA assay Massanella et al. (2018) also use the MOLT-4/CCR5 to propagate virus, but used immobilized CD3/CD28 beads to stimulate CD4 T cells and captured cell free RNA from the supernatant using magnetic beads before assaying HIV *gag* by PCR. In a recent cross-laboratory reservoir assay validation study (RAVEN), the above modification was reported to generate IUPM values that were 9.2 fold higher than traditional QVOA assays as RNA detection was thought to be more sensitive than p24 measurements (Rosenbloom et al., 2019). However, while PCR measurements as readout for the QVOA may provide more sensitivity, the potential that some of the RNA (even though released into the supernatant) detected could come from defective provirus, is not full length, and/or is not part of a viral particle should be taken into consideration (Pollack et al., 2017). RNA detection may also inherently be more prone to false positive detection due to low-level PCR product contamination.

The introduction of ultra-sensitive p24 assay platforms have ushered in additional methods to quantitate latent HIV with improved sensitivity of antigen detection in culture supernatant (Descours et al., 2017; Passaes et al., 2017; Wu et al., 2017). We have developed a modified QVOA, the Digital ELISA Viral Outgrowth or DEVO assay that takes advantage of the recently developed SIMOA platform (Quanterix), capable of femtogram detection of HIV p24 protein in contrast to the picogram limitations of traditional ELISA. In this assay, 8–10 $\times$ 10^6 purified resting CD4+ T cells from aviremic, ART-treated HIV+ participants are PHA stimulated in limiting dilution in a 96 well-format. With this assay we found that virus can be expanded using either the CD4 T cell input (i.e., addition of exogenous donor cells is not necessary), PHA blasts from an uninfected donor, or HIV permissive cell lines such as the MOLT4/CCR5. Furthermore, with the DEVO assay we obtained IUPM comparable or higher than the traditional QVOA at an earlier time point, thus reducing the overall length of the assay (Archin et al., 2018).

Finally, another modification of the QVOA reported recently involves differentiating the input memory CD4+ T cells into effector memory T cells before activation. On average, higher IUPM values were observed with the differentiated QVOA (dQVOA) compared to traditional QVOA assay methods (Wonderlich et al., 2019). This suggests that induction into the effector state prior to activation facilitates more efficient exit from latency (Kulpa et al., 2019).

REDUCING THE RESERVOIR: STABILITY AND MEANINGFUL REDUCTION

For studies that aim to deplete the reservoir, it is critical to understand how specific reservoir assay measurements (HIV DNA, QVOA, etc.) change over time on suppressive therapy without any cure intervention. Studies of reservoir stability to date have employed both bulk and intact DNA PCR (PBMCs, peripheral CD4 T cells) (Besson et al., 2014; Laanani et al., 2015; Bachmann et al., 2019; Bruner et al., 2019) and viral outgrowth (peripheral CD4 T cells) (Siliciano et al., 2003; Crooks et al., 2015). Generally, in peripheral blood CD4 T cells, QVOA and IPDA reservoir measurements have similar decay kinetics ($t_{1/2}$

TABLE 2 | Overview of modified qVOA assays.

Assay Name	Modification/Format	Readout	Reference(s)
QVOA2	PHA+ sero-negative γ-irradiated PBMC stimulation of resting CD4+ T cells; MOLT4/CCR5 or SupTI-CCR5 as targets for virus expansion	PolyA RNA qPCR or p24 ELISA	Laird et al., 2013; Fun et al., 2017
TZA	CD3/CD28 stimulated CD4+ T cells are co-cultured with TZM-bl indicator cells	B-gal activity by chemiluminescence	Sanyal et al., 2017
dQVOA	Resting CD4+ T Cells are differentiated to effector memory phenotype before activating with PHA + seronegative γ-irradiated PBMC; no targets added	p24 ELISA	Wonderlich et al., 2019
mQVOA	Immobilized CD3/CD28 simulation of CD4+ T cells; MOLT4/CCR5 targets; cell free RNA in supernatant captured by magnetic beads	*gag* or *pol* RNA qPCR	Massanella et al., 2018; Rosenbloom et al., 2019
Murine VOA (mVOA)	CD4+ T cells or PBMC from aviremic donors engrafted into immunodeficient NSG mice, followed by administration of anti- CD3/CD28 and anti-CD8 antibodies	Plasma HIV RNA detection *(gag* primers) by qPCR	Metcalf Pate et al., 2015
Humanized mouse VOA (hmVOA)	CD3/CD28 stimulated resting CD4 T cells from aviremic donors are engrafted into humanized mice	Plasma HIV RNA detection (LTR primers) by qPCR	Charlins et al., 2017
MΦ-QVOA	Myeloid cells from SIV-infected macaques are stimulated with TNF-α; co-cultured with CEMX174 as targets	SIV *gag* RNA qPCR	Avalos et al., 2016

~44 months) (Bruner et al., 2019). Measures of bulk DNA or non-intact provirus are more variable in stability (Besson et al., 2014; Laanani et al., 2015; Bachmann et al., 2019; Bruner et al., 2019). Within tissues, little is known about reservoir stability because of the difficulties with accessing tissues, especially over multiple time points in human participants. Therefore, thorough understanding of the reservoir stability within tissue may depend primarily on animal models (Henrich et al., 2017).

In addition to reservoir stability, understanding inter-assay variability and the error associated with each measurement is essential to robustly assess potential reservoir reductions. For instance, evaluation of longitudinal QVOA data suggests that a sixfold decline in the frequency of resting CD4 T cell infection would be necessary to achieve 95% confidence that the intervention resulted in the reduction of the reservoir observed (Crooks et al., 2015). For other assays, however, the decline in persistent HIV frequency to achieve 95% confidence of a reservoir reduction is unknown, and further complicated by the presence of large frequencies of non-intact proviruses. The IPDA is a promising assay to assess reservoir reductions in a high-throughput manner; however, this must be tempered with concerns about interindividual variability for false positive non-intact proviruses and the need for further understanding of the stability and reproducibility of the IPDA over multiple time points and across diverse human cohorts (Bruner et al., 2019; Gaebler et al., 2019).

There is also rationale to conduct bulk measures of HIV provirus (i.e., DNA PCR of a conserved region of a viral gene) to assess the effect of reservoir reduction interventions on global levels of HIV DNA. Although >90% of HIV provirus is replication-defective, a significant portion of proviruses can express viral proteins that may contribute to chronic immune activation and sequelae (Hunt et al., 2016; Imamichi et al., 2016; Pollack et al., 2017). Therefore, information about the effect of interventions on total persistent HIV frequency may be useful. At the same time, however, defective provirus may be more resistant to latency reversal and immune clearance interventions because of lower expression of viral RNA and/or protein. If this is the case, reservoir assays that measure intact proviruses, viral RNA/proteins, or replication-competent HIV may have a higher sensitivity to potential reservoir reductions.

For experimental medicine trials, we propose a framework where the more costly and labor intensive QVOA-based measures are employed at study beginning and as primary end points, with more intensive readouts of genetically intact DNA, bulk DNA, and/or other reservoir measurement occurring both at the start and end, as well as throughout the trial. Our reasoning behind this recommendation is that QVOA provides a direct measure of replication-competent virus that could re-establish an infection, whereas DNA and other assays all have concerns about detection of replication-deficient virus. Moreover, for QVOA, there is a defined magnitude of decline (sixfold) in reservoir frequency necessary to attribute a reservoir reduction to a specific intervention (Crooks et al., 2015), whereas for other assays this magnitude of reduction is unclear. In addition, for potential cures, it will be essential to show by QVOA-based methods over multiple time points the absence of replication-competent virus recovery. The engraftment of CD4+ T cells from individuals who are negative by QVOA into murine viral outgrowth models (mVOA or hmVOA, **Table 2**) could be used as additional metrics to ascertain the absence or reduction of replication competent virus (Metcalf Pate and Blankson, 2017).

At the same time, however, standard QVOA based measurements only provide a definitive minimal estimate of reservoir frequency, likely because of the presence of non-induced proviruses (Ho et al., 2013). Concomitant use of the IPDA overcomes this limitation because measurement of genetically intact provirus is not dependent on the transcriptional status of the cell, and may provide a maximal estimate of replication-competent provirus. Further, other reservoir measurements such as the IPDA or other assays described herein may afford a greater dynamic range and sensitivity to reservoir reductions, though this remains to be proven. As there is growing evidence for the clonality of the HIV reservoir, novel full length sequencing approaches with integration site analysis will permit the assessment of the impact of interventions on the clonality of the reservoir. Taken together, the combination of primary endpoint QVOA-based reservoir measures with more intensive, higher throughput evaluation of the reservoir using the IPDA, bulk DNA, inducible reservoir measurement(s), and/or sequencing approaches will enable a thorough evaluation of the impact of any intervention on persistent HIV in cure research trials.

SUMMARY

Assays to measure persistent HIV infection are emerging quickly. Key issues for the cure field with regard to reservoir assay development include (1) optimization of viral outgrowth assays for reproducibility, sensitivity, and dynamic range, (2) further understanding of interindividual variability in false positive intact proviruses and stability over time for the IPDA, (3) additional development of full-length/integration site sequencing approaches to understand proviral dynamics during therapy or potential interventions, and (4) advancement of DNA/RNA/p24 single and/or multiplex detection methods to better understand the dynamics and mechanisms of latency reversal with different agents.

AUTHOR CONTRIBUTIONS

SF, CC, DM, and NA conceptualized and outlined the manuscript. SF, CC, and NA wrote the first draft of the manuscript. All authors edited and approved the final version.

ACKNOWLEDGMENTS

The authors thank participants in HIV cure research studies for their collaboration.

REFERENCES

Alderson, M. R., Tough, T. W., Davis-Smith, T., Braddy, S., Falk, B., Schooley, K. A., et al. (1995). Fas ligand mediates activation-induced cell death in human T lymphocytes. *J. Exp. Med.* 181, 71–77. doi: 10.1084/jem.181.1.71

Al-Harti, L., Joseph, J., and Nath, A. (2018). Astrocytes as an HIV CNS reservoir: highlights and reflections of an NIMH-sponsored symposium. *J. Neurovirol.* 24, 665–669. doi: 10.1007/s13365-018-0691-8

Anderson, E. M., and Maldarelli, F. (2018). The role of integration and clonal expansion in HIV infection: live long and prosper. *Retrovirology* 15:71. doi: 10.1186/s12977-018-0448-8

Anderson, J. A., Archin, N. M., Ince, W., Parker, D., Wiegand, A., Coffin, J. M., et al. (2011). Clonal sequences recovered from plasma from patients with residual HIV-1 viremia and on intensified antiretroviral therapy are identical to replicating viral RNAs recovered from circulating resting CD4+ T cells. *J. Virol.* 85, 5220–5223. doi: 10.1128/JVI.00284-11

Archin, N. M., Kirchherr, J. L., Sung, J. A., Clutton, G., Sholtis, K., Xu, Y., et al. (2017). Interval dosing with the HDAC inhibitor vorinostat effectively reverses HIV latency. *J. Clin. Invest.* 127, 3126–3135. doi: 10.1172/JCI92684

Archin, N. M., Liberty, A. L., Kashuba, A. D., Choudhary, S. K., Kuruc, J. D., Crooks, A. M., et al. (2012). Administration of vorinostat disrupts HIV-1 latency in patients on antiretroviral therapy. *Nature* 487, 482–485. doi: 10.1038/nature11286

Archin, N., Stuelke, E., Sholtis, K., Kirchherr, J., and Margolis, D. (2018). A modified viral outgrowth assay incorporating ultra-sensitive P24 measurements. *J Virus Erad.* 4, 132–142.

Arrildt, K. T., LaBranche, C. C., Joseph, S. B., Dukhovlinova, E. N., Graham, W. D., Ping, L. H., et al. (2015). Phenotypic correlates of HIV-1 macrophage tropism. *J. Virol.* 89, 11294–11311. doi: 10.1128/JVI.00946-15

Avalos, C. R., Price, S. L., Forsyth, E. R., Pin, J. N., Shirk, E. N., Bullock, B. T., et al. (2016). Quantitation of productively infected monocytes and macrophages of simian immunodeficiency virus-infected macaques. *J. Virol.* 90, 5643–5656. doi: 10.1128/JVI.00290-16

Bachmann, N., von Siebenthal, C., Vongrad, V., Turk, T., Neumann, K., Beerenwinkel, N., et al. (2019). Determinants of HIV-1 reservoir size and long-term dynamics during suppressive ART. *Nat. Commun.* 10:3193. doi: 10.1038/s41467-019-10884-9

Bailey, J. R., Sedaghat, A. R., Kieffer, T., Brennan, T., Lee, P. K., Wind-Rotolo, M., et al. (2006). Residual human immunodeficiency virus type 1 viremia in some patients on antiretroviral therapy is dominated by a small number of invariant clones rarely found in circulating CD4+ T cells. *J. Virol.* 80, 6441–6457. doi: 10.1128/JVI.00591-06

Banga, R., Procopio, F. A., Noto, A., Pollakis, G., Cavassini, M., Ohmiti, K., et al. (2016). PD-1(+) and follicular helper T cells are responsible for persistent HIV-1 transcription in treated aviremic individuals. *Nat. Med.* 22, 754–761. doi: 10.1038/nm.4113

Barat, C., Proust, A., Deshiere, A., Leboeuf, M., Drouin, J., and Tremblay, M. J. (2018). Astrocytes sustain long-term productive HIV-1 infection without establishment of reactivable viral latency. *Glia* 66, 1363–1381. doi: 10.1002/glia.23310

Barton, K., Winckelmann, A., and Palmer, S. (2016). HIV-1 reservoirs during suppressive therapy. *Trends Microbiol.* 24, 345–355. doi: 10.1016/j.tim.2016.01.006

Baxter, A. E., Niessl, J., Fromentin, R., Richard, J., Porichis, F., Charlebois, R., et al. (2016). Single-cell characterization of viral translation-competent reservoirs in hiv-infected individuals. *Cell Host Microbe* 20, 368–380. doi: 10.1016/j.chom.2016.07.015

Baxter, A. E., Niessl, J., Fromentin, R., Richard, J., Porichis, F., Massanella, M., et al. (2017). Multiparametric characterization of rare HIV-infected cells using an RNA-flow FISH technique. *Nat. Protoc.* 12, 2029–2049. doi: 10.1038/nprot.2017.079

Baxter, A. E., O'Doherty, U., and Kaufmann, D. E. (2018). Beyond the replication-competent HIV reservoir: transcription and translation-competent reservoirs. *Retrovirology* 15:18. doi: 10.1186/s12977-018-0392-7

Besson, G. J., Lalama, C. M., Bosch, R. J., Gandhi, R. T., Bedison, M. A., Aga, E., et al. (2014). HIV-1 DNA decay dynamics in blood during more than a decade of suppressive antiretroviral therapy. *Clin. Infect. Dis.* 59, 1312–1321. doi: 10.1093/cid/ciu585

Boltz, V. F., Rausch, J., Shao, W., Hattori, J., Luke, B., Maldarelli, F., et al. (2016). Ultrasensitive single-genome sequencing: accurate, targeted, next generation sequencing of HIV-1 RNA. *Retrovirology* 13:87. doi: 10.1186/s12977-016-0321-6

Bosman, K. J., Nijhuis, M., van Ham, P. M., Wensing, A. M. J., Vervisch, K., Vandekerckhove, L., et al. (2015). Comparison of digital PCR platforms and semi-nested qPCR as a tool to determine the size of the HIV reservoir. *Sci. Rep.* 5:13811. doi: 10.1038/srep13811

Bozzi, G., Simonetti, F. R., Watters, S. A., Anderson, E. M., Gouzoulis, M., Kearney, M. F., et al. (2019). No evidence of ongoing HIV replication or compartmentalization in tissues during combination antiretroviral therapy: Implications for HIV eradication. *Sci. Adv.* 5:eaav2045. doi: 10.1126/sciadv.aav2045

Bruner, K. M., Hosmane, N. N., and Siliciano, R. F. (2015). Towards an HIV-1 cure: measuring the latent reservoir. *Trends Microbiol.* 23, 192–203. doi: 10.1016/j.tim.2015.01.013

Bruner, K. M., Murray, A. J., Pollack, R. A., Soliman, M. G., Laskey, S. B., Capoferri, A. A., et al. (2016). Defective proviruses rapidly accumulate during acute HIV-1 infection. *Nat. Med.* 22, 1043–1049. doi: 10.1038/nm.4156

Bruner, K. M., Wang, Z., Simonetti, F. R., Bender, A. M., Kwon, K. J., Sengupta, S., et al. (2019). A quantitative approach for measuring the reservoir of latent HIV-1 proviruses. *Nature* 566, 120–125. doi: 10.1038/s41586-019-0898-8

Siliciano, K. B. A. R. (2016). *Compositions and methods related to characterizing proviral reservoirs. US15/568,893*. Baltimore: Johns Hopkins University.

Bui, J. K., Sobolewski, M. D., Keele, B. F., Spindler, J., Musick, A., Wiegand, A., et al. (2017). Proviruses with identical sequences comprise a large fraction of the replication-competent HIV reservoir. *PLoS Pathog.* 13:e1006283. doi: 10.1371/journal.ppat.1006283

Bukrinsky, M. I., Stanwick, T. L., Dempsey, M. P., and Stevenson, M. (1991). Quiescent T lymphocytes as an inducible virus reservoir in HIV-1 infection. *Science* 254, 423–427. doi: 10.1126/science.1925601

Burel, J. G., Pomaznoy, M., Lindestam Arlehamn, C. S., Weiskopf, D., da Silva Antunes, R., Jung, Y., et al. (2019). Circulating T cell-monocyte complexes are markers of immune perturbations. *Elife* 8:e46045. doi: 10.7554/eLife.46045

Buzon, M. J., Sun, H., Li, C., Shaw, A., Seiss, K., Ouyang, Z., et al. (2014). HIV-1 persistence in CD4+ T cells with stem cell-like properties. *Nat. Med.* 20, 139–142. doi: 10.1038/nm.3445

Canaud, G., Dejucq-Rainsford, N., Avettand-Fenoel, V., Viard, J. P., Anglicheau, D., Bienaime, F., et al. (2014). The kidney as a reservoir for HIV-1 after renal transplantation. *J. Am. Soc. Nephrol.* 25, 407–419. doi: 10.1681/ASN.2013050564

Carter, C. C., Onafuwa-Nuga, A., McNamara, L. A., Riddell, J. T., Bixby, D., Savona, M. R., et al. (2010). HIV-1 infects multipotent progenitor cells causing cell death and establishing latent cellular reservoirs. *Nat. Med.* 16, 446–451. doi: 10.1038/nm.2109

Castro, B. A., Weiss, C. D., Wiviott, L. D., and Levy, J. A. (1988). Optimal conditions for recovery of the human immunodeficiency virus from peripheral blood mononuclear cells. *J. Clin. Microbiol.* 26, 2371–2376.

Cavrois, M., Banerjee, T., Mukherjee, G., Raman, N., Hussien, R., Rodriguez, B. A., et al. (2017). Mass cytometric analysis of HIV entry, replication, and remodeling in tissue CD4+ T cells. *Cell Rep.* 20, 984–998. doi: 10.1016/j.celrep.2017.06.087

Charlins, P., Schmitt, K., Remling-Mulder, L., Hogan, L. E., Hanhauser, E., Hobbs, K. S., et al. (2017). A humanized mouse-based HIV-1 viral outgrowth assay with higher sensitivity than in vitro qVOA in detecting latently infected cells from individuals on ART with undetectable viral loads. *Virology* 507, 135–139. doi: 10.1016/j.virol.2017.04.011

Chomont, N., El-Far, M., Ancuta, P., Trautmann, L., Procopio, F. A., Yassine-Diab, B., et al. (2009). HIV reservoir size and persistence are driven by T cell survival and homeostatic proliferation. *Nat. Med.* 15, 893–900. doi: 10.1038/nm.1972

Chun, T. W., Davey, R. T. Jr., Engel, D., Lane, H. C., and Fauci, A. S. (1999). Re-emergence of HIV after stopping therapy. *Nature* 401, 874–875. doi: 10.1038/44755

Chun, T. W., Engel, D., Berrey, M. M., Shea, T., Corey, L., and Fauci, A. S. (1998). Early establishment of a pool of latently infected, resting CD4(+) T cells during primary HIV-1 infection. *Proc. Natl. Acad. Sci. U.S.A.* 95, 8869–8873. doi: 10.1073/pnas.95.15.8869

Chun, T. W., Finzi, D., Margolick, J., Chadwick, K., Schwartz, D., and Siliciano, R. F. (1995). In vivo fate of HIV-1-infected T cells: quantitative analysis of the transition to stable latency. *Nat. Med.* 1, 1284–1290. doi: 10.1038/nm1295-1284

Chun, T. W., Nickle, D. C., Justement, J. S., Large, D., Semerjian, A., Curlin, M. E., et al. (2005). HIV-infected individuals receiving effective antiviral therapy for extended periods of time continually replenish their viral reservoir. *J. Clin. Invest.* 115, 3250–3255. doi: 10.1172/JCI26197

Chun, T. W., Stuyver, L., Mizell, S. B., Ehler, L. A., Mican, J. A., Baseler, M., et al. (1997). Presence of an inducible HIV-1 latent reservoir during highly active antiretroviral therapy. *Proc. Natl. Acad. Sci. U.S.A.* 94, 13193–13197. doi: 10.1073/pnas.94.24.13193

Churchill, M. J., Deeks, S. G., Margolis, D. M., Siliciano, R. F., and Swanstrom, R. (2016). HIV reservoirs: what, where and how to target them. *Nat. Rev. Microbiol.* 14, 55–60. doi: 10.1038/nrmicro.2015.5

Cillo, A. R., and Mellors, J. W. (2016). Which therapeutic strategy will achieve a cure for HIV-1? *Curr. Opin. Virol.* 18, 14–19. doi: 10.1016/j.coviro.2016.02.001

Cockerham, L. R., Siliciano, J. D., Sinclair, E., O'Doherty, U., Palmer, S., Yukl, S. A., et al. (2014). CD4+ and CD8+ T cell activation are associated with HIV DNA in resting CD4+ T cells. *PLoS One* 9:e110731. doi: 10.1371/journal.pone.0110731

Corneau, A., Cosma, A., Even, S., Katlama, C., Le Grand, R., Frachet, V., et al. (2017). Comprehensive Mass Cytometry Analysis of Cell Cycle, Activation, and Coinhibitory Receptors Expression in CD4 T Cells from Healthy and HIV-Infected Individuals. *Cytometry B Clin. Cytom.* 92, 21–32. doi: 10.1002/cyto.b.21502

Crooks, A. M., Bateson, R., Cope, A. B., Dahl, N. P., Griggs, M. K., Kuruc, J. D., et al. (2015). Precise quantitation of the latent HIV-1 reservoir: implications for eradication strategies. *J. Infect. Dis.* 212, 1361–1365. doi: 10.1093/infdis/jiv218

Das, B., Dobrowolski, C., Luttge, B., Valadkhan, S., Chomont, N., Johnston, R., et al. (2018). Estrogen receptor-1 is a key regulator of HIV-1 latency that imparts gender-specific restrictions on the latent reservoir. *Proc. Natl. Acad. Sci. U.S.A.* 115, E7795–E7804. doi: 10.1073/pnas.1803468115

Deeks, S. G., Lewin, S. R., and Bekker, L. G. (2017). The end of HIV: Still a very long way to go, but progress continues. *PLoS Med.* 14:e1002466. doi: 10.1371/journal.pmed.1002466

Deeks, S. G., Lewin, S. R., Ross, A. L., Ananworanich, J., Benkirane, M., Cannon, P., et al. (2016). International AIDS Society global scientific strategy: towards an HIV cure 2016. *Nat. Med.* 22, 839–850. doi: 10.1038/nm.4108

Deininger, P. (2011). Alu elements: know the SINEs. *Genome Biol.* 12:236. doi: 10.1186/gb-2011-12-12-236

Deleage, C., Chan, C. N., Busman-Sahay, K., and Estes, J. D. (2018). Next-generation in situ hybridization approaches to define and quantify HIV and SIV reservoirs in tissue microenvironments. *Retrovirology* 15:4. doi: 10.1186/s12977-017-0387-9

DeMaster, L. K., Liu, X., VanBelzen, D. J., Trinite, B., Zheng, L., Agosto, L. M., et al. (2015). A subset of CD4/CD8 double-negative T cells expresses HIV proteins in patients on antiretroviral therapy. *J. Virol.* 90, 2165–2179. doi: 10.1128/JVI.01913-15

Descours, B., Petitjean, G., Lopez-Zaragoza, J. L., Bruel, T., Raffel, R., Psomas, C., et al. (2017). CD32a is a marker of a CD4 T-cell HIV reservoir harbouring replication-competent proviruses. *Nature* 543, 564–567. doi: 10.1038/nature21710

Devanathan, A. S., Anderson, D. J. C., Cottrell, M. L., Burgunder, E. M., Saunders, A. C., and Kashuba, A. D. M. (2019). Contemporary drug-drug interactions in HIV treatment. *Clin. Pharmacol. Ther.* 105, 1362–1377. doi: 10.1002/cpt.1393

Di Mascio, M., Paik, C. H., Carrasquillo, J. A., Maeng, J. S., Jang, B. S., Shin, I. S., et al. (2009). Noninvasive in vivo imaging of CD4 cells in simian-human immunodeficiency virus (SHIV)-infected nonhuman primates. *Blood* 114, 328–337. doi: 10.1182/blood-2008-12-192203

Dimitrov, D. H., Melnick, J. L., and Hollinger, F. B. (1990). Microculture assay for isolation of human immunodeficiency virus type 1 and for titration of infected peripheral blood mononuclear cells. *J. Clin. Microbiol.* 28, 734–737.

Dunay, G. A., Solomatina, A., Kummer, S., Hufner, A., Bialek, J. K., Eberhard, J. M., et al. (2017). Assessment of the HIV-1 reservoir in CD4+ regulatory T cells by a droplet digital PCR based approach. *Virus Res.* 240, 107–111. doi: 10.1016/j.virusres.2017.07.008

Durand, C. M., Ghiaur, G., Siliciano, J. D., Rabi, S. A., Eisele, E. E., Salgado, M., et al. (2012). HIV-1 DNA is detected in bone marrow populations containing CD4+ T cells but is not found in purified CD34+ hematopoietic progenitor cells in most patients on antiretroviral therapy. *J. Infect. Dis.* 205, 1014–1018. doi: 10.1093/infdis/jir884

Einkauf, K. B., Lee, G. Q., Gao, C., Sharaf, R., Sun, X., Hua, S., et al. (2019). Intact HIV-1 proviruses accumulate at distinct chromosomal positions during prolonged antiretroviral therapy. *J. Clin. Invest.* 129, 988–998. doi: 10.1172/JCI124291

Eisele, E., and Siliciano, R. F. (2012). Redefining the viral reservoirs that prevent HIV-1 eradication. *Immunity* 37, 377–388. doi: 10.1016/j.immuni.2012.08.010

Elsheikh, M. M., Tang, Y., Li, D., and Jiang, G. (2019). Deep latency: a new insight into a functional HIV cure. *EBioMedicine* 45, 624–629. doi: 10.1016/j.ebiom.2019.06.020

Eriksson, S., Graf, E. H., Dahl, V., Strain, M. C., Yukl, S. A., Lysenko, E. S., et al. (2013). Comparative analysis of measures of viral reservoirs in HIV-1 eradication studies. *PLoS Pathog.* 9:e1003174. doi: 10.1371/journal.ppat.1003174

Estes, J. D., Kityo, C., Ssali, F., Swainson, L., Makamdop, K. N., Del Prete, G. Q., et al. (2017). Defining total-body AIDS-virus burden with implications for curative strategies. *Nat. Med.* 23, 1271–1276. doi: 10.1038/nm.4411

Finzi, D., Blankson, J., Siliciano, J. D., Margolick, J. B., Chadwick, K., Pierson, T., et al. (1999). Latent infection of CD4+ T cells provides a mechanism for lifelong persistence of HIV-1, even in patients on effective combination therapy. *Nat. Med.* 5, 512–517. doi: 10.1038/8394

Finzi, D., Hermankova, M., Pierson, T., Carruth, L. M., Buck, C., Chaisson, R. E., et al. (1997). Identification of a reservoir for HIV-1 in patients on highly active antiretroviral therapy. *Science* 278, 1295–1300. doi: 10.1126/science.278.5341.1295

Fischer, M., Wong, J. K., Russenberger, D., Joos, B., Opravil, M., Hirschel, B., et al. (2002). Residual cell-associated unspliced HIV-1 RNA in peripheral blood of patients on potent antiretroviral therapy represents intracellular transcripts. *Antivir. Ther.* 7, 91–103.

Fletcher, C. V., Staskus, K., Wietgrefe, S. W., Rothenberger, M., Reilly, C., Chipman, J. G., et al. (2014). Persistent HIV-1 replication is associated with lower antiretroviral drug concentrations in lymphatic tissues. *Proc. Natl. Acad. Sci. U.S.A.* 111, 2307–2312. doi: 10.1073/pnas.1318249111

Fun, A., Mok, H. P., Wills, M. R., and Lever, A. M. (2017). A highly reproducible quantitative viral outgrowth assay for the measurement of the replication-competent latent HIV-1 reservoir. *Sci. Rep.* 7:43231. doi: 10.1038/srep43231

Gaebler, C., Lorenzi, J. C. C., Oliveira, T. Y., Nogueira, L., Ramos, V., Lu, C. L., et al. (2019). Combination of quadruplex qPCR and next-generation sequencing for qualitative and quantitative analysis of the HIV-1 latent reservoir. *J. Exp. Med.* 216, 2253–2264. doi: 10.1084/jem.20190896

Gama, L., Abreu, C., Shirk, E. N., Queen, S. E., Beck, S. E., Metcalf Pate, K. A., et al. (2018). SIV latency in macrophages in the CNS. *Curr. Top. Microbiol. Immunol.* 417, 111–130. doi: 10.1007/82-2018-89

Ganor, Y., Real, F., Sennepin, A., Dutertre, C. A., Prevedel, L., Xu, L., et al. (2019). HIV-1 reservoirs in urethral macrophages of patients under suppressive antiretroviral therapy. *Nat. Microbiol.* 4, 633–644. doi: 10.1038/s41564-018-0335-z

Garrido, C., Clohosey, M. L., Whitworth, C. P., Hudgens, M., Margolis, D. M., and Soriano-Sarabia, N. (2018). Gammadelta T cells: an immunotherapeutic approach for HIV cure strategies. *JCI Insight* 3:e120121. doi: 10.1172/jci.insight.120121

GBD 2015 HIV Collaborators (2016). Estimates of global, regional, and national incidence, prevalence, and mortality of HIV, 1980-2015: the Global Burden of Disease Study 2015. *Lancet HIV* 3, e361–e387. doi: 10.1016/S2352-3018(16)30087-X

Gomez Perdiguero, E., Klapproth, K., Schulz, C., Busch, K., Azzoni, E., Crozet, L., et al. (2015). Tissue-resident macrophages originate from yolk-sac-derived erythro-myeloid progenitors. *Nature* 518, 547–551. doi: 10.1038/nature13989

Graf, E. H., and O'Doherty, U. (2013). Quantitation of integrated proviral DNA in viral reservoirs. *Curr. Opin. HIV AIDS* 8, 100–105. doi: 10.1097/COH.0b013e32835d8132

Graf, E. H., Pace, M. J., Peterson, B. A., Lynch, L. J., Chukwulebe, S. B., Mexas, A. M., et al. (2013). Gag-positive reservoir cells are susceptible to HIV-specific cytotoxic T lymphocyte mediated clearance in vitro and can be detected in vivo [corrected]. *PLoS One* 8:e71879. doi: 10.1371/journal.pone.0071879

Grau-Exposito, J., Serra-Peinado, C., Miguel, L., Navarro, J., Curran, A., Burgos, J., et al. (2017). A Novel Single-Cell FISH-Flow Assay Identifies Effector Memory CD4(+) T cells as a Major Niche for HIV-1 Transcription in HIV-Infected Patients. *MBio* 8:e876-17. doi: 10.1128/mBio.00876-17

Green, D. R., Droin, N., and Pinkoski, M. (2003). Activation-induced cell death in T cells. *Immunol. Rev.* 193, 70–81. doi: 10.1034/j.1600-065x.2003.00051.x

Hamlyn, E., Ewings, F. M., Porter, K., Cooper, D. A., Tambussi, G., Schechter, M., et al. (2012). Plasma HIV viral rebound following protocol-indicated cessation of ART commenced in primary and chronic HIV infection. *PLoS One* 7:e43754. doi: 10.1371/journal.pone.0043754

Hatano, H., Jain, V., Hunt, P. W., Lee, T. H., Sinclair, E., Do, T. D., et al. (2013). Cell-based measures of viral persistence are associated with immune activation and programmed cell death protein 1 (PD-1)-expressing CD4+ T cells. *J. Infect. Dis.* 208, 50–56. doi: 10.1093/infdis/jis630

Henrich, T. J., Deeks, S. G., and Pillai, S. K. (2017). Measuring the Size of the Latent Human Immunodeficiency Virus Reservoir: The Present and Future of Evaluating Eradication Strategies. *J. Infect. Dis.* 215(Suppl._3), S134–S141. doi: 10.1093/infdis/jiw648

Hiener, B., Horsburgh, B. A., Eden, J. S., Barton, K., Schlub, T. E., Lee, E., et al. (2017). Identification of Genetically Intact HIV-1 Proviruses in Specific CD4(+) T Cells from Effectively Treated Participants. *Cell Rep.* 21, 813–822. doi: 10.1016/j.celrep.2017.09.081

Ho, D. D., Moudgil, T., and Alam, M. (1989). Quantitation of human immunodeficiency virus type 1 in the blood of infected persons. *N. Engl. J. Med.* 321, 1621–1625. doi: 10.1056/nejm198912143212401

Ho, Y. C., Shan, L., Hosmane, N. N., Wang, J., Laskey, S. B., Rosenbloom, D. I., et al. (2013). Replication-competent noninduced proviruses in the latent reservoir increase barrier to HIV-1 cure. *Cell* 155, 540–551. doi: 10.1016/j.cell.2013.09.020

Honeycutt, J. B., Thayer, W. O., Baker, C. E., Ribeiro, R. M., Lada, S. M., Cao, Y., et al. (2017). HIV persistence in tissue macrophages of humanized myeloid-only mice during antiretroviral therapy. *Nat. Med.* 23, 638–643. doi: 10.1038/nm.4319

Hosmane, N. N., Kwon, K. J., Bruner, K. M., Capoferri, A. A., Beg, S., Rosenbloom, D. I., et al. (2017). Proliferation of latently infected CD4(+) T cells carrying replication-competent HIV-1: Potential role in latent reservoir dynamics. *J. Exp. Med.* 214, 959–972. doi: 10.1084/jem.20170193

Hunt, P. W., Lee, S. A., and Siedner, M. J. (2016). Immunologic biomarkers, morbidity, and mortality in treated HIV infection. *J. Infect. Dis.* 214(Suppl. 2), S44–S50. doi: 10.1093/infdis/jiw275

Imamichi, H., Dewar, R. L., Adelsberger, J. W., Rehm, C. A., O'Doherty, U., Paxinos, E. E., et al. (2016). Defective HIV-1 proviruses produce novel protein-coding RNA species in HIV-infected patients on combination antiretroviral therapy. *Proc. Natl. Acad. Sci. U.S.A.* 113, 8783–8788. doi: 10.1073/pnas.1609057113

Jabara, C. B., Jones, C. D., Roach, J., Anderson, J. A., and Swanstrom, R. (2011). Accurate sampling and deep sequencing of the HIV-1 protease gene using a Primer ID. *Proc. Natl. Acad. Sci. U.S.A.* 108, 20166–20171. doi: 10.1073/pnas.1110064108

Jackson, J. B., Coombs, R. W., Sannerud, K., Rhame, F. S., and Balfour, HH Jr (1988). Rapid and sensitive viral culture method for human immunodeficiency virus type 1. *J. Clin. Microbiol.* 26, 1416–1418.

Josefsson, L., Eriksson, S., Sinclair, E., Ho, T., Killian, M., Epling, L., et al. (2012). Hematopoietic precursor cells isolated from patients on long-term suppressive HIV therapy did not contain HIV-1 DNA. *J. Infect. Dis.* 206, 28–34. doi: 10.1093/infdis/jis301

Kearney, M. F., Wiegand, A., Shao, W., McManus, W. R., Bale, M. J., Luke, B., et al. (2017). Ongoing HIV Replication During ART Reconsidered. *Open Forum. Infect. Dis.* 4:ofx173. doi: 10.1093/ofid/ofx173

Kearney, M., Maldarelli, F., Shao, W., Margolick, J. B., Daar, E. S., Mellors, J. W., et al. (2009). Human immunodeficiency virus type 1 population genetics and adaptation in newly infected individuals. *J. Virol.* 83, 2715–2727. doi: 10.1128/JVI.01960-08

Kessing, C. F., Nixon, C. C., Li, C., Tsai, P., Takata, H., Mousseau, G., et al. (2017). In Vivo Suppression of HIV Rebound by Didehydro-Cortistatin A, a "Block-and-Lock" Strategy for HIV-1 Treatment. *Cell Rep.* 21, 600–611. doi: 10.1016/j.celrep.2017.09.080

Kiselinova, M., Pasternak, A. O., De Spiegelaere, W., Vogelaers, D., Berkhout, B., and Vandekerckhove, L. (2014). Comparison of droplet digital PCR and seminested real-time PCR for quantification of cell-associated HIV-1 RNA. *PLoS One* 9:e85999. doi: 10.1371/journal.pone.0085999

Ko, A., Kang, G., Hattler, J. B., Galadima, H. I., Zhang, J., Li, Q., et al. (2019). Macrophages but not astrocytes harbor HIV DNA in the brains of

HIV-1-infected aviremic individuals on suppressive antiretroviral therapy. *J. Neuroimmune Pharmacol.* 14, 110–119. doi: 10.1007/s11481-018-9809-2

Kulpa, D. A., and Chomont, N. (2015). HIV persistence in the setting of antiretroviral therapy: when, where and how does HIV hide? *J. Virus Erad.* 1, 59–66.

Kulpa, D. A., Talla, A., Brehm, J. H., Ribeiro, S. P., Yuan, S., Bebin-Blackwell, A. G., et al. (2019). Differentiation to an effector memory phenotype potentiates HIV-l latency reversal in CD4+ T cells. *J. Virol.* 93:e969-19. doi: 10.1128/JVI.00969-19

Laanani, M., Ghosn, J., Essat, A., Melard, A., Seng, R., Gousset, M., et al. (2015). Impact of the timing of initiation of antiretroviral therapy during primary HIV-1 infection on the decay of cell-associated HIV-DNA. *Clin. Infect. Dis.* 60, 1715–1721. doi: 10.1093/cid/civ171

Laird, G. M., Eisele, E. E., Rabi, S. A., Lai, J., Chioma, S., Blankson, J. N., et al. (2013). Rapid quantification of the latent reservoir for HIV-1 using a viral outgrowth assay. *PLoS Pathog.* 9:e1003398. doi: 10.1371/journal.ppat.1003398

Laird, G. M., Rosenbloom, D. I., Lai, J., Siliciano, R. F., and Siliciano, J. D. (2016). Measuring the Frequency of Latent HIV-1 in Resting CD4(+) T Cells Using a Limiting Dilution Coculture Assay. *Methods Mol. Biol.* 1354, 239–253. doi: 10.1007/978-1-4939-3046-3-16

Lee, E., Peter, B., Jeffery, M., Wei, S., Eli, B., Daniel, D., et al. (2019). Memory CD4 + T-Cells Expressing HLA-DR Contribute to HIV Persistence During Prolonged Antiretroviral Therapy. *Front. Microbiol.* 10:2214. doi: 10.3389/fmicb.2019.02214

Lee, G. Q., Orlova-Fink, N., Einkauf, K., Chowdhury, F. Z., Sun, X., Harrington, S., et al. (2017). Clonal expansion of genome-intact HIV-1 in functionally polarized Th1 CD4+ T cells. *J. Clin. Invest.* 127, 2689–2696. doi: 10.1172/JCI93289

Liszewski, M. K., Yu, J. J., and O'Doherty, U. (2009). Detecting HIV-1 integration by repetitive-sampling Alu-gag PCR. *Methods* 47, 254–260. doi: 10.1016/j.ymeth.2009.01.002

Lorenzo-Redondo, R., Fryer, H. R., Bedford, T., Kim, E. Y., Archer, J., Pond, S. L. K., et al. (2016). Persistent HIV-1 replication maintains the tissue reservoir during therapy. *Nature* 530, 51–56. doi: 10.1038/nature16933

Maldarelli, F. (2015). HIV-infected cells are frequently clonally expanded after prolonged antiretroviral therapy: implications for HIV persistence. *J. Virus Erad.* 1, 237–244.

Maldarelli, F., Wu, X., Su, L., Simonetti, F. R., Shao, W., Hill, S., et al. (2014). HIV latency. Specific HIV integration sites are linked to clonal expansion and persistence of infected cells. *Science* 345, 179–183. doi: 10.1126/science.1254194

Malnati, M. S., Scarlatti, G., Gatto, F., Salvatori, F., Cassina, G., Rutigliano, T., et al. (2008). A universal real-time PCR assay for the quantification of group-M HIV-1 proviral load. *Nat. Protoc.* 3, 1240–1248. doi: 10.1038/nprot.2008.108

Margolis, D. M., Garcia, J. V., Hazuda, D. J., and Haynes, B. F. (2016). Latency reversal and viral clearance to cure HIV-1. *Science* 353:aaf6517. doi: 10.1126/science.aaf6517

Marrack, P., Scott-Browne, J., and MacLeod, M. K. (2010). Terminating the immune response. *Immunol. Rev.* 236, 5–10. doi: 10.1111/j.1600-065X.2010.00928.x

Martinez-Picado, J., and Deeks, S. G. (2016). Persistent HIV-1 replication during antiretroviral therapy. *Curr Opin HIV AIDS* 11, 417–423. doi: 10.1097/COH.0000000000000287

Martinez-Picado, J., Zurakowski, R., Buzon, M. J., and Stevenson, M. (2018). Episomal HIV-1 DNA and its relationship to other markers of HIV-1 persistence. *Retrovirology* 15:15. doi: 10.1186/s12977-018-0398-1

Martrus, G., Niehrs, A., Cornelis, R., Rechtien, A., Garcia-Beltran, W., Lutgehetmann, M., et al. (2016). Kinetics of HIV-1 Latency Reversal Quantified on the Single-Cell Level Using a Novel Flow-Based Technique. *J. Virol.* 90, 9018–9028. doi: 10.1128/JVI.01448-16

Massanella, M., Bakeman, W., Sithinamsuwan, P., Fletcher, J. L. K., Chomchey, N., Tipsuk, S., et al. (2019). Infrequent HIV infection of circulating monocytes during antiretroviral therapy. *J. Virol.* 9:JVI.1174-19. doi: 10.1128/JVI.01174-19

Massanella, M., Yek, C., Lada, S. M., Nakazawa, M., Shefa, N., Huang, K., et al. (2018). Improved assays to measure and characterize the inducible HIV reservoir. *EBioMedicine* 36, 113–121. doi: 10.1016/j.ebiom.2018.09.036

McKinstry, K. K., Strutt, T. M., and Swain, S. L. (2010). Regulation of CD4+ T-cell contraction during pathogen challenge. *Immunol. Rev.* 236, 110–124. doi: 10.1111/j.1600-065X.2010.00921.x

Metcalf Pate, K. A., and Blankson, J. N. (2017). The mouse viral outgrowth assay: avatars for the detection of HIV-1 reservoirs. *Retrovirology* 14:52. doi: 10.1186/s12977-017-0376-z

Metcalf Pate, K. A., Pohlmeyer, C. W., Walker-Sperling, V. E., Foote, J. B., Najarro, K. M., Cryer, C. G., et al. (2015). A murine viral outgrowth assay to detect residual HIV type 1 in patients with undetectable viral loads. *J. Infect. Dis.* 212, 1387–1396. doi: 10.1093/infdis/jiv230

Miller, R. L., Ponte, R., Jones, B. R., Kinloch, N. N., Omondi, F. H., Jenabian, M. A., et al. (2019). HIV diversity and genetic compartmentalization in blood and testes during suppressive antiretroviral therapy. *J. Virol.* 93:e755-19. doi: 10.1128/JVI.00755-19

Mok, H. P., Norton, N. J., Hirst, J. C., Fun, A., Bandara, M., Wills, M. R., et al. (2018). No evidence of ongoing evolution in replication competent latent HIV-1 in a patient followed up for two years. *Sci. Rep.* 8:2639. doi: 10.1038/s41598-018-20682-w

O'Doherty, U., Swiggard, W. J., Jeyakumar, D., McGain, D., and Malim, M. H. (2002). A sensitive, quantitative assay for human immunodeficiency virus type 1 integration. *J. Virol.* 76, 10942–10950. doi: 10.1128/jvi.76.21.10942-10950.2002

Pallikkuth, S., Sharkey, M., Babic, D. Z., Gupta, S., Stone, G. W., Fischl, M. A., et al. (2015). Peripheral T Follicular Helper Cells Are the Major HIV Reservoir within Central Memory CD4 T Cells in Peripheral Blood from Chronically HIV-Infected Individuals on Combination Antiretroviral Therapy. *J. Virol.* 90, 2718–2728. doi: 10.1128/JVI.02883-15

Pardons, M., Baxter, A. E., Massanella, M., Pagliuzza, A., Fromentin, R., Dufour, C., et al. (2019). Single-cell characterization and quantification of translation-competent viral reservoirs in treated and untreated HIV infection. *PLoS Pathog.* 15:e1007619. doi: 10.1371/journal.ppat.1007619

Passaes, C. P. B., Bruel, T., Decalf, J., David, A., Angin, M., Monceaux, V., et al. (2017). Ultrasensitive HIV-1 p24 Assay Detects Single Infected Cells and Differences in Reservoir Induction by Latency Reversal Agents. *J. Virol.* 91:e2296-16. doi: 10.1128/jvi.02296-16

Pasternak, A. O., and Berkhout, B. (2018). What do we measure when we measure cell-associated HIV RNA. *Retrovirology* 15:13. doi: 10.1186/s12977-018-0397-2

Pasternak, A. O., Lukashov, V. V., and Berkhout, B. (2013). Cell-associated HIV RNA: a dynamic biomarker of viral persistence. *Retrovirology* 10:41. doi: 10.1186/1742-4690-10-41

Patro, L. D. B., Bale, M. J., Halvas, E. K., Sobolewski, M., Hasson, J., Niyongabo, A., et al. (2019). "A method to determine both the integration sites and sequences of HIV-1 proviruses," in *Proceeding of the Conference on Retroviruses and Opportunistic Infections (CROI)*, Boston, MA.

Phillips, R. E., Rowland-Jones, S., Nixon, D. F., Gotch, F. M., Edwards, J. P., Ogunlesi, A. O., et al. (1991). Human immunodeficiency virus genetic variation that can escape cytotoxic T cell recognition. *Nature* 354, 453–459. doi: 10.1038/354453a0

Pollack, R. A., Jones, R. B., Pertea, M., Bruner, K. M., Martin, A. R., Thomas, A. S., et al. (2017). Defective HIV-1 Proviruses Are Expressed and Can Be Recognized by Cytotoxic T Lymphocytes, which Shape the Proviral Landscape. *Cell Host Microbe* 21, 494–506. doi: 10.1016/j.chom.2017.03.008

Porichis, F., Hart, M. G., Griesbeck, M., Everett, H. L., Hassan, M., Baxter, A. E., et al. (2014). High-throughput detection of miRNAs and gene-specific mRNA at the single-cell level by flow cytometry. *Nat. Commun.* 5:5641. doi: 10.1038/ncomms6641

Procopio, F. A., Fromentin, R., Kulpa, D. A., Brehm, J. H., Bebin, A. G., Strain, M. C., et al. (2015). A Novel Assay to Measure the Magnitude of the Inducible Viral Reservoir in HIV-infected Individuals. *EBioMedicine* 2, 874–883. doi: 10.1016/j.ebiom.2015.06.019

Puray-Chavez, M., Tedbury, P. R., Huber, A. D., Ukah, O. B., Yapo, V., Liu, D., et al. (2017). Multiplex single-cell visualization of nucleic acids and protein during HIV infection. *Nat. Commun.* 8:1882. doi: 10.1038/s41467-017-01693-z

Rosenbloom, D. I. S., Bacchetti, P., Stone, M., Deng, X., Bosch, R. J., Richman, D. D., et al. (2019). Assessing intra-lab precision and inter-lab repeatability of outgrowth assays of HIV-1 latent reservoir size. *PLoS Comput. Biol.* 15:e1006849. doi: 10.1371/journal.pcbi.1006849

Roszer, T. (2018). Understanding the Biology of Self-Renewing Macrophages. *Cells* 7:103. doi: 10.3390/cells7080103

Rueda, S., Mitra, S., Chen, S., Gogolishvili, D., Globerman, J., Chambers, L., et al. (2016). Examining the associations between HIV-related stigma and health outcomes in people living with HIV/AIDS: a series of meta-analyses. *BMJ Open* 6:e011453. doi: 10.1136/bmjopen-2016-011453

Rutsaert, S., Bosman, K., Trypsteen, W., Nijhuis, M., and Vandekerckhove, L. (2018). Digital PCR as a tool to measure HIV persistence. *Retrovirology* 15:16. doi: 10.1186/s12977-018-0399-0

Sahu, G. K., Paar, D., Frost, S. D., Smith, M. M., Weaver, S., and Cloyd, M. W. (2009). Low-level plasma HIVs in patients on prolonged suppressive highly active antiretroviral therapy are produced mostly by cells other than CD4 T-cells. *J. Med. Virol.* 81, 9–15. doi: 10.1002/jmv.21366

Sanyal, A., Mailliard, R. B., Rinaldo, C. R., Ratner, D., Ding, M., Chen, Y., et al. (2017). Novel assay reveals a large, inducible, replication-competent HIV-1 reservoir in resting CD4(+) T cells. *Nat. Med.* 23, 885–889. doi: 10.1038/nm.4347

Sanyal, A., McGowan, I., Somsouk, M., Rinaldo, C., Sluis-Cremer, N., and Gupta, P. (2018). "Quantification Of replication competent latent Hiv-1 in galt and semen," in *Proceeding of the 25th Conference on Retroviruses and Opportunistic Infections (CROI)*, Boston, MA.

Schacker, T., Little, S., Connick, E., Gebhard-Mitchell, K., Zhang, Z. Q., Krieger, J., et al. (2000). Rapid accumulation of human immunodeficiency virus (HIV) in lymphatic tissue reservoirs during acute and early HIV infection: implications for timing of antiretroviral therapy. *J. Infect. Dis.* 181, 354–357. doi: 10.1086/315178

Sebastian, N. T., Zaikos, T. D., Terry, V., Taschuk, F., McNamara, L. A., Onafuwa-Nuga, A., et al. (2017). CD4 is expressed on a heterogeneous subset of hematopoietic progenitors, which persistently harbor CXCR4 and CCR5-tropic HIV proviral genomes in vivo. *PLoS Pathog.* 13:e1006509. doi: 10.1371/journal.ppat.1006509

Shan, L., Rabi, S. A., Laird, G. M., Eisele, E. E., Zhang, H., Margolick, J. B., et al. (2013). A novel PCR assay for quantification of HIV-1 RNA. *J. Virol.* 87, 6521–6525. doi: 10.1128/JVI.00006-13

Shen, L., and Siliciano, R. F. (2008). Viral reservoirs, residual viremia, and the potential of highly active antiretroviral therapy to eradicate HIV infection. *J. Allergy Clin. Immunol.* 122, 22–28. doi: 10.1016/j.jaci.2008.05.033

Siliciano, J. D., and Siliciano, R. F. (2005). Enhanced culture assay for detection and quantitation of latently infected, resting CD4+ T-cells carrying replication-competent virus in HIV-1-infected individuals. *Methods Mol. Biol.* 304, 3–15.

Siliciano, J. D., Kajdas, J., Finzi, D., Quinn, T. C., Chadwick, K., Margolick, J. B., et al. (2003). Long-term follow-up studies confirm the stability of the latent reservoir for HIV-1 in resting CD4+ T cells. *Nat. Med.* 9, 727–728. doi: 10.1038/nm880

Simonetta, F., and Bourgeois, C. (2013). CD4+FOXP3+ Regulatory T-Cell Subsets in Human Immunodeficiency Virus Infection. *Front. Immunol.* 4:215. doi: 10.3389/fimmu.2013.00215

Soriano-Sarabia, N., Archin, N. M., Bateson, R., Dahl, N. P., Crooks, A. M., Kuruc, J. D., et al. (2015). Peripheral Vgamma9Vdelta2 T Cells Are a Novel Reservoir of Latent HIV Infection. *PLoS Pathog* 11:e1005201. doi: 10.1371/journal.ppat.1005201

Soriano-Sarabia, N., Bateson, R. E., Dahl, N. P., Crooks, A. M., Kuruc, J. D., Margolis, D. M., et al. (2014). Quantitation of replication-competent HIV-1 in populations of resting CD4+ T cells. *J. Virol.* 88, 14070–14077. doi: 10.1128/JVI.01900-14

Spivak, A. M., Bosque, A., Balch, A. H., Smyth, D., Martins, L., and Planelles, V. (2015). Ex Vivo Bioactivity and HIV-1 Latency Reversal by Ingenol Dibenzoate and Panobinostat in Resting CD4(+) T Cells from Aviremic Patients. *Antimicrob. Agents Chemother.* 59, 5984–5991. doi: 10.1128/AAC.01077-15

Strain, M. C., Lada, S. M., Luong, T., Rought, S. E., Gianella, S., Terry, V. H., et al. (2013). Highly precise measurement of HIV DNA by droplet digital PCR. *PLoS One* 8:e55943. doi: 10.1371/journal.pone.0055943

Sun, H., Kim, D., Li, X., Kiselinova, M., Ouyang, Z., Vandekerckhove, L., et al. (2015). Th1/17 Polarization of CD4 T Cells Supports HIV-1 Persistence during Antiretroviral Therapy. *J. Virol.* 89, 11284–11293. doi: 10.1128/JVI.01595-15

Sundstrom, J. B., Ellis, J. E., Hair, G. A., Kirshenbaum, A. S., Metcalfe, D. D., Yi, H., et al. (2007). Human tissue mast cells are an inducible reservoir of persistent HIV infection. *Blood* 109, 5293–5300. doi: 10.1182/blood-2006-11-058438

Swain, S. L., Croft, M., Dubey, C., Haynes, L., Rogers, P., Zhang, X., et al. (1996). From naive to memory T cells. *Immunol. Rev.* 150, 143–167. doi: 10.1111/j.1600-065x.1996.tb00700.x

Tran, T. A., de Goer de Herve, M. G., Hendel-Chavez, H., Dembele, B., Le Nevot, E., Abbed, K., et al. (2008). Resting regulatory CD4 T cells: a site of HIV persistence in patients on long-term effective antiretroviral therapy. *PLoS One* 3:e3305. doi: 10.1371/journal.pone.0003305

van Zyl, G., Bale, M. J., and Kearney, M. F. (2018). HIV evolution and diversity in ART-treated patients. *Retrovirology* 15:14. doi: 10.1186/s12977-018-0395-4

Wagner, T. A., McLaughlin, S., Garg, K., Cheung, C. Y., Larsen, B. B., Styrchak, S., et al. (2014). HIV latency. Proliferation of cells with HIV integrated into cancer genes contributes to persistent infection. *Science* 345, 570–573. doi: 10.1126/science.1256304

Wang, X. Q., and Palmer, S. (2018). Single-molecule techniques to quantify and genetically characterise persistent HIV. *Retrovirology* 15:3. doi: 10.1186/s12977-017-0386-x

Wang, Z., Gurule, E. E., Brennan, T. P., Gerold, J. M., Kwon, K. J., Hosmane, N. N., et al. (2018a). Expanded cellular clones carrying replication-competent HIV-1 persist, wax, and wane. *Proc. Natl. Acad. Sci. U.S.A.* 115, E2575–E2584. doi: 10.1073/pnas.1720665115

Wang, Z., Simonetti, F. R., Siliciano, R. F., and Laird, G. M. (2018b). Measuring replication competent HIV-1: advances and challenges in defining the latent reservoir. *Retrovirology* 15:21. doi: 10.1186/s12977-018-0404-7

Wei, X., Decker, J. M., Wang, S., Hui, H., Kappes, J. C., Wu, X., et al. (2003). Antibody neutralization and escape by HIV-1. *Nature* 422, 307–312. doi: 10.1038/nature01470

Westermann, J., and Pabst, R. (1992). Distribution of lymphocyte subsets and natural killer cells in the human body. *Clin. Investig.* 70, 539–544.

WHO (2019). *Global Health Observatory (GHO) data*. Available at: https://www.who.int/gho/hiv/en/ (accessed July 22, 2019).

Wiegand, A., Spindler, J., Hong, F. F., Shao, W., Cyktor, J. C., Cillo, A. R., et al. (2017). Single-cell analysis of HIV-1 transcriptional activity reveals expression of proviruses in expanded clones during ART. *Proc. Natl. Acad. Sci. U.S.A.* 114, E3659–E3668. doi: 10.1073/pnas.1617961114

Wonderlich, E. R., Subramanian, K., Cox, B., Wiegand, A., Lackman-Smith, C., Bale, M. J., et al. (2019). Effector memory differentiation increases detection of replication-competent HIV-l in resting CD4+ T cells from virally suppressed individuals. *PLoS Pathog.* 15:e1008074. doi: 10.1371/journal.ppat.1008074

Wong, J. K., and Yukl, S. A. (2016). Tissue reservoirs of HIV. *Curr. Opin. HIV AIDS* 11, 362–370. doi: 10.1097/COH.0000000000000293

Wong, J. K., Gunthard, H. F., Havlir, D. V., Zhang, Z. Q., Haase, A. T., Ignacio, C. C., et al. (1997a). Reduction of HIV-1 in blood and lymph nodes following potent antiretroviral therapy and the virologic correlates of treatment failure. *Proc. Natl. Acad. Sci. U.S.A.* 94, 12574–12579. doi: 10.1073/pnas.94.23.12574

Wong, J. K., Hezareh, M., Gunthard, H. F., Havlir, D. V., Ignacio, C. C., Spina, C. A., et al. (1997b). Recovery of replication-competent HIV despite prolonged suppression of plasma viremia. *Science* 278, 1291–1295. doi: 10.1126/science.278.5341.1291

Wong, M. E., Jaworowski, A., and Hearps, A. C. (2019). The HIV reservoir in monocytes and macrophages. *Front. Immunol.* 10:1435. doi: 10.3389/fimmu.2019.01435

Wu, G., Swanson, M., Talla, A., Graham, D., Strizki, J., Gorman, D., et al. (2017). HDAC inhibition induces HIV-1 protein and enables immune-based clearance following latency reversal. *JCI Insight* 2:92901. doi: 10.1172/jci.insight.92901

Yucha, R. W., Hobbs, K. S., Hanhauser, E., Hogan, L. E., Nieves, W., Ozen, M. O., et al. (2017). High-throughput Characterization of HIV-1 Reservoir Reactivation Using a Single-Cell-in-Droplet PCR Assay. *EBioMedicine* 20, 217–229. doi: 10.1016/j.ebiom.2017.05.006

Yukl, S. A., and Wong, J. K. (2015). "Anatomic compartments as a barrier to HIV cure," in *Encyclopedia of AIDS*, eds D. D. R. Thomas, and J. Hope, (New York, NY: Springer).

Yukl, S. A., Kaiser, P., Kim, P., Telwatte, S., Joshi, S. K., Vu, M., et al. (2018). HIV latency in isolated patient CD4(+) T cells may be due to blocks in HIV transcriptional elongation, completion, and splicing. *Sci. Transl. Med.* 10:eaa9927. doi: 10.1126/scitranslmed.aap9927

Yukl, S. A., Shergill, A. K., Ho, T., Killian, M., Girling, V., Epling, L., et al. (2013). The distribution of HIV DNA and RNA in cell subsets differs in gut and blood of HIV-positive patients on ART: implications for viral persistence. *J. Infect. Dis.* 208, 1212–1220. doi: 10.1093/infdis/jit308

Zaikos, T. D., Terry, V. H., Sebastian Kettinger, N. T., Lubow, J., Painter, M. M., Virgilio, M. C., et al. (2018). Hematopoietic Stem and Progenitor Cells Are a

Distinct HIV Reservoir that Contributes to Persistent Viremia in Suppressed Patients. *Cell Rep.* 25, 3759–3773. doi: 10.1016/j.celrep.2018.11.104

Zerbato, J. M., McMahon, D. K., Sobolewski, M. D., Mellors, J. W., and Sluis-Cremer, N. (2019). Naive CD4+ T Cells Harbor a Large Inducible Reservoir of Latent, Replication-Competent HIV-1. *Clin. Infect. Dis.* 69, 1919–1925. doi: 10.1093/cid/ciz108

Zhang, W., Svensson Akusjarvi, S., Sonnerborg, A., and Neogi, U. (2018). Characterization of Inducible Transcription and Translation-Competent HIV-1 Using the RNAscope ISH Technology at a Single-Cell Resolution. *Front. Microbiol.* 9:2358. doi: 10.3389/fmicb.2018.02358

Zhou, S., Bednar, M. M., Sturdevant, C. B., Hauser, B. M., and Swanstrom, R. (2016). Deep Sequencing of the HIV-1 env Gene Reveals Discrete X4 Lineages and Linkage Disequilibrium between X4 and R5 Viruses in the V1/V2 and V3 Variable Regions. *J. Virol.* 90, 7142–7158. doi: 10.1128/JVI.00441-16

Zhou, S., Jones, C., Mieczkowski, P., and Swanstrom, R. (2015). Primer ID Validates Template Sampling Depth and Greatly Reduces the Error Rate of Next-Generation Sequencing of HIV-1 Genomic RNA Populations. *J. Virol.* 89, 8540–8555. doi: 10.1128/JVI.00522-15

4

Does B Cell Follicle Exclusion of CD8+ T Cells Make Lymph Nodes Sanctuaries of HIV Replication?

Sarah E. Beck[1]*, Rebecca T. Veenhuis*[1] *and Joel N. Blankson*[1,2*]

[1] *Department of Molecular and Comparative Pathobiology, Johns Hopkins University School of Medicine, Baltimore, MD, United States,* [2] *Department of Medicine, Johns Hopkins University School of Medicine, Baltimore, MD, United States*

***Correspondence:**
Joel N. Blankson
jblanks@jhmi.edu

As we learn more about the HIV latent reservoir, we continue to discover that the viral reservoir is more complicated than just a pool of infected resting memory CD4+ T cells in peripheral blood. Evidence increasingly points to both certain tissues and certain types of cells as potential viral reservoirs. T follicular helper cells (T_{FH}) are prime targets of HIV infection—this creates a sanctuary for infected cells because CD8+ T cells generally do not enter lymph node follicles unless they express CXCR5, and are not as effective at killing infected CD4+ T cells as peripheral CD8+ T cells. In this review, we summarize the current state of research on T_{FH} cell infection in peripheral lymphoid tissues and focus on the question of whether CD8+ T cell exclusion from B cell follicles is responsible, at least in part, for establishing secondary lymphoid tissue B cell follicles as an anatomic site of HIV transcription and replication.

Keywords: CD8+ lymphocytes, HIV, lymph nodes, B cell follicle sanctuary, reservoir

INTRODUCTION

As we approach the 5th decade of the HIV pandemic and after years of intensive cure study, we continue to find a cure for HIV outside the reach of natural immunity due to the persistence of the latent reservoir found in resting memory CD4+ T cells. Retrovirus replication has several unique properties that have made eradication a challenge. Recent evidence suggests that the HIV reservoir is established in the very early stages of HIV infection (1, 2). As CD4+ T cells are the preferred target of HIV, a massive depletion of memory CD4+ T cells occurs in acute HIV infection but not all infected cells die (3–5). Because CD4+ T cells can transition to relatively transcriptionally inactive memory cells, HIV is able to "hide" from the immune system in these cells for long periods of time. In addition, because of a lack of ongoing viral replication, suppressive antiretroviral therapy (ART) does not effectively target latently infected CD4+ T cells and a study by Siliciano et al. estimated that it will take more than 73 years for an HIV-infected individual to clear the latent reservoir with ART alone (6).

Most studies of the latent reservoir have been done exclusively using peripheral blood mononuclear cells (PBMCs). This presents a problem for accurate estimation of the size of the reservoir as many lymphocytes in the body reside in the lymphatic system and tissues. Therefore, throughout the body there are likely other reservoirs and sanctuaries for HIV which may have different characteristics from the peripheral blood reservoir (7).

CD8+ T Cell Immunity Is Critical to Controlling HIV Infection

Studies in people living with HIV (PLWH) and *Simian immunodeficiency virus* (SIV)-infected primates support the hypothesis that CD8+ T cell immunity is critical to natural control of HIV infection. An early HIV-specific CD8+ T cell immune response is associated with increased viral control compared to patients that lack an early cytotoxic T lymphocyte (CTL) response (8, 9). SIV-infected macaques that are pharmacologically depleted of CD8+ T cells go on to develop higher viremia and more rapidly progressive disease compared to those SIV-infected macaques that are not CD8+ depleted, providing more evidence for the importance of CD8+ T cell-mediated HIV control (10–12).

A small subset of PLWH are able to control viral levels below the limit of detection in the absence of ART (13, 14). Elite Controllers (EC) are individuals that maintain a viral load below 50 copies of HIV-1 and extremely rare (<1% of the HIV infected human population). ECs have provided a great deal of insight as to the importance of CD8+ T cells in naturally controlling HIV disease progression (13). Certain human leukocyte antigen (HLA) alleles, such as HLA-B*57 and HLA-B*27 are significantly overrepresented in ECs (15, 16). Since T cell immunity is HLA allele restricted, this provides compelling evidence of the importance of CTL-mediated control of HIV replication. On a population scale, viral CTL escape mutations track along with expression of certain HLA alleles (17), demonstrating that HIV has developed a crucial mechanism of immune evasion via the development of CTL escape mutations. Additionally, multiple studies have also shown that the quality of CD8+ T cell response is associated with viral control in ECs (18–21).

Despite the importance of CD8+ CTL-mediated control of viral replication in ECs, CTLs alone are incapable of completely eliminating HIV and reservoirs of replication-competent virus are present in these subjects (22). Bailey et al. sequenced plasma virus and peripheral CD4+ T cell proviral DNA from HLA-B*57 ECs and found a striking discordance in sequences present in the HLA-B*57 restricted epitopes (23). Escape mutations were rare in CD4+ T cells but present in every single plasma virus sequenced. This suggested that CD8+ T cells were exerting strong selective pressure in these patients and that the plasma virions were not being produced from peripheral CD4+ T cells. This led to two question; how is HIV able to still replicate in the face of effective CTL immunity in these subjects? And where is this viral replication occurring? In this review, we hope to explore some answers to these questions as they will be important to understand if we are to develop CTL-mediated strategies to induce HIV remission in patients with progressive disease on ART.

Follicular Tissue as a Sanctuary Site for HIV Replication

As we learn more about the HIV latent reservoir, we continue to discover that the viral reservoir is more complicated than just infected resting memory CD4+ T cells in peripheral blood. Evidence increasingly points to both certain tissues and certain types of cells as potential sites of latent reservoir maintenance. There is evidence that multiple tissues, including the brain (24–26), spinal cord (27), and reproductive organs (28, 29) could be sanctuary sites for HIV, possibly because of their immune privileged status. Other tissues, such as the spleen, lung, and adipose tissue have also been suggested as sites of HIV persistence (30–32).

However, secondary lymphoid tissue is likely one of the largest potential sites for HIV replication and persistence throughout the course of infection (33–36).

Some studies suggest that HIV continues to replicate in lymphoid tissues in PLWH on fully-suppressive ART regimens, albeit at a lower level than untreated viremic individuals (36) and data suggestive of ongoing replication have also been seen in studies using ART-treated SIV-infected macaques (37, 38). However, other studies have not found evidence of ongoing viral replication in lymphoid tissue and have suggested that HIV is maintained by clonal expansion of infected CD4 T cells in LN tissues rather than ongoing viral replication (39). Regardless of the mechanism, it is clear that a potential reservoir exists in lymphoid tissue and the inability of the immune system to eliminate these infected cells needs further investigation.

While primary lymphoid tissue, the bone marrow and thymus, are considered the birthing sites for T and B cells, it is within secondary lymphoid tissues that activation and lineage maturation occur. Secondary lymphoid organs include the spleen, tonsils, and adenoids, bronchiolar-associated lymphoid tissue (BALT), gut-associated lymphoid tissue (GALT), and all lymph nodes. Secondary lymphoid tissues contain large numbers of CD4+ lymphocytes susceptible to infection, and recent studies continue to support the hypothesis that follicles within secondary lymphoid tissues represent a major site of viral persistence. Using inguinal lymph nodes collected from viremic HIV patients, Folkvord et al. showed that CD4+ T cells within follicles are 31 times more likely to be positive for HIV RNA than CD4+ T cells in extrafollicular sites (35). The same group later showed that CD4+ T cells within follicles are 40 times more likely to produce HIV RNA compared to extrafollicular tissues (40).

Over the last several decades, multiple studies in primates have also provided compelling evidence that lymphoid follicles are a focal point for SIV replication in chronic infection. By morphologic studies using *in situ* hybridization, there are consistently higher concentrations of SIV+ RNA in follicular than extrafollicular zones in multiple secondary lymphoid organs, including peripheral lymph nodes, the spleen, and GALT in multiple sites (41, 42). Early studies pointed to follicular dendritic cells (FDCs) as the major source of maintenance of HIV in B cell follicles of secondary lymphoid tissues (43, 44), and it certainly seems likely that these cells play a major role in infecting CD4+ T helper cells in secondary lymphoid tissue, contributing to CD4+ depletion and immunodeficiency (45). However, in the presence of undetectable viral loads, FDCs would not be capable of continuously infecting CD4 T cells, suggesting that the latent reservoir is mostly comprised of quiescently infected CD4+ helper T cells in lymphoid follicles. Therefore, it has been proposed that CD4 T cells can become infected outside of the lymph node prior to entering the follicle and subsequently differentiating into T_{FH}. Regardless, all mechanisms point to one central issue that remains: the immune system is not capable of acting on infected cells within the LN.

Follicular Helper T Cells in Secondary Lymphoid Tissue as a Viral Reservoir

How has HIV been able to "hide" in lymphoid tissues so effectively? Much of the answer likely lies with the follicular helper T cell subset (T_{FH} cells), located within germinal centers of secondary lymphoid tissues. A brief review of lymph node (LN) structure and function is provided in **Figure 1** to help illustrate how T_{FH} cells may contribute to the reservoir. LNs are secondary lymphoid tissues that are dispersed throughout the body along the lymphatic vasculature. Since they number in the hundreds, these are relatively easy sites of secondary lymphoid tissue to surgically biopsy, and so they are some of the most commonly studied secondary lymphoid tissue in HIV infection.

T_{FH} cells are a unique CD4+ T cell subset within secondary lymphoid tissues that interact with B cells at the T:B zone. They are characterized by high expression of the B cell follicle-homing chemokine receptor CXCR5, allowing T_{FH} cells to migrate to the site of T cell-mediated B cell activation in secondary lymphoid tissues (47–49). CD4+ CXCR5+ T_{FH} cells have also been found in the peripheral blood, although it is not yet clear if these cells are really the same population as the follicular T_{FH} cells or if they represent a completely different T_{FH} population, and there remains debate as to their significance is in respect to the latent reservoir (47, 51, 52). Recent evidence even suggests that a proportion of circulating T_{FH} cells originate in lymph nodes and subsequently traffic to the periphery via the lymphatics (53).

Using lymph nodes isolated from HIV viremic individuals, Perreau et al. previously showed that T_{FH} cells in lymph nodes are a potential sanctuary for viral replication within the CD4+ T cell compartment. By flow cytometry, follicular T_{FH} cells were identified as the largest subcategory of CD4+ T cells to be positive for HIV DNA, and *in vitro* these cells were more permissive to HIV infection than other CD4+ T cell subsets (54). These studies were in concordance with data collected from SIV-infected rhesus macaques (38, 42). Recent studies have found higher levels of inducible virus and cell-associated HIV-1 RNA in T_{FH} cells than in other memory cells in both viremic subjects and patients on long-term ART and concluded that there is ongoing viral transcription in these cells (55, 56). The mechanism for ongoing transcription was unclear but some studies have found reduced concentrations of antiretroviral drugs in lymph nodes cells in humans (57) and in NHPs (58). However, in contrast to these studies, a recent study found that the concentration of antiretroviral drugs in lymph nodes in humans and NHPs exceeded that found in plasma (59).

Studies utilizing both native and non-native SIV hosts have been instrumental in supporting that T_{FH} cell infection in germinal centers plays a major role in maintaining the viral reservoir. Native host species of SIV, such as the sooty mangaby, develop chronic viremia but do not develop immunosuppression and progression to AIDS (60, 61). Brenchley et al. demonstrated that untreated sooty mangabys and rhesus macaques (a non-native host for SIV) both have HIV-infected CD4+ T_{FH} cells within lymph nodes, but that rhesus macaques, as non-native hosts for SIV that develop progressive disease, have far more infected T_{FH} cells compared to the non-progressor sooty mangabys (42). This suggests that the level of CD4+ T_{FH} cell HIV infection is a critical difference between non-progressive, native SIV host species and progressive, non-native macaques, but the immunologic mechanism behind this difference is unclear.

Similar to human ECs, there are a small proportion of SIV-infected macaques that naturally control infection, and, like human ECs, certain MHC class I alleles are overexpressed in these animals (62, 63). Fukazawa et al. recently demonstrated that SIV infection was restricted to CD4 T_{FH} cells within the lymphoid follicle of SIV-infected EC macaques but not progressor macaques (38). They also showed that viral RNA in CD4+ T_{FH} cells was higher than non T_{FH} CD4+ memory cells in EC macaques (38), further supporting for the theory that T_{FH} cells within the lymphoid follicle represent a potential reservoir for HIV and SIV latency. Boritz et al. also found evidence of ongoing viral replication in lymphoid tissue in untreated PLWH who had low level viremia (64). Sequence analysis revealed that the reservoir in lymphoid tissue was distinct from the reservoir in peripheral CD4+ T cells suggesting that lymphoid tissue may be the source of the plasma escape mutants seen in ECs in prior studies (24).

CD8+ T Cell Exclusion From Follicles

Why does HIV continue to replicate in follicular T_{FH} cells even with robust and effective CD8+ T cell mediated viral control? It is likely that CD8+ T cells are, for a variety of possible reasons, unable to control HIV replication in T_{FH} cells, but the exact mechanisms of this CTL failure are still unclear. However, there are now several proposed mechanisms for why CD8+ T cells may be unable to effectively target HIV-infected follicular CD4+ cells. Lymphocytes in secondary lymphoid tissues are phenotypically and functionally distinct from their counterparts found in peripheral blood (65), and these different effector functions that may also extend to CD8+ T cell cytotoxicity. In fact, CTLs have been shown to have altered cytolytic activity in lymphoid tissue, potentially reducing their effectiveness in eliminating HIV-infected CD4 cells in follicles (66). Compared to their peripheral blood counterparts, CD8+ T cells within secondary lymphoid tissue have altered expression of cytolytic markers, including dysregulated and low expression of the granzyme B and perforin (66). However, this conclusion is somewhat controversial and other studies have suggested that these lymphoid CD8+ T cells are functional by cytolytic assays (40).

One hypothesis that could explain the lack of CD8+ T cell control of low level viral replication in germinal centers is the theory that B cell follicles represent immunologically privileged sites due the exclusion of CD8+ T cells. While one study showed that PLWH have more CD8+ T cells in lymph nodes than HIV negative subjects (67), multiple groups have shown that CD8+ T cells fail to accumulate at the site of infected

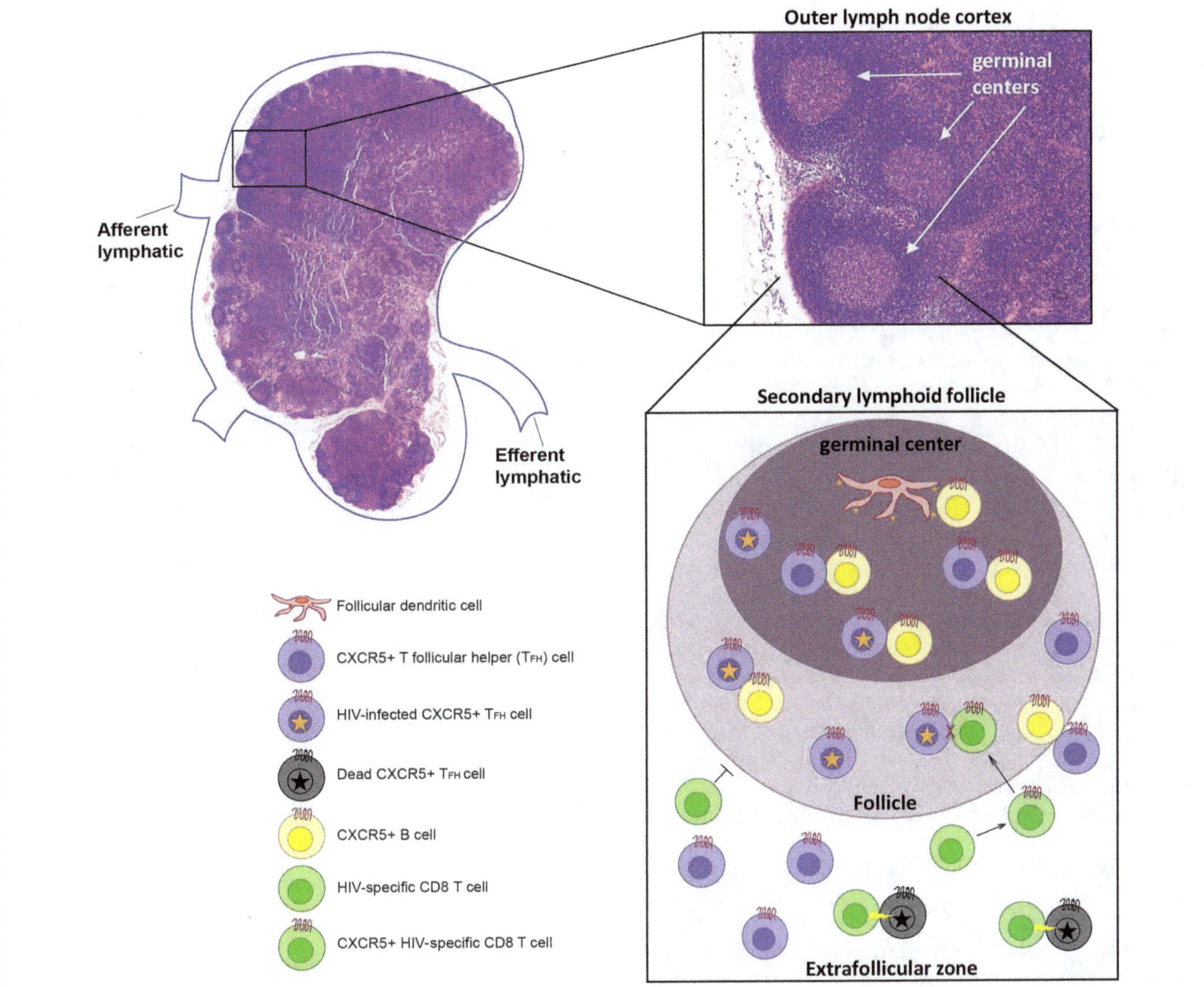

FIGURE 1 | Afferent lymph fluid enters at the cortex of the node, and efferent lymph fluid leaves at the hilus through lymphatic vessels. The lymph node (LN) itself consists of immune cells of both lymphocytic and myeloid lineage arranged on an interlacing lymphoreticular network that organizes these immune cells, promoting activation and clonal expansion (46). The LN cortex is divided into an outer cortex, containing primary and secondary lymphoid follicles, and an inner cortex. Primary follicles consist mostly of B cells and do not contain a germinal center, while secondary follicles, which form after immune activation, consist of a mantle of B cells surrounding a central germinal center consisting of centroblasts and follicular dendritic cells (FDCs). T follicular helper (T_{FH}) cells can be found in the extrafollicular zone (T cell zone) and B cell follicles. T_{FH} cells are a unique CD4+ T cell subset within secondary lymphoid tissues that interact with B cells at the T:B zone. They are characterized by high expression of the B cell follicle-homing chemokine receptor CXCR5, allowing T_{FH} cells to migrate to the site of T cell-mediated B cell activation in secondary lymphoid tissues (47–49). Follicular dendritic cells (FDC) can present infectious HIV virions for long periods of time which leads to the infection of T_{FH} within the germinal center (50). It is also possible that CD4 T cells are infected outside the follicle and differentiate into T_{FH} within the follicles. Infected T_{FH} cells are primarily located within B cell follicle and germinal centers because CTLs cannot enter these regions unless they express CXCR5. If CTLs do express CXCR5 they are able to enter the follicle but have been shown to be incapable of killing HIV infected T_{FH} cells. However, infected T_{FH} that leave the follicle can be killed by HIV-specific CTLs.

T_{FH} helper cells in chronic HIV infection and both acute and chronic SIV infection (38, 40, 68, 69). And it has been shown that the lack of the B cell follicle homing marker CXCR5 on many CD8+ T cells exclude these CTLs effectively from B cell follicles, preventing CTLs from effectively killing HIV-infected T_{FH} cells in follicles (38, 40). Early work assessing lymph node biopsies untreated PLWH suggested that CD8+ T cells failed to specifically localize adjacent to HIV-producing cells in lymphoid tissues (69). Using lymph node biopsies from HIV viremic patients, Connick et al. showed that, although there are a large number of HIV-specific tetramer positive CD8+ T cells in the lymph node, these cells were largely not present in lymphoid follicles where HIV is predominantly replicating in CD4+ cells (40). More recently, a study by Fukazawa et al. confirmed that not only is SIV infection is restricted largely to T_{FH} cells in GCs of SIV-infected rhesus macaque ECs, but the depletion of

CD8+ cells relocated HIV-production to non-T_{FH} cells within lymphoid tissue (38). Once CD8+ cells recovered, SIV-infection was once again restricted to T_{FH} cells within GCs of lymphoid tissue (38). These studies provide compelling support for the hypothesis that B cell follicles are indeed sanctuaries for HIV replication, and that this sanctuary is largely mediated by the inability of CD8+ T cells to effectively kill T_{FH} in sequestered in GCs.

Although the studies mentioned have shown CD8+ T cell exclusion in chronic infection, until recently, there was little work looking at follicular CD8+ T cell exclusion and killing of T_{FH} cells in acute infection. Using SIV-infected rhesus macaques, Li et al. has shown that CD8+ T cell exclusion from follicles appears to start as early as several weeks after infection (68).

CD8+ T Cell Functionality in Lymphoid Follicles

However, CD8+ T cell exclusion from B cell follicles may not be the only explanation for the maintenance of an HIV reservoir in lymphoid tissues, as there is conflicting data as to how much CD8+ T cell-exclusion from the B cell follicles actually occurs. Several studies have demonstrated a population of CXCR5 + CD8+ T cells within B cell follicles. These cells have been shown to have different transcriptional profiles from their CXR5-CD8+ T cell counterparts and their role in controlling viral replication has been the subject of many recent studies (70, 71). It has been shown that increased CXCR5+ effector CD8+ T cells in secondary lymphoid tissue is associated with increased control of chronic viral infections, including HIV (66, 72, 73).

Several groups have studied the functionality of follicular CXCR5+ CD8+ T cells in the context of lymphocytic choriomeningitis virus (LCMV) infected mice, a frequently used mouse model of chronic viral infection with some similarities to HIV infection (72, 73). These murine studies have shown that virus specific CXCR5+ CD8+ T cells become activated and migrate into B cell follicles and were able to control viral replication in chronic infection (72, 73). Similar findings have been shown in PLWH, where an inverse correlation was found between viral loads and the frequency of virus-specific CXCR5+ CD8+ T cells in the B cell follicle (72). Interestingly, in another study, there was no correlation between viral loads and granzyme B and perforin expression by CXCR5+ effector CD8+ T cells (66), raising some questions about the true killing capacity of follicular CXCR5+ CD8+ T cells. Clearly more research into this area is needed to answer the question of if follicular CD8+ T cells represent a distinct subset of CD8+ T cells that are less efficient at killing HIV-infected CD4+ T cells.

Targeting CD8+ T Cells to HIV-Infected CD4+ T Cells in the Lymphoid Follicle

How do we reconcile the need for CD8+ T cell immune responses within B cell follicles to target HIV-infected T_{FH} cells with the possible inability of these CD8+ T cells to either access or kill infected cells within B cell follicles? There are several groups that are working on strategies to specifically direct CD8+ T cells into follicles at the site of smoldering HIV infection of T_{FH} cells. One possibly strategy uses pharmacologic chemokines to direct CD8+ T cells into the B cell follicles. The cytokine IL-15 is important for maintenance of memory CD8+ T cells, so IL-15 agonists are an attractive pharmacologic target to boost CD8+ T cell-mediated HIV-1 immunity. Webb et al. showed recently that the IL-15 superagonist ALT-803 both activates and induces migration of CD8+ T cells into B cell follicles (74). ALT-803 treatment was effective in reducing the amount of SIV RNA and DNA in B cell follicles in ALT-803 treated EC macaques (74). Watson et al. used heterodimeric IL-15 in rhesus macaques to successfully increase CD8+ T cells within lymph node follicles and decrease HIV-1 viremia (75). Taking a different approach, Ayala et al. genetically engineered rhesus CD8+ T cells to overexpress CXCR5 which resulted in increased CD8+ T cell trafficking to rhesus B cell follicles (76). Conversely, Ferrando-Martiez et al. have employed anti-HIV/anti-CD3 biphasic antibodies to redirect follicular CD8+ T cells to kill HIV-infected CD4+ T cells *in vitro* (77), indicating that, at least with the help of biphasic antibody stimulation, follicular CD8+ T cells are capable of effective killing. Based on these studies, genetic engineering of CD8 T cells or treatment with immunotherapy compounds show promise as an avenue to specifically target LN sanctuaries and reduce long-term viral reservoirs in HIV-1 infected individuals.

However, it should be noted that, immunologically speaking, having follicular CD8+ T cells capable of killing within a lymphoid follicle could lead to the disruption of the follicle and the immune response itself. It seems that the existence of a mechanism to exclude activated CD8+ T cells or prevent killing within follicles may be necessary to maintain the integrity of the immune response, but further studies in this area are sorely needed.

DISCUSSION

Years of HIV and SIV latency research has revealed several important conclusions, first that lymphoid tissues represent a major site for HIV replication in viremic individuals and a significant reservoir of inducible virus in patients on ART. Secondly, CD4+ helper T cells are more likely to be productively infected within lymphoid follicles compared to extrafollicular sites. And finally, cytotoxic CD8+ T cells appear to be unable to effectively target these HIV infected cells when localized to a lymphoid follicle. The mechanisms behind the inability of CD8+ T cells to kill productively infected CD4+ cells in follicles are not completely understood. There is evidence that lymphoid CD8+ T cells have deficient cytolytic capabilities compared to CD8+ T cells in peripheral blood, other studies suggest that the CD8+ T cells are unable to target HIV infected CD4+ cells in follicles because of the lack of expression of appropriate chemokine homing receptors, therefore excluding the CD8+ T cells from trafficking to follicular sites of HIV replication. Regardless of the exact mechanism, ineffective CD8+ T cell killing of HIV-infected CD4+ helper T cells in secondary lymphoid tissue follicles is a major barrier to any strategy of HIV cure that relies on CTL-mediated eradication of infected CD4+ T cells. Further studies are needed to clarify the functionality of follicular CD8+ T cells in chronic HIV infection, to discover new ways of targeting CD8+ cells effectively to a major site of ongoing HIV replication as well as to determine if CTL killing within a follicle will alter the integrity of the immune response. Hopefully these future studies will enable scientists to effectively target and eliminate an important sanctuary of infected CD4+ T cells.

AUTHOR CONTRIBUTIONS

SB wrote the manuscript. RV and JB reviewed and edited the manuscript.

REFERENCES

Henrich TJ, Hatano H, Bacon O, Hogan LE, Rutishauser R, Hill A, et al. HIV- 1 persistence following extremely early initiation of antiretroviral therapy (ART) during acute HIV-1 infection: an observational study. *PLoS Med.* (2017) 14:e1002417. doi: 10.1371/journal.pmed.1002417

Ananworanich J, Chomont N, Eller LA, Kroon E, Tovanabutra S, Bose M, et al. HIV DNA set point is rapidly established in acute HIV infection and dramatically reduced by early ART. *EBioMed.* (2016) 11:68–72. doi: 10.1016/j.ebiom.2016.07.024

Schnittman SM, Lane HC, Greenhouse J, Justement JS, Baseler M, Fauci AS. Preferential infection of CD4+ memory T cells by human immunodeficiency virus type 1: evidence for a role in the selective T-cell functional defects observed in infected individuals. *Proc Natl Acad Sci USA.* (1990) 87:6058–62. doi: 10.1073/pnas.87.16.6058

Mattapallil JJ, Douek DC, Hill B, Nishimura Y, Martin M, Roederer M. Massive infection and loss of memory CD4+ T cells in multiple tissues during acute SIV infection. *Nature.* (2005) 434:1093–7. doi: 10.1038/nature03501

Brenchley JM, Schacker TW, Ruff LE, Price DA, Taylor JH, Beilman GJ, et al. CD4+ T cell depletion during all stages of HIV disease occurs predominantly in the gastrointestinal tract. *J Exp Med.* (2004) 200:749–59. doi: 10.1084/jem.20040874

Siliciano JD, Kajdas J, Finzi D, Quinn TC, Chadwick K, Margolick JB, et al. Long-term follow-up studies confirm the stability of the latent reservoir for HIV-1 in resting CD4+ T cells. *Nat Med.* (2003) 9:727–8. doi: 10.1038/nm880

Svicher V, Ceccherini-Silberstein F, Antinori A, Aquaro S, Perno CF. Understanding HIV compartments and reservoirs. *Curr HIV/AIDS Rep.* (2014) 11:186–94. doi: 10.1007/s11904-014-0207-y

Koup RA, Safrit JT, Cao Y, Andrews CA, McLeod G, Borkowsky W, et al. Temporal association of cellular immune responses with the initial control of viremia in primary human immunodeficiency virus type 1 syndrome. *J Virol.* (1994) 68:4650–5.

Borrow P, Lewicki H, Hahn BH, Shaw GM, Oldstone MB. Virus-specific CD8+ cytotoxic T-lymphocyte activity associated with control of viremia in primary human immunodeficiency virus type 1 infection. *J Virol.* (1994) 68:6103–10.

Jin X, Bauer DE, Tuttleton SE, Lewin S, Gettie A, Blanchard J, et al. Dramatic rise in plasma viremia after CD8(+) T cell depletion in *Simian immunodeficiency virus*-infected macaques. *J Exp Med.* (1999) 189:991–8. doi: 10.1084/jem.189.6.991

Matano T, Shibata R, Siemon C, Connors M, Lane HC, Martin MA. Administration of an anti-CD8 monoclonal antibody interferes with the clearance of chimeric simian/human immunodeficiency virus during primary infections of rhesus macaques. *J Virol.* (1998) 72:164–9.

Schmitz JE, Kuroda MJ, Santra S, Sasseville VG, Simon MA, Lifton MA, et al. Control of viremia in *Simian immunodeficiency virus* infection by CD8+ lymphocytes. *Science.* (1999) 283:857–60. doi: 10.1126/science.283.5403.857

Migueles SA, Connors M. Success and failure of the cellular immune response against HIV-1. *Nat Immunol.* (2015) 16:563–70. doi: 10.1038/ni.3161

O'Connell KA, Bailey JR, Blankson JN. Elucidating the elite: mechanisms of control in HIV-1 infection. *Trends Pharmacol Sci.* (2009) 30:631–7. doi: 10.1016/j.tips.2009.09.005

Migueles SA, Sabbaghian MS, Shupert WL, Bettinotti MP, Marincola FM, Martino L, et al. HLA B*5701 is highly associated with restriction of virus replication in a subgroup of HIV-infected long term nonprogressors. *Proc Natl Acad Sci USA.* (2000) 97:2709–14. doi: 10.1073/pnas.050567397

Pereyra F, Addo MM, Kaufmann DE, Liu Y, Miura T, Rathod A, et al. Genetic and immunologic heterogeneity among persons who control HIV infection in the absence of therapy. *J Infect Dis.* (2008) 197:563–71. doi: 10.1086/526786

Moore CB, John M, James IR, Christiansen FT, Witt CS, Mallal SA. Evidence of HIV-1 adaptation to HLA-restricted immune responses at a population level. *Science.* (2002) 296:1439–43. doi: 10.1126/science.1069660

Betts MR, Nason MC, West SM, De Rosa SC, Migueles SA, Abraham J, et al. HIV nonprogressors preferentially maintain highly functional HIV-specific CD8+ T cells. *Blood.* (2006) 107:4781–9. doi: 10.1182/blood-2005-12-4818

Migueles SA, Laborico AC, Shupert WL, Sabbaghian MS, Rabin R, Hallahan CW, et al. HIV-specific CD8+ T cell proliferation is coupled to perforin expression and is maintained in nonprogressors. *Nat Immunol.* (2002) 3:1061–8. doi: 10.1038/ni845

Migueles SA, Osborne CM, Royce C, Compton AA, Joshi RP, Weeks KA, et al. Lytic granule loading of CD8+ T cells is required for HIV-infected cell elimination associated with immune control. *Immunity.* (2008) 29:1009–21. doi: 10.1016/j.immuni.2008.10.010

Sáez-Cirión A, Lacabaratz C, Lambotte O, Versmisse P, Urrutia A, Boufassa F, et al. HIV controllers exhibit potent CD8 T cell capacity to suppress HIV infection *ex vivo* and peculiar cytotoxic T lymphocyte activation phenotype. *Proc Natl Acad Sci USA.* (2007) 104:6776–81. doi: 10.1073/pnas.0611244104

Blankson JN, Bailey JR, Thayil S, Yang HC, Lassen K, Lai J, et al. Isolation and characterization of replication-competent human immunodeficiency virus type 1 from a subset of elite suppressors. *J Virol.* (2007) 81:2508–18. doi: 10.1128/JVI.02165-06

Bailey JR, Williams TM, Siliciano RF, Blankson JN. Maintenance of viral suppression in HIV-1-infected HLA-B* 57+ elite suppressors despite CTL escape mutations. *J Exp Med.* (2006) 203:1357–69. doi: 10.1084/jem.20052319

Avalos CR, Abreu CM, Queen SE, Li M, Price S, Shirk EN, et al. Brain macrophages in *Simian immunodeficiency virus*-Infected, antiretroviral-suppressed macaques: a functional latent reservoir. *MBio.* (2017) 8:e01186-17. doi: 10.1128/mBio.01186-17

Chahroudi A, Wagner TA, Persaud D. CNS persistence of HIV-1 in children: the untapped reservoir. *Curr HIV/AIDS Rep.* (2018) 15:382–7. doi: 10.1007/s11904-018-0412-1

Abreu C, Shirk EN, Queen SE, Mankowski JL, Gama L, Clements JE. A quantitative approach to SIV functional latency in brain macrophages. *J Neuroimmune Pharmacol.* (2019) 14:23–32. doi: 10.1007/s11481-018-9803-8

Mangus LM, Dorsey JL, Laast VA, Hauer P, Queen SE, Adams RJ, et al. Neuroinflammation and virus replication in the spinal cord of *Simian immunodeficiency virus*-infected macaques. *J Neuropathol Exp Neurol.* (2015) 74:38–47. doi: 10.1097/NEN.0000000000000148

Fiscus SA, Cu-Uvin S, Eshete AT, Hughes MD, Bao Y, Hosseinipour M, et al. Changes in HIV-1 subtypes B and C genital tract RNA in women and men after initiation of antiretroviral therapy. *Clin Infect Dis.* (2013) 57:290–7. doi: 10.1093/cid/cit195

Jenabian MA, Costiniuk CT, Mehraj V, Ghazawi FM, Fromentin R, Brousseau J, et al. Immune tolerance properties of the testicular tissue as a viral sanctuary site in ART-treated HIV-infected adults. *AIDS.* (2016) 30:2777–86. doi:10.1097/QAD.0000000000001282

Couturier J, Lewis DE. HIV persistence in adipose tissue reservoirs. *Curr HIV/AIDS Rep.* (2018) 15:60–71. doi: 10.1007/s11904-018-0378-z

Nolan DJ, Rose R, Rodriguez PH, Salemi M, Singer EJ, Lamers SL, et al. The spleen is an HIV-1 sanctuary during combined antiretroviral therapy. *AIDS Res Hum Retroviruses.* (2018) 34:123–5. doi: 10.1089/aid.2017.0254

Nayak DK, Zhou F, Xu M, Huang J, Tsuji M, Hachem R, et al. Long- term persistence of donor alveolar macrophages in human lung transplant recipients that influences donor-specific immune responses. *Am J Transplant.* (2016) 16:2300–11. doi: 10.1111/ajt.13819

Haase AT, Henry K, Zupancic M, Sedgewick G, Faust RA, Melroe H, et al. Quantitative image analysis of HIV-1 infection in lymphoid tissue. *Science.* (1996) 274:985–9. doi: 10.1126/science.274.5289.985

Pantaleo G, Graziosi C, Butini L, Pizzo PA, Schnittman SM, Kotler DP, et al. Lymphoid organs function as major reservoirs for human immunodeficiency virus. *Proc Natl Acad Sci USA.* (1991) 88:9838–42. doi:10.1073/pnas.88.21.9838

Folkvord JM, Armon C, Connick E. Lymphoid follicles are sites of heightened human immunodeficiency virus type 1 (HIV-1) replication and reduced antiretroviral effector mechanisms. *AIDS Res Hum Retroviruses.* (2005) 21:363–70. doi: 10.1089/aid.2005.21.363

Lorenzo-Redondo R, Fryer HR, Bedford T, Kim EY, Archer J, Pond SLK, et al. Persistent HIV-1 replication maintains the tissue reservoir during therapy. *Nature.* (2016) 530:51–6. doi: 10.1038/nature16933

Deleage C, Wietgrefe SW, Del Prete G, Morcock DR, Hao XP, Piatak M, et al. Defining HIV and SIV reservoirs in lymphoid tissues. *Pathog Immun.* (2016) 1:68–106. doi: 10.20411/pai.v1i1.100

Fukazawa Y, Lum R, Okoye AA, Park H, Matsuda K, Bae JY, et al. B cell follicle sanctuary permits persistent productive *Simian immunodeficiency virus* infection in elite controllers. *Nat Med.* (2015) 21:132–9. doi: 10.1038/nm.3781

McManus WR, Bale MJ, Spindler J, Wiegand A, Musick A, Patro SC, et al. HIV-1 in lymph nodes is maintained by cellular proliferation during antiretroviral therapy. *J Clin Invest.* (2019) 130:126714. doi: 10.1172/JCI126714

Connick E, Mattila T, Folkvord JM, Schlichtemeier R, Meditz AL, Ray MG, et al. CTL fail to accumulate at sites of HIV-1 replication in lymphoid tissue. *J Immunol.* (2007) 178:6975–83. doi: 10.4049/jimmunol.178.11.6975

Connick E, Folkvord JM, Lind KT, Rakasz EG, Miles B, Wilson NA, et al. Compartmentalization of *Simian immunodeficiency virus* replication within secondary lymphoid tissues of rhesus macaques is linked to disease stage and inversely related to localization of virus-specific CTL. *J Immunol.* (2014) 193:5613–25. doi: 10.4049/jimmunol.1401161

Brenchley JM, Vinton C, Tabb B, Hao XP, Connick E, Paiardini M, et al. Differential infection patterns of CD4+ T cells and lymphoid tissue viral burden distinguish progressive and nonprogressive lentiviral infections. *Blood.* (2012) 120:4172–81. doi: 10.1182/blood-2012-06-437608

Spiegel H, Herbst H, Niedobitek G, Foss HD, Stein H. Follicular dendritic cells are a major reservoir for human immunodeficiency virus type 1 in lymphoid tissues facilitating infection of CD4+ T-helper cells. *Am J Pathol.* (1992) 140:15–22.

Tenner-Racz K, Racz P. Follicular dendritic cells initiate and maintain infection of the germinal centers by human immunodeficiency virus. *Curr Top Microbiol Immunol.* (1995) 201:141–59. doi: 10.1007/978-3-642-79603-6_9

Embretson J, Zupancic M, Ribas JL, Burke A, Racz P, Tenner-Racz K, et al. Massive covert infection of helper T lymphocytes and macrophages by HIV during the incubation period of AIDS. *Nature.* (1993) 362:359–62. doi:10.1038/362359a0

Brown FD, Turley SJ. Fibroblastic reticular cells: organization and regulation of the T lymphocyte life cycle. *J Immunol.* (2015) 194:1389–94. doi: 10.4049/jimmunol.1402520

Sánchez-Vargas LA, Mathew A. Peripheral follicular helper T cells in acute viral diseases: a perspective on dengue. *Future Virol.* (2019) 14:161–9. doi: 10.2217/fvl-2018-0197

Breitfeld D, Ohl L, Kremmer E, Ellwart J, Sallusto F, Lipp M, et al. Follicular B helper T cells express CXC chemokine receptor 5, localize to B cell follicles, and support immunoglobulin production. *J Exp Med.* (2000) 192:1545–52. doi: 10.1084/jem.192.11.1545

Lindqvist M, van Lunzen J, Soghoian DZ, Kuhl BD, Ranasinghe S, Kranias G, et al. Expansion of HIV-specific T follicular helper cells in chronic HIV infection. *J Clin Invest.* (2012) 122:3271–80. doi: 10.1172/JCI64314

Heesters BA, Myers RC, Carroll MC. Follicular dendritic cells: dynamic antigen libraries. *Nat Rev Immunol.* (2014) 14:495–504. doi: 10.1038/nri3689

Boswell KL, Paris R, Boritz E, Ambrozak D, Yamamoto T, Darko S, et al. Loss of circulating CD4 T cells with B cell helper function during chronic HIV infection. *PLoS Pathog.* (2014) 10:e1003853. doi:10.1371/journal.ppat.1003853

Claireaux M, Galperin M, Benati D, Nouël A, Mukhopadhyay M, Klingler J, et al. A high frequency of HIV-specific circulating follicular helper T cells is associated with preserved memory B cell responses in HIV controllers. *MBio.* (2018) 9:e00317–18. doi: 10.1128/mBio.00317-18

Vella LA, Buggert M, Manne S, Herati RS, Sayin I, Kuri-Cervantes L, et al. T follicular helper cells in human efferent lymph retain lymphoid characteristics. *J Clin Invest.* (2019) 129:3185–200. doi: 10.1172/JCI125628

Perreau M, Savoye AL, De Crignis E, Corpataux JM, Cubas R, Haddad EK, et al. Follicular helper T cells serve as the major CD4 T cell compartment for HIV-1 infection, replication, and production. *J Exp Med.* (2013) 210:143–56. doi: 10.1084/jem.20121932

Banga R, Procopio FA, Noto A, Pollakis G, Cavassini M, Ohmiti K, et al. PD-1(+) and follicular helper T cells are responsible for persistent HIV- 1 transcription in treated aviremic individuals. *Nat Med.* (2016) 22:754–61. doi: 10.1038/nm.4113

Noto A, Procopio FA, Banga R, Suffiotti M, Corpataux JM, Cavassini M, et al. CD32+ and PD-1+ lymph node CD4 T cells support persistent HIV- 1 transcription in treated aviremic individuals. *J Virol.* (2018) 92:e00901–18. doi: 10.1128/JVI.00901-18

Fletcher CV, Staskus K, Wietgrefe SW, Rothenberger M, Reilly C, Chipman JG, et al. Persistent HIV-1 replication is associated with lower antiretroviral drug concentrations in lymphatic tissues. *Proc Natl Acad Sci USA.* (2014) 111:2307–12. doi: 10.1073/pnas.1318249111

Estes JD, Kityo C, Ssali F, Swainson L, Makamdop KN, Del Prete GQ, et al. Defining total-body AIDS-virus burden with implications for curative strategies. *Nat Med.* (2017) 23:1271–6. doi: 10.1038/nm.4411

Burgunder E, Fallon JK, White N, Schauer AP, Sykes C, Remling-Mulder L, et al. Antiretroviral drug concentrations in lymph nodes: a cross-species comparison of the effect of drug transporter expression, viral infection, and sex in humanized mice, nonhuman primates, and humans. *J Pharmacol Exp Ther.* (2019) 370:360–8. doi: 10.1124/jpet.119.259150

Silvestri G, Sodora DL, Koup RA, Paiardini M, O'Neil SP, McClure HM, et al. Nonpathogenic SIV infection of sooty mangabeys is characterized by limited bystander immunopathology despite chronic high-level viremia. *Immunity.* (2003) 18:441–52. doi: 10.1016/S1074-7613(03)00060-8

Goldstein S, Brown CR, Ourmanov I, Pandrea I, Buckler-White A, Erb C, et al. Comparison of *Simian immunodeficiency virus* SIVagmVer replication and CD4+ T-cell dynamics in vervet and sabaeus African green monkeys. *J Virol.* (2006) 80:4868–77. doi: 10.1128/JVI.80.10.4868-4877.2006

Loffredo JT, Maxwell J, Qi Y, Glidden CE, Borchardt GJ, Soma T, et al. Mamu- B* 08-positive macaques control *Simian immunodeficiency virus* replication. *J Virol.* (2007) 81:8827–32. doi: 10.1128/JVI.00895-07

Mudd PA, Ericsen AJ, Burwitz BJ, Wilson NA, O'Connor DH, Hughes AL, et al. Escape from CD8(+) T cell responses in Mamu-B* 00801(+) macaques differentiates progressors from elite controllers. *J Immunol.* (2012) 188:3364– 70. doi: 10.4049/jimmunol.1102470

Boritz EA, Darko S, Swaszek L, Wolf G, Wells D, Wu X, et al. Multiple origins of virus persistence during natural control of HIV infection. *Cell.* (2016) 166:1004–15. doi: 10.1016/j.cell.2016.06.039

Kim CH, Rott LS, Clark-Lewis I, Campbell DJ, Wu L, Butcher EC. Subspecialization of CXCR5+ T cells: B helper activity is focused in a germinal center-localized subset of CXCR5+ T cells. *J Exp Med.* (2001) 193:1373–81. doi: 10.1084/jem.193.12.1373

Reuter MA, Del Rio Estrada PM, Buggert M, Petrovas C, Ferrando-Martinez S, Nguyen S, et al. HIV-specific CD8+ T cells exhibit reduced and differentially regulated cytolytic activity in lymphoid tissue. *Cell Rep.* (2017) 21:3458–70. doi: 10.1016/j.celrep.2017.11.075

Shen J, Luo X, Wu Q, Huang J, Xiao G, Wang L, et al. A subset of CXCR5+CD8+ T cells in the germinal centers from human tonsils and lymph nodes help B cells produce immunoglobulins. *Front Immunol.* (2018) 9:2287. doi: 10.3389/fimmu.2018.02287

Li S, Folkvord JM, Kovacs KJ, Wagstaff RK, Mwakalundwa G, Rendahl AK, et al. Low levels of SIV-specific CD8+ T cells in germinal centers characterizes acute SIV infection. *PLoS Pathog.* (2019) 15:e1007311. doi: 10.1371/journal.ppat.1007311

Folkvord JM, Anderson DM, Arya J, MaWhinney S, Connick E. Microanatomic relationships between CD8+ cells and HIV-1-producing cells in human lymphoid tissue *in vivo*. *J Acquir Immune Defic Syndr.* (2003) 32:469–76. doi: 10.1097/00126334-200304150-00001

Perdomo-Celis F, Taborda NA, Rugeles MT. Follicular CD8+ T cells: origin, function and importance during HIV infection. *Front Immunol.* (2017) 8:1241. doi: 10.3389/fimmu.2017.01241

Valentine KM, Hoyer KK. CXCR5+ CD8 T cells: protective or pathogenic? *Front Immunol.* (2019) 10:1322. doi: 10.3389/fimmu.2019.01322

He R, Hou S, Liu C, Zhang A, Bai Q, Han M, et al. Follicular CXCR5-expressing CD8(+) T cells curtail chronic viral infection. *Nature.* (2016) 537:412–28. doi: 10.1038/nature19317

Leong YA, Chen Y, Ong HS, Wu D, Man K, Deleage C, et al. CXCR5(+) follicular cytotoxic T cells control viral infection in B cell follicles. *Nat Immunol.* (2016) 17:1187–96. doi: 10.1038/ni.3543

Webb GM, Li S, Mwakalundwa G, Folkvord JM, Greene JM, Reed JS, et al. The human IL-15 superagonist ALT- 803 directs SIV-specific CD8+ T cells into B-cell follicles. *Blood Adv.* (2018) 2:76–84. doi: 10.1182/bloodadvances.20170 12971

Watson DC, Moysi E, Valentin A, Bergamaschi C, Devasundaram S, Fortis SP, et al. Treatment with native heterodimeric IL-15 increases cytotoxic lymphocytes and reduces SHIV RNA in lymph nodes. *PLoS Pathog.* (2018) 14:e1006902. doi: 10.1371/journal.ppat.1006902

Ayala VI, Deleage C, Trivett MT, Jain S, Coren LV, Breed MW, et al. CXCR5-Dependent entry of CD8 T cells into rhesus macaque B-cell follicles achieved through T-cell engineering. *J Virol.* (2017) 91:e02507–16. doi: 10.1128/JVI.02507-16

Petrovas C, Ferrando-Martinez S, Gerner MY, Casazza JP, Pegu A, Deleage C, et al. Follicular CD8 T cells accumulate in HIV infection and can kill infected cells *in vitro* via bispecific antibodies. *Sci Transl Med.* (2017) 9:eaag2285. doi: 10.1126/scitranslmed.aag2285

5

Impacts of HIV Cure Interventions on Viral Reservoirs in Tissues

Paul W. Denton[1]*, *Ole S. Søgaard*[2,3] *and Martin Tolstrup*[2,3]

[1] *Department of Biology, University of Nebraska Omaha, Omaha, NE, United States,* [2] *Institute of Clinical Medicine, Aarhus University, Aarhus, Denmark,* [3] *Department of Infectious Diseases, Aarhus University Hospital, Aarhus, Denmark*

***Correspondence:**
Paul W. Denton
pdenton@unomaha.edu

HIV reservoirs persist in infected individuals despite combination antiretroviral therapy and can be identified in secondary lymphoid tissues, in intestinal tissues, in the central nervous system as well as in blood. Clinical trials have begun to explore effects of small molecule interventions to perturb the latent viral infection, but only limited information is available regarding the impacts of HIV cure-related clinical interventions on viral reservoirs found in tissues. Of the 14 HIV cure-related clinical trials since 2012 that have evaluated the effects of small molecule interventions *in vivo*, four trials have examined the impacts of the interventions in peripheral blood as well as other tissues that harbor persistent HIV. The additional tissues examined include cerebral spinal fluid, intestines and lymph nodes. We provide a comparison contrast analyses of the data across anatomical compartments tested in these studies to reveal where peripheral blood analyses reflect outcomes in other tissues as well as where the data reveal differences between tissue outcomes. We also summarize the current knowledge on these topics and highlight key open questions that need to be addressed experimentally to move the HIV cure research field closer to the development of an intervention strategy capable of eliciting long-term antiretroviral free remission of HIV disease.

Keywords: HIV cure, viral persistence, latency, tissues, interventional clinical trials

INTRODUCTION

Despite years of successful combination antiretroviral therapy (cART), viral replication rebounds almost inevitably in all HIV infected individuals upon cART cessation (Deeks et al., 2016; Margolis et al., 2016; Wong and Yukl, 2016). This is due to the presence of persistent viral reservoirs which are the greatest barrier to an HIV cure. Because of the relative ease with which peripheral blood can be collected, this is the most common anatomical compartment analyzed in clinical HIV studies (Archin et al., 2012, 2014, 2017; Elliott et al., 2014, 2015; Rasmussen et al., 2014; Spivak et al., 2014; Mothe et al., 2015; Søgaard et al., 2015; Gutierrez et al., 2016; Leth et al., 2016; Vibholm et al., 2017, 2019a; Saxena et al., 2019; **Table 1**). However, it is known that HIV (and SIV in non-human primates) persists in multiple organ systems throughout the body during cART and that peripheral blood reservoir findings may not accurately reflect reservoirs in tissue (Costiniuk and Jenabian, 2014; Lamers et al., 2016; Rose et al., 2016, 2018; Estes et al., 2017; Nolan et al., 2018). Thus, it is essential that the impacts of curative strategies in all relevant organ systems be defined.

There are many unanswered questions regarding the impacts of HIV cure-related interventions on systemic HIV persistence. Among these are: Do findings in peripheral blood reflect outcomes in other tissues like the intestines and lymph nodes? and Do persistent viruses move freely between anatomical compartments? Studies have indicated that compartmentalization of HIV-infected cells into specific anatomical compartment and/or immunological sanctuaries occurs in untreated infections and that this compartmentalization persists during suppressive cART (Blackard, 2012). In addition, some of the drugs that have been tested in HIV cure trials may have reduced penetration into these compartments which may impede HIV cure efforts (Berg et al., 2004; Rasmussen et al., 2015). Therefore, we have focused this review on the impacts of HIV cure-related strategies onto clinical studies dosing small molecule interventions [e.g., histone deacetylase inhibitors, PKC agonist, disulfiram and *toll*-like receptor (TLR) agonists] and examining HIV persistence in tissues. Specifically, we review the impacts of such interventions on mechanisms that regulate HIV persistence *in vivo* as well as the immunological and virological impacts of these interventions in tissues other than peripheral blood. Other HIV cure related interventions including gene therapy approaches, stem cell transplants, antiretroviral intensification, therapeutic vaccines and broadly neutralizing antibody infusions have recently been reviewed elsewhere (Rasmussen and Sogaard, 2018; Caskey et al., 2019). Similarly, we callout several key animal model findings but do not elaborate upon animal model studies of HIV cure-related interventions as these data have also recently been reviewed elsewhere (Micci et al., 2015; Denton et al., 2016; Policicchio et al., 2016; Nixon et al., 2017; Honeycutt and Garcia, 2018; Whitney and Brad Jones, 2018).

EFFECTS OF HIV CURE INTERVENTIONS IN THE CENTRAL NERVOUS SYSTEM, INTESTINES, AND LYMPH NODES

We and others have made efforts to complement peripheral blood analyses by defining the effects of various HIV cure-related interventions on HIV persistence within key tissues. In these trials, the intervention were either suberoylanilide hydroxamic acid (SAHA), panobinostat or the TLR9 agonist MGN1703 (Elliott et al., 2014; Rasmussen et al., 2014; Vibholm et al., 2017, 2019a). In the trial exploring SAHA as a latency reversing agent (LRA), the Lewin group examined rectal tissue biopsies (Elliott et al., 2014). In our panobinostat trial, we examined cerebral spinal fluid and sigmoid biopsies (Christensen et al., 2015; Rasmussen et al., 2015). And in our MGN1703 trials, we examined sigmoid biopsies and lymph nodes (Krarup et al., 2017; Schleimann et al., 2019). All these anatomical reservoir studies were longitudinal in design as they included analyses of samples at baseline as well as near the end of the dosing period for the interventional drug in the respective study.

Human and animal study data highlight the potential for the central nervous system to function as an HIV reservoir or sanctuary site for the virus during treatment (Clements et al., 2005; Barber et al., 2006; Churchill et al., 2009; Zink et al., 2010; Queen et al., 2011; Gray et al., 2014; Honeycutt et al., 2017, 2018). Investigators have examined the toxicity and latency reversal effects of multiple agents including panobinostat and romidepsin on primary astrocytes *ex vivo* (Gray et al., 2016). These agents were found to be non-toxic and capable of inducing viral transcription at therapeutic concentrations. Our study provides the only published *in vivo* human data on central nervous system effects of a latency reversal agent to date (Rasmussen et al., 2015). We found that repeated, cyclic treatment with panobinostat did not lead to central nervous system adverse effects according to cerebral spinal fluid biomarkers of inflammation and neurodegeneration. We also found that panobinostat did not sufficiently penetrate the central nervous system to detectable levels and that there were no treatment-associated changes in HIV reservoir detection in the cerebral spinal fluid (Rasmussen et al., 2015). This study represents a single foray into determining the *in vivo* effects of HIV cure interventions in the cerebral spinal fluid for one intervention. However, this finding may not be specific for panobinostat since it has been shown in non-human primates that the concentration of another latency reversal agent romidepsin in cerebral spinal fluid is only approximately 2% of the level found in plasma (Berg et al., 2004). Given the scarcity of data, drawing conclusions about distinct HIV cure-related intervention impacts in the central nervous system is premature.

The role of intestines in HIV persistence has been researched extensively in humans as well as non-human primates (Anton et al., 2003; Guadalupe et al., 2003; Brenchley et al., 2004; Mehandru et al., 2004; Li et al., 2005; Mattapallil et al., 2005; van Marle et al., 2007; Chun et al., 2008; Ciccone et al., 2010; North et al., 2010; Yukl et al., 2010a,b; Chege et al., 2011; Lerner et al., 2011; Evering et al., 2012; Horiike et al., 2012; Kline et al., 2013; Deere et al., 2014; Estes et al., 2017). In a clinical study of 14 days of repeated administration of the histone deacetylase inhibitor SAHA, HIV RNA levels in rectal CD4 + T cells were modestly increased and HIV DNA levels were unchanged (Elliott et al., 2014). This outcome was also realized in our studies of the sigmoid colon during panobinostat as well as MGN1703 dosing given that we did not observe cohort wide changes in the size of the HIV reservoir in either study (Christensen et al., 2015; Krarup et al., 2017). While SAHA had no impact on T cell activation in rectal tissue, panobinostat dosing was associated with a decreased frequency of CD69+ intestinal T cells (Elliott et al., 2014; Christensen et al., 2015). This was in contrast to findings in peripheral blood where T cell activation (CD69+) was found to be increased following the first doses of panobinostat (Brinkmann et al., 2018). Additionally, we observed that panobinostat increased IL-17A expression in the intestinal epithelium and IL-17a is known to induce the production of antimicrobial peptides that may help to maintain the intestinal epithelial barrier which is damaged during HIV infection (Brenchley et al., 2006; Liang et al., 2006; Christensen et al., 2015). With dosing of the TLR9 agonist MGN1703, a robust interferon response was noted in the sigmoid colon (Krarup et al., 2017). This interferon response in the intestine was quite distinct from that observed in the

TABLE 1 | Overview of tissue analyses in clinical studies dosing small molecule interventions in HIV cure-related context.

Drug class	Drug	Trial identifier	Intervention	Tissues (other than peripheral blood) examined and analyses performed	Primary study citation	Sub-study citations
Histone deacetylase inhibitors	Vorinostat	NCT01319383	Single dose of vorinostat	No other tissues examined	Archin et al., 2012	Wu et al., 2017
			22 cyclical doses of vorinostat over 12–16 weeks	No other tissues examined	Archin et al., 2014	Wu et al., 2017; Garrido et al., 2019
			Up to 10 doses of vorinostat given at 72-h intervals	No other tissues examined	Archin et al., 2017	Wu et al., 2017
		NCT01365065	Daily vorinostat for 14 days	Rectal biopsies: CA US HIV RNA#; HIV DNA; T cell activation	Elliott et al., 2014	Mota et al., 2017
	Panobinostat	NCT01680094	Panobinostat dosed three times per week every other week for 8 weeks	Cerebral Spinal Fluid: HIV RNA; levels of biomarkers of neurodegeneration Sigmoid Biopsies: HIV DNA; T cell activation; T cell cytokine production; virus clonality	Rasmussen et al., 2014	Christensen et al., 2015; Hogh Kolbaek Kjaer et al., 2015; Olesen et al., 2015; Rasmussen et al., 2015; Barton et al., 2016; Lee et al., 2017; Wu et al., 2017; Brinkmann et al., 2018; Garrido et al., 2019
	Romidepsin	NCT02092116	3 romidepsin infusions once weekly for 3 weeks	No other tissues examined	Søgaard et al., 2015	Jorgensen et al., 2018
			6-Vacc4x$^{\Delta}$ immunizations followed by 3 romidepsin infusions	No other tissues examined	Leth et al., 2016	Tapia et al., 2017; Jorgensen et al., 2018
Aldehyde Dehydrogenase Inhibitor	Disulfiram	NCT01286259	Daily disulfiram for 14 days	No other tissues examined	Spivak et al., 2014	None indexed in PubMed
		NCT01944371	3-day course of disulfiram	No other tissues examined	Elliott et al., 2015	Lee et al., 2019
		NCT01571466	3 immunizations of MVA-B* $\pm$ 3 months once daily disulfiram	No other tissues examined	Mothe et al., 2015	None indexed in PubMed
PKC‡ Agonist	Bryostatin-1	NCT02269605	Single dose of bryostatin-1	No other tissues examined	Gutierrez et al., 2016	None Indexed in Pubmed
TLR3§ agonist	Poly-ICLC‡‡	NCT02071095	2 consecutive daily doses	No other tissues examined	Saxena et al., 2019	None indexed in PubMed
TLR9§§ Agonist	MGN1703	NCT02443935	Twice-weekly dosing for 4 weeks	Sigmoid Biopsies: HIV DNA; T cell activation; microbiome diversity; RNASeq, IHC† for interferon response	Vibholm et al., 2017	Krarup et al., 2017
			Twice-weekly dosing for 24 weeks	Inguinal Lymph Nodes: CA US HIV RNA#; HIV DNA; immune cell activation; B cell differentiation and maturation; antibody production, glycan status and HIV-specificity; RNASeq; IHC† for interferon response; IF†† for follicles; ISH††† for HIV RNA; virus clonality	Vibholm et al., 2019a	Schleimann et al., 2019; Vibholm et al., 2019b

*#CA US HIV RNA: Cell-associated unspliced HIV RNA; $^{\Delta}$Vacc-4x: a synthetic p24 gag peptide vaccine; *MVA-B: modified vaccinia Ankara-based HIV-1 vaccine; ‡PKC: Protein kinase C; ‡‡Poly-ICLC: Polyinosinic-polycytidylic acid, and poly-L-lysine; § TLR3: Toll-like receptor 3; §§ TLR9: Toll-like receptor 9; †IHC: Immunohistochemistry; ††IF: Immunofluorescence; †††ISH: In situ hybridization*

peripheral blood of the same individuals (Vibholm et al., 2017). Specifically, we observed that both type I and type II interferons were generated in the periphery of treated individuals but only a type I interferon response was detected in the sigmoid colon. The type I interferon response in the colon was associated with a trend toward improved intestinal microbiome species composition. Furthermore, we found that higher baseline levels of TLR9 expression in the intestine was associated with greater reductions in levels of integrated HIV DNA during MGN1703 treatment (Krarup et al., 2017). This result suggests that tissue-specific biomarkers may help determine which individuals will exhibit the strongest response to HIV cure-related interventions in future studies. Overall, these analyses examining the intestines of participants taking HIV cure-related interventions show that the intestines are an important anatomical site for study as the peripheral blood and intestines did not always exhibit similar responses to treatment in the examined parameters. Future studies will benefit from incorporating comprehensive intestinal biopsy analyses into the study plan.

The importance of lymphoid tissues, particularly lymph nodes, in HIV persistence is clear (Shen et al., 2003; Dinoso et al., 2009; Fukazawa et al., 2015; Banga et al., 2016; Deleage et al., 2016; Lorenzo-Redondo et al., 2016; Estes et al., 2017). Beyond the observation that lymph node tissues showed no changes in SIV reservoirs in non-human primates given SAHA (Del Prete et al., 2014), there has been no published data on the impacts of HIV cure-related interventions *in vivo* in lymph node tissues. To begin addressing this major knowledge gap in the field, we undertook a longitudinal study of inguinal lymph nodes in participants taking the TLR9 agonist MGN1703 for 24 weeks (Schleimann et al., 2019). We found that lymph nodes exhibited a potent interferon response to MGN1703 dosing as was observed in peripheral blood (Vibholm et al., 2019a). We also observed similarities between the lymph nodes and peripheral blood regarding significant changes in B cell differentiation and maturation levels in response to TLR9 agonist treatment. Related to these observations, we found that MGN1703 increased plasma IgG levels as well as increased AID expression in lymph nodes (Schleimann et al., 2019). Furthermore, after 24 weeks of MGN1703 dosing, plasma and lymph node IgG glycosylation patterns were significantly altered. Changes in glycosylation were associated with reductions in viral reservoir. This study revealing similarities between the peripheral blood and lymph node responses to MGN1703 is a beginning in the process of understanding the lymphoid tissue effects of HIV cure-related interventions.

NO EVIDENCE OF VIRAL COMPARTMENTALIZATION IN TLR9 AGONIST THERAPY TRIAL

While the direct *in vivo* impacts of HIV cure-related clinical interventions on latency controlling mechanisms have not been fully elucidated, there are multiple analyses that have focused on determining whether such interventions impact only clonal HIV isolates or reactivate a broad spectrum of persistent HIV isolates. These phylogenetic analyses performed with clinical trial samples have revealed that the histone deacetylase inhibitors SAHA, panobinostat and romidepsin reactivate latent viruses with unique sequence signatures as well as families of virus clones (Barton et al., 2016; Winckelmann et al., 2017, 2018). The panobinostat study also provided the first *in vivo* observation of a tissue-derived cell (i.e., a sigmoid colon lamina propria mononuclear cell) harboring an HIV provirus that matched plasma-derived rebound viruses isolated following analytical treatment interruption (Barton et al., 2016). Thus, these HIV cure-related interventions have broad latency reversing capacity *in vivo* in HIV infected individuals.

We recently examined the clonality of persistent virus in lymph nodes and compared these sequences to replication competent viruses that rebounded during an analytical treatment interruption (Vibholm et al., 2019b). We examined samples from our clinical trial in which participants received 24 weeks of repeated TLR9 agonist treatment. When we compared the latent viruses obtained from CD4+ T cells in peripheral blood and lymph nodes to viruses emerging during treatment interruption, we found there was no overlap between latent reservoir and rebound sequences. This was true even though 98% of intact or replication competent clonal sequences overlapped between these two anatomical compartments. Although rebound viruses were not derived from reservoirs detected in either blood or lymph node, we were able to show that rebound viruses were generated by recombination events between viruses within these two compartments (Vibholm et al., 2019b). This observation is consistent with peripheral blood data showing that recombination events are important during the emergence of rebound viremia (Lu et al., 2018). Whether the recombination events are due to improved viral fitness or escape of immune pressure is not yet known (Streeck et al., 2008; Ritchie et al., 2014). Overall, these data indicate that CD4+ T cells harboring latent HIV circulate between blood and lymphoid tissues during cART.

CONCLUSION

Understanding the regulation of HIV reservoir persistence is a high priority in the HIV cure research field. Since 2012, 14 HIV cure-related clinical trials have been published where the objective was to test the impacts of small molecule interventions designed to either cause infected cells to become visible to the immune system for clearance or to improve the ability of the immune system to clear infected cells. These clinical studies have yielded new insights into the effects of the interventions on the regulation of HIV persistence, particularly related to clonal populations of latently infected cells. In four of the trials, efforts were made to define the impacts of the respective intervention in the central nervous system, intestinal tissues and/or lymph nodes. Data from these four trials reveal key similarities between the peripheral blood and the organs. Furthermore, they highlight that observations made in peripheral blood are not always fully representative of the impacts made by interventions in the organs which also harbor persistent HIV reservoirs. Such differential responses highlight the importance of defining the impacts of curative strategies in all relevant organ systems including those reviewed herein as well as other applicable tissues such as spleen and bone marrow. With improved methods for analyzing tissue reservoirs, investigators will begin to overcome the limitations in studies that are due to the extreme rarity and heterogeneity of HIV infected cells *in vivo* in the setting of cART.

Advancement of the HIV cure research agenda will benefit from a continued push to seek detailed explorations of infected cells both derived from peripheral blood as well as from organ sources. Thus, there is strong impetus to continue examining multiple organs in such trials.

AUTHOR CONTRIBUTIONS

PD wrote the first draft the manuscript. OS and MT helped to wrote the manuscript. All authors read and approved the final manuscript.

REFERENCES

Anton, P. A., Mitsuyasu, R. T., Deeks, S. G., Scadden, D. T., Wagner, B., Huang, C., et al. (2003). Multiple measures of HIV burden in blood and tissue are correlated with each other but not with clinical parameters in aviremic subjects. *AIDS* 17, 53–63. doi: 10.1097/00002030-200301030-00008

Archin, N. M., Bateson, R., Tripathy, M. K., Crooks, A. M., Yang, K. H., Dahl, N. P., et al. (2014). HIV-1 expression within resting CD4+ T cells after multiple doses of vorinostat. *J. Infect. Dis.* 210, 728–735. doi: 10.1093/infdis/jiu155

Archin, N. M., Kirchherr, J. L., Sung, J. A., Clutton, G., Sholtis, K., Xu, Y., et al. (2017). Interval dosing with the HDAC inhibitor vorinostat effectively reverses HIV latency. *J. Clin. Invest.* 127, 3126–3135. doi: 10.1172/JCI92684

Archin, N. M., Liberty, A. L., Kashuba, A. D., Choudhary, S. K., Kuruc, J. D., Crooks, A. M., et al. (2012). Administration of vorinostat disrupts HIV-1 latency in patients on antiretroviral therapy. *Nature* 487, 482–485. doi: 10.1038/nature11286

Banga, R., Procopio, F. A., Noto, A., Pollakis, G., Cavassini, M., Ohmiti, K., et al. (2016). PD-1(+) and follicular helper T cells are responsible for persistent HIV-1 transcription in treated aviremic individuals. *Nat. Med.* 22, 754–761. doi: 10.1038/nm.4113

Barber, S. A., Gama, L., Dudaronek, J. M., Voelker, T., Tarwater, P. M., and Clements, J. E. (2006). Mechanism for the establishment of transcriptional HIV latency in the brain in a simian immunodeficiency virus-macaque model. *J. Infect. Dis.* 193, 963–970. doi: 10.1086/500983

Barton, K., Hiener, B., Winckelmann, A., Rasmussen, T. A., Shao, W., Byth, K., et al. (2016). Broad activation of latent HIV-1 in vivo. *Nat. Commun.* 7:12731. doi: 10.1038/ncomms12731

Berg, S. L., Stone, J., Xiao, J. J., Chan, K. K., Nuchtern, J., Dauser, R., et al. (2004). Plasma and cerebrospinal fluid pharmacokinetics of depsipeptide (FR901228) in nonhuman primates. *Cancer Chemother. Pharmacol.* 54, 85–88. doi: 10.1007/s00280-004-0766-5

Blackard, J. T. (2012). HIV compartmentalization: a review on a clinically important phenomenon. *Curr. HIV Res.* 10, 133–142. doi: 10.2174/157016212799937245

Brenchley, J. M., Price, D. A., Schacker, T. W., Asher, T. E., Silvestri, G., Rao, S., et al. (2006). Microbial translocation is a cause of systemic immune activation in chronic HIV infection. *Nat. Med.* 12, 1365–1371.

Brenchley, J. M., Schacker, T. W., Ruff, L. E., Price, D. A., Taylor, J. H., Beilman, G. J., et al. (2004). CD4+ T cell depletion during all stages of HIV disease occurs predominantly in the gastrointestinal tract. *J. Exp. Med.* 200, 749–759. doi: 10.1084/jem.20040874

Brinkmann, C. R., Hojen, J. F., Rasmussen, T. A., Kjaer, A. S., Olesen, R., Denton, P. W., et al. (2018). Treatment of HIV-infected individuals with the histone deacetylase inhibitor panobinostat results in increased numbers of regulatory t cells and limits ex vivo lipopolysaccharide-induced inflammatory responses. *mSphere* 3:e00616-17. doi: 10.1128/mSphere.00616-17

Caskey, M., Klein, F., and Nussenzweig, M. C. (2019). Broadly neutralizing anti-HIV-1 monoclonal antibodies in the clinic. *Nat. Med.* 25, 547–553. doi: 10.1038/s41591-019-0412-8

Chege, D., Sheth, P. M., Kain, T., Kim, C. J., Kovacs, C., Loutfy, M., et al. (2011). Sigmoid Th17 populations, the HIV latent reservoir, and microbial translocation in men on long-term antiretroviral therapy. *AIDS* 25, 741–749. doi: 10.1097/QAD.0b013e328344cefb

Christensen, A. B., Dige, A., Vad-Nielsen, J., Brinkmann, C. R., Bendix, M., Ostergaard, L., et al. (2015). Administration of panobinostat is associated with increased IL-17A mRNA in the intestinal epithelium of HIV-1 patients. *Mediators Inflamm.* 2015:120605. doi: 10.1155/2015/120605

Chun, T. W., Nickle, D. C., Justement, J. S., Meyers, J. H., Roby, G., Hallahan, C. W., et al. (2008). Persistence of HIV in gut-associated lymphoid tissue despite long-term antiretroviral therapy. *J. Infect. Dis.* 197, 714–720. doi: 10.1086/527324

Churchill, M. J., Wesselingh, S. L., Cowley, D., Pardo, C. A., Mcarthur, J. C., Brew, B. J., et al. (2009). Extensive astrocyte infection is prominent in human immunodeficiency virus-associated dementia. *Ann. Neurol.* 66, 253–258. doi: 10.1002/ana.21697

Ciccone, E. J., Read, S. W., Mannon, P. J., Yao, M. D., Hodge, J. N., Dewar, R., et al. (2010). Cycling of gut mucosal CD4+ T cells decreases after prolonged anti-retroviral therapy and is associated with plasma LPS levels. *Mucosal Immunol.* 3, 172–181. doi: 10.1038/mi.2009.129

Clements, J. E., Li, M., Gama, L., Bullock, B., Carruth, L. M., Mankowski, J. L., et al. (2005). The central nervous system is a viral reservoir in simian immunodeficiency virus–infected macaques on combined antiretroviral therapy: a model for human immunodeficiency virus patients on highly active antiretroviral therapy. *J. Neurovirol.* 11, 180–189. doi: 10.1080/13550280590922829

Costiniuk, C. T., and Jenabian, M. A. (2014). The lungs as anatomical reservoirs of HIV infection. *Rev. Med. Virol.* 24, 35–54. doi: 10.1002/rmv.1772

Deeks, S. G., Lewin, S. R., Ross, A. L., Ananworanich, J., Benkirane, M., Cannon, P., et al. (2016). International AIDS Society global scientific strategy: towards an HIV cure 2016. *Nat. Med.* 22, 839–850. doi: 10.1038/nm.4108

Deere, J. D., Kauffman, R. C., Cannavo, E., Higgins, J., Villalobos, A., Adamson, L., et al. (2014). Analysis of multiply spliced transcripts in lymphoid tissue reservoirs of rhesus macaques infected with RT-SHIV during HAART. *PLoS One* 9:e87914. doi: 10.1371/journal.pone.0087914

Del Prete, G. Q., Shoemaker, R., Oswald, K., Lara, A., Trubey, C. M., Fast, R., et al. (2014). Effect of suberoylanilide hydroxamic acid (SAHA) administration on the residual virus pool in a model of combination antiretroviral therapy-mediated suppression in SIVmac239-infected indian rhesus macaques. *Antimicrob. Agents Chemother.* 58, 6790–6806. doi: 10.1128/AAC.03746-14

Deleage, C., Wietgrefe, S. W., Del Prete, G., Morcock, D. R., Hao, X. P., Piatak, M., et al. (2016). Defining HIV and SIV reservoirs in lymphoid tissues. *Pathog. Immun.* 1, 68–106.

Denton, P. W., Sogaard, O. S., and Tolstrup, M. (2016). Using animal models to overcome temporal, spatial and combinatorial challenges in HIV persistence research. *J. Transl. Med.* 14:44. doi: 10.1186/s12967-016-0807-y

Dinoso, J. B., Rabi, S. A., Blankson, J. N., Gama, L., Mankowski, J. L., Siliciano, R. F., et al. (2009). A simian immunodeficiency virus-infected macaque model to study viral reservoirs that persist during highly active antiretroviral therapy. *J. Virol.* 83, 9247–9257. doi: 10.1128/JVI.00840-09

Elliott, J. H., Mcmahon, J. H., Chang, C. C., Lee, S. A., Hartogensis, W., Bumpus, N., et al. (2015). Short-term administration of disulfiram for reversal of latent HIV infection: a phase 2 dose-escalation study. *Lancet HIV* 2, e520–e529. doi: 10.1016/S2352-3018(15)00226-X

Elliott, J. H., Wightman, F., Solomon, A., Ghneim, K., Ahlers, J., Cameron, M. J., et al. (2014). Activation of HIV transcription with short-course vorinostat in HIV-infected patients on suppressive antiretroviral therapy. *PLoS Pathog.* 10:e1004473. doi: 10.1371/journal.ppat.1004473

Estes, J. D., Kityo, C., Ssali, F., Swainson, L., Makamdop, K. N., Del Prete, G. Q., et al. (2017). Defining total-body AIDS-virus burden with implications for curative strategies. *Nat. Med.* 23, 1271–1276. doi: 10.1038/nm.4411

Evering, T. H., Mehandru, S., Racz, P., Tenner-Racz, K., Poles, M. A., Figueroa, A., et al. (2012). Absence of HIV-1 evolution in the gut-associated lymphoid tissue from patients on combination antiviral therapy initiated during primary infection. *PLoS Pathog.* 8:e1002506. doi: 10.1371/journal.ppat.1002506

Fukazawa, Y., Lum, R., Okoye, A. A., Park, H., Matsuda, K., Bae, J. Y., et al. (2015). B cell follicle sanctuary permits persistent productive simian immunodeficiency virus infection in elite controllers. *Nat. Med.* 21, 132–139. doi: 10.1038/nm.3781

Garrido, C., Tolstrup, M., Sogaard, O. S., Rasmussen, T. A., Allard, B., Soriano-Sarabia, N., et al. (2019). In-vivo administration of histone deacetylase inhibitors does not impair natural killer cell function in HIV+ individuals. *AIDS* 33, 605–613. doi: 10.1097/qad.0000000000002112

Gray, L. R., On, H., Roberts, E., Lu, H. K., Moso, M. A., Raison, J. A., et al. (2016). Toxicity and in vitro activity of HIV-1 latency-reversing agents in primary CNS cells. *J. Neurovirol.* 22, 455–463. doi: 10.1007/s13365-015-0413-4

Gray, L. R., Roche, M., Flynn, J. K., Wesselingh, S. L., Gorry, P. R., and Churchill, M. J. (2014). Is the central nervous system a reservoir of HIV-1? *Curr. Opin. HIV AIDS* 9, 552–558. doi: 10.1097/COH.0000000000000108

Guadalupe, M., Reay, E., Sankaran, S., Prindiville, T., Flamm, J., Mcneil, A., et al. (2003). Severe CD4+ T-cell depletion in gut lymphoid tissue during primary human immunodeficiency virus type 1 infection and substantial delay in restoration following highly active antiretroviral therapy. *J. Virol.* 77, 11708–11717. doi: 10.1128/jvi.77.21.11708-11717.2003

Gutierrez, C., Serrano-Villar, S., Madrid-Elena, N., Perez-Elias, M. J., Martin, M. E., Barbas, C., et al. (2016). Bryostatin-1 for latent virus reactivation in HIV-infected patients on antiretroviral therapy. *AIDS* 30, 1385–1392. doi: 10.1097/QAD.0000000000001064

Hogh Kolbaek Kjaer, A. S., Brinkmann, C. R., Dinarello, C. A., Olesen, R., Ostergaard, L., Sogaard, O. S., et al. (2015). The histone deacetylase inhibitor panobinostat lowers biomarkers of cardiovascular risk and inflammation in HIV patients. *AIDS* 29, 1195–1200. doi: 10.1097/QAD.0000000000000678

Honeycutt, J. B., and Garcia, J. V. (2018). Humanized mice: models for evaluating NeuroHIV and cure strategies. *J. Neurovirol.* 24, 185–191. doi: 10.1007/s13365-017-0567-3

Honeycutt, J. B., Liao, B., Nixon, C. C., Cleary, R. A., Thayer, W. O., Birath, S. L., et al. (2018). T cells establish and maintain CNS viral infection in HIV-infected humanized mice. *J. Clin. Invest.* 128, 2862–2876. doi: 10.1172/JCI98968

Honeycutt, J. B., Thayer, W. O., Baker, C. E., Ribeiro, R. M., Lada, S. M., Cao, Y., et al. (2017). HIV persistence in tissue macrophages of humanized myeloid-only mice during antiretroviral therapy. *Nat. Med.* 23, 638–643. doi: 10.1038/nm.4319

Horiike, M., Iwami, S., Kodama, M., Sato, A., Watanabe, Y., Yasui, M., et al. (2012). Lymph nodes harbor viral reservoirs that cause rebound of plasma viremia in SIV-infected macaques upon cessation of combined antiretroviral therapy. *Virology* 423, 107–118. doi: 10.1016/j.virol.2011.11.024

Jorgensen, S., Leth, S., Sommerfelt, M., Ostergaard, L., Tolstrup, M., and Sogaard, O. S. (2018). Differences in antiretroviral regimens do not impact safety or level of latency reversal in persons receiving romidepsin. *AIDS* 32, 1729–1731. doi: 10.1097/qad.0000000000001904

Kline, C., Ndjomou, J., Franks, T., Kiser, R., Coalter, V., Smedley, J., et al. (2013). Persistence of viral reservoirs in multiple tissues after antiretroviral therapy suppression in a macaque RT-SHIV model. *PLoS One* 8:e84275. doi: 10.1371/journal.pone.0084275

Krarup, A. R., Abdel-Mohsen, M., Schleimann, M. H., Vibholm, L., Engen, P. A., Dige, A., et al. (2017). The TLR9 agonist MGN1703 triggers a potent type I interferon response in the sigmoid colon. *Mucosal Immunol.* 11, 449–461. doi: 10.1038/mi.2017.59

Lamers, S. L., Rose, R., Maidji, E., Agsalda-Garcia, M., Nolan, D. J., Fogel, G. B., et al. (2016). HIV DNA is frequently present within pathologic tissues evaluated at autopsy from combined antiretroviral therapy-treated patients with undetectable viral loads. *J. Virol.* 90, 8968–8983. doi: 10.1128/JVI.00674-16

Lee, S. A., Elliott, J. H., Mcmahon, J., Hartogenesis, W., Bumpus, N. N., Lifson, J. D., et al. (2019). Population pharmacokinetics and pharmacodynamics of disulfiram on inducing latent HIV-1 transcription in a phase IIb trial. *Clin. Pharmacol. Ther.* 105, 692–702. doi: 10.1002/cpt.1220

Lee, W. S., Kristensen, A. B., Rasmussen, T. A., Tolstrup, M., Ostergaard, L., Sogaard, O. S., et al. (2017). Anti-HIV-1 ADCC antibodies following latency reversal and treatment interruption. *J. Virol.* 91: e00603-17. doi: 10.1128/JVI.00603-17

Lerner, P., Guadalupe, M., Donovan, R., Hung, J., Flamm, J., Prindiville, T., et al. (2011). The gut mucosal viral reservoir in HIV-infected patients is not the major source of rebound plasma viremia following interruption of highly active antiretroviral therapy. *J. Virol.* 85, 4772–4782. doi: 10.1128/jvi.02409-10

Leth, S., Schleimann, M. H., Nissen, S. K., Hojen, J. F., Olesen, R., Graversen, M. E., et al. (2016). Combined effect of Vacc-4x, recombinant human granulocyte macrophage colony-stimulating factor vaccination, and romidepsin on the HIV-1 reservoir (REDUC): a single-arm, phase 1B/2A trial. *Lancet HIV* 3, e463–e472. doi: 10.1016/S2352-3018(16)30055-8

Li, Q., Duan, L., Estes, J. D., Ma, Z. M., Rourke, T., Wang, Y., et al. (2005). Peak SIV replication in resting memory CD4+ T cells depletes gut lamina propria CD4+ T cells. *Nature* 434, 1148–1152. doi: 10.1038/nature03513

Liang, S. C., Tan, X. Y., Luxenberg, D. P., Karim, R., Dunussi-Joannopoulos, K., Collins, M., et al. (2006). Interleukin (IL)-22 and IL-17 are coexpressed by Th17 cells and cooperatively enhance expression of antimicrobial peptides. *J. Exp. Med.* 203, 2271–2279. doi: 10.1084/jem.20061308

Lorenzo-Redondo, R., Fryer, H. R., Bedford, T., Kim, E. Y., Archer, J., Kosakovsky Pond, S. L., et al. (2016). Persistent HIV-1 replication maintains the tissue reservoir during therapy. *Nature* 530, 51–56. doi: 10.1038/nature16933

Lu, C. L., Pai, J. A., Nogueira, L., Mendoza, P., Gruell, H., Oliveira, T. Y., et al. (2018). Relationship between intact HIV-1 proviruses in circulating CD4(+) T cells and rebound viruses emerging during treatment interruption. *Proc. Natl. Acad. Sci. U.S.A.* 115, E11341–E11348. doi: 10.1073/pnas.1813512115

Margolis, D. M., Garcia, J. V., Hazuda, D. J., and Haynes, B. F. (2016). Latency reversal and viral clearance to cure HIV-1. *Science* 353:aaf6517. doi: 10.1126/science.aaf6517

Mattapallil, J. J., Douek, D. C., Hill, B., Nishimura, Y., Martin, M., and Roederer, M. (2005). Massive infection and loss of memory CD4+ T cells in multiple tissues during acute SIV infection. *Nature* 434, 1093–1097. doi: 10.1038/nature03501

Mehandru, S., Poles, M. A., Tenner-Racz, K., Horowitz, A., Hurley, A., Hogan, C., et al. (2004). Primary HIV-1 infection is associated with preferential depletion of CD4+ T lymphocytes from effector sites in the gastrointestinal tract. *J. Exp. Med.* 200, 761–770. doi: 10.1084/jem.20041196

Micci, L., Mcgary, C. S., and Paiardini, M. (2015). Animal models in HIV cure research. *J. Virus Erad.* 1, 17–22.

Mota, T. M., Rasmussen, T. A., Rhodes, A., Tennakoon, S., Dantanarayana, A., Wightman, F., et al. (2017). No adverse safety or virological changes 2 years following vorinostat in HIV-infected individuals on antiretroviral therapy. *AIDS* 31, 1137–1141. doi: 10.1097/QAD.0000000000001442

Mothe, B., Climent, N., Plana, M., Rosas, M., Jimenez, J. L., Munoz-Fernandez, M. A., et al. (2015). Safety and immunogenicity of a modified vaccinia Ankara-based HIV-1 vaccine (MVA-B) in HIV-1-infected patients alone or in combination with a drug to reactivate latent HIV-1. *J. Antimicrob. Chemother.* 70, 1833–1842. doi: 10.1093/jac/dkv046

Nixon, C. C., Mavigner, M., Silvestri, G., and Garcia, J. V. (2017). In vivo models of human immunodeficiency virus persistence and cure strategies. *J. Infect. Dis.* 215, S142–S151. doi: 10.1093/infdis/jiw637

Nolan, D. J., Rose, R., Rodriguez, P. H., Salemi, M., Singer, E. J., Lamers, S. L., et al. (2018). The spleen is an HIV-1 sanctuary during combined antiretroviral therapy. *AIDS Res. Hum. Retroviruses* 34, 123–125. doi: 10.1089/AID.2017.0254

North, T. W., Higgins, J., Deere, J. D., Hayes, T. L., Villalobos, A., Adamson, L., et al. (2010). Viral sanctuaries during highly active antiretroviral therapy in a nonhuman primate model for AIDS. *J. Virol.* 84, 2913–2922. doi: 10.1128/JVI.02356-09

Olesen, R., Vigano, S., Rasmussen, T. A., Sogaard, O. S., Ouyang, Z., Buzon, M., et al. (2015). Innate immune activity correlates with CD4 T cell-associated HIV-1 DNA decline during latency-reversing treatment with panobinostat. *J. Virol.* 89, 10176–10189. doi: 10.1128/JVI.01484-15

Policicchio, B. B., Pandrea, I., and Apetrei, C. (2016). Animal models for HIV cure research. *Front. Immunol.* 7:12. doi: 10.3389/fimmu.2016.00012

Queen, S. E., Mears, B. M., Kelly, K. M., Dorsey, J. L., Liao, Z., Dinoso, J. B., et al. (2011). Replication-competent simian immunodeficiency virus (SIV) gag escape mutations archived in latent reservoirs during antiretroviral treatment of SIV-infected macaques. *J. Virol.* 85, 9167–9175. doi: 10.1128/JVI.00366-11

Rasmussen, T. A., and Sogaard, O. S. (2018). Clinical interventions in HIV cure research. *Adv. Exp. Med. Biol.* 1075, 285–318. doi: 10.1007/978-981-13-0484-2_12

Rasmussen, T. A., Tolstrup, M., Brinkmann, C. R., Olesen, R., Erikstrup, C., Solomon, A., et al. (2014). Panobinostat, a histone deacetylase inhibitor, for latent-virus reactivation in HIV-infected patients on suppressive antiretroviral therapy: a phase 1/2, single group, clinical trial. *Lancet HIV* 1, e13–e21. doi: 10.1016/S2352-3018(14)70014-1

Rasmussen, T. A., Tolstrup, M., Moller, H. J., Brinkmann, C. R., Olesen, R., Erikstrup, C., et al. (2015). Activation of latent human immunodeficiency virus by the histone deacetylase inhibitor panobinostat: a pilot study to assess effects on the central nervous system. *Open Forum Infect. Dis.* 2:ofv037. doi: 10.1093/ofid/ofv037

Ritchie, A. J., Cai, F., Smith, N. M., Chen, S., Song, H., Brackenridge, S., et al. (2014). Recombination-mediated escape from primary CD8+ T cells in acute HIV-1 infection. *Retrovirology* 11:69. doi: 10.1186/s12977-014-0069-9

Rose, R., Lamers, S. L., Nolan, D. J., Maidji, E., Faria, N. R., Pybus, O. G., et al. (2016). HIV maintains an evolving and dispersed population in multiple tissues during suppressive combined antiretroviral therapy in individuals with cancer. *J. Virol.* 90, 8984–8993. doi: 10.1128/JVI.00684-16

Rose, R., Nolan, D. J., Maidji, E., Stoddart, C. A., Singer, E. J., Lamers, S. L., et al. (2018). Eradication of HIV from tissue reservoirs: challenges for the cure. *AIDS Res. Hum. Retroviruses* 34, 3–8. doi: 10.1089/AID.2017.0072

Saxena, M., Sabado, R. L., La Mar, M., Mohri, H., Salazar, A. M., Dong, H., et al. (2019). Poly-ICLC, a tlr3 agonist, induces transient innate immune responses in patients with treated HIV-Infection: a randomized double-blinded placebo controlled trial. *Front. Immunol.* 10:725. doi: 10.3389/fimmu.2019.00725

Schleimann, M. H., Kobberø, M. L., Vibholm, L. K., Kjaer, K., Giron, L. B., Busman-Sahay, K., et al. (2019). TLR9 agonist MGN1703 enhances B cell differentiation and function in lymph nodes. *EBioMedicine* 45, 328–340. doi: 10.1016/j.ebiom.2019.07.005

Shen, A., Zink, M. C., Mankowski, J. L., Chadwick, K., Margolick, J. B., Carruth, L. M., et al. (2003). Resting CD4+ T lymphocytes but not thymocytes provide a latent viral reservoir in a simian immunodeficiency virus-*Macaca nemestrina* model of human immunodeficiency virus type 1-infected patients on highly active antiretroviral therapy. *J. Virol.* 77, 4938–4949. doi: 10.1128/jvi.77.8.4938-4949.2003

Søgaard, O. S., Graversen, M. E., Leth, S., Olesen, R., Brinkmann, C. R., Nissen, S. K., et al. (2015). The depsipeptide romidepsin reverses HIV-1 latency in vivo. *PLoS Pathog.* 11:e1005142. doi: 10.1371/journal.ppat.1005142

Spivak, A. M., Andrade, A., Eisele, E., Hoh, R., Bacchetti, P., Bumpus, N. N., et al. (2014). A pilot study assessing the safety and latency-reversing activity of disulfiram in HIV-1-infected adults on antiretroviral therapy. *Clin. Infect. Dis.* 58, 883–890. doi: 10.1093/cid/cit813

Streeck, H., Li, B., Poon, A. F., Schneidewind, A., Gladden, A. D., Power, K. A., et al. (2008). Immune-driven recombination and loss of control after HIV superinfection. *J. Exp. Med.* 205, 1789–1796. doi: 10.1084/jem.20080281

Tapia, G., Hojen, J. F., Okvist, M., Olesen, R., Leth, S., Nissen, S. K., et al. (2017). Sequential Vacc-4x and romidepsin during combination antiretroviral therapy (cART): immune responses to Vacc-4x regions on p24 and changes in HIV reservoirs. *J. Infect.* 75, 555–571. doi: 10.1016/j.jinf.2017.09.004

van Marle, G., Gill, M. J., Kolodka, D., Mcmanus, L., Grant, T., and Church, D. L. (2007). Compartmentalization of the gut viral reservoir in HIV-1 infected patients. *Retrovirology* 4:87. doi: 10.1186/1742-4690-4-87

Vibholm, L., Schleimann, M. H., Hojen, J. F., Benfield, T., Offersen, R., Rasmussen, K., et al. (2017). Short-course toll-like receptor 9 agonist treatment impacts innate immunity and plasma viremia in individuals with human immunodeficiency virus infection. *Clin. Infect. Dis.* 64, 1686–1695. doi: 10.1093/cid/cix201

Vibholm, L. K., Konrad, C. V., Schleimann, M. H., Frattari, G., Winckelmann, A., Klastrup, V., et al. (2019a). Effects of 24 week toll-like receptor 9 agonist treatment in HIV-1+ individuals: a single-arm, phase 1B/2A trial. *AIDS* 33, 1315–1325. doi: 10.1097/QAD.0000000000002213

Vibholm, L. K., Lorenzi, J. C. C., Pai, J. A., Cohen, Y. Z., Oliveira, T. Y., Barton, J. P., et al. (2019b). Characterization of intact proviruses in blood and lymph node from HIV-infected individuals undergoing analytical treatment interruption. *J. Virol.* 93, e1920–18. doi: 10.1128/JVI.01920-18

Whitney, J. B., and Brad Jones, R. (2018). In vitro and in vivo models of HIV latency. *Adv. Exp. Med. Biol.* 1075, 241–263. doi: 10.1007/978-981-13-0484-2_10

Winckelmann, A., Barton, K., Hiener, B., Schlub, T. E., Shao, W., Rasmussen, T. A., et al. (2017). Romidepsin-induced HIV-1 viremia during effective antiretroviral therapy contains identical viral sequences with few deleterious mutations. *AIDS* 31, 771–779. doi: 10.1097/QAD.0000000000001400

Winckelmann, A., Morcilla, V., Shao, W., Schleimann, M. H., Hojen, J. F., Schlub, T. E., et al. (2018). Genetic characterization of the HIV-1 reservoir after Vacc-4x and romidepsin therapy in HIV-1 infected individuals. *AIDS* 32, 1793–1802. doi: 10.1097/QAD.0000000000001861

Wong, J. K., and Yukl, S. A. (2016). Tissue reservoirs of HIV. *Curr. Opin. HIV AIDS* 11, 362–370. doi: 10.1097/coh.0000000000000293

Wu, G., Swanson, M., Talla, A., Graham, D., Strizki, J., Gorman, D., et al. (2017). HDAC inhibition induces HIV-1 protein and enables immune-based clearance following latency reversal. *JCI Insight* 2:e92901. doi: 10.1172/jci.insight.92901

Yukl, S. A., Gianella, S., Sinclair, E., Epling, L., Li, Q., Duan, L., et al. (2010a). Differences in HIV burden and immune activation within the gut of HIV-positive patients receiving suppressive antiretroviral therapy. *J. Infect. Dis.* 202, 1553–1561. doi: 10.1086/656722

Yukl, S. A., Shergill, A. K., Mcquaid, K., Gianella, S., Lampiris, H., Hare, C. B., et al. (2010b). Effect of raltegravir-containing intensification on HIV burden and T-cell activation in multiple gut sites of HIV-positive adults on suppressive antiretroviral therapy. *AIDS* 24, 2451–2460. doi: 10.1097/QAD.0b013e32833ef7bb

Zink, M. C., Brice, A. K., Kelly, K. M., Queen, S. E., Gama, L., Li, M., et al. (2010). Simian immunodeficiency virus-infected macaques treated with highly active antiretroviral therapy have reduced central nervous system viral replication and inflammation but persistence of viral DNA. *J. Infect. Dis.* 202, 161–170. doi: 10.1086/653213

6

Persistent HIV-1 Viremia on Antiretroviral Therapy: Measurement and Mechanisms

Jana L. Jacobs, Elias K. Halvas, Melissa A. Tosiano and John W. Mellors*

Division of Infectious Diseases, Department of Medicine, University of Pittsburgh School of Medicine, Pittsburgh, PA, United States

***Correspondence:**
Jana L. Jacobs
jlj90@pitt.edu

HIV-1 viremia persists at low-levels despite clinically effective antiretroviral therapy (ART). Here we review new methods to quantify and characterize persistent viremia at the single genome level, and discuss the mechanisms of persistence including clonal expansion of infected cells and tissue origins of viremia. A deeper understanding of how viremia persists on ART is critically important to the design of therapies to eliminate viremia and achieve a functional cure for HIV-1.

Keywords: HIV-1 persistence, HIV-1 cure, low-level viremia, antiretroviral therapy, plasma viremia, plasma HIV-1 RNA

INTRODUCTION

Over the last 30 years there have been great strides made in the diagnosis and treatment of HIV-1 infection. The broad implementation of antiretroviral therapy (ART) has saved the lives of many millions of persons with HIV (Palella et al., 1998), but has also uncovered the persistence of HIV-1 on ART, both as a latent reservoir and as an expression of low-level viremia (Chun et al., 1995, 1997a,b; Finzi et al., 1997; Wong et al., 1997; Dornadula et al., 1999). Studies of patients on ART revealed two sources of plasma viremia: (1) short-lived, productively infected CD4+ T-cells that produce bursts of virus and then die; and (2) long-lived cells capable of producing viremia that is below the limit of detection of commercial assays (Ho et al., 1995; Wei et al., 1995; Perelson et al., 1996, 1997; Dornadula et al., 1999). Longitudinal studies of persistent plasma HIV-1 viremia below the limit of detection of commercial assays in persons on long-term ART have provided a biphasic model of viremia decay, including an initial decay phase with a half-life of 39 weeks and a more slowly decaying phase with a half-life of 11 years (Maldarelli et al., 2007; Palmer et al., 2008; Riddler et al., 2016). These studies showed a positive association between persistent plasma viremia and pre-ART plasma HIV-1 RNA. Riddler et al. (2016) reported that persistent plasma viremia was associated with higher CD8 T-cell counts and a lower CD4/CD8 ratio on ART, both markers of incomplete immune recovery. The source(s) and mechanisms of persistent HIV-1 plasma viremia are still largely uncharacterized despite improved detection methods. Because persistent viremia represents a major barrier to HIV-1 cure, its characterization and clearance remain a high priority. Here we review some recent advances in measuring and identifying the origins of persistent viremia.

PERSISTENT HIV-1 VIREMIA ON ART

Measurement and Recent Improvements

The development of more sensitive, reverse-transcriptase initiated quantitative PCR (RT qPCR) assays revealed that more than half of individuals on ART with plasma HIV-1 RNA suppressed below the limit of detection of commercial assays (20–40 copies/ml) still have detectable HIV-1

RNA in plasma, averaging around 1–3 copies/mL (Dornadula et al., 1999; Palmer et al., 2003, 2008; Maldarelli et al., 2007; Zheng et al., 2013; Riddler et al., 2016). Recent innovations have improved the measurement of this low-level plasma HIV-1 RNA. The first-generation two-step qRT-PCR assay with single copy sensitivity targeted HIV-1 *gag* (gSCA) and required 6–7 mL of plasma (Palmer et al., 2003). A subsequent single copy qRT-PCR assay targeted a highly conserved region of integrase in HIV-1 pol (iSCA v1.0) and enhanced nucleic acid recovery from a smaller volume of plasma (Cillo et al., 2014). Despite highly successful implementation in many clinical studies, iSCA v1.0 required ultracentrifugation and only assayed about half of the total extracted nucleic acid for HIV-1 RNA. In the most recent iteration of a single-copy assay (iSCA v2.0), ultracentrifugation is replaced with tabletop centrifugation and a greater proportion (~80%) of the total extracted nucleic acid is tested for HIV-1 RNA. Importantly, when equal volumes of the same donor plasma were tested using versions of iSCA, 55% of the samples that had no HIV-1 RNA detected by iSCA v1.0 had HIV-1 RNA detected by iSCA v2.0 (Tosiano et al., 2019a).

Automated, next-generation commercial platforms can reproducibly measure HIV-1 RNA in plasma above the limit of quantification (20–200 copies/mL depending on the platform) (Wiesmann et al., 2018). Although individual measurements using commercial platforms do not provide the sensitivity of manual single copy assays, automated platforms have potential as a screening tool. For example, results reported by either Roche or Abbott automated platforms as <20 or <40 copies/mL respectively (also known as "detected but not quantifiable") are almost always detected and quantified by manual single copy assay (Margot et al., 2018; Tosiano et al., 2019b), whereas automated platform results indicating "no target detected" are associated with a significantly lower frequency of HIV-1 RNA detection by manual single copy assays. In addition, Bakkour et al. (2019) have reported that reasonable estimates of HIV-1 RNA copies/mL below the limit of quantification can be obtained using automated platforms to test multiple replicates of plasma to generate a combination of detected, non-detected, and detected but not quantifiable results. Each sample can be assigned a value for HIV-1 RNA by applying a mathematical algorithm based upon the qualitative readouts. Comparisons are in progress of HIV-1 RNA levels obtained by manual single copy assays versus multiple replicates on automated platforms. An automated platform with single copy sensitivity would have distinct advantages over more labor intensive and lower throughput, manual single copy assays.

Association of Persistent Viremia With Cell-Associated HIV-1 DNA

The half-life of persistent plasma viremia on stable ART, calculated using decay dynamics modeling, is more than 11 years (Riddler et al., 2016). Interestingly, decay of HIV-1 proviral DNA-containing cells on ART was recently reported to have a similar half-life of 13 years (Gandhi et al., 2017). Although it is enticing to suggest that the similar half-lives of total cell-associated HIV-1 DNA and plasma HIV-1 RNA on ART represent a direct association between infected cells and persistent plasma viremia, it is important to note that proviral DNA-containing cells rarely contain full-length, intact proviruses. In fact, less than 1–10% of proviruses that persist on ART are capable of producing infectious virus (Fourati et al., 2012; Ho et al., 2013; Bruner et al., 2019). Despite this data, many have reported direct associations of varying degrees between qPCR measures of the proviral reservoir (total cell-associated HIV-1 DNA) and persistent plasma viremia, suggesting that they are related (Chun et al., 2011; Mexas et al., 2012; Hong et al., 2018). The recent development of an assay capable of quantifying intact proviral DNA (Intact Proviral DNA Assay, IPDA) will help address questions regarding the degree of correlation between total and intact cell-associated DNA and plasma viremia (Bruner et al., 2019). Intact proviral DNA correlated modestly with *ex vivo* measurements of inducible, infectious virus outgrowth. However, such quantitative viral outgrowth assays (qVOAs) have not correlated with levels of persistent plasma viremia in individuals on ART (Siliciano et al., 2003; Eriksson et al., 2013). qVOAs have also been shown to underestimate the size of the reservoir by missing the fraction of intact provirus that is non-inducible *ex vivo*; this fraction could contribute to plasma viremia *in vivo* (Ho et al., 2013; Bruner et al., 2019). As such, assays that quantify intact proviruses may show stronger correlations with plasma viremia than total HIV-1 DNA. Studies are currently in progress to assess this possibility.

Association of Persistent Viremia With Cell-Associated HIV-1 RNA

Measurements of various forms of cell-associated bulk HIV-1 RNA have been used to estimate proviral transcriptional activity, both at steady-state and in response to latency reversal agents (Pasternak et al., 2008; Strain and Richman, 2013; Kiselinova et al., 2014; Kearney et al., 2015; Procopio et al., 2015; Hong et al., 2016; Li et al., 2016; Yukl et al., 2018). Whether cell-associated HIV-1 RNA correlates with production of plasma virus is debated. Typically, PCR-based approaches have targeted a single small region of bulk HIV-1 RNA. Although important information about HIV-1 pathogenesis has been garnered from these assays, their utility for assessing latency reversal or changes in viremia have been questioned (Eriksson et al., 2013; Archin et al., 2014; Elliott et al., 2014). In a recent study, cell-associated unspliced HIV-1 RNA strongly correlated with plasma viremia in untreated individuals, but not in individuals on ART (Hong et al., 2018). These conflicting results could be attributed to the accumulation of defective provirus after ART initiation (Bruner et al., 2016) leading to production of defective transcripts that do not result in virion production (Imamichi et al., 2016; Pollack et al., 2017; Wiegand et al., 2017). Interestingly, an analysis of various forms of cell-associated HIV-1 RNA transcripts that are expressed following treatment with latency reversal agents showed very different expression profiles depending upon the conditions and agent used, most of which did not lead to production of full-length polyadenylated transcripts (Yukl et al., 2018; Moron-Lopez et al., 2019). Given the uncertain value of measuring cell-associated HIV-1 RNA in all infected cells, assays that measure HIV-1 RNA transcribed only from intact proviruses (and therefore more likely to produce plasma virus) are likely to be more useful for assessing interventions aimed at perturbing and/or eliminating the HIV-1 reservoir (Wiegand et al., 2017; Yucha et al., 2017).

SOURCES OF PERSISTENT HIV-1 VIREMIA ON ART

Cell and Tissue Sources

Understanding the source of persistent viremia is critically important for the design of interventions to eliminate it. While the source of persistent viremia is likely multi-faceted and variable across individuals, ongoing studies are seeking common sources of viremia that could serve as more specific therapeutic targets. In virologically suppressed individuals, most HIV-1 proviral DNA is found in resting CD4+ T-cells (Chun et al., 1997a; Finzi et al., 1997; Wong et al., 1997). Though not considered a major contribution to the reservoir, other cells types such as monocytes, macrophages, and hematopoietic stem cells have been reported to harbor proviral DNA (Sonza et al., 2001; Zhu et al., 2002; Zaikos et al., 2018; Mitchell et al., 2019). The propensity for white blood cells to circulate throughout the body and penetrate various tissues and lymphoid organs provides an opportunity for infected cells to access ordinarily anatomically protected and/or immune-privileged sites. As such, HIV-1 RNA and/or DNA have been detected widely across tissues in virologically suppressed individuals, including in lymph nodes (Perreau et al., 2013), cerebrospinal fluid (Dahl et al., 2014; Spudich et al., 2019), adipose tissue (Couturier et al., 2015; Damouche et al., 2015), gut-associated lymphoid tissue (GALT) (Lampinen et al., 2000; Anton et al., 2003; Belmonte et al., 2007); and most recently, in the urethra (Ganor et al., 2019).

By contrast, the cellular and/or tissue reservoir(s) that contribute to persistent plasma viremia have not been clearly identified. It is possible that multiple sources contribute to variable degrees, and that sources vary between individuals. Historically, comparison of sequences of persistent plasma virus and total cell-associated proviral DNA in circulating CD4+ T-cells have rarely identified matches. This finding is likely because limited sequencing methods may not detect rare intact provirus that are producing virus. Indeed, in a study in which intensive sampling and single genome sequencing were performed, proviral sequences were detected that did match persistent plasma virus (Bailey et al., 2006). Another likely explanation for the discrepancy between proviral and plasma viral sequences is that most of the cellular reservoir of HIV-1 is found in anatomically protected and immune-privileged sites and is absent from the peripheral CD4+ T-cells. A combination of assays that can detect and characterize intact proviruses and HIV-1 mRNA in both tissues and blood samples should help identify the likely source(s) of persistent viremia.

Viral Replication or Proviral Expression as the Major Source of Persistent Viremia?

A longstanding debate is whether low-level viremia on ART results from ongoing, complete cycles of viral replication or is from clonally expanded infected T cells that produce virions but that do not infect new cells because they are protected by antiretrovirals (Finzi et al., 1997; Wong et al., 1997; Lorenzo-Redondo et al., 2016). As shown in **Figure 1**, complete cycles of viral replication give rise to rapid accumulation of mutations attributed to the error-prone nature of reverse transcriptase. An additional consequence of productive cycles of viral replication is multiple integrations of proviral DNA into different locations in chromosomal DNA. Conversely, expansion of infected cells through cellular proliferation produces identical HIV proviral sequences and identical integration sites in cell progeny. Importantly, a subset of these cell progeny can contain transcriptionally active proviruses that produce virions (**Figure 1**; Bailey et al., 2006; Wagner et al., 2014, Wiegand et al., 2017). For example, Simonetti et al. (2016) reported the detection of a highly expanded CD4+ T-cell clone containing an intact provirus that was a source of persistent viremia on ART.

It has been reported that anatomical sanctuary sites such as the lymph nodes can allow residual viral replication on ART, contributing to maintenance of the HIV reservoir (Lorenzo-Redondo et al., 2016). However, a reanalysis of this data revealed (1) a limited data set after adjusting for PCR resampling and hyper-mutated sequences, (2) limited unique HIV RNA and DNA sequences that were available (median of 5 per sample, range 0–37), (3) sampling time points that may not have taken into account the shifting dynamics of the HIV DNA population within the first year of ART, and (4) inconsistent evidence of viral evolution using more complex analyses (Kearney et al., 2017). These results, along with previous studies reporting no evidence of HIV-1 evolution on suppressive ART in chronically infected adults, as well as in children treated shortly after birth when viral diversity is low, argue against active viral replication being the major source of persistent viremia (Joos et al., 2008; Kearney et al., 2014; van Zyl et al., 2017). Additionally, the presence of invariant sequences and the absence of sequence divergence during prolonged ART, or during and after analytical treatment interruption, is indicative of long-lived cells infected and argues against viral replication. As there have been additional reports of viral replication on ART due to low drug penetration and exclusion of immune cells in anatomical sanctuary sites (Buzón et al., 2010, 2011; Sigal et al., 2011; Hatano et al., 2013; Luo et al., 2013; Patterson et al., 2013; Cardozo et al., 2014; Fletcher et al., 2014; Piovoso and Zurakowski, 2014; Puertas et al., 2014), some residual low-level viral replication on ART cannot be definitively ruled out. Nevertheless, the weight of the evidence discussed above argues against viral replication as the major source of persistent viremia.

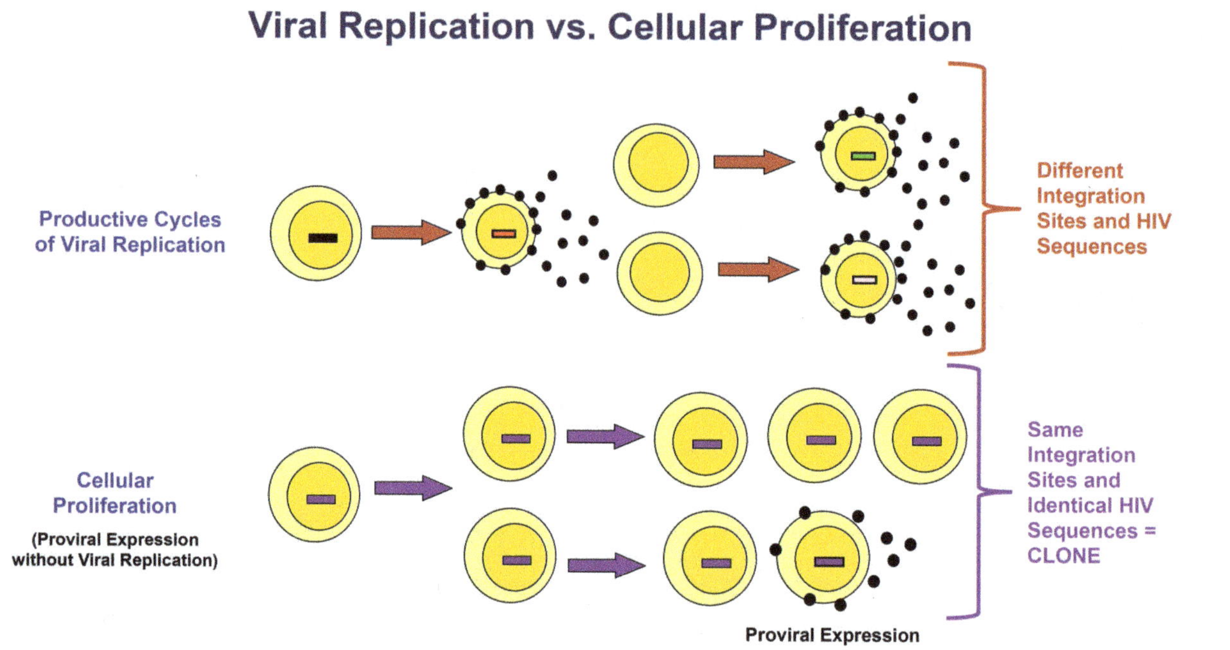

FIGURE 1 | Differentiating Viral Replication From Clonal Expansion with Proviral Expression as the Source of Persistent Viremia on ART. Integration site and HIV sequence analyses can be used to assess the origin of proviral expansion and/or viremia. Productive cycles of viral replication result in both genetic heterogeneity due to errors introduced by reverse transcriptase, and variation in the chromosomal integration site of the HIV provirus. Conversely, clonal expansion results in identical chromosomal HIV integration sites in cell progeny, identical proviral sequences, and identical viral sequences from the subset of cell in the clone that produce virus. See text for more details.

Finally, the recent discovery by multiple groups that most of the inducible, infectious virus comes from clonally expanded T-cells argues for cellular proliferation and against ongoing viral replication as the major mechanism for persistence of HIV-1 reservoirs (Lorenzi et al., 2016; Bui et al., 2017; Hosmane et al., 2017). Additional studies are in progress to determine whether most persistent viremia is of clonal cell origin, as has already been described in one instance of an individual with advanced malignancy (Simonetti et al., 2016). Identifying the clonal origin of viremia requires in depth analyses, including full-length single genome sequencing of HIV-1 RNA from plasma and viral outgrowth cultures, and HIV DNA from infected cells, to identify possible clones, with confirmation of clonality by integration site analyses (Palmer et al., 2005; Maldarelli et al., 2014; Bui et al., 2017).

Clearing Persistent Viremia

Many interventions are being investigated for their ability to clear the HIV-1 reservoir and achieve a functional or sterilizing cure. Among the strategies being studied are: (1) latency reversal to induce viral protein production and expose infected cells to the immune system; (2) engineering immune cells for artificial priming of an HIV-specific immune response or targeted killing of infected cells; (3) gene therapy for alteration of target cell susceptibility to prevent HIV-1 infection; (4) passive immunotherapy with antibodies identified as broadly HIV neutralizing (bnAbs) to clear viremia and infected cells; and combinations of these approaches. These diverse strategies are reviewed elsewhere (Deeks et al., 2016). A promising monoclonal bnAb targeting the CD4 binding site of the HIV-1 envelope (VRC01) has been extensively evaluated for safety, neutralization capacity and pre-existence or development of resistance. Given its high efficacy in neutralizing free virus and the property of bnAbs to promote antibody-dependent cell-mediated cytotoxicity, VRC01 was evaluated in individuals on long-term ART for its effect on persistent plasma viremia and infected cells. Intravenous infusions of VRC01 in individuals on long-term ART did not lead to any change in markers of the reservoir such as cell-associated proviral DNA and RNA, or in levels of persistent plasma viremia (Lynch et al., 2015; Riddler et al., 2018). These disappointing results suggest that persistent virus is either resistant to VRC01 binding or VRC01 effector functions are impaired, such as Fc-mediated clearance or antibody-dependent cellular cytoxicity (ADCC). Work is ongoing to identify the reason(s) for the lack of effect of VRC01 on reservoir markers and on improving the breadth and effector function of bnAbs.

UNANSWERED QUESTIONS AND CONCLUDING REMARKS

Whether persistent plasma viremia in individuals on long-term ART consists of infectious virus remains unclear. It has been shown, at least in some instances, that a portion of the persistent viremia produced by infected cell clones is infectious and contributes to rebound virus when ART is stopped (Simonetti et al., 2016; Kearney et al., 2017). Since only an intact *gag* gene is required for virion production and budding (Delchambre et al., 1989), a scenario in which non-infectious virus is released into the plasma and contributes to persistent plasma viremia is also possible. This possibility may help explain the lack of correlation between levels of persistent plasma viremia and the quantity of inducible, infectious virus *ex vivo* (Siliciano et al., 2003; Eriksson et al., 2013; van Zyl et al., 2018). Studies evaluating the ability of virions present in persistent plasma viremia to infect target cells would be useful to address this question.

It is also unclear whether viremia that rebounds following ART interruption is coming from the same source as that producing persistent viremia on ART. Interestingly, a recent study linked clonal proviral populations in infected cells to clonal sequences in rebounding viremia after treatment interruption, showing that infected cell clones are an important viral reservoir (De Scheerder et al., 2019). The report also described preliminary evidence of linkage between virus in plasma and rebound virus in a subset of individuals. Additional studies examining sequences from persistent viremia and rebound virus will further inform the question of the relevance of persistent viremia to rebound off ART.

In conclusion, although unanswered questions remain, remarkable progress has been made toward measuring and characterizing persistent plasma viremia in individuals on ART since it was first reported in 1999. Mounting evidence indicates that persistent HIV-1 viremia on ART largely arises from clonally expanded CD4+ T-cells, although some contribution of ongoing viral replication cannot be excluded. Future and ongoing studies to further characterize clonal populations producing low-level viremia and their mechanisms of escape from immune clearance will be important to achieve a functional cure.

AUTHOR CONTRIBUTIONS

All authors listed have made a substantial, direct and intellectual contribution to the work, and approved it for publication.

ACKNOWLEDGMENTS

The authors wish to thank the study volunteers and investigators who contributed to the work cited in this review, and to Lorraine Pollini for her excellent editorial assistance.

REFERENCES

Anton, P. A., Mitsuyasu, R. T., Deeks, S. G., Scadden, D. T., Wagner, B., Huang, C., et al. (2003). Multiple measures of HIV burden in blood and tissue are correlated with each other but not with clinical parameters in aviremic subjects. *AIDS* 17, 53–63. doi: 10.1097/00002030-200301030-00008

Archin, N. M., Bateson, R., Tripathy, M. K., Crooks, A. M., Yang, K. H., Dahl, N. P., et al. (2014). HIV-1 expression within resting CD4+ T cells after multiple doses of vorinostat. *J. Infect. Dis.* 210, 728–735. doi: 10.1093/infdis/jiu155

Bailey, J. R., Sedaghat, A. R., Kieffer, T., Brennan, T., Lee, P. K., Wind-Rotolo, M., et al. (2006). Residual human immunodeficiency virus type 1 viremia in some patients on antiretroviral therapy is dominated by a small number of invariant clones rarely found in circulating CD4+ T cells. *J. Virol.* 80, 6441–6457. doi: 10.1128/jvi.00591-06

Bakkour, S., Deng, X., Bacchetti, P., Stone, M., Worlock, A., Hauenstein, S., et al. (2019). "Replicate Aptima Assay For Quantifying Residual Plasma Viremia In Individuals On ART," in *Proceedings of the Conference on Retroviruses and Opportunistic Infections (CROI)*, Seattle, WA.

Belmonte, L., Olmos, M., Fanin, A., Parodi, C., Bare, P., Concetti, H., et al. (2007). The intestinal mucosa as a reservoir of HIV-1 infection after successful HAART. *AIDS* 21, 2106–2108. doi: 10.1097/qad.0b013e3282efb74b

Bruner, K. M., Murray, A. J., Pollack, R. A., Soliman, M. G., Laskey, S. B., Capoferri, A. A., et al. (2016). Defective proviruses rapidly accumulate during acute HIV-1 infection. *Nat. Med.* 2, 1043–1049. doi: 10.1038/nm.4156

Bruner, K. M., Wang, Z., Simonetti, F. R., Bender, A. M., Kwon, K. J., Sengupta, S., et al. (2019). A quantitative approach for measuring the reservoir of latent HIV-1 proviruses. *Nature* 566, 120–125. doi: 10.1038/s41586-019-0898-8

Bui, J. K., Sobolewski, M. D., Keele, B. F., Spindler, J., Musick, A., Wiegand, A., et al. (2017). Proviruses with identical sequences comprise a large fraction of the replication-competent HIV reservoir. *PLoS Pathog.* 13:e1006283. doi: 10.1371/journal.ppat.1006283

Buzón, M. J., Codoñer, F. M., Frost, S. D., Pou, C., Puertas, M. C., Massanella, M., et al. (2011). Deep molecular characterization of HIV-1 dynamics under suppressive HAART. *PLoS Pathog.* 7:e1002314. doi: 10.1371/journal.ppat.1002314

Buzón, M. J., Massanella, M., Llibre, J. M., Esteve, A., Dahl, V., Puertas, M. C., et al. (2010). HIV-1 replication and immune dynamics are affected by raltegravir intensification of HAART-suppressed subjects. *Nat. Med.* 16, 460–465. doi: 10.1038/nm.2111

Cardozo, E. F., Luo, R., Piovoso, M. J., and Zurakowski, R. (2014). Spatial modeling of HIV cryptic viremia and 2-LTR formation during raltegravir intensification. *J. Theor. Biol.* 345, 61–69. doi: 10.1016/j.jtbi.2013.12.020

Chun, T. W., Carruth, L., Finzi, D., Shen, X., Digiuseppe, J. A., Taylor, H., et al. (1997a). Quantification of latent tissue reservoirs and total body viral load in HIV-1 infection. *Nature* 387, 183–188. doi: 10.1038/387183a0

Chun, T. W., Stuyver, L., Mizell, S. B., Ehler, L. A., Mican, J. A., Baseler, M., et al. (1997b). Presence of an inducible HIV-1 latent reservoir during highly active antiretroviral therapy. *Proc. Natl. Acad. Sci. U.S.A.* 94, 13193–13197. doi: 10.1073/pnas.94.24.13193

Chun, T. W., Finzi, D., Margolick, J., Chadwick, K., Schwartz, D., and Siliciano, R. F. (1995). In vivo fate of HIV-1-infected T cells: quantitative analysis of the transition to stable latency. *Nat. Med.* 1, 1284–1290. doi: 10.1038/nm1295-1284

Chun, T. W., Murray, D., Justement, J. S., Hallahan, C. W., Moir, S., Kovacs, C., et al. (2011). Relationship between residual plasma viremia and the size of HIV proviral DNA reservoirs in infected individuals receiving effective antiretroviral therapy. *J. Infect. Dis.* 204, 135–138. doi: 10.1093/infdis/jir208

Cillo, A. R., Vagratian, D., Bedison, M. A., Anderson, E. M., Kearney, M. F., Fyne, E., et al. (2014). Improved single-copy assays for quantification of persistent HIV-1 viremia in patients on suppressive antiretroviral therapy. *J. Clin. Microbiol.* 52, 3944–3951. doi: 10.1128/JCM.02060-14

Couturier, J., Suliburk, J. W., Brown, J. M., Luke, D. J., Agarwal, N., Yu, X., et al. (2015). Human adipose tissue as a reservoir for memory CD4+ T cells and HIV. *AIDS* 29, 667–674. doi: 10.1097/QAD.0000000000000599

Dahl, V., Peterson, J., Fuchs, D., Gisslen, M., Palmer, S., and Price, R. W. (2014). Low levels of HIV-1 RNA detected in the cerebrospinal fluid after up to 10 years of suppressive therapy are associated with local immune activation. *AIDS* 28, 2251–2258. doi: 10.1097/QAD.0000000000000400

Damouche, A., Lazure, T., Avettand-Fenoel, V., Huot, N., Dejucq-Rainsford, N., Satie, A. P., et al. (2015). Adipose tissue is a neglected viral reservoir and an inflammatory site during chronic HIV and SIV infection. *PLoS Pathog.* 11:e1005153. doi: 10.1371/journal.ppat.1005153

De Scheerder, M. A., Vrancken, B., Dellicour, S., Schlub, T., Lee, E., Shao, W., et al. (2019). HIV rebound is predominantly fueled by genetically identical viral expansions from diverse reservoirs. *Cell Host Microbe* 26, 347–358.e7. doi: 10.1016/j.chom.2019.08.003

Deeks, S. G., Lewin, S. R., Ross, A. L., Ananworanich, J., Benkirane, M., Cannon, P., et al. (2016). International AIDS society global scientific strategy: towards an HIV cure 2016. *Nat. Med.* 22, 839–850. doi: 10.1038/nm.4108

Delchambre, M., Gheysen, D., Thines, D., Thiriart, C., Jacobs, E., Verdin, E., et al. (1989). The GAG precursor of simian immunodeficiency virus assembles into virus-like particles. *EMBO J.* 8, 2653–2660. doi: 10.1002/j.1460-2075.1989.tb08405.x

Dornadula, G., Zhang, H., VanUitert, B., Stern, J., Livornese, L., Jr, Ingerman, M. J., et al. (1999). Residual HIV-1 RNA in blood plasma of patients taking suppressive highly active antiretroviral therapy. *JAMA* 282, 1627–1632.

Elliott, J. H., Wightman, F., Solomon, A., Ghneim, K., Ahlers, J., Cameron, M. J., et al. (2014). Activation of HIV transcription with short-course vorinostat in HIV-infected patients on suppressive antiretroviral therapy. *PLoS Pathog.* 10:e1004473. doi: 10.1371/journal.ppat.1004473

Eriksson, S., Graf, E. H., Dahl, V., Strain, M. C., Yukl, S. A., Lysenko, E. S., et al. (2013). Comparative analysis of measures of viral reservoirs in HIV-1 eradication studies. *PLoS Pathog.* 9:e1003174. doi: 10.1371/journal.ppat.1003174

Finzi, D., Hermankova, M., Pierson, T., Carruth, L. M., Buck, C., Chaisson, R. E., et al. (1997). Identification of a reservoir for HIV-1 in patients on highly active antiretroviral therapy. *Science* 278, 1295–1300. doi: 10.1126/science.278.5341.1295

Fletcher, C. V., Staskus, K., Wietgrefe, S. W., Rothenberger, M., Reilly, C., Chipman, J. G., et al. (2014). Persistent HIV-1 replication is associated with lower antiretroviral drug concentrations in lymphatic tissues. *Proc. Natl. Acad. Sci. U.S.A.* 111, 2307–2312. doi: 10.1073/pnas.1318249111

Fourati, S., Lambert-Niclot, S., Soulie, C., Malet, I., Valantin, M. A., Descours, B., et al. (2012). HIV-1 genome is often defective in PBMCs and rectal tissues after long-term HAART as a result of APOBEC3 editing and correlates with the size of reservoirs. *J. Antimicrob. Chemother.* 67, 2323–2326. doi: 10.1093/jac/dks219

Gandhi, R. T., Mcmahon, D. K., Bosch, R. J., Lalama, C. M., Cyktor, J. C., Macatangay, B. J., et al. (2017). Levels of HIV-1 persistence on antiretroviral therapy are not associated with markers of inflammation or activation. *PLoS Pathog.* 13:e1006285. doi: 10.1371/journal.ppat.1006285

Ganor, Y., Real, F., Sennepin, A., Dutertre, C. A., Prevedel, L., Xu, L., et al. (2019). HIV-1 reservoirs in urethral macrophages of patients under suppressive antiretroviral therapy. *Nat. Microbiol.* 4, 633–644. doi: 10.1038/s41564-018-0335-z

Hatano, H., Strain, M. C., Scherzer, R., Bacchetti, P., Wentworth, D., Hoh, R., et al. (2013). Increase in 2-long terminal repeat circles and decrease in D-dimer after raltegravir intensification in patients with treated HIV infection: a randomized, placebo-controlled trial. *J. Infect. Dis.* 208, 1436–1442. doi: 10.1093/infdis/jit453

Ho, D. D., Neumann, A. U., Perelson, A. S., Chen, W., Leonard, J. M., and Markowitz, M. (1995). Rapid turnover of plasma virions and CD4 lymphocytes in HIV-1 infection. *Nature* 373, 123–126. doi: 10.1038/373123a0

Ho, Y. C., Shan, L., Hosmane, N. N., Wang, J., Laskey, S. B., Rosenbloom, D. I., et al. (2013). Replication-competent noninduced proviruses in the latent reservoir increase barrier to HIV-1 cure. *Cell* 155, 540–551. doi: 10.1016/j.cell.2013.09.020

Hong, F., Aga, E., Cillo, A., Yates, A. L., Besson, G., Fyne, E., et al. (2016). Novel assays to measure total cell-associated HIV-1 DNA and RNA. *J. Clin. Microbiol.* 54, 902–911. doi: 10.1128/JVI.01763-08

Hong, F., Jacobs, J. L., Aga, E., Cillo, A. R., Fyne, E., Koontz, D. L., et al. (2018). Associations between HIV-1 DNA copy number, proviral transcriptional activity, and plasma viremia in individuals off or on suppressive antiretroviral therapy. *Virology* 521, 51–57. doi: 10.1016/j.virol.2018.05.018

Hosmane, N. N., Kwon, K. J., Bruner, K. M., Capoferri, A. A., Beg, S., Rosenbloom, D. I., et al. (2017). Proliferation of latently infected CD4(+) T cells carrying replication-competent HIV-1: potential role in latent reservoir dynamics. *J. Exp. Med.* 214, 959–972. doi: 10.1084/jem.20170193

Imamichi, H., Dewar, R. L., Adelsberger, J. W., Rehm, C. A., O'doherty, U., Paxinos, E. E., et al. (2016). Defective HIV-1 proviruses produce novel protein-coding RNA species in HIV-infected patients on combination antiretroviral therapy. *Proc. Natl. Acad. Sci. U.S.A.* 113, 8783–8788. doi: 10.1073/pnas.1609057113

Joos, B., Fischer, M., Kuster, H., Pillai, S. K., Wong, J. K., Boni, J., et al. (2008). HIV rebounds from latently infected cells, rather than from continuing low-level replication. *Proc. Natl. Acad. Sci. U.S.A.* 105, 16725–16730. doi: 10.1073/pnas.0804192105

Kearney, M. F., Spindler, J., Shao, W., Yu, S., Anderson, E. M., O'shea, A., et al. (2014). Lack of detectable HIV-1 molecular evolution during suppressive antiretroviral therapy. *PLoS Pathog.* 10:e1004010. doi: 10.1371/journal.ppat.1004010

Kearney, M. F., Wiegand, A., Shao, W., Coffin, J. M., Mellors, J. W., Lederman, M., et al. (2015). Origin of rebound plasma HIV includes cells with identical proviruses that are transcriptionally active before stopping antiretroviral therapy. *J. Virol.* 90, 1369–1376. doi: 10.1128/JVI.02139-15

Kearney, M. F., Wiegand, A., Shao, W., Mcmanus, W. R., Bale, M. J., Luke, B., et al. (2017). Ongoing HIV replication during ART reconsidered. *Open Forum Infect. Dis.* 4:ofx173. doi: 10.1093/ofid/ofx173

Kiselinova, M., Pasternak, A. O., De Spiegelaere, W., Vogelaers, D., Berkhout, B., and Vandekerckhove, L. (2014). Comparison of droplet digital PCR and seminested real-time PCR for quantification of cell-associated HIV-1 RNA. *PLoS One* 9:e85999. doi: 10.1371/journal.pone.0085999

Lampinen, T. M., Critchlow, C. W., Kuypers, J. M., Hurt, C. S., Nelson, P. J., Hawes, S. E., et al. (2000). Association of antiretroviral therapy with detection of HIV-1 RNA and DNA in the anorectal mucosa of homosexual men. *AIDS* 14, F69–F75.

Li, J. Z., Etemad, B., Ahmed, H., Aga, E., Bosch, R. J., Mellors, J. W., et al. (2016). The size of the expressed HIV reservoir predicts timing of viral rebound after treatment interruption. *AIDS* 30, 343–353. doi: 10.1097/QAD.0000000000000953

Lorenzi, J. C., Cohen, Y. Z., Cohn, L. B., Kreider, E. F., Barton, J. P., Learn, G. H., et al. (2016). Paired quantitative and qualitative assessment of the replication-competent HIV-1 reservoir and comparison with integrated proviral DNA. *Proc. Natl. Acad. Sci. U.S.A.* 113, E7908–E7916.

Lorenzo-Redondo, R., Fryer, H. R., Bedford, T., Kim, E. Y., Archer, J., Pond, S. L. K., et al. (2016). Persistent HIV-1 replication maintains the tissue reservoir during therapy. *Nature* 530, 51–56. doi: 10.1038/nature16933

Luo, R., Cardozo, E. F., Piovoso, M. J., Wu, H., Buzón, M. J., Martinez-Picado, J., et al. (2013). Modelling HIV-1 2-LTR dynamics following raltegravir intensification. *J. R. Soc. Interface* 10:20130186. doi: 10.1098/rsif.2013.0186

Lynch, R. M., Boritz, E., Coates, E. E., Dezure, A., Madden, P., Costner, P., et al. (2015). Virologic effects of broadly neutralizing antibody VRC01 administration during chronic HIV-1 infection. *Sci. Transl. Med.* 7:319ra206. doi: 10.1126/scitranslmed.aad5752

Maldarelli, F., Palmer, S., King, M. S., Wiegand, A., Polis, M. A., Mican, J., et al. (2007). ART suppresses plasma HIV-1 RNA to a stable set point predicted by pretherapy viremia. *PLoS Pathog.* 3:e46. doi: 10.1371/journal.ppat.0030046

Maldarelli, F., Wu, X., Su, L., Simonetti, F. R., Shao, W., Hill, S., et al. (2014). HIV latency. Specific HIV integration sites are linked to clonal expansion and persistence of infected cells. *Science* 345, 179–183. doi: 10.1126/science.1254194

Margot, N., Koontz, D., Mccallister, S., Mellors, J. W., and Callebaut, C. (2018). Measurement of plasma HIV-1 RNA below the limit of quantification (<20 copies/mL) of commercial assays with the integrase HIV RNA single-copy assay. *J. Clin. Virol.* 108, 50–52. doi: 10.1016/j.jcv.2018.09.003

Mexas, A. M., Graf, E. H., Pace, M. J., Yu, J. J., Papasavvas, E., Azzoni, L., et al. (2012). Concurrent measures of total and integrated HIV DNA monitor reservoirs and ongoing replication in eradication trials. *AIDS* 26, 2295–2306. doi: 10.1097/QAD.0b013e32835a5c2f

Mitchell, B. I., Laws, E. I., and Ndhlovu, L. C. (2019). Impact of myeloid reservoirs in HIV cure trials. *Curr. HIV/AIDS Rep.* 16, 129–140. doi: 10.1007/s11904-019-00438-5

Moron-Lopez, S., Kim, P., Sogaard, O. S., Tolstrup, M., Wong, J. K., and Yukl, S. A. (2019). Characterization of the HIV-1 transcription profile after romidepsin administration in ART-suppressed individuals. *AIDS* 33, 425–431. doi: 10.1097/QAD.0000000000002083

Palella, F. J., Jr, Delaney, K. M., Moorman, A. C., Loveless, M. O., Fuhrer, J., Satten, G. A., et al. (1998). Declining morbidity and mortality among patients with advanced human immunodeficiency virus infection. HIV Outpatient Study Investigators. *N. Engl. J. Med.* 338, 853–860. doi: 10.1056/nejm199803263381301

Palmer, S., Kearney, M., Maldarelli, F., Halvas, E. K., Bixby, C. J., Bazmi, H., et al. (2005). Multiple, linked human immunodeficiency virus type 1 drug resistance mutations in treatment-experienced patients are missed by standard genotype analysis. *J. Clin. Microbiol.* 43, 406–413. doi: 10.1128/jcm.43.1.406-413.2005

Palmer, S., Maldarelli, F., Wiegand, A., Bernstein, B., Hanna, G. J., Brun, S. C., et al. (2008). Low-level viremia persists for at least 7 years in patients on suppressive antiretroviral therapy. *Proc. Natl. Acad. Sci. U.S.A.* 105, 3879–3884. doi: 10.1073/pnas.0800050105

Palmer, S., Wiegand, A. P., Maldarelli, F., Bazmi, H., Mican, J. M., Polis, M., et al. (2003). New real-time reverse transcriptase-initiated PCR assay with single-copy sensitivity for human immunodeficiency virus type 1 RNA in plasma. *J. Clin. Microbiol.* 41, 4531–4536. doi: 10.1128/jcm.41.10.4531-4536.2003

Pasternak, A. O., Adema, K. W., Bakker, M., Jurriaans, S., Berkhout, B., Cornelissen, M., et al. (2008). Highly sensitive methods based on seminested real-time reverse transcription-PCR for quantitation of human immunodeficiency virus type 1 unspliced and multiply spliced RNA and proviral DNA. *J. Clin. Microbiol.* 46, 2206–2211. doi: 10.1128/JCM.00055-08

Patterson, K. B., Prince, H. A., Stevens, T., Shaheen, N. J., Dellon, E. S., Madanick, R. D., et al. (2013). Differential penetration of raltegravir throughout gastrointestinal tissue: implications for eradication and cure. *AIDS* 27, 1413–1419. doi: 10.1097/QAD.0b013e32835f2b49

Perelson, A. S., Essunger, P., Cao, Y., Vesanen, M., Hurley, A., Saksela, K., et al. (1997). Decay characteristics of HIV-1-infected compartments during combination therapy. *Nature* 387, 188–191. doi: 10.1038/387188a0

Perelson, A. S., Neumann, A. U., Markowitz, M., Leonard, J. M., and Ho, D. D. (1996). HIV-1 dynamics in vivo: virion clearance rate, infected cell life-span, and viral generation time. *Science* 271, 1582–1586. doi: 10.1126/science.271.5255.1582

Perreau, M., Savoye, A. L., De Crignis, E., Corpataux, J. M., Cubas, R., Haddad, E. K., et al. (2013). Follicular helper T cells serve as the major CD4 T cell compartment for HIV-1 infection, replication, and production. *J. Exp. Med.* 210, 143–156. doi: 10.1084/jem.20121932

Piovoso, M. J., and Zurakowski, R. (2014). "Evaluation of HIV 2-LTR formation models using monotone system theory," in *Proceedings of the American Control Conference (ACC)*, Portland, OR, 2747–2752.

Pollack, R. A., Jones, R. B., Pertea, M., Bruner, K. M., Martin, A. R., Thomas, A. S., et al. (2017). Defective HIV-1 proviruses are expressed and can be recognized by cytotoxic T lymphocytes, which shape the proviral landscape. *Cell Host Microbe* 21:e494. doi: 10.1016/j.chom.2017.03.008

Procopio, F. A., Fromentin, R., Kulpa, D. A., Brehm, J. H., Bebin, A. G., Strain, M. C., et al. (2015). A novel assay to measure the magnitude of the inducible viral reservoir in hiv-infected individuals. *Ebiomedicine* 2, 874–883. doi: 10.1016/j.ebiom.2015.06.019

Puertas, M. C., Massanella, M., Llibre, J. M., Ballestero, M., Buzón, M. J., Ouchi, D., et al. (2014). Intensification of a raltegravir-based regimen with maraviroc in early HIV-1 infection. *AIDS* 28, 325–334. doi: 10.1097/QAD.0000000000000066

Riddler, S. A., Aga, E., Bosch, R. J., Bastow, B., Bedison, M., Vagratian, D., et al. (2016). Continued slow decay of residual plasma viremia in HIV-1-infected adults receiving long term antiretroviral therapy. *J. Infect. Dis.* 213, 556–560. doi: 10.1093/infdis/jiv433

Riddler, S. A., Zheng, L., Durand, C. M., Ritz, J., Koup, R. A., Ledgerwood, J., et al. (2018). Randomized clinical trial to assess the impact of the broadly neutralizing HIV-1 monoclonal antibody VRC01 on HIV-1 persistence in individuals on effective ART. *Open Forum Infect. Dis.* 5:ofy242. doi: 10.1093/ofid/ofy242

Sigal, A., Kim, J. T., Balazs, A. B., Dekel, E., Mayo, A., Milo, R., et al. (2011). Cell-to-cell spread of HIV permits ongoing replication despite antiretroviral therapy. *Nature* 477, 95–98. doi: 10.1038/nature10347

Siliciano, J. D., Kajdas, J., Finzi, D., Quinn, T. C., Chadwick, K., Margolick, J. B., et al. (2003). Long-term follow-up studies confirm the stability of the latent reservoir for HIV-1 in resting CD4+ T cells. *Nat. Med.* 9, 727–728. doi: 10.1038/nm880

Simonetti, F. R., Sobolewski, M. D., Fyne, E., Shao, W., Spindler, J., Hattori, J., et al. (2016). Clonally expanded CD4+ T cells can produce infectious HIV-1 in vivo. *Proc. Natl. Acad. Sci. U.S.A.* 113, 1883–1888. doi: 10.1073/pnas.1522675113

Sonza, S., Mutimer, H. P., Oelrichs, R., Jardine, D., Harvey, K., Dunne, A., et al. (2001). Monocytes harbour replication-competent, non-latent HIV-1 in patients on highly active antiretroviral therapy. *AIDS* 15, 17–22. doi: 10.1097/00002030-200101050-00005

Spudich, S., Robertson, K., Bosch, R. J., Gandhi, R. T., Cyktor, J. C., Mar, H., et al. (2019). Persistent HIV-infected cells in cerebrospinal fluid are associated with poorer neurocognitive performance. *J. Clin. Invest.* 129, 3339–3346. doi: 10.1172/JCI127413

Strain, M. C., and Richman, D. D. (2013). New assays for monitoring residual HIV burden in effectively treated individuals. *Curr. Opin. HIV AIDS* 8, 106–110. doi: 10.1097/COH.0b013e32835d811b

Tosiano, M. A., Jacobs, J. L., Shutt, K. A., Cyktor, J. C., and Mellors, J. W. (2019a). A simpler and more sensitive single-copy HIV-1 RNA assay for quantification of persistent HIV-1 viremia in individuals on suppressive antiretroviral therapy. *J. Clin. Microbiol.* 57, e1714–e1718. doi: 10.1128/JCM.01714-18

Tosiano, M. A., Mar, H., Cyktor, J. C., Koontz, D. L., Eron, J. J., Gandhi, R. T., et al. (2019b). "HIV-1 RNA Detection By Abbott M2000 Correlates With Integrase Single Copy Assay," in *Proceedings of the Conference on Retroviruses and Opportunistic Infections (CROI)*, Seattle, WA.

van Zyl, G., Bale, M. J., and Kearney, M. F. (2018). HIV evolution and diversity in ART-treated patients. *Retrovirology* 15:14. doi: 10.1186/s12977-018-0395-4

van Zyl, G. U., Katusiime, M. G., Wiegand, A., Mcmanus, W. R., Bale, M. J., Halvas, E. K., et al. (2017). No evidence of HIV replication in children on antiretroviral therapy. *J. Clin. Invest.* 127, 3827–3834. doi: 10.1172/JCI94582

Wagner, T. A., Mclaughlin, S., Garg, K., Cheung, C. Y., Larsen, B. B., Styrchak, S., et al. (2014). HIV latency. Proliferation of cells with HIV integrated into cancer genes contributes to persistent infection. *Science* 345, 570–573. doi: 10.1126/science.1256304

Wei, X., Ghosh, S. K., Taylor, M. E., Johnson, V. A., Emini, E. A., Deutsch, P., et al. (1995). Viral dynamics in human immunodeficiency virus type 1 infection. *Nature* 373, 117–122.

Wiegand, A., Spindler, J., Hong, F. F., Shao, W., Cyktor, J. C., Cillo, A. R., et al. (2017). Single-cell analysis of HIV-1 transcriptional activity reveals expression of proviruses in expanded clones during ART. *Proc. Natl. Acad. Sci. U.S.A.* 114, E3659–E3668. doi: 10.1073/pnas.1617961114

Wiesmann, F., Ehret, R., Naeth, G., Daumer, M., Fuhrmann, J., Kaiser, R., et al. (2018). Multicenter evaluation of two next-generation HIV-1 quantitation assays, aptima quant Dx and Cobas 6800, in comparison to the realtime HIV-1 reference assay. *J. Clin. Microbiol.* 56, e292–e218. doi: 10.1128/JCM.00292-18

Wong, J. K., Hezareh, M., Gunthard, H. F., Havlir, D. V., Ignacio, C. C., Spina, C. A., et al. (1997). Recovery of replication-competent HIV despite prolonged suppression of plasma viremia. *Science* 278, 1291–1295. doi: 10.1126/science.278.5341.1291

Yucha, R. W., Hobbs, K. S., Hanhauser, E., Hogan, L. E., Nieves, W., Ozen, M. O., et al. (2017). High-throughput characterization of HIV-1 reservoir reactivation using a single-cell-in-droplet PCR assay. *Ebiomedicine* 20, 217–229. doi: 10.1016/j.ebiom.2017.05.006

Yukl, S. A., Kaiser, P., Kim, P., Telwatte, S., Joshi, S. K., Vu, M., et al. (2018). HIV latency in isolated patient CD4(+) T cells may be due to blocks in

HIV transcriptional elongation, completion, and splicing. *Sci. Transl. Med.* 10:eaa9927. doi: 10.1126/scitranslmed.aap9927

Zaikos, T. D., Terry, V. H., Sebastian Kettinger, N. T., Lubow, J., Painter, M. M., Virgilio, M. C., et al. (2018). Hematopoietic stem and progenitor cells are a distinct hiv reservoir that contributes to persistent viremia in suppressed patients. *Cell Rep* 25, 3759–3773.e9. doi: 10.1016/j.celrep.2018.11.104

Zheng, L., Bosch, R. J., Chan, E. S., Read, S., Kearney, M., Margolis, D. M., et al. (2013). Predictors of residual viraemia in patients on long-term suppressive antiretroviral therapy. *Antivir. Ther.* 18, 39–43. doi: 10.3851/IMP2323

Zhu, T., Muthui, D., Holte, S., Nickle, D., Feng, F., Brodie, S., et al. (2002). Evidence for human immunodeficiency virus type 1 replication in vivo in CD14(+) monocytes and its potential role as a source of virus in patients on highly active antiretroviral therapy. *J. Virol.* 76, 707–716. doi: 10.1128/jvi.76.2.707-716.2002

7

The Role of Macrophages in HIV-1 Persistence and Pathogenesis

*Zita Kruize and Neeltje A. Kootstra**

Laboratory for Viral Immune Pathogenesis, Department of Experimental Immunology, Amsterdam UMC, Amsterdam Infection & Immunity Institute, University of Amsterdam, Amsterdam, Netherlands

Correspondence:
Neeltje A. Kootstra
n.a.kootstra@amsterdamumc.nl;
n.a.kootstra@amc.uva.nl

Current antiretroviral therapy (ART) effectively suppresses Human Immunodeficiency Virus type 1 (HIV-1) in infected individuals. However, even long term ART does not eradicate HIV-1 infected cells and the virus persists in cellular reservoirs. Beside memory $CD4^+$ T cells, cells of the myeloid lineage, especially macrophages, are believed to be an important sanctuary for HIV-1. Monocytes and macrophages are key players in the innate immune response to pathogens and are recruited to sites of infection and inflammation. Due to their long life span and ability to reside in virtually every tissue, macrophages have been proposed to play a critical role in the establishment and persistence of the HIV-1 reservoir. Current HIV-1 cure strategies mainly focus on the concept of "shock and kill" to purge the viral reservoir. This approach aims to reactivate viral protein production in latently infected cells, which subsequently are eliminated as a consequence of viral replication, or recognized and killed by the immune system. Macrophage susceptibility to HIV-1 infection is dependent on the local microenvironment, suggesting that molecular pathways directing differentiation and polarization are involved. Current latency reversing agents (LRA) are mainly designed to reactivate the HIV-1 provirus in CD4+ T cells, while their ability to abolish viral latency in macrophages is largely unknown. Moreover, the resistance of macrophages to HIV-1 mediated kill and the presence of infected macrophages in immune privileged regions including the central nervous system (CNS), may pose a barrier to elimination of infected cells by current "shock and kill" strategies. This review focusses on the role of monocytes/macrophages in HIV-1 persistence. We will discuss mechanisms of viral latency and persistence in monocytes/macrophages. Furthermore, the role of these cells in HIV-1 tissue distribution and pathogenesis will be discussed.

Keywords: HIV-1, monocytes/macrophages, latency, pathogenesis, reservoir

INTRODUCTION

Antiretroviral therapy (ART) has dramatically improved the clinical outcome of Human Immunodeficiency Virus type 1 (HIV-1) infection. However, eradication of HIV-1 is not achieved due to persistence of a viral reservoir that harbors latent provirus that is reactivated upon discontinuation of ART. This latent viral reservoir is a major hurdle in curative treatment of HIV-1 infection and therefore new therapeutic approaches that aim to eliminate or reduce the viral reservoir are explored.

CD4+ T cells and cells from the monocyte/macrophage lineage are considered as the most important target cells for HIV-1, and play an important role in viral persistence and the formation of the viral reservoir. While the major viral reservoir in treated HIV-1 infection is comprised of CD4+ T cells, the distribution and characteristics of the monocyte/macrophage reservoir remain largely unknown.

Monocytes and macrophages are part of the innate immune system and respond to different signals which will direct macrophage differentiation, polarization and function. Monocytes/macrophages sense and clear pathogens, serve as antigen presenting cells priming the adaptive immune response, are involved in both pro- and anti-inflammatory responses, and tissue repair. Macrophages are found in all lymphoid as well as non-lymphoid tissues and their origin was originally described to be dependent on circulating monocytes, which would replenish the tissue-resident macrophage pool if needed. Recent studies in mice showed that the majority of tissue-resident macrophages are embryonically derived and have been implicated to be self-renewing, with the exception of the mucosal/border tissues like the intestine, the dermis and the heart, where bone marrow-derived circulating monocytes constantly replenish the aging tissue-resident macrophage pool (Ginhoux et al., 2010; Schulz et al., 2012; Hashimoto et al., 2013; Yona et al., 2013; Bain et al., 2014; Hoeffel et al., 2015; Mass et al., 2016). The proportion between the pool of tissue-resident macrophages and the pool of monocytes-derived macrophages vary during a state of homeostasis or inflammation (Wang and Kubes, 2016).

Upon differentiation of monocytes into macrophages, these cells become susceptible to HIV-1 infection and due to their ability to migrate into tissues, they contribute to the spread of viral infection to nearly every tissue of the body including gut, semen, lung, gut-associated lymphoid tissue, brain, liver, urethra, and lymph nodes (Zhang et al., 1998; Mayer et al., 1999; Lambotte et al., 2005; Guadalupe et al., 2006; Poles et al., 2006; Chun et al., 2008; Zalar et al., 2010; Deleage et al., 2011; Abbas et al., 2014; Yukl et al., 2014; Cribbs et al., 2015; Hansen et al., 2016; Rose et al., 2016; Kandathil et al., 2018; Tso et al., 2018; Ganor et al., 2019; Ko et al., 2019). Furthermore, macrophages are considered long lived, resistant to virally induced cytopathic effects, and can reside in anatomical sanctuaries with restricted penetration of ART, which will support viral persistent even during ART (Ho et al., 1986; Nicholson et al., 1986; Lafeuillade et al., 1998; Solas et al., 2003; Estes et al., 2017; Clayton et al., 2018).

In this review we will discuss the role of monocytes/macrophages in HIV-1 pathogenesis, HIV-1 persistence and viral reservoir.

MONOCYTES AND MACROPHAGES IN HIV-1 PATHOGENESIS

HIV-1 Transmission

Human Immunodeficiency Virus type 1 enters the body mostly through mucosal surfaces of the genital or gastrointestinal tract. The underlying lamina propria is populated with high populations of lymphocytes and macrophages, which express CD4 in combination with the coreceptor C-C chemokine receptor type 5 (CCR5) and serve as targets for HIV-1 infection. Although the CD4+ T cells in the lamina propria are considered the major target for HIV-1 (Zhang et al., 1999; Greenhead et al., 2000; Gupta et al., 2002; Guadalupe et al., 2003; Brenchley et al., 2004; Hladik et al., 2007), infection of macrophages located in the lamina propria of the intestinal, penile urethral and vaginal mucosa has been described (Shen et al., 2009; Zalar et al., 2010; Ganor et al., 2013; Josefsson et al., 2013; Yukl et al., 2014). This confirms a role for macrophages during the early phases of infection, however, it remains under debate whether these mucosal macrophages support HIV-1 replication and spread the infection. Indeed, HIV-1 RNA has been demonstrated to be present in macrophages located in the vagina (Shen et al., 2009), but not in the gut, indicating that local environmental signals required for efficient viral replication in macrophages can be lacking in local mucosal tissues under homeostatic conditions.

Monocytes in HIV-1 Infection

Human Immunodeficiency Virus type 1 infection is characterized by high immune activation and inflammation, caused by high levels of HIV-1 replication, bacterial translocation, coinfection with other viruses (e.g., CMV, HCV, HBV) and, immune dysregulation (Brenchley and Douek, 2008; Deeks, 2011). ART strongly reduces HIV-1 associated inflammation and immune activation, however, residual immune activation and inflammation is still observed even in effectively treated individuals (Brenchley and Douek, 2008; Deeks, 2011). During HIV-1 infection, increased activation and differentiation of peripheral blood monocytes is also observed (Allen et al., 1990; Thieblemont et al., 1995; Pulliam et al., 1997; Ancuta et al., 2008; Hearps et al., 2012; Williams et al., 2012; Westhorpe et al., 2014; Booiman et al., 2017), which may affect their susceptibility to HIV-1 infection and their ability to migrate into the tissues, thus contributing to HIV-1 pathogenesis.

In the peripheral blood, three monocyte subpopulations can be distinguished based on the expression of the LPS receptor CD14 and the FcγIII receptor CD16. The majority of the peripheral blood monocytes (>85%) are classical monocytes that express high levels of CD14 (CD14++CD16-), whereas CD16 is co-expressed on the intermediate (CD14++CD16+) and non-classical monocytes (CD14+CD16+) (Passlick et al., 1989; Ziegler-Heitbrock et al., 2010; Wong et al., 2011). Murine studies and more recently a humanized mouse study showed that monocyte precursors differentiate first into classical monocytes in bone marrow for a maturation phase of ~ 38 h. This classical monocyte population is retained in the bone marrow and can respond to acute systemic inflammation. Most classical monocytes remain in the circulation for approximately 1–3 day before migration into the tissues. However, a small proportion matures further into intermediate monocytes within the circulation and most of these cells finally mature into non-classical monocytes before leaving the circulation (Sunderkotter et al., 2004; Varol et al., 2007; Yona et al., 2013; Gamrekelashvili et al., 2016; Patel et al., 2017). In HIV-1 infected individuals, an expansion of CD16 expressing monocytes or intermediate monocytes (CD14+CD16+) is evident during all phases of infection, especially in viremic individuals, which is normalized after initiation of ART in at least part of the patients (Allen et al., 1990; Thieblemont et al., 1995; Pulliam et al., 1997; Ancuta et al., 2008; Hearps et al., 2012; Williams et al., 2012; Westhorpe et al., 2014; Booiman et al., 2017). Moreover, monocytes express increased levels of activation markers (e.g., CD163, HLA-DR, CD69), T-cell costimulatory molecules (e.g., CD40 and CD86), adhesion molecules (e.g., CD11b, CD11c, CD91, CX3CR1), and chemokine receptors (e.g., C-C chemokine receptor type 2 (CCR2), CCR5), which is also observed during ART (Pulliam et al., 1997; Ancuta et al., 2008; Hearps et al., 2012; Westhorpe et al., 2014; Booiman et al., 2017).

In the peripheral blood, a small population (<0.1%) of the monocytes harbor replication competent HIV-1 provirus (Furtado et al., 1999; Crowe and Sonza, 2000; Sonza et al., 2001; Shiramizu et al., 2005; Ellery et al., 2007). While classical monocytes are relatively resistant to HIV-1 infection most likely due to low CCR5 expression, CD16+ or intermediate monocytes express higher levels of CCR5 and can be infected by HIV-1 (Ellery et al., 2007; Ancuta et al., 2008). Indeed, CD16+ or intermediate monocytes have been demonstrated to harbor proviral DNA in untreated as well as treated HIV-1 infection (Shiramizu et al., 2005; Jaworowski et al., 2006, 2007; Ellery et al., 2007).

Tissue Macrophages as HIV-1 Reservoirs

Macrophages can be found in all lymphoid as well as non-lymphoid tissues and could therefore serve as a tissue reservoir for HIV-1 (**Figure 1**). In the lamina propria of mucosal tissues like the gastro intestinal tract, penile urethra and vagina, HIV-1 infection of local macrophages has been demonstrated in tissues from healthy individuals *in vitro* (Shen et al., 2009; Ganor et al., 2013), and *in vivo* in HIV-1 infected untreated (Josefsson et al., 2013) and ART treated individuals (Zalar et al., 2010; Josefsson et al., 2013; Yukl et al., 2014; Ganor et al., 2019). Although, HIV-1 DNA has been readily detected in these mucosal tissues, viral RNA has been demonstrated only in vaginal and urethral macrophages (Shen et al., 2009; Ganor et al., 2019). Moreover, replication competent HIV-1 could be isolated from urethral macrophages (Ganor et al., 2019). In contrast, HIV-1 proviral integration could not be detected in macrophages from colon of ART treated HIV-1 infected individuals (Cattin et al., 2019), and therefore it seems unlikely that these cells contribute to the replication competent HIV-1 reservoir (Shen et al., 2011).

In lymphoid tissues like spleen and lymph node, CD4+ T cells (resting memory cells) are the predominant reservoir, however, latently infected resident macrophages have been detected at low frequencies in lymph nodes (Embretson et al., 1993; Orenstein et al., 1997). HIV-1 residing in lymphoid tissues does not genetically differ from variants circulating in the blood, which suggest that there is no compartmentalization of HIV-1 in lymphoid tissue (Ball et al., 1994; van't Wout et al., 1998). However, genetic diversity of HIV-1 and independent viral evolution in monocytes and CD4+ T cells during the course of infection in treated and untreated patients suggests cellular compartmentalization (Fulcher et al., 2004; Llewellyn et al., 2006).

Tissue resident macrophages like Kupffer cells in the liver have been demonstrated to be susceptible to HIV-1 infection, and persistence of HIV-1 in Kupffer cells has been demonstrated in HIV-1 infected individuals on ART (Schmitt et al., 1990; Hufert et al., 1993; Mosoian et al., 2017; Kandathil et al., 2018). However, virus particles produced by Kupffer cells could not be propagated *in vitro* using CEMx174 cells (Kandathil et al., 2018). Phylogenetic analysis of the viral quasi-species showed distinct clustering of viral variants in the liver, evident of compartmentalization of HIV-1 in the liver (Penton and Blackard, 2014). Also alveolar macrophages in the lung have been identified as HIV-1 targets, and HIV-1 persistence as determined by the presence of HIV-1 DNA and HIV-1 RNA has been demonstrated in patients, even during effective ART (Sierra-Madero et al., 1994; Jambo et al., 2014; Cribbs et al., 2015). Analysis of the HIV quasi-species also suggested compartmentalization of macrophage tropic HIV-1 variants in the lung (van't Wout et al., 1998).

The central nervous system (CNS) has been identified as an important viral reservoir. HIV-1 enters the CNS through trafficking of infected cells across the blood brain barrier (BBB) which occurs already shortly after primary infection. Indeed, HIV-1 associated monocyte activation increases migratory abilities of peripheral monocytes by the upregulation of adhesion molecules and chemokine receptors, in response to for instance the monocyte chemoattractant protein 1 (MCP1) (Ancuta et al., 2004; Williams et al., 2013, 2014). In the CNS, HIV-1 persists predominantly in resident macrophages, like microglial cells and perivascular macrophages (Stoler et al., 1986; Wiley et al., 1986; Neuen-Jacob et al., 1993; Fischer-Smith et al., 2001; Cosenza et al., 2002; Ko et al., 2019). Genetic analysis of the viral quasi-species revealed compartmentalized viral replication in the CNS (Korber et al., 1994; van't Wout et al., 1998; Schnell et al., 2009).

Although HIV-1 infection of macrophages has been demonstrated in different tissue, their role as a replication-competent reservoir remains under debate (**Figure 1**). Macrophages are terminally differentiated and their contribution to the viral reservoir is mainly dependent on their lifespan, whereas latently infected resting CD4+ memory T cells which are also long lived cells, contribute to the viral reservoir through homeostatic or antigen specific proliferation. However, recent reports have clearly demonstrated that macrophages can be infected *in vivo* and contribute to the viral reservoir (**Figure 1**; Micci et al., 2014; Clayton et al., 2017; DiNapoli et al., 2017). In SHIV infected rhesus macaques, *in vivo* viral replication was sustained by tissue macrophages upon CD4 T cell depletion (Igarashi et al., 2001). Moreover, HIV-1 persistence in macrophages was confirmed in HIV-1 infected humanized myeloid only mice in which viral rebound was observed in 33% of the animals following treatment interruption (Honeycutt et al., 2017).

Macrophages in HIV-1 Related Comorbidities

Monocytes and macrophages play a crucial role in several HIV-1 related comorbidities including neurological disorders,

Mucosal tissues			
HIV-1:	DNA	RNA	Replication competent
Urethral macrophage	+	+	+
Vaginal macrophage	+	+	+
Intestinal macrophage	+/-		

CNS			
HIV-1:	DNA	RNA	Replication competent
Microglial cell	+	+	+
Perivascular macrophage	+	+	+

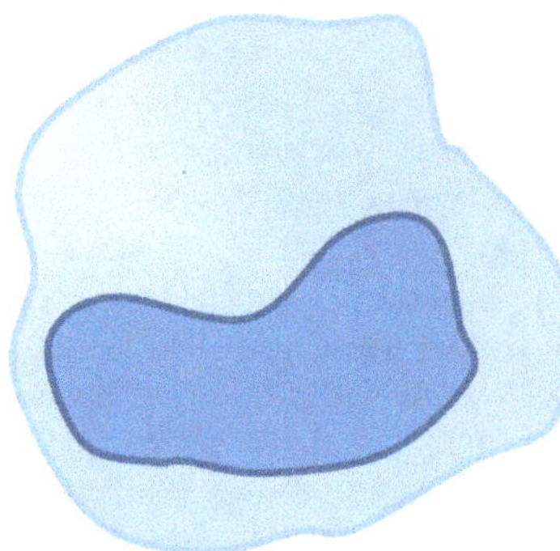

Liver			
HIV-1:	DNA	RNA	Replication competent
Kupffer cell	+	+	-
		<1 year ART	

Lymphoid tissues			
HIV-1:	DNA	RNA	Replication competent
Macrophage	+	+	+
	No compartmentalization		

Lung			
HIV-1:	DNA	RNA	Replication competent
Alveolar macrophage	+	+	+

FIGURE 1 | Tissue distribution and anatomical sanctuaries of latently infected macrophages. Macrophages can be found in all lymphoid as well as non-lymphoid tissues and could therefore serve as a tissue reservoir for Human Immunodeficiency Virus type 1(HIV-1). This figure summarizes findings on HIV-1 latency in monocytes/macrophages *in vivo*, showing anatomical sanctuaries, the presence of HV-1 DNA and RNA and whether the virus was replication competent or not.

atherosclerosis and cardiovascular disease (CVD). HIV-1 associated neurocognitive disorders (HAND) describe a broad range of neurocognitive disorders from asymptomatic neurocognitive impairment, mild neurocognitive disorders (MND), and HIV-1 associated dementia (HAD). Although the use of ART has dramatically reduced development of HAD, milder forms of HAND are still highly prevalent amongst effectively treated HIV-1 infected individuals (Robertson et al., 2007; Heaton et al., 2010; Simioni et al., 2010). In HIV-1 infection, activated peripheral blood monocytes have increased migratory ability (Ancuta et al., 2004; Williams et al., 2013, 2014) and can cross the BBB, and therefore it is generally believed that HIV-1 infected peripheral monocytes are the main source of HIV-1 infection in the brain. Increased monocyte activation, expansion of the activated monocyte population as well as the level of HIV-1 DNA positive monocytes (CD14+/CD16+) have been associated with HIV-1 associated neuroinflammation and HAND (Pulliam et al., 1997, 2004; Shiramizu et al., 2005; Williams et al., 2014; Booiman et al., 2017). The ongoing neuroinflammation caused by monocyte activation and migration, is considered a strong mediator of neuronal damage in HAND. Moreover, persistent HIV-1 replication in resident macrophages and microglial cells of the brain, contributes to the ongoing neuroinflammation and neuronal damage. In particular the viral envelope protein gp120 (Giulian et al., 1993; Meucci et al., 1998; Kaul and Lipton, 1999; Ohagen et al., 1999), the HIV-1 accessory protein

Vpr (Piller et al., 1998; Patel et al., 2000) and the HIV-1 transcriptional activator Tat (Liu et al., 2000; Park et al., 2001; Andras et al., 2003; Song et al., 2003) have been identified to contribute directly or indirectly to neurotoxicity.

HIV-1 associated inflammation and immune activation, both risk factors in the onset of atherosclerosis and CVD, likely contribute to the increased risk of CVD in the HIV-1 infected population (Nou et al., 2016; Triant and Grinspoon, 2017). In early stages of atherosclerosis development, hyperlipidemia [(cholesterol, triglyceride, and low-density lipoprotein (LDL)] promotes the retention and uptake of LDL in the sub-endothelial space (Fogelstrand and Boren, 2012), which results in activation of endothelial cells and smooth muscle cells by the upregulation of adhesion molecules [intercellular adhesion molecule 1 (ICAM-1) and vascular cell adhesion protein 1 (VCAM-1)] and secretion of chemokines [MCP-1 and macrophage colony-stimulating factor (M-CSF)] in the arterial wall (Frostegard et al., 1991). Cells of the immune system expressing the MCP-1 receptor CCR2, are recruited and can infiltrate the lesion (Frostegard et al., 1991). During HIV-1 infection, circulating activated monocytes express increased levels of CCR2, and have an increased ability to migrate in response to MCP1 into the arterial wall (Ancuta et al., 2004; Williams et al., 2013, 2014). These infiltrating monocytes further increase arterial inflammation by cytokine production [interleukin 1ß (IL-1ß) and IL-6] and uptake of (modified) lipoproteins, thereby accelerating atherosclerosis and CVD progression (Hansson, 2005). Indeed, it has been shown that aortic inflammation as measured by ^{18}fluorodeoxyglucose uptake (^{18}F-fluorodexoyglucose Positron Emission Tomography - Computed Tomography: ^{18}F-FDG PET-CT) was increased in effectively treated HIV-1 infected patients to a degree resembling that of uninfected individuals with known CVD. Furthermore, ^{18}F-FDG PET-CT activity was associated with serum levels of soluble CD163 (sCD163), a marker of monocyte/macrophage activation (Subramanian et al., 2012; Tawakol et al., 2017), clearly indicating a role of these cells in accelerated onset of atherosclerosis and CVD in HIV-1 infection.

MECHANISMS OF HIV-1 LATENCY

Macrophage Differentiation and Polarization

Human Immunodeficiency Virus type 1 infection in macrophages and their role in the viral reservoir are difficult to study *in vivo* and therefore *in vitro* culture models have been developed. In these models, monocytes are isolated from peripheral blood and differentiated in an *in vitro* culture system toward monocyte derived macrophages. In addition, different stimuli or cytokines can be added to the cultures in order to obtain phenotypically and functionally distinct macrophages. An advantage of this *in vitro* culture system is that large number of cells are available for analysis and macrophage activation, differentiation, polarization and function can easily be directed. A major disadvantage is that conditions in the culture system are not representative of the local environment in the different tissues, as tissue resident macrophages continuously respond to local signals influencing their function and phenotype resulting in a heterogeneous resident macrophage population. Recently, macrophages isolated from tissues of HIV-1 infected individuals have provided a better insight in the *in vivo* relevance and the state of the viral reservoir (latent, activated) (Zalar et al., 2010; Yukl et al., 2014; Cribbs et al., 2015; Kandathil et al., 2018; Ganor et al., 2019; Ko et al., 2019). However, these materials are difficult to obtain and invasive for the patient.

In vitro, monocytes become highly susceptible to HIV-1 infection upon differentiation into macrophages (Rich et al., 1992; Schuitemaker et al., 1992; Sonza et al., 1996; Peng et al., 2007; Wang et al., 2009; Cobos Jimenez et al., 2012). Macrophages respond to different stimuli in their environment which will shape their physiology and function. Interferon-γ (IFN-γ) and tumor necrosis factor-α (TNF-α) polarize macrophages into an M1 or pro-inflammatory phenotype (Mosser, 2003). M2 or alternatively activated macrophages are generated upon exposure to IL-4 or IL-13 (M2a), immunoglobulin G (IgG) immune complexes and toll-like receptor (TLR) agonists (M2b) or IL-10 or glucocorticoids (M2c) (Mosser, 2003; Mantovani et al., 2004; Mosser and Edwards, 2008; Martinez et al., 2009). Polarization toward a M2a phenotype results in resistance to HIV-1 infection due to restrictions at the level of reverse transcription (Schuitemaker et al., 1992; Montaner et al., 1997; Wang et al., 1998; Cobos Jimenez et al., 2012), whereas polarization toward M1 or M2c inhibits viral replication at a transcriptional or post-transcriptional level (Kootstra et al., 1994; Montaner et al., 1994; Naif et al., 1996; Perez-Bercoff et al., 2003; David et al., 2006; Cassol et al., 2009, 2010; Cobos Jimenez et al., 2012). This data suggests that polarizing signals can induce viral latency in macrophages at both a pre- or post-integration level (**Table 1**).

Mechanisms of Pre-integration Latency

Integration of HIV-1 proviral DNA into the host genome is essential for viral replication. Upon entry into the cell, HIV-1 RNA is reverse transcribed, and subsequently the pre-integration complex (PIC), consisting of viral proteins (integrase, matrix, Vpr, capsid) and double stranded DNA (dsDNA) is assembled (Greene and Peterlin, 2002). The PIC is transported into the nucleus and where the proviral DNA integrates into the host cell genome. Pre-integration latency results when the viral replication cycle is partially or completely blocked at steps prior to integration (**Table 1**). Pre-integration latency is frequently observed in CD4+ T cells but was assumed not to be clinically relevant, because *in vitro* studies demonstrated that the unintegrated proviral DNA only persists for 1 day in these cells (Pierson et al., 2002; Zhou et al., 2005). However, in patients treated with ART, including an integrase inhibitor, unintegrated HIV-1 DNA subspecies where shown to persist in CD4+ T cells and can potentially integrate when integrase inhibitor medication is discontinued (Murray et al., 2014). Moreover, metabolically active macrophages can contain large quantities of unintegrated viral DNA, which remains stable and biologically

TABLE 1 | Cellular/viral factors involved in pre- and post-integration latency.

Latency level	Block in viral replication cycle	Cellular/viral factor involved	Cell type	References
Pre-integration	Reverse transcription	APOBEC3A	Monocytes/macrophages, monocytic cell line	Peng et al., 2007; Miyagi et al., 2008; Berger G. et al., 2011
		Low dNTPs pool	Macrophages, monocytic cell line;	Kootstra et al., 2000; Lahouassa et al., 2012
			CD4+ T cells	Korin and Zack, 1999
		SAMHD1	Macrophages, monocytic cell lines;	Berger A. et al., 2011; Hrecka et al., 2011; Laguette et al., 2011; Lahouassa et al., 2012
			CD4+ T cells	Baldauf et al., 2012; Descours et al., 2012
		PAF1	Monocytes/macrophages;	Liu et al., 2011; Tyagi and Kashanchi, 2012
			CD4+ T cells	Liu et al., 2011; Tyagi and Kashanchi, 2012
	Nuclear import	MX2	Macrophages, monocytic cell lines;	Goujon et al., 2013; Kane et al., 2013; Wang et al., 2017; Buffone et al., 2019
			CD4+ T cells	Goujon et al., 2013; Kane et al., 2013
Post-integration	Transcriptional regulation	SP1, CTIP2, SUV39H1, HDACs, c-myc, and HP1 in complex	Monocytes/macrophages, monocytic cell lines	Rohr et al., 2003; Marban et al., 2005, 2007; du Chene et al., 2007; Desplats et al., 2013; Gray et al., 2016
			CD4+ T cells, T cell lines	du Chene et al., 2007; Jiang et al., 2007
		HDACs, CTIP2, YY1, CBF-1 and LSF in complex	Monocytes/macrophages, monocytic cell line	Buescher et al., 2009
			T cell lines	Margolis et al., 1994; Coull et al., 2000; He and Margolis, 2002; Tyagi and Karn, 2007
		CTIP2, LSD1, and hSET1/WDR5 in complex	Monocytes/macrophages monocytic cell line	Le Douce et al., 2012
		DYRK1A and NFAT	Macrophages	Bol et al., 2011
			CD4+ T cells, T cell line	Booiman et al., 2015; Heffern et al., 2019
		TCF-4, β-catenin, and SMAR1 complex	Monocytes/macrophages, monocytic cell line, PBMCs	Kumar et al., 2008; Henderson et al., 2012; Aljawai et al., 2014
		CTIP2, Tat, and P-TEFb	Monocytes/macrophages, monocytic T cells	Herrmann et al., 1998; Liou et al., 2002; Rice and Herrmann, 2003; Cherrier et al., 2013
			CD4+ T cells	Herrmann et al., 1998; Rice and Herrmann, 2003
	Transcription/Translation	miRNAs (miR-17/92, miR-28, miR-150, miR-223 and miR-382)	Monocytes/macrophages, monocytic cell line	Sung and Rice, 2009; Wang et al., 2009; Lodge et al., 2017
			CD4+ T cells, T cell line, PBMCs	Huang et al., 2007; Triboulet et al., 2007
	Nuclear export	MATR3, PSF and Rev	CD4+ T cells	Sarracino et al., 2018
	Translation	G3BP1	Monocytes/macrophages	Cobos Jimenez et al., 2015
			CD4+ T cell	Cobos Jimenez et al., 2015

active in non-dividing macrophages for up to 2 months (Gillim-Ross et al., 2005; Kelly et al., 2008). Therefore, unintegrated HIV-1 DNA in macrophages may contribute to the viral reservoir in HIV-1 pathogenesis. Indeed, some studies have reported detection of unintegrated HIV-1 DNA in macrophages from patients, mostly in the brain (Pang et al., 1990; Teo et al., 1997). In monocytes/macrophages pre-integration latency could be a consequence of poor reverse transcription efficiency due to a reduced deoxynucleotide triphosphates (dNTP) pool or inhibition of nuclear transport of the PIC as a consequence of low adenosine triphosphate (ATP) levels (Bukrinsky et al., 1992; Kootstra et al., 2000;

Kennedy et al., 2010; Lahouassa et al., 2012). Several cellular factors have been implicated to play a role in the observed restriction in monocytes/macrophages: apolipoprotein B mRNA editing enzyme catalytic subunit 3G (APOBEC3G) and subunit 3A (APOBEC3A), a cellular deoxycytidine deaminases which induces G to A hypermutation and degradation of the HIV-1 genome (Peng et al., 2007; Miyagi et al., 2008; Berger G. et al., 2011); Sterile α-motif/histidine-aspartate domain-containing protein 1 (SAMHD1) which hydrolyses dNTPs into their precursors (nucleosides and triphosphates), in turn reducing the dNTPs pool and thereby limiting the reverse transcriptase activity (Berger A. et al., 2011; Hrecka et al., 2011; Laguette et al., 2011; Lahouassa et al., 2012); Myxovirus-resistance protein 2 (MX2) which inhibits HIV-1 replication post entry by hindering the nuclear accumulation and integration of proviral DNA into host chromatin (Goujon et al., 2013; Kane et al., 2013; Wang et al., 2017; Buffone et al., 2019); and members of the RNA polymerase II-associated factor 1 (PAF1) family, which are expressed in monocytes/macrophages and repress HIV-1 reverse transcription and proviral DNA integration (Liu et al., 2011; Tyagi and Kashanchi, 2012).

Mechanisms of Post-integration Latency

Post-integration latency, which is established after integration of the HIV-1 proviral DNA into the host chromatin, is in contrast to pre-integration latency very stable and only limited by the lifespan of the infected cell. Mechanisms underlying HIV-1 latency *in vivo* are incompletely understood, however, it is a multifactorial phenomenon. Post-integration viral latency may be maintained at a transcriptional or a post-transcriptional level inhibiting HIV-1 protein production and virus formation. Several mechanisms acting at transcriptional and post-transcriptional level inducing HIV-1 latency in CD4+ T cells are well described. However, it is unknown whether these mechanism are also effective in cells of the monocyte/macrophage lineage. Nevertheless, several mechanisms inducing HIV-1 post-integration latency have been described in monocytes/macrophages, including chromatin environment, the absence of transcriptional activation, presence of transcriptional repressors and host antiviral processes. However, not all of these mechanisms are specific for post-integration latency in monocytes/macrophages (**Table 1**).

Site of Integration and Chromatin Remodeling

The host chromatin is organized into heterochromatin which is densely packed and transcriptionally silent and euchromatin which is loosely packed and transcriptionally active (Demeret et al., 2001). After nuclear import a transcriptional co-activator, lens epithelium-derived growth factor (LEDGF)/p75, which interacts with HIV-1 integrase (Vandegraaff et al., 2006; Meehan et al., 2009), targets the PIC mainly to intronic regions of actively transcribed genes (Schroder et al., 2002; Lewinski et al., 2006). The majority of silent HIV-1 provirus is integrated into the euchromatin, which seems paradoxical considering the fact that euchromatin is transcriptionally active (Han et al., 2004). Different mechanisms of transcriptional interference (e.g., steric hindrance, promotor occlusion and enhancer trapping) have been suggested as possible explanation for integrated proviral DNA expression suppression (Lassen et al., 2004; Bisgrove et al., 2005; Taube and Peterlin, 2013). Most of the data on HIV-1 integration and latency has been derived from CD4+ T cells. However, the integration of HIV-1 proviruses has also been studied in primary macrophages. Barr et al., for instance, studied HIV-1 DNA integration sites in primary macrophages by sequencing 754 unique integration sites and found that, similar to CD4+ T cells, HIV-1 also integrates preferentially into the transcriptionally active regions in macrophages (Mack et al., 2003; Barr et al., 2006; Wellensiek et al., 2009). In CD4+ T cells transcription gene silencing is the most favored mechanism for the establishment and maintenance of HIV-1 latency, whether this is also the case in monocytes/macrophages still has to be determined. However, it is well established that chromatin organization and reorganization influences the gene expression and that HIV-1 proviral DNA follows the same rules that apply to host genes. The role of histone H3 lysine 9 trimethylation (H3K9me3) in heterochromatin formation and the transcriptional silencing of integrated HIV-1 has been described (Grewal and Moazed, 2003; Stewart et al., 2005; du Chene et al., 2007; Marban et al., 2007). In addition, there are two nucleosomes, nuc-0 and nuc-1, that interact with the HIV-1 promoter irrespective of the HIV-1 integration site in the host genome. HIV-1 gene transcription from proviral DNA is only possible with the displacement of nuc-1 (Verdin et al., 1993). These studies were performed in the monocytic U1 cell line and collectively suggest that chromatin remodeling is an essential mechanism of HIV-1 latency establishment and regulation in monocytes/macrophages, however, these observations have not yet been confirmed in primary monocytes/macrophages.

Transcriptional Regulation

The integrated HIV-1 proviral DNA is flanked by the long terminal repeats (LTR). The 5′LTR has binding sites for several transcription factors including specificity protein 1 (Sp1), activator protein 1 (AP1), nuclear factor of activated T-cells (NFAT), nuclear factor-κB (NF-κB), c-myc, chicken ovalbumin upstream promoter (COUP), upstream stimulatory factor (USF), CCAAT box transcription factor/nuclear factor 1 (CTF/NF1), T cell factor 1α (TCF-1α) and the glucocorticoid receptor (Verdin et al., 1993). These transcription factors act together to regulate HIV-1 proviral DNA expression (**Table 1**). Sp1, for instance, recruits c-myc to the 5′LTR of proviral DNA, which in turn recruits histone deacetylase 1 (HDAC1). HDAC1 then induces chromatin remodeling, which results in the suppression of HIV-1 gene expression (Jiang et al., 2007; Gray et al., 2016). In addition, HDACs were also shown to be recruited to the proviral promoter by COUP transcription factor interacting protein 2 (CTIP2), Ying Yang 1 (YY1), C-promoter binding factor-1 (CBF-1) and Late SV40 Factor (LSF), thereby promoting the establishment of latency (Coull et al., 2000; He and Margolis, 2002; Tyagi and Karn, 2007; Buescher et al., 2009; Le Douce et al., 2010). Similar results were observed in microglial cells, where CTIP2 has been shown to recruit both HDAC1 and HDAC2 to the 5′LTR of HIV-1 proviral

DNA (Marban et al., 2007). Moreover, CTIP2 also interacts with suppressor of variegation 3–9 homolog 1 (SUV39H1), a methyl transferase for H3K9me3 which subsequently promotes the recruitment of heterochromatin protein 1 (HP1) leading to local heterochromatization and induction of viral latency (Rohr et al., 2003; Marban et al., 2005; du Chene et al., 2007). The role of CTIP2 was further confirmed by Desplats et al. (2013) who analyzed the expression of CTIP2 in postmortem brain tissue of HIV-1 infected patients with HIV-1 encephalitis (HIV-1 DNA and RNA positive) and HIV-1 positive patients with latent HIV-1 (HIV-1 DNA positive and HIV-1 RNA negative) and no detectable HIV-1 (HIV-1 DNA negative) in the CNS. Higher amounts of CTIP2 were observed in the HIV-1 patients with latent HIV-1 in the CNS as compared to the other groups. Notably, CTIP2 was detected in microglial cells of patients with latent HIV-1, indicating that CTIP2 may play an important role in the regulation of viral latency in microglial cells (Desplats et al., 2013). Furthermore, lysine-specific demethylase 1 (LSD1) was found to regulate HIV-1 gene expression in a synergistic way with CTIP2 in microglial cells (Le Douce et al., 2012). LSD1 also assists in the recruitment of CTIP2 and human SET1/WD40-repeat protein 5 (hSET1/WDR5) at the Sp-1 binding sites of the HIV-1 proximal promoter, resulting in increased H3K4 trimethylation (H3K4me3), which in turn represses viral gene expression (Le Douce et al., 2012). This property of LSD1 seems to be highly specific for cells of the monocyte/macrophage lineage.

Recently, the host factor dual specificity tyrosine-phosphorylation-regulated kinase 1A (DYRK1A) was shown to control HIV-1 replication by regulating HIV-1 provirus transcription in macrophages and CD4+ T cells (Bol et al., 2011; Booiman et al., 2015). DYRK1A was shown to regulate HIV-1 transcription via phosphorylation of the NFAT, thereby promoting NFAT translocation from the nucleus to the cytoplasm resulting in decreased viral transcription and latency. Chemical inhibition of DYRK1A resulted in an increased NFAT binding to the viral LTR and reactivating latent provirus (Bol et al., 2011; Booiman et al., 2015).

Furthermore, it has been reported the 5′LTR of the HIV-1 provirus contains multiple T cell factor 4 (TCF-4) binding sites. TCF-4 interacts with β-catenin and the scaffold matrix attachment region-binding protein 1 (SMAR1) at the 5′LTR and this complex has been shown to repress HIV-1 proviral gene expression in different cell types including lymphocytes and astrocytes (Kumar et al., 2008; Henderson et al., 2012). β-catenin/TCF4 signaling has also been demonstrated to regulate HIV-1 replication in cells of the monocyte/macrophage lineage (Aljawai et al., 2014), which makes it plausible that these proteins also play a role in viral latency in these cells (Kumar et al., 2008).

Apart from cellular factors, HIV-1 latency is also influenced by viral factors. HIV-1 replication requires the viral *trans*-activator protein Tat for efficient transcription and virus production. In the absence of Tat, only low level of HIV-1 transcription of mostly short abortive transcripts is observed (Karn, 2011). These short RNA transcripts contain a *trans*-activation response (TAR) element which is the binding site for the Tat protein (Berkhout et al., 1989). The positive transcription elongation factor (P-TEFb) is a critical cellular cofactor of Tat, that favors the generation of complete transcripts from HIV-1 proviral DNA (Price, 2000; Karn, 2011). P-TEFb is composed of a catalytic subunit, cyclin-dependent kinase 9 (CDK9), and a regulatory subunit, cyclin T1 (CycT1) (Herrmann et al., 1998; Rice and Herrmann, 2003; Bres et al., 2008). Tat binds to the TAR region of the RNA transcript and directs P-TEFb to the RNA polymerase II resulting in transcription of full-length HIV-1 RNA (Berkhout et al., 1989; Karn, 2011; Cherrier et al., 2013). The CDK2 can phosphorylate Ser90 on CDK9, thereby assisting in HIV-1 transcription (Ammosova et al., 2005; Breuer et al., 2012). Monocytes express very low levels of CycT1, which transiently increases during differentiation into macrophages. In contrast CDK9 expression levels remain constant in monocytes and macrophages (Liou et al., 2002). The low levels of CycT1 in monocytes result in low functional levels of P-TEFb, resulting in low HIV-1 transcription and thus viral latency in monocytes (Liou et al., 2002).

Post-transcriptional Regulation

Human Immunodeficiency Virus type 1 latency can also be regulated at a post-transcriptional level (**Table 1**). miRNAs are small single stranded non-coding RNAs that can regulate host gene expression at a post-transcriptional level. miRNAs have also been reported to influence HIV-1 gene expression (Huang et al., 2007; Sung and Rice, 2009; Haasnoot and Berkhout, 2011; Narayanan et al., 2011; Lodge et al., 2017). For instance, the miRNA cluster miR-17/92 is actively inhibited by HIV-1 to support efficient replication in different cell types including lymphocytes, monocytes and macrophages (Triboulet et al., 2007). Furthermore, miR-28; miR-150; miR-223; and miR-382 have been demonstrated to target HIV-1 and play a role in HIV-1 susceptibility of monocytes and macrophages. Inhibition of these miRNAs in monocytes results in increased HIV-1 replication, while increased expression of these miRNAs in macrophages decrease of HIV-1 replication (Huang et al., 2007; Wang et al., 2009). These data indicate that miRNAs can play an important role in viral latency in macrophages.

RNA binding host proteins like GTPase-activating protein-(SH3 domain)-binding protein 1 (G3BP1) and the matrix-associated RNA binding protein Matrin 3 (MATR3), have been shown to play a role in the post-transcriptional regulation of HIV-1 latency. G3BP1 is a single-strand-specific endonuclease that binds mRNA transcripts at the 3′UTR inside stress granules to control mRNA translation during cellular stress (Tourriere et al., 2001; Ortega et al., 2010). G3BP1 was shown to interact with HIV-1 mRNA transcripts thus preventing viral protein translation and restricting HIV-1 replication in T cells and macrophages (Cobos Jimenez et al., 2015). Resting T cells and IFNγ and TNFα polarized macrophages, express high levels of G3BP1 indicating a role of this host factor in HIV-1 latency (Cobos Jimenez et al., 2015). MATR3 is a nuclear matrix protein that has the ability to bind DNA and RNA, and is involved in the regulation of gene expression and controls mRNA export from the nucleus. MATR3 also plays an essential role in Rev-mediated export of HIV-1 mRNA transcript from the nucleus (Kula et al., 2011; Yedavalli and Jeang, 2011), through the interaction with the polypyrimidine tract binding protein and associated splicing factor (PSF) and the viral protein Rev (Zolotukhin et al., 2003). Depletion of MATR3 was demonstrated to inhibit nuclear export of Rev responsive element (RRE)-containing viral RNAs resulting in decreased HIV-1 replication (Sarracino et al., 2018). Resting T cells only express low levels of MATR3 which increases upon activation, indicating a role of this protein in the establishment of latency in resting cells (Sarracino et al., 2018). Since MATR3 is also expressed in monocytes (Ancuta et al., 2009), it can be expected that it is also involved in the posttranscriptional regulation of HIV-1 in these cells.

ERADICATION STRATEGIES TARGETING THE TRANSCRIPTIONALLY LATENT RESERVOIR

Even though ART has significantly increased life expectancy of HIV-1 infected individuals, complete eradication of the virus is not achievable without targeting the HIV-1 latent reservoirs. Currently, several therapeutic strategies are explored and early findings suggest that different strategies may be required to eliminate the different cellular viral reservoirs: memory CD4+ T cells which importantly maintain the viral reservoir through homeostatic- or antigen specific proliferation, and long lived cells like macrophages residing in the tissue.

Latency Reversal

The latent viral reservoir is not recognized by the immune system and therefore these cells are not eliminated. The "shock and kill" strategy aims to induce viral protein production by reactivation of the latent HIV-1 provirus to prompt elimination of the infected cells through recognition by the immune system or cell death as a result of viral replication (Matalon et al., 2011; Badley et al., 2013). The "shock and kill" strategy has been investigated primarily using CD4+ T cells and T cell lines. Histone deacetylases (HDACs), for instance, are important for suppression of HIV-1 proviral DNA expression, and several HDAC inhibitors including SAHA, vorinostat, oxamflatin, metacept-1, and metacept-3 (Shehu-Xhilaga et al., 2009; Badley et al., 2013) have been studied for their ability to reactivate and eliminate latently infected cells. Although HDAC inhibitors have shown activity to reactivate HIV-1 from latent reservoirs in patients on ART, no decline in HIV-1 proviral DNA in CD4+ T cells was observed (Archin et al., 2009a,b, 2012, 2017). In contrast, *in vitro* studies in both the monocytic U1 cell line and monocyte-derived macrophages show that HDAC inhibitors not only reactivate and decrease HIV-1 release, but also degrades the viral particles through the canonical autophagy pathway (Shehu-Xhilaga et al., 2009; Rasmussen et al., 2013; Campbell et al., 2015). Moreover, several other compounds targeting different pathways have also been shown to effectively reactivate latent HIV-1, these include protein kinase C agonists (*in vitro* in both monocytic and T cell lines) (e.g., prostratin and ingenols) (Gulakowski et al., 1997; Korin and Zack, 1999; Warrilow et al., 2006; Colin and Van Lint, 2009; Abreu et al., 2014; Jiang et al., 2014, 2015; Darcis et al., 2015), histone methyltransferases inhibitors (*in vitro* in T cell lines and primary monocytes/macrophages and CD4+ T cells from HIV-1 infected ART treated patients) (Greiner et al., 2005; Miranda et al., 2009; Bernhard et al., 2011; Bouchat et al., 2012), anti-miRNA inhibitors (Zhang, 2009), NF-κB activators (Fernandez et al., 2013; Kumar et al., 2013), and cytokine therapy *in vitro* and *in vivo* in CD4+ T cells as well as in cells of the monocyte/macrophage lineage (Chun et al., 1999; Scripture-Adams et al., 2002; Oguariri et al., 2007). Although the efficacy of the majority of these latency reversing agents (LRAs) has been demonstrated, a major hurdle in this treatment approach is that HIV-1 reactivation only occurs in a small subset of the latently infected cells, which might be overcome at least in part by the use of combinations of these LRAs. Furthermore, targeting of cellular factors and pathways identified to be involved in the regulation of HIV-1 latency at a transcription or post-transcription level, such as DYRK1A, β-catenin/TCF4 and Tat/pTEFb (Kumar et al., 2008; Aljawai et al., 2014; Booiman et al., 2015; Wu et al., 2017; Abner et al., 2018; **Table 1**) may improve the efficacy of latency reversal. Moreover, LRAs alone are mostly not sufficient to induce cell death and therefore an effective immune response is essential for the elimination of the reactivated cells and this is lacking in the majority of HIV-1 infected patients. Furthermore, HIV-1 infected macrophages can reside in immune privileged compartments like the CNS and can therefore not be reached by cytotoxic T cells (Shan et al., 2012; Badley et al., 2013).

Apoptosis Inducing Agents

Recently more research is done into the "Prime, Shock, and Kill" method, where latent reservoirs are made sensitive to apoptosis (Prime), followed by reactivation of HIV-1 (Shock) and subsequently leading to cell death of the infected cell (Kill) (Badley et al., 2013). HIV-1 infection of CD4+ T cells and macrophages have been shown to induce an anti-apoptotic gene profile and resistance to apoptosis (Olivares et al., 2009). Several viral proteins have been associated with the resistance to apoptosis (Tanaka et al., 1999; Fernandez Larrosa et al., 2008): Vpr upregulates expression of anti-apoptotic proteins like B-cell lymphoma 2 (Bcl-2) in T cells only, thereby promoting cell survival (Conti et al., 1998). In monocytes/macrophages vpr facilitates HIV-1 replication (Connor et al., 1995). Tat, however, does upregulate Bcl-2 and X-linked inhibitor of apoptosis protein (XIAP) in both monocytes/macrophages and CD4+ T cells (Zhang et al., 2002; Lopez-Huertas et al., 2013); Nef upregulates the anti-apoptotic protein B-cell lymphoma-extra large (Bcl-Xl) in macrophages (Choi and Smithgall, 2004), while nef inactivates the Bcl-2-associated death promoter protein (BAD), a pro-apoptotic Bcl-2 family member, in a phosphoinositide 3-kinase (PI3K)- and p21-activated kinase (PAK)-dependent manner in T cells (Wolf et al., 2001); Furthermore, gp120 has been demonstrated to increase in expression of M-CSF in HIV-1 infected macrophages resulting in the upregulation of anti-apoptotic proteins [e.g., induced myeloid leukemia cell differentiation protein 1 (Mcl-1) and Bcl-2-related protein A1 (Bfl-1)] (Swingler et al., 2007). Therefore, targeting of the HIV-1 induced anti-apoptotic pathways during proviral reactivation strategies may promote cell death of the latently infected cells. Multiple agents targeting the anti-apoptotic pathways including PI3K/Protein kinase B (AKT) inhibitors, Bcl2 inhibitors and second mitochondria-derived activator of caspase (SMAC) mimetics/XIAP inhibitors, are explored for their ability to clear latently infected cells (Busca et al., 2012; Badley et al., 2013; Kim et al., 2018). SMAC mimetics/XIAP inhibitors, for instance, function by sensitizing macrophages to Vpr-induced cell death (Busca et al., 2012). In addition, SMAC mimetics/XIAP inhibitors can trigger transcription of latent proviruses via the non-canonical NF-κB pathway. Furthermore, *in vitro* studies showed that combinations of HDAC inhibitors and SMAC/XIAP mimetics have synergistic activities in T cells (Pache et al., 2015). However, all these compounds do not specifically target the viral reservoir, and targeting of non-HIV-1 infected bystander cells will likely occur especially in ART-treated individuals with increased levels of immune activation, inflammation, and high prevalence of coinfections.

Indeed, an apoptosis resistant gene expression signature was observed in monocytes from HIV-1 infected individuals (Giri et al., 2009). The circulating monocyte population is largely uninfected, which indicates that the anti-apoptotic expression profile may not be due to direct effects of viral infection. Moreover, *in vitro* infection of monocytes/macrophages demonstrated that HIV-1 infection, as well as exposure to HIV-1 or immune modulators increased apoptosis resistance (Giri et al., 2009).

CONCLUDING REMARKS

Despite effective treatment, HIV-1 infected patients are not cured because the virus is not eradicated and latently infected cells persist. The latent viral reservoir mainly resides in resting CD4+ T cells, however, latent HIV-1 proviruses have also been detected in cells of the monocyte/macrophage lineage. HIV-1 infected macrophages can be found in virtually every tissue including the CNS. Viral latency in cells of the monocyte/macrophage lineage can be regulated by diverse molecular mechanisms either at a transcriptional or post-transcriptional level and this is most likely dependent on the activation and differentiation state of these cells. Current eradication strategies rely on reactivation of the latent virus and subsequent kill of the infected cell. The majority of LRAs under study, have been shown to reactivate only small proportions of the latent HIV-1 reservoir, and therefore there is an urgent need for the development of new compounds that target different mechanisms of viral latency both in CD4+ T cells and monocytes/macrophages. Another hurdle is the lack of kill of latently infected cells upon reactivation, which is mainly due to an inefficient antiviral immune response and HIV-1 induced resistance to apoptosis. Apoptosis inducing compounds have been developed for cancer therapy, and their efficacy to specifically induce apoptosis in HIV-1 infected cells is currently under study.

Cure research has mainly focused on CD4+ T cells, because these cells contribute to maintenance pf the viral reservoir through their long lifespan as well as their ability to proliferate under homeostatic conditions or in response to antigens. In contrast, macrophages are terminally differentiated and their contribution to the viral reservoir is mainly dependent on their lifespan and distribution to immune privileged tissues like the CNS. Although, these terminally differentiated latently infected macrophages cannot proliferate, they could be able to spread HIV-1 infection to CD4+ T cells upon reactivation of the virus by LRAs. Therefore, development of eradication strategies combining both novel LRAs and apoptosis inducing agents, targeting either specific cell types or ideally target both latently infected CD4+ T cells and monocytes/macrophages are needed.

AUTHOR CONTRIBUTIONS

ZK and NK wrote and edited the review.

REFERENCES

Abbas, W., Khan, K. A., Kumar, A., Tripathy, M. K., Dichamp, I., Keita, M., et al. (2014). Blockade of BFA-mediated apoptosis in macrophages by the HIV-1 Nef protein. *Cell Death Dis.* 5:e1080. doi: 10.1038/cddis.2014.16

Abner, E., Stoszko, M., Zeng, L., Chen, H. C., Izquierdo-Bouldstridge, A., Konuma, T., et al. (2018). A new quinoline BRD4 inhibitor targets a distinct latent HIV-1 reservoir for reactivation from other "Shock" drugs. *J. Virol.* 92:e2056-17. doi: 10.1128/JVI.02056-17

Abreu, C. M., Price, S. L., Shirk, E. N., Cunha, R. D., Pianowski, L. F., Clements, J. E., et al. (2014). Dual role of novel ingenol derivatives from Euphorbia tirucalli in HIV replication: inhibition of de novo infection and activation of viral LTR. *PLoS One* 9:e97257. doi: 10.1371/journal.pone.0097257

Aljawai, Y., Richards, M. H., Seaton, M. S., Narasipura, S. D., and Al-Harthi, L. (2014). beta-Catenin/TCF-4 signaling regulates susceptibility of macrophages and resistance of monocytes to HIV-1 productive infection. *Curr. HIV Res.* 12, 164–173. doi: 10.2174/1570162x12666140526122249

Allen, J. B., McCartney-Francis, N., Smith, P. D., Simon, G., Gartner, S., Wahl, L. M., et al. (1990). Expression of interleukin 2 receptors by monocytes from patients with acquired immunodeficiency syndrome and induction of monocyte interleukin 2 receptors by human immunodeficiency virus in vitro. *J. Clin. Invest.* 85, 192–199. doi: 10.1172/JCI114412

Ammosova, T., Berro, R., Kashanchi, F., and Nekhai, S. (2005). RNA interference directed to CDK2 inhibits HIV-1 transcription. *Virology* 341, 171–178. doi: 10.1016/j.virol.2005.06.041

Ancuta, P., Kamat, A., Kunstman, K. J., Kim, E. Y., Autissier, P., Wurcel, A., et al. (2008). Microbial translocation is associated with increased monocyte activation and dementia in AIDS patients. *PLoS One* 3:e2516. doi: 10.1371/journal.pone.0002516

Ancuta, P., Liu, K. Y., Misra, V., Wacleche, V. S., Gosselin, A., Zhou, X., et al. (2009). Transcriptional profiling reveals developmental relationship and distinct biological functions of CD16+ and CD16- monocyte subsets. *BMC Genomics* 10:403. doi: 10.1186/1471-2164-10-403

Ancuta, P., Moses, A., and Gabuzda, D. (2004). Transendothelial migration of CD16+ monocytes in response to fractalkine under constitutive and inflammatory conditions. *Immunobiology* 209, 11–20. doi: 10.1016/j.imbio.2004.04.001

Andras, I. E., Pu, H., Deli, M. A., Nath, A., Hennig, B., and Toborek, M. (2003). HIV-1 Tat protein alters tight junction protein expression and distribution in cultured brain endothelial cells. *J. Neurosci. Res.* 74, 255–265. doi: 10.1002/jnr.10762

Archin, N. M., Espeseth, A., Parker, D., Cheema, M., Hazuda, D., and Margolis, D. M. (2009a). Expression of latent HIV induced by the potent HDAC inhibitor suberoylanilide hydroxamic acid. *AIDS Res. Hum. Retrovirus.* 25, 207–212. doi: 10.1089/aid.2008.0191

Archin, N. M., Keedy, K. S., Espeseth, A., Dang, H., Hazuda, D. J., and Margolis, D. M. (2009b). Expression of latent human immunodeficiency type 1 is induced by novel and selective histone deacetylase inhibitors. *AIDS* 23, 1799–1806. doi: 10.1097/QAD.0b013e32832ec1dc

Archin, N. M., Kirchherr, J. L., Sung, J. A., Clutton, G., Sholtis, K., Xu, Y., et al. (2017). Interval dosing with the HDAC inhibitor vorinostat effectively reverses HIV latency. *J. Clin. Invest.* 127, 3126–3135. doi: 10.1172/JCI92684

Archin, N. M., Liberty, A. L., Kashuba, A. D., Choudhary, S. K., Kuruc, J. D., Crooks, A. M., et al. (2012). Administration of vorinostat disrupts HIV-1 latency in patients on antiretroviral therapy. *Nature* 487, 482–485. doi: 10.1038/nature11286

Badley, A. D., Sainski, A., Wightman, F., and Lewin, S. R. (2013). Altering cell death pathways as an approach to cure HIV infection. *Cell Death Dis.* 4:e718. doi: 10.1038/cddis.2013.248

Bain, C. C., Bravo-Blas, A., Scott, C. L., Perdiguero, E. G., Geissmann, F., Henri, S., et al. (2014). Constant replenishment from circulating monocytes maintains the macrophage pool in the intestine of adult mice. *Nat. Immunol.* 15, 929–937. doi: 10.1038/ni.2967

Baldauf, H. M., Pan, X., Erikson, E., Schmidt, S., Daddacha, W., Burggraf, M., et al. (2012). SAMHD1 restricts HIV-1 infection in resting CD4(+) T cells. *Nat. Med.* 18, 1682–1687. doi: 10.1038/nm.2964

Ball, J. K., Holmes, E. C., Whitwell, H., and Desselberger, U. (1994). Genomic variation of human immunodeficiency virus type 1 (HIV-1): molecular analyses of HIV-1 in sequential blood samples and various organs obtained at autopsy. *J. Gen. Virol.* 75(Pt 4), 67–79. doi: 10.1099/0022-1317-75-4-867

Barr, S. D., Ciuffi, A., Leipzig, J., Shinn, P., Ecker, J. R., and Bushman, F. D. (2006). HIV integration site selection: targeting in macrophages and the effects of different routes of viral entry. *Mol. Ther.* 14, 218–225. doi: 10.1016/j.ymthe.2006.03.012

Berger, A., Sommer, A. F., Zwarg, J., Hamdorf, M., Welzel, K., Esly, N., et al. (2011). SAMHD1-deficient CD14+ cells from individuals with Aicardi-Goutieres syndrome are highly susceptible to HIV-1 infection. *PLoS Pathog.* 7:e1002425. doi: 10.1371/journal.ppat.1002425

Berger, G., Durand, S., Fargier, G., Nguyen, X. N., Cordeil, S., Bouaziz, S., et al. (2011). APOBEC3A is a specific inhibitor of the early phases of HIV-1 infection in myeloid cells. *PLoS Pathog.* 7:e1002221. doi: 10.1371/journal.ppat.1002221

Berkhout, B., Silverman, R. H., and Jeang, K. T. (1989). Tat trans-activates the human immunodeficiency virus through a nascent RNA target. *Cell* 59, 273–282. doi: 10.1016/0092-8674(89)90289-4

Bernhard, W., Barreto, K., Saunders, A., Dahabieh, M. S., Johnson, P., and Sadowski, I. (2011). The Suv39H1 methyltransferase inhibitor chaetocin causes induction of integrated HIV-1 without producing a T cell response. *FEBS Lett.* 585, 3549–3554. doi: 10.1016/j.febslet.2011.10.018

Bisgrove, D., Lewinski, M., Bushman, F., and Verdin, E. (2005). Molecular mechanisms of HIV-1 proviral latency. *Expert Rev. Anti Infect. Ther.* 3, 805–814. doi: 10.1586/14787210.3.5.805

Bol, S. M., Moerland, P. D., Limou, S., van Remmerden, Y., Coulonges, C., van Manen, D., et al. (2011). Genome-wide association study identifies single nucleotide polymorphism in DYRK1A associated with replication of HIV-1 in monocyte-derived macrophages. *PLoS One* 6:e17190. doi: 10.1371/journal.pone.0017190

Booiman, T., Loukachov, V. V., van Dort, K. A., van 't Wout, A. B., and Kootstra, N. A. (2015). DYRK1A controls HIV-1 replication at a transcriptional level in an NFAT dependent manner. *PLoS One* 10:e0144229. doi: 10.1371/journal.pone.0144229

Booiman, T., Wit, F. W., Maurer, I., De Francesco, D., Sabin, C. A., Harskamp, A. M., et al. (2017). High cellular monocyte activation in people living with human immunodeficiency virus on combination antiretroviral therapy and lifestyle-matched controls is associated with greater inflammation in Cerebrospinal Fluid. *Open Forum Infect. Dis.* 4:ofx108. doi: 10.1093/ofid/ofx108

Bouchat, S., Gatot, J. S., Kabeya, K., Cardona, C., Colin, L., Herbein, G., et al. (2012). Histone methyltransferase inhibitors induce HIV-1 recovery in resting CD4(+) T cells from HIV-1-infected HAART-treated patients. *AIDS* 26, 1473–1482. doi: 10.1097/QAD.0b013e32835535f5

Brenchley, J. M., and Douek, D. C. (2008). The mucosal barrier and immune activation in HIV pathogenesis. *Curr. Opin. HIV AIDS* 3, 356–361. doi: 10.1097/COH.0b013e3282f9ae9c

Brenchley, J. M., Schacker, T. W., Ruff, L. E., Price, D. A., Taylor, J. H., Beilman, G. J., et al. (2004). CD4+ T cell depletion during all stages of HIV disease occurs predominantly in the gastrointestinal tract. *J. Exp. Med.* 200, 749–759. doi: 10.1084/jem.20040874

Bres, V., Yoh, S. M., and Jones, K. A. (2008). The multi-tasking P-TEFb complex. *Curr. Opin. Cell Biol.* 20, 334–340. doi: 10.1016/j.ceb.2008.04.008

Breuer, D., Kotelkin, A., Ammosova, T., Kumari, N., Ivanov, A., Ilatovskiy, A. V., et al. (2012). CDK2 regulates HIV-1 transcription by phosphorylation of CDK9 on serine 90. *Retrovirology* 9:94. doi: 10.1186/1742-4690-9-94

Buescher, J. L., Martinez, L. B., Sato, S., Okuyama, S., and Ikezu, T. (2009). YY1 and FoxD3 regulate antiretroviral zinc finger protein OTK18 promoter activation induced by HIV-1 infection. *J. Neuroimmune Pharmacol.* 4, 103–115. doi: 10.1007/s11481-008-9139-x

Buffone, C., Kutzner, J., Opp, S., Martinez-Lopez, A., Selyutina, A., Coggings, S. A., et al. (2019). The ability of SAMHD1 to block HIV-1 but not SIV requires expression of MxB. *Virology* 531, 260–268. doi: 10.1016/j.virol.2019.03.018

Bukrinsky, M. I., Sharova, N., Dempsey, M. P., Stanwick, T. L., Bukrinskaya, A. G., Haggerty, S., et al. (1992). Active nuclear import of human immunodeficiency virus type 1 preintegration complexes. *Proc. Natl. Acad. Sci. U.S.A.* 89, 6580–6584. doi: 10.1073/pnas.89.14.6580

Busca, A., Saxena, M., and Kumar, A. (2012). Critical role for antiapoptotic Bcl-xL and Mcl-1 in human macrophage survival and cellular IAP1/2 (cIAP1/2) in resistance to HIV-Vpr-induced apoptosis. *J. Biol. Chem.* 287, 15118–15133. doi: 10.1074/jbc.M111.312660

Campbell, G. R., Bruckman, R. S., Chu, Y. L., and Spector, S. A. (2015). Autophagy induction by histone deacetylase inhibitors inhibits HIV type 1. *J. Biol. Chem.* 290, 5028–5040. doi: 10.1074/jbc.M114.605428

Cassol, E., Cassetta, L., Alfano, M., and Poli, G. (2010). Macrophage polarization and HIV-1 infection. *J. Leukoc. Biol.* 87, 599–608. doi: 10.1189/jlb.1009673

Cassol, E., Cassetta, L., Rizzi, C., Alfano, M., and Poli, G. (2009). M1 and M2a polarization of human monocyte-derived macrophages inhibits HIV-1 replication by distinct mechanisms. *J. Immunol.* 182, 6237–6246. doi: 10.4049/jimmunol.0803447

Cattin, A., Wiche Salinas, T. R., Gosselin, A., Planas, D., Shacklett, B., Cohen, E. A., et al. (2019). HIV-1 is rarely detected in blood and colon myeloid cells during viral-suppressive antiretroviral therapy. *AIDS* 33, 1293–1306. doi: 10.1097/QAD.0000000000002195

Cherrier, T., Le Douce, V., Eilebrecht, S., Riclet, R., Marban, C., Dequiedt, F., et al. (2013). CTIP2 is a negative regulator of P-TEFb. *Proc. Natl. Acad. Sci. U.S.A.* 110, 12655–12660. doi: 10.1073/pnas.1220136110

Choi, H. J., and Smithgall, T. E. (2004). HIV-1 Nef promotes survival of TF-1 macrophages by inducing Bcl-XL expression in an extracellular signal-regulated kinase-dependent manner. *J. Biol. Chem.* 279, 51688–51696. doi: 10.1074/jbc.M410068200

Chun, T. W., Engel, D., Mizell, S. B., Hallahan, C. W., Fischette, M., Park, S., et al. (1999). Effect of interleukin-2 on the pool of latently infected, resting CD4+ T cells in HIV-1-infected patients receiving highly active anti-retroviral therapy. *Nat. Med.* 5, 651–655. doi: 10.1038/9498

Chun, T. W., Nickle, D. C., Justement, J. S., Meyers, J. H., Roby, G., Hallahan, C. W., et al. (2008). Persistence of HIV in gut-associated lymphoid tissue despite long-term antiretroviral therapy. *J. Infect. Dis.* 197, 714–720. doi: 10.1086/527324

Clayton, K. L., Collins, D. R., Lengieza, J., Ghebremichael, M., Dotiwala, F., Lieberman, J., et al. (2018). Resistance of HIV-infected macrophages to CD8(+) T lymphocyte-mediated killing drives activation of the immune system. *Nat. Immunol.* 19, 475–486. doi: 10.1038/s41590-018-0085-3

Clayton, K. L., Garcia, J. V., Clements, J. E., and Walker, B. D. (2017). HIV infection of macrophages: implications for pathogenesis and cure. *Pathog. Immun.* 2, 179–192. doi: 10.20411/pai.v2i2.204

Cobos Jimenez, V., Booiman, T., de Taeye, S. W., van Dort, K. A., Rits, M. A., Hamann, J., et al. (2012). Differential expression of HIV-1 interfering factors in monocyte-derived macrophages stimulated with polarizing cytokines or interferons. *Sci. Rep.* 2:763. doi: 10.1038/srep00763

Cobos Jimenez, V., Martinez, F. O., Booiman, T., van Dort, K. A., van de Klundert, M. A., Gordon, S., et al. (2015). G3BP1 restricts HIV-1 replication in macrophages and T-cells by sequestering viral RNA. *Virology* 486, 94–104. doi: 10.1016/j.virol.2015.09.007

Colin, L., and Van Lint, C. (2009). Molecular control of HIV-1 postintegration latency: implications for the development of new therapeutic strategies. *Retrovirology* 6:111. doi: 10.1186/1742-4690-6-111

Connor, R. I., Chen, B. K., Choe, S., and Landau, N. R. (1995). Vpr is required for efficient replication of human immunodeficiency virus type-1 in mononuclear phagocytes. *Virology* 206, 935–944. doi: 10.1006/viro.1995.1016

Conti, L., Rainaldi, G., Matarrese, P., Varano, B., Rivabene, R., Columba, S., et al. (1998). The HIV-1 vpr protein acts as a negative regulator of apoptosis in a human lymphoblastoid T cell line: possible implications for the pathogenesis of AIDS. *J. Exp. Med.* 187, 403–413. doi: 10.1084/jem.187.3.403

Cosenza, M. A., Zhao, M. L., Si, Q., and Lee, S. C. (2002). Human brain parenchymal microglia express CD14 and CD45 and are productively infected by HIV-1 in HIV-1 encephalitis. *Brain Pathol.* 12, 442–455. doi: 10.1111/j.1750-3639.2002.tb00461.x

Coull, J. J., Romerio, F., Sun, J. M., Volker, J. L., Galvin, K. M., Davie, J. R., et al. (2000). The human factors YY1 and LSF repress the human immunodeficiency virus type 1 long terminal repeat via recruitment of histone deacetylase 1. *J. Virol.* 74, 6790–6799. doi: 10.1128/jvi.74.15.6790-6799.2000

Cribbs, S. K., Lennox, J., Caliendo, A. M., Brown, L. A., and Guidot, D. M. (2015). Healthy HIV-1-infected individuals on highly active antiretroviral therapy harbor HIV-1 in their alveolar macrophages. *AIDS Res. Hum. Retroviruses* 31, 64–70. doi: 10.1089/AID.2014.0133

Crowe, S. M., and Sonza, S. (2000). HIV-1 can be recovered from a variety of cells including peripheral blood monocytes of patients receiving highly active antiretroviral therapy: a further obstacle to eradication. *J. Leukoc. Biol.* 68, 345–350.

Darcis, G., Kula, A., Bouchat, S., Fujinaga, K., Corazza, F., Ait-Ammar, A., et al. (2015). An in-depth comparison of latency-reversing agent combinations in various in vitro and ex vivo HIV-1 latency models identified Bryostatin-1+JQ1 and ingenol-B+JQ1 to potently reactivate viral gene expression. *PLoS Pathog.* 11:e1005063. doi: 10.1371/journal.ppat.1005063

David, A., Saez-Cirion, A., Versmisse, P., Malbec, O., Iannascoli, B., Herschke, F., et al. (2006). The engagement of activating FcgammaRs inhibits primate lentivirus replication in human macrophages. *J. Immunol.* 177, 6291–6300. doi: 10.4049/jimmunol.177.9.6291

Deeks, S. G. (2011). HIV infection, inflammation, immunosenescence, and aging. *Annu. Rev. Med.* 62, 141–155. doi: 10.1146/annurev-med-042909-093756

Deleage, C., Moreau, M., Rioux-Leclercq, N., Ruffault, A., Jegou, B., and Dejucq-Rainsford, N. (2011). Human immunodeficiency virus infects human seminal vesicles in vitro and in vivo. *Am. J. Pathol.* 179, 2397–2408. doi: 10.1016/j.ajpath.2011.08.005

Demeret, C., Vassetzky, Y., and Mechali, M. (2001). Chromatin remodelling and DNA replication: from nucleosomes to loop domains. *Oncogene* 20, 3086–3093. doi: 10.1038/sj.onc.1204333

Descours, B., Cribier, A., Chable-Bessia, C., Ayinde, D., Rice, G., Crow, Y., et al. (2012). SAMHD1 restricts HIV-1 reverse transcription in quiescent CD4(+) T-cells. *Retrovirology* 9:87. doi: 10.1186/1742-4690-9-87

Desplats, P., Dumaop, W., Smith, D., Adame, A., Everall, I., Letendre, S., et al. (2013). Molecular and pathologic insights from latent HIV-1 infection in the human brain. *Neurology* 80, 1415–1423. doi: 10.1212/WNL.0b013e31828c2e9e

DiNapoli, S. R., Ortiz, A. M., Wu, F., Matsuda, K., Twigg, H. L. III, Hirsch, V. M., et al. (2017). Tissue-resident macrophages can contain replication-competent virus in antiretroviral-naive, SIV-infected Asian macaques. *JCI Insight* 2:e91214. doi: 10.1172/jci.insight.91214

du Chene, I., Basyuk, E., Lin, Y. L., Triboulet, R., Knezevich, A., Chable-Bessia, C., et al. (2007). Suv39H1 and HP1gamma are responsible for chromatin-mediated HIV-1 transcriptional silencing and post-integration latency. *EMBO J.* 26, 424–435. doi: 10.1038/sj.emboj.7601517

Ellery, P. J., Tippett, E., Chiu, Y. L., Paukovics, G., Cameron, P. U., Solomon, A., et al. (2007). The CD16+ monocyte subset is more permissive to infection and preferentially harbors HIV-1 in vivo. *J. Immunol.* 178, 6581–6589. doi: 10.4049/jimmunol.178.10.6581

Embretson, J., Zupancic, M., Ribas, J. L., Burke, A., Racz, P., Tenner-Racz, K., et al. (1993). Massive covert infection of helper T lymphocytes and macrophages by HIV during the incubation period of AIDS. *Nature* 362, 359–362. doi: 10.1038/362359a0

Estes, J. D., Kityo, C., Ssali, F., Swainson, L., Makamdop, K. N., Del Prete, G. Q., et al. (2017). Defining total-body AIDS-virus burden with implications for curative strategies. *Nat. Med.* 23, 1271–1276. doi: 10.1038/nm.4411

Fernandez, G., Zaikos, T. D., Khan, S. Z., Jacobi, A. M., Behlke, M. A., and Zeichner, S. L. (2013). Targeting IkappaB proteins for HIV latency activation: the role of individual IkappaB and NF-kappaB proteins. *J. Virol.* 87, 3966–3978. doi: 10.1128/JVI.03251-12

Fernandez Larrosa, P. N., Croci, D. O., Riva, D. A., Bibini, M., Luzzi, R., Saracco, M., et al. (2008). Apoptosis resistance in HIV-1 persistently-infected cells is independent of active viral replication and involves modulation of the apoptotic mitochondrial pathway. *Retrovirology* 5:19. doi: 10.1186/1742-4690-5-19

Fischer-Smith, T., Croul, S., Sverstiuk, A. E., Capini, C., L'Heureux, D., Regulier, E. G., et al. (2001). CNS invasion by CD14+/CD16+ peripheral blood-derived monocytes in HIV dementia: perivascular accumulation and reservoir of HIV infection. *J. Neurovirol.* 7, 528–541. doi: 10.1080/135502801753248114

Fogelstrand, P., and Boren, J. (2012). Retention of atherogenic lipoproteins in the artery wall and its role in atherogenesis. *Nutr. Metab. Cardiovasc. Dis.* 22, 1–7. doi: 10.1016/j.numecd.2011.09.007

Frostegard, J., Haegerstrand, A., Gidlund, M., and Nilsson, J. (1991). Biologically modified LDL increases the adhesive properties of endothelial cells. *Atherosclerosis* 90, 119–126. doi: 10.1016/0021-9150(91)90106-d

Fulcher, J. A., Hwangbo, Y., Zioni, R., Nickle, D., Lin, X., Heath, L., et al. (2004). Compartmentalization of human immunodeficiency virus type 1 between blood monocytes and CD4+ T cells during infection. *J. Virol.* 78, 7883–7893. doi: 10.1128/JVI.78.15.7883-7893.2004

Furtado, M. R., Callaway, D. S., Phair, J. P., Kunstman, K. J., Stanton, J. L., Macken, C. A., et al. (1999). Persistence of HIV-1 transcription in peripheral-blood mononuclear cells in patients receiving potent antiretroviral therapy. *N. Engl. J. Med.* 340, 1614–1622. doi: 10.1056/NEJM199905273402102

Gamrekelashvili, J., Giagnorio, R., Jussofie, J., Soehnlein, O., Duchene, J., Briseno, C. G., et al. (2016). Regulation of monocyte cell fate by blood vessels mediated by Notch signalling. *Nat. Commun.* 7:12597. doi: 10.1038/ncomms12597

Ganor, Y., Real, F., Sennepin, A., Dutertre, C. A., Prevedel, L., Xu, L., et al. (2019). HIV-1 reservoirs in urethral macrophages of patients under suppressive antiretroviral therapy. *Nat. Microbiol.* 4, 633–644. doi: 10.1038/s41564-018-0335-z

Ganor, Y., Zhou, Z., Bodo, J., Tudor, D., Leibowitch, J., Mathez, D., et al. (2013). The adult penile urethra is a novel entry site for HIV-1 that preferentially targets resident urethral macrophages. *Mucosal. Immunol.* 6, 776–786. doi: 10.1038/mi.2012.116

Gillim-Ross, L., Cara, A., and Klotman, M. E. (2005). HIV-1 extrachromosomal 2-LTR circular DNA is long-lived in human macrophages. *Viral Immunol.* 18, 190–196. doi: 10.1089/vim.2005.18.190

Ginhoux, F., Greter, M., Leboeuf, M., Nandi, S., See, P., Gokhan, S., et al. (2010). Fate mapping analysis reveals that adult microglia derive from primitive macrophages. *Science* 330, 841–845. doi: 10.1126/science.1194637

Giri, M. S., Nebozyhn, M., Raymond, A., Gekonge, B., Hancock, A., Creer, S., et al. (2009). Circulating monocytes in HIV-1-infected viremic subjects exhibit an antiapoptosis gene signature and virus- and host-mediated apoptosis resistance. *J. Immunol.* 182, 4459–4470. doi: 10.4049/jimmunol.0801450

Giulian, D., Wendt, E., Vaca, K., and Noonan, C. A. (1993). The envelope glycoprotein of human immunodeficiency virus type 1 stimulates release of neurotoxins from monocytes. *Proc. Natl. Acad. Sci. U.S.A.* 90, 2769–2773. doi: 10.1073/pnas.90.7.2769

Goujon, C., Moncorge, O., Bauby, H., Doyle, T., Ward, C. C., Schaller, T., et al. (2013). Human MX2 is an interferon-induced post-entry inhibitor of HIV-1 infection. *Nature* 502, 559–562. doi: 10.1038/nature12542

Gray, L. R., Cowley, D., Welsh, C., Lu, H. K., Brew, B. J., Lewin, S. R., et al. (2016). CNS-specific regulatory elements in brain-derived HIV-1 strains affect responses to latency-reversing agents with implications for cure strategies. *Mol. Psychiatry* 21, 574–584. doi: 10.1038/mp.2015.111

Greene, W. C., and Peterlin, B. M. (2002). Charting HIV's remarkable voyage through the cell: Basic science as a passport to future therapy. *Nat. Med.* 8, 673–680. doi: 10.1038/nm0702-673

Greenhead, P., Hayes, P., Watts, P. S., Laing, K. G., Griffin, G. E., and Shattock, R. J. (2000). Parameters of human immunodeficiency virus infection of human cervical tissue and inhibition by vaginal virucides. *J. Virol.* 74, 5577–5586. doi: 10.1128/jvi.74.12.5577-5586.2000

Greiner, D., Bonaldi, T., Eskeland, R., Roemer, E., and Imhof, A. (2005). Identification of a specific inhibitor of the histone methyltransferase SU(VAR)3-9. *Nat. Chem. Biol.* 1, 143–145. doi: 10.1038/nchembio721

Grewal, S. I., and Moazed, D. (2003). Heterochromatin and epigenetic control of gene expression. *Science* 301, 798–802. doi: 10.1126/science.1086887

Guadalupe, M., Reay, E., Sankaran, S., Prindiville, T., Flamm, J., McNeil, A., et al. (2003). Severe CD4+ T-cell depletion in gut lymphoid tissue during primary human immunodeficiency virus type 1 infection and substantial delay in restoration following highly active antiretroviral therapy. *J. Virol.* 77, 11708–11717. doi: 10.1128/jvi.77.21.11708-11717.2003

Guadalupe, M., Sankaran, S., George, M. D., Reay, E., Verhoeven, D., Shacklett, B. L., et al. (2006). Viral suppression and immune restoration in the gastrointestinal mucosa of human immunodeficiency virus type 1-infected patients initiating therapy during primary or chronic infection. *J. Virol.* 80, 8236–8247. doi: 10.1128/JVI.00120-06

Gulakowski, R. J., McMahon, J. B., Buckheit, R. W. Jr., Gustafson, K. R., and Boyd, M. R. (1997). Antireplicative and anticytopathic activities of prostratin, a non-tumor-promoting phorbol ester, against human immunodeficiency virus (HIV). *Antiviral Res.* 33, 87–97. doi: 10.1016/s0166-3542(96)01004-2

Gupta, P., Collins, K. B., Ratner, D., Watkins, S., Naus, G. J., Landers, D. V., et al. (2002). Memory CD4(+) T cells are the earliest detectable human immunodeficiency virus type 1 (HIV-1)-infected cells in the female genital mucosal tissue during HIV-1 transmission in an organ culture system. *J. Virol.* 76, 9868–9876. doi: 10.1128/jvi.76.19.9868-9876.2002

Haasnoot, J., and Berkhout, B. (2011). RNAi and cellular miRNAs in infections by mammalian viruses. *Methods Mol. Biol.* 721, 23–41. doi: 10.1007/978-1-61779-037-9_2

Han, Y., Lassen, K., Monie, D., Sedaghat, A. R., Shimoji, S., Liu, X., et al. (2004). Resting CD4+ T cells from human immunodeficiency virus type 1 (HIV-1)-infected individuals carry integrated HIV-1 genomes within actively transcribed host genes. *J. Virol.* 78, 6122–6133. doi: 10.1128/JVI.78.12.6122-6133.2004

Hansen, E. C., Ransom, M., Hesselberth, J. R., Hosmane, N. N., Capoferri, A. A., Bruner, K. M., et al. (2016). Diverse fates of uracilated HIV-1 DNA during infection of myeloid lineage cells. *eLife* 5:e18447. doi: 10.7554/eLife.18447

Hansson, G. K. (2005). Inflammation, atherosclerosis, and coronary artery disease. *N. Engl. J. Med.* 352, 1685–1695. doi: 10.1056/NEJMra043430

Hashimoto, D., Chow, A., Noizat, C., Teo, P., Beasley, M. B., Leboeuf, M., et al. (2013). Tissue-resident macrophages self-maintain locally throughout adult life with minimal contribution from circulating monocytes. *Immunity* 38, 792–804. doi: 10.1016/j.immuni.2013.04.004

He, G., and Margolis, D. M. (2002). Counterregulation of chromatin deacetylation and histone deacetylase occupancy at the integrated promoter of human immunodeficiency virus type 1 (HIV-1) by the HIV-1 repressor YY1 and HIV-1 activator Tat. *Mol. Cell Biol.* 22, 2965–2973. doi: 10.1128/mcb.22.9.2965-2973.2002

Hearps, A. C., Maisa, A., Cheng, W. J., Angelovich, T. A., Lichtfuss, G. F., Palmer, C. S., et al. (2012). HIV infection induces age-related changes to monocytes and innate immune activation in young men that persist despite combination antiretroviral therapy. *AIDS* 26, 843–853. doi: 10.1097/QAD.0b013e328351f756

Heaton, R. K., Clifford, D. B., Franklin, DR Jr., Woods, S. P., Ake, C., Vaida, F., et al. (2010). HIV-associated neurocognitive disorders persist in the era of potent antiretroviral therapy: CHARTER Study. *Neurology* 75, 2087–2096. doi: 10.1212/WNL.0b013e318200d727

Heffern, E. F., Ramani, R., Marshall, G., and Kyei, G. B. (2019). Identification of isoform-selective hydroxamic acid derivatives that potently reactivate HIV from latency. *J. Virus Erad.* 5, 84–91.

Henderson, L. J., Narasipura, S. D., Adarichev, V., Kashanchi, F., and Al-Harthi, L. (2012). Identification of novel T cell factor 4 (TCF-4) binding sites on the HIV long terminal repeat which associate with TCF-4, beta-catenin, and SMAR1 to repress HIV transcription. *J. Virol.* 86, 9495–9503. doi: 10.1128/JVI.00486-12

Herrmann, C. H., Carroll, R. G., Wei, P., Jones, K. A., and Rice, A. P. (1998). Tat-associated kinase, TAK, activity is regulated by distinct mechanisms in peripheral blood lymphocytes and promonocytic cell lines. *J. Virol.* 72, 9881–9888.

Hladik, F., Sakchalathorn, P., Ballweber, L., Lentz, G., Fialkow, M., Eschenbach, D., et al. (2007). Initial events in establishing vaginal entry and infection by human immunodeficiency virus type-1. *Immunity* 26, 257–270. doi: 10.1016/j.immuni.2007.01.007

Ho, D. D., Rota, T. R., and Hirsch, M. S. (1986). Infection of monocyte/macrophages by human T lymphotropic virus type III. *J. Clin. Invest.* 77, 1712–1715. doi: 10.1172/JCI112491

Hoeffel, G., Chen, J., Lavin, Y., Low, D., Almeida, F. F., See, P., et al. (2015). C-Myb(+) erythro-myeloid progenitor-derived fetal monocytes give rise to adult tissue-resident macrophages. *Immunity* 42, 665–678. doi: 10.1016/j.immuni.2015.03.011

Honeycutt, J. B., Thayer, W. O., Baker, C. E., Ribeiro, R. M., Lada, S. M., Cao, Y., et al. (2017). HIV persistence in tissue macrophages of humanized myeloid-only mice during antiretroviral therapy. *Nat. Med.* 23, 638–643. doi: 10.1038/nm.4319

Hrecka, K., Hao, C., Gierszewska, M., Swanson, S. K., Kesik-Brodacka, M., Srivastava, S., et al. (2011). Vpx relieves inhibition of HIV-1 infection of macrophages mediated by the SAMHD1 protein. *Nature* 474, 658–661. doi: 10.1038/nature10195

Huang, J., Wang, F., Argyris, E., Chen, K., Liang, Z., Tian, H., et al. (2007). Cellular microRNAs contribute to HIV-1 latency in resting primary CD4+ T lymphocytes. *Nat. Med.* 13, 1241–1247. doi: 10.1038/nm1639

Hufert, F. T., Schmitz, J., Schreiber, M., Schmitz, H., Racz, P., and von Laer, D. D. (1993). Human Kupffer cells infected with HIV-1 in vivo. *J. Acquir. Immune Defic. Syndr.* 6, 772–777.

Igarashi, T., Brown, C. R., Endo, Y., Buckler-White, A., Plishka, R., Bischofberger, N., et al. (2001). Macrophage are the principal reservoir and sustain high virus loads in rhesus macaques after the depletion of CD4+ T cells by a highly pathogenic simian immunodeficiency virus/HIV type 1 chimera (SHIV): Implications for HIV-1 infections of humans. *Proc. Natl. Acad. Sci. U.S.A.* 98, 658–663. doi: 10.1073/pnas.021551798

Jambo, K. C., Banda, D. H., Kankwatira, A. M., Sukumar, N., Allain, T. J., Heyderman, R. S., et al. (2014). Small alveolar macrophages are infected preferentially by HIV and exhibit impaired phagocytic function. *Mucosal. Immunol.* 7, 1116–1126. doi: 10.1038/mi.2013.127

Jaworowski, A., Ellery, P., Maslin, C. L., Naim, E., Heinlein, A. C., Ryan, C. E., et al. (2006). Normal CD16 expression and phagocytosis of Mycobacterium avium complex by monocytes from a current cohort of HIV-1-infected patients. *J. Infect. Dis.* 193, 693–697. doi: 10.1086/500367

Jaworowski, A., Kamwendo, D. D., Ellery, P., Sonza, S., Mwapasa, V., Tadesse, E., et al. (2007). CD16+ monocyte subset preferentially harbors HIV-1 and is expanded in pregnant Malawian women with *Plasmodium falciparum* malaria and HIV-1 infection. *J. Infect. Dis.* 196, 38–42. doi: 10.1086/518443

Jiang, G., Espeseth, A., Hazuda, D. J., and Margolis, D. M. (2007). c-Myc and Sp1 contribute to proviral latency by recruiting histone deacetylase 1 to the human immunodeficiency virus type 1 promoter. *J. Virol.* 81, 10914–10923. doi: 10.1128/JVI.01208-07

Jiang, G., Mendes, E. A., Kaiser, P., Sankaran-Walters, S., Tang, Y., Weber, M. G., et al. (2014). Reactivation of HIV latency by a newly modified Ingenol derivative via protein kinase Cdelta-NF-kappaB signaling. *AIDS* 28, 1555–1566. doi: 10.1097/QAD.0000000000000289

Jiang, G., Mendes, E. A., Kaiser, P., Wong, D. P., Tang, Y., Cai, I., et al. (2015). Synergistic Reactivation of Latent HIV Expression by Ingenol-3-Angelate, PEP005, Targeted NF-kB Signaling in Combination with JQ1 Induced p-TEFb Activation. *PLoS Pathog.* 11:e1005066. doi: 10.1371/journal.ppat.1005066

Josefsson, L., von Stockenstrom, S., Faria, N. R., Sinclair, E., Bacchetti, P., Killian, M., et al. (2013). The HIV-1 reservoir in eight patients on long-term suppressive antiretroviral therapy is stable with few genetic changes over time. *Proc. Natl. Acad. Sci. U.S.A.* 110, E4987–E4996. doi: 10.1073/pnas.1308313110

Kandathil, A. J., Sugawara, S., Goyal, A., Durand, C. M., Quinn, J., Sachithanandham, J., et al. (2018). No recovery of replication-competent HIV-1 from human liver macrophages. *J. Clin. Invest.* 128, 4501–4509. doi: 10.1172/JCI121678

Kane, M., Yadav, S. S., Bitzegeio, J., Kutluay, S. B., Zang, T., Wilson, S. J., et al. (2013). MX2 is an interferon-induced inhibitor of HIV-1 infection. *Nature* 502, 563–566. doi: 10.1038/nature12653

Karn, J. (2011). The molecular biology of HIV latency: breaking and restoring the Tat-dependent transcriptional circuit. *Curr. Opin. HIV AIDS* 6, 4–11. doi: 10.1097/COH.0b013e328340ffbb

Kaul, M., and Lipton, S. A. (1999). Chemokines and activated macrophages in HIV gp120-induced neuronal apoptosis. *Proc. Natl. Acad. Sci. U.S.A.* 96, 8212–8216. doi: 10.1073/pnas.96.14.8212

Kelly, J., Beddall, M. H., Yu, D., Iyer, S. R., Marsh, J. W., and Wu, Y. (2008). Human macrophages support persistent transcription from unintegrated HIV-1 DNA. *Virology* 372, 300–312. doi: 10.1016/j.virol.2007.11.007

Kennedy, E. M., Gavegnano, C., Nguyen, L., Slater, R., Lucas, A., Fromentin, E., et al. (2010). Ribonucleoside triphosphates as substrate of human immunodeficiency virus type 1 reverse transcriptase in human macrophages. *J. Biol. Chem.* 285, 39380–39391. doi: 10.1074/jbc.M110.178582

Kim, Y., Anderson, J. L., and Lewin, S. R. (2018). Getting the "Kill" into "Shock and Kill": Strategies to Eliminate Latent HIV. *Cell Host Microbe* 23, 14–26. doi: 10.1016/j.chom.2017.12.004

Ko, A., Kang, G., Hattler, J. B., Galadima, H. I., Zhang, J., Li, Q., et al. (2019). Macrophages but not astrocytes harbor HIV DNA in the brains of HIV-1-infected aviremic individuals on suppressive antiretroviral therapy. *J. Neuroimmune Pharmacol.* 14, 110–119. doi: 10.1007/s11481-018-9809-2

Kootstra, N. A., van 't Wout, A., Huisman, H. G., Miedema, F., and Schuitemaker, H. (1994). Interference of interleukin-10 with human immunodeficiency virus type 1 replication in primary monocyte-derived macrophages. *J. Virol.* 68, 6967–6975.

Kootstra, N. A., Zwart, B. M., and Schuitemaker, H. (2000). Diminished human immunodeficiency virus type 1 reverse transcription and nuclear transport in primary macrophages arrested in early G(1) phase of the cell cycle. *J. Virol.* 74, 1712–1717. doi: 10.1128/jvi.74.4.1712-1717.2000

Korber, B. T., Kunstman, K. J., Patterson, B. K., Furtado, M., McEvilly, M. M., Levy, R., et al. (1994). Genetic differences between blood- and brain-derived viral sequences from human immunodeficiency virus type 1-infected patients: evidence of conserved elements in the V3 region of the envelope protein of brain-derived sequences. *J. Virol.* 68, 7467–7481.

Korin, Y. D., and Zack, J. A. (1999). Nonproductive human immunodeficiency virus type 1 infection in nucleoside-treated G0 lymphocytes. *J. Virol.* 73, 6526–6532.

Kula, A., Guerra, J., Knezevich, A., Kleva, D., Myers, M. P., and Marcello, A. (2011). Characterization of the HIV-1 RNA associated proteome identifies Matrin 3 as a nuclear cofactor of Rev function. *Retrovirology* 8:60. doi: 10.1186/1742-4690-8-60

Kumar, A., Abbas, W., and Herbein, G. (2013). TNF and TNF receptor superfamily members in HIV infection: new cellular targets for therapy? *Mediators Inflamm.* 2013:484378. doi: 10.1155/2013/484378

Kumar, A., Zloza, A., Moon, R. T., Watts, J., Tenorio, A. R., and Al-Harthi, L. (2008). Active beta-catenin signaling is an inhibitory pathway for human immunodeficiency virus replication in peripheral blood mononuclear cells. *J. Virol.* 82, 2813–2820. doi: 10.1128/JVI.02498-07

Lafeuillade, A., Chollet, L., Hittinger, G., Profizi, N., Costes, O., and Poggi, C. (1998). Residual human immunodeficiency virus type 1 RNA in lymphoid tissue of patients with sustained plasma RNA of <200 copies/mL. *J. Infect. Dis.* 177, 235–238. doi: 10.1086/517362

Laguette, N., Sobhian, B., Casartelli, N., Ringeard, M., Chable-Bessia, C., Segeral, E., et al. (2011). SAMHD1 is the dendritic- and myeloid-cell-specific HIV-1 restriction factor counteracted by Vpx. *Nature* 474, 654–657. doi: 10.1038/nature10117

Lahouassa, H., Daddacha, W., Hofmann, H., Ayinde, D., Logue, E. C., Dragin, L., et al. (2012). SAMHD1 restricts the replication of human immunodeficiency virus type 1 by depleting the intracellular pool of deoxynucleoside triphosphates. *Nat. Immunol.* 13, 223–228. doi: 10.1038/ni.2236

Lambotte, O., Chaix, M. L., Gasnault, J., Goujard, C., Lebras, P., Delfraissy, J. F., et al. (2005). Persistence of replication-competent HIV in the central nervous system despite long-term effective highly active antiretroviral therapy. *AIDS* 19, 217–218. doi: 10.1097/00002030-200501280-00018

Lassen, K., Han, Y., Zhou, Y., Siliciano, J., and Siliciano, R. F. (2004). The multifactorial nature of HIV-1 latency. *Trends Mol. Med.* 10, 525–531. doi: 10.1016/j.molmed.2004.09.006

Le Douce, V., Colin, L., Redel, L., Cherrier, T., Herbein, G., Aunis, D., et al. (2012). LSD1 cooperates with CTIP2 to promote HIV-1 transcriptional silencing. *Nucleic Acids Res.* 40, 1904–1915. doi: 10.1093/nar/gkr857

Le Douce, V., Herbein, G., Rohr, O., and Schwartz, C. (2010). Molecular mechanisms of HIV-1 persistence in the monocyte-macrophage lineage. *Retrovirology* 7:32. doi: 10.1186/1742-4690-7-32

Lewinski, M. K., Yamashita, M., Emerman, M., Ciuffi, A., Marshall, H., Crawford, G., et al. (2006). Retroviral DNA integration: viral and cellular determinants of target-site selection. *PLoS Pathog.* 2:e60. doi: 10.1371/journal.ppat.0020060

Liou, L. Y., Herrmann, C. H., and Rice, A. P. (2002). Transient induction of cyclin T1 during human macrophage differentiation regulates human immunodeficiency virus type 1 Tat transactivation function. *J. Virol.* 76, 10579–10587. doi: 10.1128/jvi.76.21.10579-10587.2002

Liu, L., Oliveira, N. M., Cheney, K. M., Pade, C., Dreja, H., Bergin, A. M., et al. (2011). A whole genome screen for HIV restriction factors. *Retrovirology* 8:94. doi: 10.1186/1742-4690-8-94

Liu, Y., Jones, M., Hingtgen, C. M., Bu, G., Laribee, N., Tanzi, R. E., et al. (2000). Uptake of HIV-1 tat protein mediated by low-density lipoprotein receptor-related protein disrupts the neuronal metabolic balance of the receptor ligands. *Nat. Med.* 6, 1380–1387. doi: 10.1038/82199

Llewellyn, N., Zioni, R., Zhu, H., Andrus, T., Xu, Y., Corey, L., et al. (2006). Continued evolution of HIV-1 circulating in blood monocytes with antiretroviral therapy: genetic analysis of HIV-1 in monocytes and CD4+ T cells of patients with discontinued therapy. *J. Leukoc. Biol.* 80, 1118–1126. doi: 10.1189/jlb.0306144

Lodge, R., Ferreira Barbosa, J. A., Lombard-Vadnais, F., Gilmore, J. C., Deshiere, A., Gosselin, A., et al. (2017). Host MicroRNAs-221 and -222 inhibit HIV-1 entry in macrophages by targeting the CD4 viral receptor. *Cell Rep.* 21, 141–153. doi: 10.1016/j.celrep.2017.09.030

Lopez-Huertas, M. R., Mateos, E., Sanchez Del Cojo, M., Gomez-Esquer, F., Diaz-Gil, G., Rodriguez-Mora, S., et al. (2013). The presence of HIV-1 Tat protein second exon delays fas protein-mediated apoptosis in CD4+ T lymphocytes: a potential mechanism for persistent viral production. *J. Biol. Chem.* 288, 7626–7644. doi: 10.1074/jbc.M112.408294

Mack, K. D., Jin, X., Yu, S., Wei, R., Kapp, L., Green, C., et al. (2003). HIV insertions within and proximal to host cell genes are a common finding in tissues containing high levels of HIV DNA and macrophage-associated p24 antigen expression. *J. Acquir. Immune Defic. Syndr.* 33, 308–320. doi: 10.1097/00126334-200307010-00004

Mantovani, A., Sica, A., Sozzani, S., Allavena, P., Vecchi, A., and Locati, M. (2004). The chemokine system in diverse forms of macrophage activation and polarization. *Trends Immunol.* 25, 677–686. doi: 10.1016/j.it.2004.09.015

Marban, C., Redel, L., Suzanne, S., Van Lint, C., Lecestre, D., Chasserot-Golaz, S., et al. (2005). COUP-TF interacting protein 2 represses the initial phase of HIV-1 gene transcription in human microglial cells. *Nucleic Acids Res.* 33, 2318–2331. doi: 10.1093/nar/gki529

Marban, C., Suzanne, S., Dequiedt, F., de Walque, S., Redel, L., Van Lint, C., et al. (2007). Recruitment of chromatin-modifying enzymes by CTIP2 promotes HIV-1 transcriptional silencing. *EMBO J.* 26, 412–423. doi: 10.1038/sj.emboj.7601516

Margolis, D. M., Somasundaran, M., and Green, M. R. (1994). Human transcription factor YY1 represses human immunodeficiency virus type 1 transcription and virion production. *J. Virol.* 68, 905–910.

Martinez, F. O., Helming, L., and Gordon, S. (2009). Alternative activation of macrophages: an immunologic functional perspective. *Annu. Rev. Immunol.* 27, 451–483. doi: 10.1146/annurev.immunol.021908.132532

Mass, E., Ballesteros, I., Farlik, M., Halbritter, F., Gunther, P., Crozet, L., et al. (2016). Specification of tissue-resident macrophages during organogenesis. *Science* 353:aaf4238. doi: 10.1126/science.aaf4238

Matalon, S., Rasmussen, T. A., and Dinarello, C. A. (2011). Histone deacetylase inhibitors for purging HIV-1 from the latent reservoir. *Mol. Med.* 17, 466–472. doi: 10.2119/molmed.2011.00076

Mayer, K. H., Boswell, S., Goldstein, R., Lo, W., Xu, C., Tucker, L., et al. (1999). Persistence of human immunodeficiency virus in semen after adding indinavir to combination antiretroviral therapy. *Clin. Infect. Dis.* 28, 1252–1259. doi: 10.1086/514775

Meehan, A. M., Saenz, D. T., Morrison, J. H., Garcia-Rivera, J. A., Peretz, M., Llano, M., et al. (2009). LEDGF/p75 proteins with alternative chromatin tethers are functional HIV-1 cofactors. *PLoS Pathog.* 5:e1000522. doi: 10.1371/journal.ppat.1000522

Meucci, O., Fatatis, A., Simen, A. A., Bushell, T. J., Gray, P. W., and Miller, R. J. (1998). Chemokines regulate hippocampal neuronal signaling and gp120 neurotoxicity. *Proc. Natl. Acad. Sci. U.S.A.* 95, 14500–14505. doi: 10.1073/pnas.95.24.14500

Micci, L., Alvarez, X., Iriele, R. I., Ortiz, A. M., Ryan, E. S., McGary, C. S., et al. (2014). CD4 depletion in SIV-infected macaques results in macrophage and microglia infection with rapid turnover of infected cells. *PLoS Pathog.* 10:e1004467. doi: 10.1371/journal.ppat.1004467

Miranda, T. B., Cortez, C. C., Yoo, C. B., Liang, G., Abe, M., Kelly, T. K., et al. (2009). DZNep is a global histone methylation inhibitor that reactivates developmental genes not silenced by DNA methylation. *Mol. Cancer Ther.* 8, 1579–1588. doi: 10.1158/1535-7163.MCT-09-0013

Miyagi, E., Schwartzkopff, F., Plishka, R., Buckler-White, A., Clouse, K. A., and Strebel, K. (2008). APOBEC3G-independent reduction in virion infectivity during long-term HIV-1 replication in terminally differentiated macrophages. *Virology* 379, 266–274. doi: 10.1016/j.virol.2008.06.033

Montaner, L. J., Bailer, R. T., and Gordon, S. (1997). IL-13 acts on macrophages to block the completion of reverse transcription, inhibit virus production, and reduce virus infectivity. *J. Leukoc. Biol.* 62, 126–132. doi: 10.1002/jlb.62.1.126

Montaner, L. J., Griffin, P., and Gordon, S. (1994). Interleukin-10 inhibits initial reverse transcription of human immunodeficiency virus type 1 and mediates a virostatic latent state in primary blood-derived human macrophages in vitro. *J. Gen. Virol.* 75(Pt 12), 3393–3400. doi: 10.1099/0022-1317-75-12-3393

Mosoian, A., Zhang, L., Hong, F., Cunyat, F., Rahman, A., Bhalla, R., et al. (2017). Frontline science: HIV infection of Kupffer cells results in an amplified proinflammatory response to LPS. *J. Leukoc. Biol.* 101, 1083–1090. doi: 10.1189/jlb.3HI0516-242R

Mosser, D. M. (2003). The many faces of macrophage activation. *J. Leukoc. Biol.* 73, 209–212. doi: 10.1189/jlb.0602325

Mosser, D. M., and Edwards, J. P. (2008). Exploring the full spectrum of macrophage activation. *Nat. Rev. Immunol.* 8, 958–969. doi: 10.1038/nri2448

Murray, J. M., Zaunders, J. J., McBride, K. L., Xu, Y., Bailey, M., Suzuki, K., et al. (2014). HIV DNA subspecies persist in both activated and resting memory CD4+ T cells during antiretroviral therapy. *J. Virol.* 88, 3516–3526. doi: 10.1128/JVI.03331-13

Naif, H. M., Chang, J., Ho-Shon, M., Li, S., and Cunningham, A. L. (1996). Inhibition of human immunodeficiency virus replication in differentiating monocytes by interleukin 10 occurs in parallel with inhibition of cellular RNA expression. *AIDS Res. Hum. Retroviruses* 12, 1237–1245. doi: 10.1089/aid.1996.12.1237

Narayanan, A., Kehn-Hall, K., Bailey, C., and Kashanchi, F. (2011). Analysis of the roles of HIV-derived microRNAs. *Expert Opin. Biol. Ther.* 11, 17–29. doi: 10.1517/14712598.2011.540564

Neuen-Jacob, E., Arendt, G., Wendtland, B., Jacob, B., Schneeweis, M., and Wechsler, W. (1993). Frequency and topographical distribution of CD68-positive macrophages and HIV-1 core proteins in HIV-associated brain lesions. *Clin. Neuropathol.* 12, 315–324.

Nicholson, J. K., Cross, G. D., Callaway, C. S., and McDougal, J. S. (1986). In vitro infection of human monocytes with human T lymphotropic virus type III/lymphadenopathy-associated virus (HTLV-III/LAV). *J. Immunol.* 137, 323–329.

Nou, E., Lo, J., and Grinspoon, S. K. (2016). Inflammation, immune activation, and cardiovascular disease in HIV. *AIDS* 30, 1495–1509. doi: 10.1097/QAD.0000000000001109

Oguariri, R. M., Brann, T. W., and Imamichi, T. (2007). Hydroxyurea and interleukin-6 synergistically reactivate HIV-1 replication in a latently infected promonocytic cell line via SP1/SP3 transcription factors. *J. Biol. Chem.* 282, 3594–3604. doi: 10.1074/jbc.M608150200

Ohagen, A., Ghosh, S., He, J., Huang, K., Chen, Y., Yuan, M., et al. (1999). Apoptosis induced by infection of primary brain cultures with diverse human immunodeficiency virus type 1 isolates: evidence for a role of the envelope. *J. Virol.* 73, 897–906.

Olivares, I., Ballester, A., Lombardia, L., Dominguez, O., and Lopez-Galindez, C. (2009). Human immunodeficiency virus type 1 chronic infection is associated with different gene expression in MT-4, H9 and U937 cell lines. *Virus Res.* 139, 22–31. doi: 10.1016/j.virusres.2008.09.010

Orenstein, J. M., Fox, C., and Wahl, S. M. (1997). Macrophages as a source of HIV during opportunistic infections. *Science* 276, 1857–1861. doi: 10.1126/science.276.5320.1857

Ortega, A. D., Willers, I. M., Sala, S., and Cuezva, J. M. (2010). Human G3BP1 interacts with beta-F1-ATPase mRNA and inhibits its translation. *J. Cell Sci.* 123(Pt 16), 2685–2696. doi: 10.1242/jcs.065920

Pache, L., Dutra, M. S., Spivak, A. M., Marlett, J. M., Murry, J. P., Hwang, Y., et al. (2015). BIRC2/cIAP1 is a negative regulator of HIV-1 transcription and can be targeted by smac mimetics to promote reversal of viral latency. *Cell Host Microbe* 18, 345–353. doi: 10.1016/j.chom.2015.08.009

Pang, S., Koyanagi, Y., Miles, S., Wiley, C., Vinters, H. V., and Chen, I. S. (1990). High levels of unintegrated HIV-1 DNA in brain tissue of AIDS dementia patients. *Nature* 343, 85–89. doi: 10.1038/343085a0

Park, I. W., Wang, J. F., and Groopman, J. E. (2001). HIV-1 Tat promotes monocyte chemoattractant protein-1 secretion followed by transmigration of monocytes. *Blood* 97, 352–358. doi: 10.1182/blood.v97.2.352

Passlick, B., Flieger, D., and Ziegler-Heitbrock, H. W. (1989). Identification and characterization of a novel monocyte subpopulation in human peripheral blood. *Blood* 74, 2527–2534. doi: 10.1182/blood.v74.7.2527.2527

Patel, A. A., Zhang, Y., Fullerton, J. N., Boelen, L., Rongvaux, A., Maini, A. A., et al. (2017). The fate and lifespan of human monocyte subsets in steady state and systemic inflammation. *J. Exp. Med.* 214, 1913–1923. doi: 10.1084/jem.20170355

Patel, C. A., Mukhtar, M., and Pomerantz, R. J. (2000). Human immunodeficiency virus type 1 Vpr induces apoptosis in human neuronal cells. *J. Virol.* 74, 9717–9726. doi: 10.1128/jvi.74.20.9717-9726.2000

Peng, G., Greenwell-Wild, T., Nares, S., Jin, W., Lei, K. J., Rangel, Z. G., et al. (2007). Myeloid differentiation and susceptibility to HIV-1 are linked to APOBEC3 expression. *Blood* 110, 393–400. doi: 10.1182/blood-2006-10-051763

Penton, P. K., and Blackard, J. T. (2014). Analysis of HIV quasispecies suggests compartmentalization in the liver. *AIDS Res. Hum. Retroviruses* 30, 394–402. doi: 10.1089/AID.2013.0146

Perez-Bercoff, D., David, A., Sudry, H., Barre-Sinoussi, F., and Pancino, G. (2003). Fcgamma receptor-mediated suppression of human immunodeficiency virus type 1 replication in primary human macrophages. *J. Virol.* 77, 4081–4094. doi: 10.1128/jvi.77.7.4081-4094.2003

Pierson, T. C., Zhou, Y., Kieffer, T. L., Ruff, C. T., Buck, C., and Siliciano, R. F. (2002). Molecular characterization of preintegration latency in human immunodeficiency virus type 1 infection. *J. Virol.* 76, 8518–8531. doi: 10.1128/jvi.76.17.8518-8513.2002

Piller, S. C., Jans, P., Gage, P. W., and Jans, D. A. (1998). Extracellular HIV-1 virus protein R causes a large inward current and cell death in cultured hippocampal neurons: implications for AIDS pathology. *Proc. Natl. Acad. Sci. U.S.A.* 95, 4595–4600. doi: 10.1073/pnas.95.8.4595

Poles, M. A., Boscardin, W. J., Elliott, J., Taing, P., Fuerst, M. M., McGowan, I., et al. (2006). Lack of decay of HIV-1 in gut-associated lymphoid tissue reservoirs in maximally suppressed individuals. *J. Acquir. Immune Defic. Syndr.* 43, 65–68. doi: 10.1097/01.qai.0000230524.71717.14

Price, D. H. (2000). P-TEFb, a cyclin-dependent kinase controlling elongation by RNA polymerase II. *Mol. Cell Biol.* 20, 2629–2634. doi: 10.1128/mcb.20.8.2629-2634.2000

Pulliam, L., Gascon, R., Stubblebine, M., McGuire, D., and McGrath, M. S. (1997). Unique monocyte subset in patients with AIDS dementia. *Lancet* 349, 692–695. doi: 10.1016/S0140-6736(96)10178-1

Pulliam, L., Sun, B., and Rempel, H. (2004). Invasive chronic inflammatory monocyte phenotype in subjects with high HIV-1 viral load. *J. Neuroimmunol.* 157, 93–98. doi: 10.1016/j.jneuroim.2004.08.039

Rasmussen, T. A., Schmeltz Sogaard, O., Brinkmann, C., Wightman, F., Lewin, S. R., Melchjorsen, J., et al. (2013). Comparison of HDAC inhibitors in clinical development: effect on HIV production in latently infected cells and T-cell activation. *Hum. Vaccin. Immunother.* 9, 993–1001. doi: 10.4161/hv.23800

Rice, A. P., and Herrmann, C. H. (2003). Regulation of TAK/P-TEFb in CD4+ T lymphocytes and macrophages. *Curr. HIV Res.* 1, 395–404. doi: 10.2174/1570162033485159

Rich, E. A., Chen, I. S., Zack, J. A., Leonard, M. L., and O'Brien, W. A. (1992). Increased susceptibility of differentiated mononuclear phagocytes to productive infection with human immunodeficiency virus-1 (HIV-1). *J. Clin. Invest.* 89, 176–183. doi: 10.1172/JCI115559

Robertson, K. R., Smurzynski, M., Parsons, T. D., Wu, K., Bosch, R. J., Wu, J., et al. (2007). The prevalence and incidence of neurocognitive impairment in the HAART era. *AIDS* 21, 1915–1921. doi: 10.1097/QAD.0b013e32828e4e27

Rohr, O., Lecestre, D., Chasserot-Golaz, S., Marban, C., Avram, D., Aunis, D., et al. (2003). Recruitment of Tat to heterochromatin protein HP1 via interaction with CTIP2 inhibits human immunodeficiency virus type 1 replication in microglial cells. *J. Virol.* 77, 5415–5427. doi: 10.1128/jvi.77.9.5415-5427.2003

Rose, R., Lamers, S. L., Nolan, D. J., Maidji, E., Faria, N. R., Pybus, O. G., et al. (2016). HIV maintains an evolving and dispersed population in multiple tissues during suppressive combined antiretroviral therapy in individuals with cancer. *J. Virol.* 90, 8984–8993. doi: 10.1128/JVI.00684-16

Sarracino, A., Gharu, L., Kula, A., Pasternak, A. O., Avettand-Fenoel, V., Rouzioux, C., et al. (2018). Posttranscriptional Regulation of HIV-1 Gene Expression during Replication and Reactivation from Latency by Nuclear Matrix Protein MATR3. *mBio* 9:e2158-18. doi: 10.1128/mBio.02158-18

Schmitt, M. P., Gendrault, J. L., Schweitzer, C., Steffan, A. M., Beyer, C., Royer, C., et al. (1990). Permissivity of primary cultures of human Kupffer cells for HIV-1. *AIDS Res. Hum. Retroviruses* 6, 987–991. doi: 10.1089/aid.1990.6.987

Schnell, G., Spudich, S., Harrington, P., Price, R. W., and Swanstrom, R. (2009). Compartmentalized human immunodeficiency virus type 1 originates from long-lived cells in some subjects with HIV-1-associated dementia. *PLoS Pathog.* 5:e1000395. doi: 10.1371/journal.ppat.1000395

Schroder, A. R., Shinn, P., Chen, H., Berry, C., Ecker, J. R., and Bushman, F. (2002). HIV-1 integration in the human genome favors active genes and local hotspots. *Cell* 110, 521–529. doi: 10.1016/s0092-8674(02)00864-4

Schuitemaker, H., Kootstra, N. A., Koppelman, M. H., Bruisten, S. M., Huisman, H. G., Tersmette, M., et al. (1992). Proliferation-dependent HIV-1 infection of monocytes occurs during differentiation into macrophages. *J. Clin. Invest.* 89, 1154–1160. doi: 10.1172/JCI115697

Schulz, C., Gomez Perdiguero, E., Chorro, L., Szabo-Rogers, H., Cagnard, N., Kierdorf, K., et al. (2012). A lineage of myeloid cells independent of Myb and hematopoietic stem cells. *Science* 336, 86–90. doi: 10.1126/science.1219179

Scripture-Adams, D. D., Brooks, D. G., Korin, Y. D., and Zack, J. A. (2002). Interleukin-7 induces expression of latent human immunodeficiency virus type 1 with minimal effects on T-cell phenotype. *J. Virol.* 76, 13077–13082. doi: 10.1128/jvi.76.24.13077-13082.2002

Shan, L., Deng, K., Shroff, N. S., Durand, C. M., Rabi, S. A., Yang, H. C., et al. (2012). Stimulation of HIV-1-specific cytolytic T lymphocytes facilitates elimination of latent viral reservoir after virus reactivation. *Immunity* 36, 491–501. doi: 10.1016/j.immuni.2012.01.014

Shehu-Xhilaga, M., Rhodes, D., Wightman, F., Liu, H. B., Solomon, A., Saleh, S., et al. (2009). The novel histone deacetylase inhibitors metacept-1 and metacept-3 potently increase HIV-1 transcription in latently infected cells. *AIDS* 23, 2047–2050. doi: 10.1097/QAD.0b013e328330342c

Shen, R., Meng, G., Ochsenbauer, C., Clapham, P. R., Grams, J., Novak, L., et al. (2011). Stromal down-regulation of macrophage CD4/CCR5 expression and NF-kappaB activation mediates HIV-1 non-permissiveness in intestinal macrophages. *PLoS Pathog.* 7:e1002060. doi: 10.1371/journal.ppat.1002060

Shen, R., Richter, H. E., Clements, R. H., Novak, L., Huff, K., Bimczok, D., et al. (2009). Macrophages in vaginal but not intestinal mucosa are monocyte-like and permissive to human immunodeficiency virus type 1 infection. *J. Virol.* 83, 3258–3267. doi: 10.1128/JVI.01796-08

Shiramizu, B., Gartner, S., Williams, A., Shikuma, C., Ratto-Kim, S., Watters, M., et al. (2005). Circulating proviral HIV DNA and HIV-associated dementia. *AIDS* 19, 45–52. doi: 10.1097/00002030-200501030-00005

Sierra-Madero, J. G., Toossi, Z., Hom, D. L., Finegan, C. K., Hoenig, E., and Rich, E. A. (1994). Relationship between load of virus in alveolar macrophages from human immunodeficiency virus type 1-infected persons, production of cytokines, and clinical status. *J. Infect. Dis.* 169, 18–27. doi: 10.1093/infdis/169.1.18

Simioni, S., Cavassini, M., Annoni, J. M., Rimbault Abraham, A., Bourquin, I., Schiffer, V., et al. (2010). Cognitive dysfunction in HIV patients despite long-standing suppression of viremia. *AIDS* 24, 1243–1250. doi: 10.1097/QAD.0b013e3283354a7b

Solas, C., Lafeuillade, A., Halfon, P., Chadapaud, S., Hittinger, G., and Lacarelle, B. (2003). Discrepancies between protease inhibitor concentrations and viral load in reservoirs and sanctuary sites in human immunodeficiency virus-infected patients. *Antimicrob. Agents Chemother.* 47, 238–243. doi: 10.1128/aac.47.1.238-243.2003

Song, L., Nath, A., Geiger, J. D., Moore, A., and Hochman, S. (2003). Human immunodeficiency virus type 1 Tat protein directly activates neuronal N-methyl-D-aspartate receptors at an allosteric zinc-sensitive site. *J. Neurovirol.* 9, 399–403. doi: 10.1080/13550280390201704

Sonza, S., Maerz, A., Deacon, N., Meanger, J., Mills, J., and Crowe, S. (1996). Human immunodeficiency virus type 1 replication is blocked prior to reverse transcription and integration in freshly isolated peripheral blood monocytes. *J. Virol.* 70, 3863–3869.

Sonza, S., Mutimer, H. P., Oelrichs, R., Jardine, D., Harvey, K., Dunne, A., et al. (2001). Monocytes harbour replication-competent, non-latent HIV-1 in patients on highly active antiretroviral therapy. *AIDS* 15, 17–22. doi: 10.1097/00002030-200101050-00005

Stewart, M. D., Li, J., and Wong, J. (2005). Relationship between histone H3 lysine 9 methylation, transcription repression, and heterochromatin protein 1 recruitment. *Mol. Cell Biol.* 25, 2525–2538. doi: 10.1128/MCB.25.7.2525-2538.2005

Stoler, M. H., Eskin, T. A., Benn, S., Angerer, R. C., and Angerer, L. M. (1986). Human T-cell lymphotropic virus type III infection of the central nervous system. A preliminary in situ analysis. *JAMA* 256, 2360–2364. doi: 10.1001/jama.256.17.2360

Subramanian, S., Tawakol, A., Burdo, T. H., Abbara, S., Wei, J., Vijayakumar, J., et al. (2012). Arterial inflammation in patients with HIV. *JAMA* 308, 379–386. doi: 10.1001/jama.2012.6698

Sunderkotter, C., Nikolic, T., Dillon, M. J., Van Rooijen, N., Stehling, M., Drevets, D. A., et al. (2004). Subpopulations of mouse blood monocytes differ in maturation stage and inflammatory response. *J. Immunol.* 172, 4410–4417. doi: 10.4049/jimmunol.172.7.4410

Sung, T. L., and Rice, A. P. (2009). miR-198 inhibits HIV-1 gene expression and replication in monocytes and its mechanism of action appears to involve repression of cyclin T1. *PLoS Pathog.* 5:e1000263. doi: 10.1371/journal.ppat.1000263

Swingler, S., Mann, A. M., Zhou, J., Swingler, C., and Stevenson, M. (2007). Apoptotic killing of HIV-1-infected macrophages is subverted by the viral envelope glycoprotein. *PLoS Pathog.* 3:e0030134. doi: 10.1371/journal.ppat.0030134

Tanaka, Y., Kameoka, M., Ota, K., Itaya, A., Ikuta, K., and Yoshihara, K. (1999). Establishment of persistent infection with HIV-1 abrogates the caspase-3-dependent apoptotic signaling pathway in U937 cells. *Exp. Cell Res.* 247, 514–524. doi: 10.1006/excr.1998.4376

Taube, R., and Peterlin, M. (2013). Lost in transcription: molecular mechanisms that control HIV latency. *Viruses* 5, 902–927. doi: 10.3390/v5030902

Tawakol, A., Ishai, A., Li, D., Takx, R. A., Hur, S., Kaiser, Y., et al. (2017). Association of arterial and lymph node inflammation with distinct inflammatory pathways in human immunodeficiency virus infection. *JAMA Cardiol.* 2, 163–171. doi: 10.1001/jamacardio.2016.4728

Teo, I., Veryard, C., Barnes, H., An, S. F., Jones, M., Lantos, P. L., et al. (1997). Circular forms of unintegrated human immunodeficiency virus type 1 DNA and high levels of viral protein expression: association with dementia and multinucleated giant cells in the brains of patients with AIDS. *J. Virol.* 71, 2928–2933.

Thieblemont, N., Weiss, L., Sadeghi, H. M., Estcourt, C., and Haeffner-Cavaillon, N. (1995). CD14lowCD16high: a cytokine-producing monocyte subset which expands during human immunodeficiency virus infection. *Eur. J. Immunol.* 25, 3418–3424. doi: 10.1002/eji.1830251232

Tourriere, H., Gallouzi, I. E., Chebli, K., Capony, J. P., Mouaikel, J., van der Geer, P., et al. (2001). RasGAP-associated endoribonuclease G3Bp: selective RNA degradation and phosphorylation-dependent localization. *Mol. Cell Biol.* 21, 7747–7760. doi: 10.1128/MCB.21.22.7747-7760.2001

Triant, V. A., and Grinspoon, S. K. (2017). Epidemiology of ischemic heart disease in HIV. *Curr. Opin. HIV AIDS* 12, 540–547. doi: 10.1097/COH.0000000000000410

Triboulet, R., Mari, B., Lin, Y. L., Chable-Bessia, C., Bennasser, Y., Lebrigand, K., et al. (2007). Suppression of microRNA-silencing pathway by HIV-1 during virus replication. *Science* 315, 1579–1582. doi: 10.1126/science.1136319

Tso, F. Y., Kang, G., Kwon, E. H., Julius, P., Li, Q., West, J. T., et al. (2018). Brain is a potential sanctuary for subtype C HIV-1 irrespective of ART treatment outcome. *PLoS One* 13:e0201325. doi: 10.1371/journal.pone.0201325

Tyagi, M., and Karn, J. (2007). CBF-1 promotes transcriptional silencing during the establishment of HIV-1 latency. *EMBO J.* 26, 4985–4995. doi: 10.1038/sj.emboj.7601928

Tyagi, M., and Kashanchi, F. (2012). New and novel intrinsic host repressive factors against HIV-1: PAF1 complex, HERC5 and others. *Retrovirology* 9:19. doi: 10.1186/1742-4690-9-19

Vandegraaff, N., Devroe, E., Turlure, F., Silver, P. A., and Engelman, A. (2006). Biochemical and genetic analyses of integrase-interacting proteins lens epithelium-derived growth factor (LEDGF)/p75 and hepatoma-derived growth factor related protein 2 (HRP2) in preintegration complex function and HIV-1 replication. *Virology* 346, 415–426. doi: 10.1016/j.virol.2005.11.022

van't Wout, A. B., Ran, L. J., Kuiken, C. L., Kootstra, N. A., Pals, S. T., and Schuitemaker, H. (1998). Analysis of the temporal relationship between human immunodeficiency virus type 1 quasispecies in sequential blood samples and various organs obtained at autopsy. *J. Virol.* 72, 488–496.

Varol, C., Landsman, L., Fogg, D. K., Greenshtein, L., Gildor, B., Margalit, R., et al. (2007). Monocytes give rise to mucosal, but not splenic, conventional dendritic cells. *J. Exp. Med.* 204, 171–180. doi: 10.1084/jem.20061011

Verdin, E., Paras, P. Jr., and Van Lint, C. (1993). Chromatin disruption in the promoter of human immunodeficiency virus type 1 during transcriptional activation. *EMBO J.* 12, 3249–3259. doi: 10.1002/j.1460-2075.1993.tb05994.x

Wang, J., and Kubes, P. (2016). A reservoir of mature cavity macrophages that can rapidly invade visceral organs to affect tissue repair. *Cell* 165, 668–678. doi: 10.1016/j.cell.2016.03.009

Wang, J., Roderiquez, G., Oravecz, T., and Norcross, M. A. (1998). Cytokine regulation of human immunodeficiency virus type 1 entry and replication in human monocytes/macrophages through modulation of CCR5 expression. *J. Virol.* 72, 7642–7647.

Wang, X., Wang, H., Liu, M. Q., Li, J. L., Zhou, R. H., Zhou, Y., et al. (2017). IFN-lambda inhibits drug-resistant HIV infection of macrophages. *Front. Immunol.* 8:210. doi: 10.3389/fimmu.2017.00210

Wang, X., Ye, L., Hou, W., Zhou, Y., Wang, Y. J., Metzger, D. S., et al. (2009). Cellular microRNA expression correlates with susceptibility of monocytes/macrophages to HIV-1 infection. *Blood* 113, 671–674. doi: 10.1182/blood-2008-09-175000

Warrilow, D., Gardner, J., Darnell, G. A., Suhrbier, A., and Harrich, D. (2006). HIV type 1 inhibition by protein kinase C modulatory compounds. *AIDS Res. Hum. Retroviruses* 22, 854–864. doi: 10.1089/aid.2006.22.854

Wellensiek, B. P., Ramakrishnan, R., Sundaravaradan, V., Mehta, R., Harris, D. T., and Ahmad, N. (2009). Differential HIV-1 integration targets more actively transcribed host genes in neonatal than adult blood mononuclear cells. *Virology* 385, 28–38. doi: 10.1016/j.virol.2008.10.052

Westhorpe, C. L., Maisa, A., Spelman, T., Hoy, J. F., Dewar, E. M., Karapanagiotidis, S., et al. (2014). Associations between surface markers on blood monocytes and carotid atherosclerosis in HIV-positive individuals. *Immunol. Cell Biol.* 92, 133–138. doi: 10.1038/icb.2013.84

Wiley, C. A., Schrier, R. D., Nelson, J. A., Lampert, P. W., and Oldstone, M. B. (1986). Cellular localization of human immunodeficiency virus infection within the brains of acquired immune deficiency syndrome patients. *Proc. Natl. Acad. Sci. U.S.A.* 83, 7089–7093. doi: 10.1073/pnas.83.18.7089

Williams, D. W., Byrd, D., Rubin, L. H., Anastos, K., Morgello, S., and Berman, J. W. (2014). CCR2 on CD14(+)CD16(+) monocytes is a biomarker of HIV-associated neurocognitive disorders. *Neurol. Neuroimmunol. Neuroinflamm.* 1:e36. doi: 10.1212/NXI.0000000000000036

Williams, D. W., Calderon, T. M., Lopez, L., Carvallo-Torres, L., Gaskill, P. J., Eugenin, E. A., et al. (2013). Mechanisms of HIV entry into the CNS: increased sensitivity of HIV infected CD14+CD16+ monocytes to CCL2 and key roles of CCR2, JAM-A, and ALCAM in diapedesis. *PLoS One* 8:e69270. doi: 10.1371/journal.pone.0069270

Williams, D. W., Eugenin, E. A., Calderon, T. M., and Berman, J. W. (2012). Monocyte maturation, HIV susceptibility, and transmigration across the blood brain barrier are critical in HIV neuropathogenesis. *J. Leukoc. Biol.* 91, 401–415. doi: 10.1189/jlb.0811394

Wolf, D., Witte, V., Laffert, B., Blume, K., Stromer, E., Trapp, S., et al. (2001). HIV-1 Nef associated PAK and PI3-kinases stimulate Akt-independent Bad-phosphorylation to induce anti-apoptotic signals. *Nat. Med.* 7, 1217–1224. doi: 10.1038/nm1101-1217

Wong, K. L., Tai, J. J., Wong, W. C., Han, H., Sem, X., Yeap, W. H., et al. (2011). Gene expression profiling reveals the defining features of the classical, intermediate, and nonclassical human monocyte subsets. *Blood* 118, e16–e31. doi: 10.1182/blood-2010-12-326355

Wu, J., Ao, M. T., Shao, R., Wang, H. R., Yu, D., Fang, M. J., et al. (2017). A chalcone derivative reactivates latent HIV-1 transcription through activating P-TEFb and promoting Tat-SEC interaction on viral promoter. *Sci. Rep.* 7:10657. doi: 10.1038/s41598-017-10728-w

Yedavalli, V. S., and Jeang, K. T. (2011). Matrin 3 is a co-factor for HIV-1 Rev in regulating post-transcriptional viral gene expression. *Retrovirology* 8:61. doi: 10.1186/1742-4690-8-61

Yona, S., Kim, K. W., Wolf, Y., Mildner, A., Varol, D., Breker, M., et al. (2013). Fate mapping reveals origins and dynamics of monocytes and tissue macrophages under homeostasis. *Immunity* 38, 79–91. doi: 10.1016/j.immuni.2012.12.001

Yukl, S. A., Sinclair, E., Somsouk, M., Hunt, P. W., Epling, L., Killian, M., et al. (2014). A comparison of methods for measuring rectal HIV levels suggests that HIV DNA resides in cells other than CD4+ T cells, including myeloid cells. *AIDS* 28, 439–442. doi: 10.1097/QAD.0000000000000166

Zalar, A., Figueroa, M. I., Ruibal-Ares, B., Bare, P., Cahn, P., de Bracco, M. M., et al. (2010). Macrophage HIV-1 infection in duodenal tissue of patients on long term HAART. *Antiviral Res.* 87, 269–271. doi: 10.1016/j.antiviral.2010.05.005

Zhang, H. (2009). Reversal of HIV-1 latency with anti-microRNA inhibitors. *Int. J. Biochem. Cell Biol.* 41, 451–454. doi: 10.1016/j.biocel.2008.07.016

Zhang, H., Dornadula, G., Beumont, M., Livornese, L. Jr., Van Uitert, B., Henning, K., et al. (1998). Human immunodeficiency virus type 1 in the semen of men receiving highly active antiretroviral therapy. *N. Engl. J. Med.* 339, 1803–1809. doi: 10.1056/NEJM199812173392502

Zhang, M., Li, X., Pang, X., Ding, L., Wood, O., Clouse, K. A., et al. (2002). Bcl-2 upregulation by HIV-1 Tat during infection of primary human macrophages in culture. *J. Biomed. Sci.* 9, 133–139. doi: 10.1007/bf02256024

Zhang, Z., Schuler, T., Zupancic, M., Wietgrefe, S., Staskus, K. A., Reimann, K. A., et al. (1999). Sexual transmission and propagation of SIV and HIV in resting and activated CD4+ T cells. *Science* 286, 1353–1357. doi: 10.1126/science.286.5443.1353

Zhou, Y., Zhang, H., Siliciano, J. D., and Siliciano, R. F. (2005). Kinetics of human immunodeficiency virus type 1 decay following entry into resting CD4+ T cells. *J. Virol.* 79, 2199–2210. doi: 10.1128/JVI.79.4.2199-2210.2005

Ziegler-Heitbrock, L., Ancuta, P., Crowe, S., Dalod, M., Grau, V., Hart, D. N., et al. (2010). Nomenclature of monocytes and dendritic cells in blood. *Blood* 116, e74–e80. doi: 10.1182/blood-2010-02-258558

Zolotukhin, A. S., Michalowski, D., Bear, J., Smulevitch, S. V., Traish, A. M., Peng, R., et al. (2003). PSF acts through the human immunodeficiency virus type 1 mRNA instability elements to regulate virus expression. *Mol. Cell Biol.* 23, 6618–6630. doi: 10.1128/mcb.23.18.6618-6630.2003

8

Improving HIV Outgrowth by Optimizing Cell-Culture Conditions and Supplementing with *all-trans* Retinoic Acid

*Yuwei Zhang[1,2], Delphine Planas[1,2], Laurence Raymond Marchand[2], Marta Massanella[1,2], Huicheng Chen[1,2], Vanessa Sue Wacleche[1,2], Annie Gosselin[2], Jean-Philippe Goulet[3], Mario Filion[4], Jean-Pierre Routy[5], Nicolas Chomont[1,2] and Petronela Ancuta[1,2]**

[1] *Département de microbiologie, infectiologie et immunologie, Faculté de Médecine, Université de Montréal, Montreal, QC, Canada,* [2] *Centre hospitalier de l'Université de Montréal (CHUM)-Research Centre, Montreal, QC, Canada,* [3] *Caprion, Montreal, QC, Canada,* [4] *Alethia Biotherapeutics, Montreal, QC, Canada,* [5] *McGill University Health Centre, Montreal, QC, Canada*

Correspondence:
Petronela Ancuta
petronela.ancuta@umontreal.ca

The persistence of replication-competent HIV reservoirs in people living with HIV (PLWH) receiving antiretroviral therapy (ART) is a barrier to cure. Therefore, their accurate quantification is essential for evaluating the efficacy of new therapeutic interventions and orienting the decision to interrupt ART. Quantitative viral outgrowth assays (QVOAs) represent the "*gold standard*" for measuring the size of replication-competent HIV reservoirs. However, they require large numbers of cells and are technically challenging. This justifies the need for the development of novel simplified methods adapted for small biological samples. Herein, we sought to simplify the viral outgrowth procedure (VOP) by (*i*) using memory CD4$^+$ T-cells, documented to be enriched in HIV reservoirs (*ii*) optimizing cell-culture conditions, and (*iii*) supplementing with *all-trans* retinoic acid (ATRA), a positive regulator of HIV replication. Memory CD4$^+$ T-cells were sorted from the peripheral blood of ART-treated (HIV+ART; n = 14) and untreated (HIV+; n = 5) PLWH. The VOP was first performed with one original replicate of 1×10^6 cells/well in 48-well plates. Cells were stimulated *via* CD3/CD28 for 3 days, washed to remove residual CD3/CD28 Abs, split every 3 days for optimal cell density, and cultured in the presence or the absence of ATRA for 12 days. Soluble and intracellular HIV-p24 levels were quantified by ELISA and flow cytometry, respectively. Optimal cell-culture density achieved by splitting improved HIV outgrowth detection. ATRA promoted superior/accelerated detection of replication-competent HIV in all HIV+ART individuals tested, including those with low/undetectable viral outgrowth in the absence of ATRA. Finally, this VOP was used to design a simplified ATRA-based QVOA by including 4 and 6 original replicates of 1×10^6 cells/well in 48-well plates and 2×10^5 cells/well in 96-well plates, respectively. Consistently, the number of infectious units per million cells (IUPM) was significantly increased in the presence of ATRA. In conclusion, we demonstrate that memory CD4$^+$ T-cell splitting for optimal density in culture and ATRA supplementation significantly improved the efficacy of HIV outgrowth in a simplified ATRA-based QVOA performed in the absence of feeder/target cells or indicator cell lines.

Keywords: memory CD4$^+$ T-cells, ART, HIV-1 reservoirs, ATRA, QVOAs

INTRODUCTION

Antiretroviral therapy (ART) significantly reduces the morbidity and mortality associated with HIV-1 infection (Barre-Sinoussi et al., 2013). Although ART reduces plasma viral load below the limit of detection of current clinical tests (<40 copies HIV-RNA/ml plasma), viral rebound occurs in most HIV-infected individuals upon treatment interruption, including those receiving ART at a very early stage of primary infection (Ho and Zhang, 2000; Gianella et al., 2015; Henrich et al., 2017; Colby et al., 2018). The persistence of viral reservoirs during ART is well-established to represent a major barrier for HIV eradication (Chomont et al., 2011; Chun et al., 2015; Churchill et al., 2016; Deeks et al., 2016; Martin and Siliciano, 2016). Therefore, major efforts are invested toward the development of HIV cure/remission strategies (Margolis et al., 2016; Goulder and Deeks, 2018; Sengupta and Siliciano, 2018).

Replication-competent HIV reservoirs are established in long-lived memory $CD4^+$ T-cells, with a frequency estimated as low as one infected cell *per* 1×10^6 $CD4^+$ T-cells (Finzi et al., 1997; Eisele and Siliciano, 2012; Massanella et al., 2018; Siliciano and Siliciano, 2018). Multiple groups, including ours, documented the fact that HIV-DNA reservoirs are enriched in $CD4^+$ T-cells with unique phenotypes and functions, including central memory (T_{CM}) (Chomont et al., 2009), stem cell memory (T_{SCM}) (Buzon et al., 2014), helper (Th) type 17 (Th17) (Sun et al., 2015; Khoury et al., 2016; Gosselin et al., 2017; Planas et al., 2017, 2018; Anderson et al., 2019), Th1 (Lee et al., 2017), and/or follicular helper T-cells (Tfh) (Banga et al., 2016; Miles and Connick, 2016). Different HIV cure strategies have been proposed and/or are under pre-clinical evaluation, including "*shock and kill*" strategies using latency reversing agents (LRAs), gene therapy, and most recently "*block and lock*" strategies using Tat inhibitors (Buzon et al., 2010; Archin et al., 2012; Archin and Margolis, 2014; Chun et al., 2015; Mousseau et al., 2015a; Margolis et al., 2016; Kessing et al., 2017; Kim et al., 2017). To evaluate the efficacy of such strategies, progress has been made in the field of HIV reservoir quantification (Eriksson et al., 2013; Bruner et al., 2015, 2019; Massanella and Richman, 2016; Massanella et al., 2018). Despite these advances, the accurate quantification of clinically-relevant replication-competent HIV reservoirs using standardized assays remains a key research priority for orienting treatment interruption upon HIV curative interventions.

To quantify HIV reservoirs, the assays developed to date include PCR/RT-PCR-based and cell-culture based approaches (Bruner et al., 2015; Massanella and Richman, 2016; Massanella et al., 2018; Siliciano and Siliciano, 2018; Wang et al., 2018). Among PCR-based assays, the quantification of integrated HIV-DNA using HIV/Alu primers and FRET-based nested real-time PCR provides an estimate of the frequency of cells carrying HIV proviruses (Brussel and Sonigo, 2003; Chomont et al., 2009; Pinzone and O'Doherty, 2018). Although this method allows a simple, scalable, and low cost estimation of viral reservoir size, a large proportion of integrated HIV-DNA is defective (Eriksson et al., 2013; Ho et al., 2013; Cohn et al., 2015; Bruner et al., 2016; Deeks et al., 2016; Kiselinova et al., 2016; Lorenzi et al., 2016); therefore, such approaches largely over-estimate the size of replication-competent HIV reservoirs (Bruner et al., 2015; Deeks et al., 2016). Most recently, a multiplex PCR-based approach, entitled intact proviral DNA assay (IPDA), was established to quantify intact versus defective HIV proviruses (Bruner et al., 2019).

To quantify transcriptionally-competent HIV proviruses, one approach is to measure levels of cell-associated HIV-RNA upon short-term activation *in vitro*, where the fractional provirus expression (fPVE) upon TCR triggering and/or LRAs stimulation is measured (Cillo et al., 2014). To this aim, the Tat/Rev Induced Limiting Dilution Assay (TILDA) was developed to quantify the frequency of $CD4^+$ T-cells expressing multiply spliced HIV-RNA upon short-term PMA/Ionomycin stimulation *in vitro* (Procopio et al., 2015). One step further in the quantification of HIV reservoirs at a single-cell level is now offered by HIV-Flow (Pardons et al., 2019) and the flow cytometry-based intracellular staining and *in situ* hybridization assay (Flow-FISH) that quantifies transcription/translation-competent HIV reservoirs *via* the detection of cells co-expressing HIV-RNA and the HIV capsid protein (HIV-p24) (Baxter et al., 2016, 2017, 2018). Similar to the PCR methods, the fPVE, TILDA, HIV-Flow, and Flow-FISH assays also overestimate the size of HIV reservoirs considering the fact that not all transcription/translation events lead to the production of infectious virions.

Quantitative viral outgrowth assays (QVOAs) estimate the frequency of resting $CD4^+$ T-cells harboring replication-competent proviruses in the peripheral blood of ART-treated individuals (Finzi et al., 1997; Eriksson et al., 2013; Bullen et al., 2014; Bruner et al., 2015; Martin and Siliciano, 2016). The frequency of such reservoirs is significantly lower compared to the frequency of cells carrying integrated HIV-DNA, in line with findings demonstrating that a large proportion of proviruses is defective (Wong et al., 1997; Eriksson et al., 2013; Ho et al., 2013; Cohn et al., 2015; Bruner et al., 2016; Deeks et al., 2016; Kiselinova et al., 2016; Lorenzi et al., 2016; Siliciano and Siliciano, 2018). Classical QVOAs are labor intensive and time consuming, requiring multiple replicates in serial dilution and co-culture with irradiated PBMCs as feeder cells and/or CD8-depleted lymphoblasts from uninfected individuals as target cells for efficient amplification of replication-competent virions (Siliciano and Siliciano, 2005; Bruner et al., 2015; Laird et al., 2016; Massanella and Richman, 2016). Simplified versions of QVOAs use the indicator HIV-permissive cell lines MOLT-4/CCR5 (Laird et al., 2013) or Sup T1 $CCR5^+$ (Fun et al., 2017). The sensitivity of the QVOA was improved by introducing the RT-PCR measurement of viral RNA (Laird et al., 2013) instead of the measurement of HIV-p24 in cell-culture supernatants by ELISA (Finzi et al., 1997). Despite these improvements, the sensitivity of QVOAs remains suboptimal, as reflected by the inability to detect HIV outgrowth in all tested samples even by using large numbers of $CD4^+$ T-cells in multiple replicates (Laird et al., 2013; Siliciano and Siliciano, 2018). Indeed, several rounds of reactivation are needed to reverse latency in specific $CD4^+$ T-cell subsets (Laird et al., 2013; Bruner et al., 2015; Hosmane et al., 2017; Siliciano and Siliciano, 2018; Wang et al., 2018), indicative that current cell activation strategies are suboptimal for efficient viral reactivation/outgrowth. These are critical limitations, especially for studies on small blood samples (e.g., pediatric samples), as well as cells isolated from deep tissue upon biopsy and/or autopsy.

In this manuscript, we provide new insights into the optimization of a simplified viral outgrowth procedure (VOP), in which memory CD4$^+$ T-cells of ART-treated PLWH were stimulated *via* the TCR, cultured in the presence of *all-trans* retinoic acid (ATRA), and maintained at optimal density by regular splitting into new wells. Noteworthy, the viral outgrowth was robustly detected in the absence of feeder/target cells or indicator cell lines upon 12 days of culture. Finally, the culture of the cells in four original replicates of 1×10^6 cells/well in 48-well plates and six original replicates of 2×10^5 cells/well in 96-well plates allowed the calculation of the number of infectious units per million (IUPM) (Rosenbloom et al., 2015), with the detection of IUPMs being significantly increased by ATRA. These insights emerged from our experience in reactivating HIV reservoirs in rare subsets of CCR6$^+$ Th17 cells (Wacleche et al., 2016), as well as the evidence generated by our group (Monteiro et al., 2011; Gosselin et al., 2017; Planas et al., 2017) and others (Cicala et al., 2009; Martinelli et al., 2011; Li et al., 2016) that ATRA increases HIV permissiveness *in vitro* and viral outgrowth *ex vivo*. In conclusion, cell-culture strategies presented in this manuscript are important to simplify current QVOAs for scalable viral reservoir quantifications in clinical trials using small biological samples.

MATERIALS AND METHODS

Subjects

HIV-infected study participants were recruited at the McGill University Health Centre and at the Centre Hospitalier de l'Université de Montréal (CHUM, Montreal, Québec, Canada). Large quantities of peripheral blood mononuclear cells (PBMCs) (10^9–10^{10}) were collected by leukapheresis (Boulassel et al., 2003) and cryopreserved until use, as previously reported (Chomont et al., 2009; Wacleche et al., 2016; Gosselin et al., 2017; Planas et al., 2017). The clinical characteristics of HIV-infected study participants treated or not with ART at the time of blood collection are listed in **Supplementary Table S1**.

Ethics Statement

This study, using PBMC samples from HIV-infected subjects, was conducted in compliance with the principles included in the Declaration of Helsinki. This study received approval from the Institutional Review Board of the McGill University Health Centre and the CHUM-Research Centre, Montreal, QC, Canada. Written informed consents and agreement to publish the results were obtained from all study participants.

Flow-Cytometry Analysis

Surface staining for flow cytometry analysis was performed with the following fluorochrome-conjugated antibodies (Abs): CD3 Pacific blue (clone UCHT1), CD4 Alexa700 (clone RPA-T4; BD Biosciences), and CD45RA APC-eFluor 780 (clone HI100; eBioscience). Intracellular staining was performed with FITC-conjugated HIV-p24 Abs (clone KC57; Beckman Coulter) and the Fixation/Permeabilization Kit (BD). The LIVE/DEAD Fixable Aqua Dead Cell Stain Kit (Invitrogen) was used to exclude dead cells. Flow-cytometry analysis was performed using a LSRII cytometer, Diva version 8 (BD Biosciences, San Jose, CA, United States), and FlowJo version 10.0.6 (Tree Star, Inc.). Flow cytometry gates were defined using the *fluorescence minus one* (FMO) strategy (Roederer, 2002; Gosselin et al., 2010).

Cell Sorting

Highly pure (>95%) total memory (CD45RA$^-$) CD4$^+$ T-cells were enriched from PBMCs by negative selection using magnetic beads (MACS, Miltenyi) (Monteiro et al., 2011; Gosselin et al., 2017). Memory CCR6$^+$ and CCR6$^-$ CD4$^+$ T-cells were further isolated by flow cytometry (BD Aria III), using specific procedures and antibodies previously described (Planas et al., 2017).

Quantification of Integrated HIV-DNA

The quantification of integrated HIV-DNA levels was performed in triplicates on 0.5–1 $\times 10^5$ CD4 T-cells by nested real-time PCR, as we previously described (Chomont et al., 2009; Gosselin et al., 2017). To ensure accurate integrated HIV-DNA quantification for non-clade B HIV, primers were designed to amplify viral genomes from a larger number of HIV clades (A, B, C, D, and CRF01A_E), as we previously described (Vandergeeten et al., 2014).

Viral Outgrowth Procedure (VOP)

Memory CD4$^+$ T-cells were cultured at 1×10^6 cells/well in 1 ml of media (RPMI, 10% FBS, 1% Penicillin/Streptomycin) in a 48-well plate (Costar) coated with CD3 Abs (1 μg/ml, Clone UCHT1) and in the presence of soluble CD28 Abs (1 μg/ml) (BD Biosciences, Clone CD28.2). At day 3, cells from each original replicate were individually washed with media, split into two new CD3 Abs-uncoated 48-well plate wells, and cultured in media containing IL-2 (5 ng/ml; R&D Systems), in the presence or in the absence of ATRA (10, 100, 1,000, and 10,000 nM; SIGMA). The equivalent volume of DMSO was used as a control for ATRA. Cells from each well were further split into two new wells (without washing) at day 6 and 9 post-stimulation, with half of the media being refreshed with IL-2 with/without ATRA. Thus, each original replicate generated eight splitting replicates at days 9–12. At day 12, cells from all of the splitting replicates were individually harvested and the intracellular expression of HIV-p24 was measured by flow-cytometry, with the percentage of cells expressing intracellular HIV-p24 reflecting viral outgrowth in culture but not the size of the initial viral reservoir. In parallel, soluble HIV-p24 levels were quantified in cell-culture supernatants collected every three days post-stimulation using a previously described home-made ELISA assay (limit of detection: 5 pg/ml HIV-p24) (Bounou et al., 2002). ELISA optical density (OD) values for samples were considered positive only when they exceeded two times the OD value of the blank.

ATRA-Based Quantitative Viral Outgrowth Assay (ATRA-QVOA)

To render the VOP quantitative, memory CD4$^+$ T-cells isolated from ART-treated PLWH were cultured in multiple original replicates of 1 × 10^6 cells/well in 48-well plates (four original replicates at day 0, generating 32 splitting replicates at days 9–12) and 2 × 10^5 cells/well in 96-well plates (6 original replicates at day 0, generating 48 splitting replicates at days 9–12) using the VOP described above, as depicted in **Figure 4A**. Cultures were performed in the presence or in the absence of ATRA (100 nM). The control for ATRA was medium instead of DMSO; this simplification of the protocol for the VOP as described above was based on preliminary results demonstrating that an equivalent volume of DMSO (0.01 μl/ml) had no impact on the magnitude and the kinetics of HIV replication *in vitro* (data not shown). At day 12, HIV-p24 levels were measured by ELISA in cell-culture supernatants collected separately from all individual splitting replicates. For the calculation of IUPM one original replicate was considered positive if the HIV-p24 values were positive for at least two consecutive time points (typically days 9 and 12) and in one/multiple splitting replicates (**Supplementary Figure S5**). The IUPM values were calculated using the formula established by the group of Dr. Siliciano (https://silicianolab.johnshopkins.edu) (Rosenbloom et al., 2015).

Statistical Analysis

Figures were generated using the Prism 7 (GraphPad) software. Specifications relative to the statistical tests used are included in the results and figure legends. Briefly, statistical analysis were performed using R [R Core Team (2017); R: A language and environment for statistical computing. R Foundation for Statistical Computing, Vienna, Austria (https://www.R-project.org/)]. We used R packages lme4 to fit the linear mixed regression (**Supplementary Tables 3A,B, 4A,B**) model and glmmTMB package to fit the negative binomial generalized regression model (**Supplementary Tables S5A,B**). The aov() and pairwise t.test() functions implemented in the R package stats were used for the paired ANOVA analysis (**Supplementary Tables S2A,B**).

RESULTS

A Simplified Viral Outgrowth Procedure Using Memory CD4$^+$ T-Cells of ART-Treated PLWH

Our goal was to optimize a new simplified VOP suitable for relatively small blood volumes collected from ART-treated PLWH. This VOP was performed in the absence of allergenic feeder cells, lymphoblast target cells, or HIV-permissive indicator cell lines. This VOP is based on our previous reports demonstrating successful HIV outgrowth from as low as 0.5 × 10^6 flow-cytometry-sorted memory CCR6$^+$ Th17 subsets from ART-treated PLWH (Wacleche et al., 2016). Briefly, one original replicate of 1 × 10^6 memory CD4$^+$ T-cells/well were cultured in 48-well plates coated with CD3 Abs (iCD3) and cultured in the presence of soluble CD28 (sCD28) Abs (1 μg/ml), a T-cell activation strategy that proved to be optimal for promoting HIV outgrowth in other studies (Spina et al., 2013; Cillo et al., 2014; Beliakova-Bethell et al., 2017). Of note, although increased T-cell activation (i.e., CD25 expression) and proliferative potential (i.e., Ki67 expression) were observed by increasing the concentration of CD3/CD28 Abs (>1 μg/ml) or upon activation with CD3/CD28-coated Dynal beads, unexpectedly, this strong T-cell activation led to decreased HIV outgrowth; this result is indicative that a low/moderate TCR triggering is required for optimal HIV outgrowth (data not shown). The VOP was performed as illustrated in **Figure 1A** and detailed in section Materials and Methods.

To test the efficacy of this VOP, a first set of experiments was performed with memory CD4$^+$ T-cells from five untreated PLWH with detectable plasma viral load (**Supplementary Table S1**; HIV+ #14–18). Regardless of inter individual differences in integrated HIV-DNA levels (**Supplementary Figure S1A**), robust HIV outgrowth from 1 × 10^6 memory CD4$^+$ T cells was detected in all 5/5 donors tested, as early as at day 6 post-stimulation (**Supplementary Figures S1B,C**). Thus, this VOP allowed the detection of replication-competent HIV in as low as 1 × 10^6 memory CD4$^+$ T-cells from 5/5 ART-untreated PLWH tested.

Further, the same VOP was performed using memory CD4$^+$ T-cells from a cohort of virally-suppressed ART-treated PLWH (HIV+ART), with clinical parameters listed in **Supplementary Table S1**. Although relatively high levels of integrated HIV-DNA were detected in memory CD4$^+$ T-cells from all 10/10 HIV+ART individuals (**Figure 1B**), HIV-p24 levels in the cell-culture supernatant were only detected by ELISA in cells from 8/10 individuals (**Figure 1C**). Similarly, the presence of HIV-p24$^+$ T-cells at various frequencies was detected by flow-cytometry in cells from the same 8/10 individuals at day 12 post-stimulation (**Figures 1D,E**), indicative of efficient cell-to-cell spread of virions *in vitro*. Of note, viral outgrowth was undetectable in T-cells from donors ART#9 and ART#10 (**Figures 1C–E**), despite relatively high levels of integrated HIV-DNA detected in these donors (**Figure 1B**). These findings are consistent with the knowledge that replication-incompetent HIV proviruses exist in ART-treated individuals (Eisele and Siliciano, 2012; Eriksson et al., 2013; Ho et al., 2013; Bruner et al., 2016). Thus, this VOP allowed the successful detection of replication-competent HIV reservoirs in 80% of HIV+ART individuals tested using one original replicate of 1 × 10^6 memory CD4$^+$ T-cells and cell-culture for 12 days.

Optimal Cell Density in Culture Is Key for HIV Outgrowth

The decision to wash cells at day 3 post-TCR triggering and to split cells every 3 days is justified by our previous observations that Th17 viability, proliferation, and production of lineage-specific cytokines are well-maintained under such experimental settings in long-term culture *in vitro* (Wacleche et al., 2016).

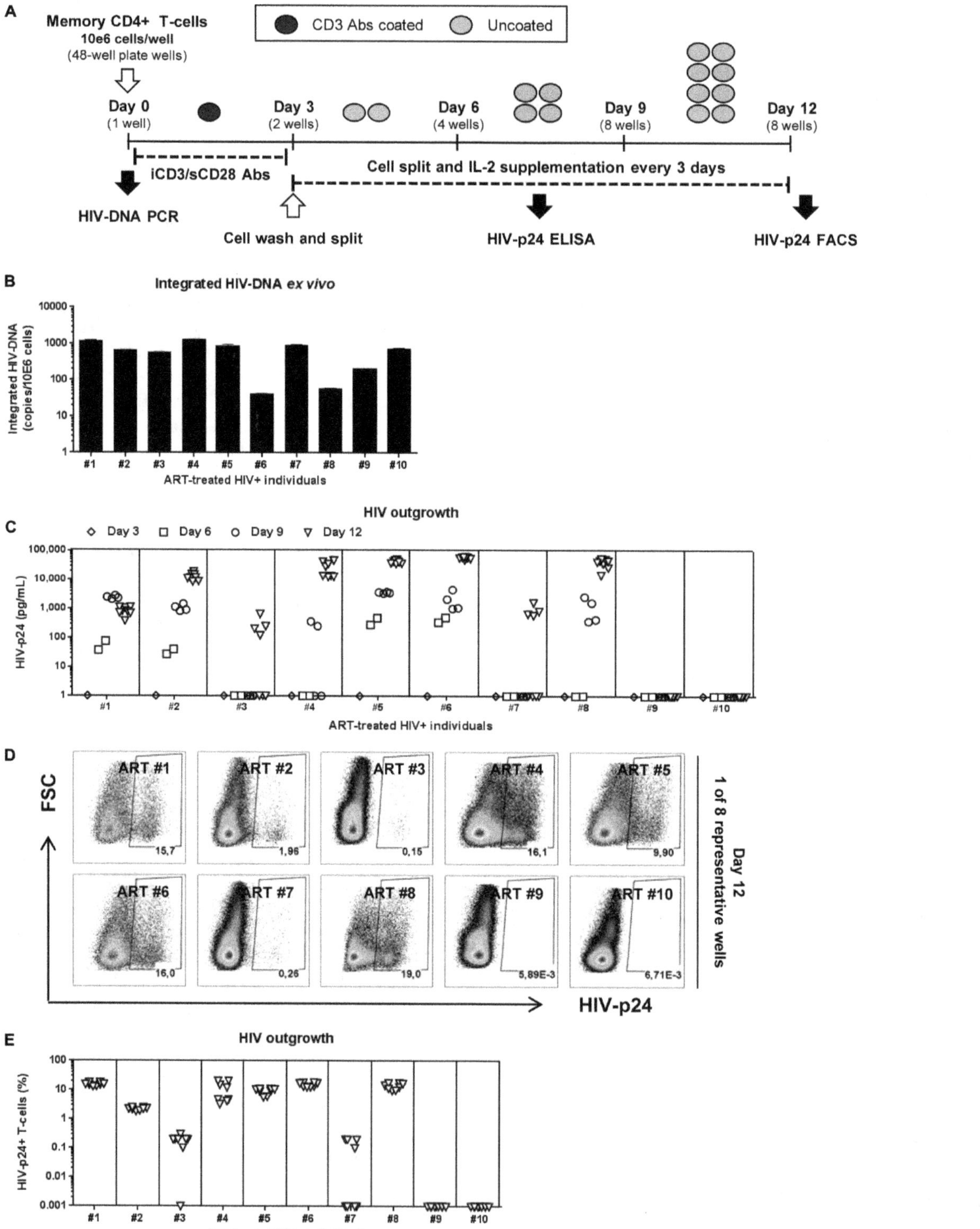

FIGURE 1 | HIV reservoir outgrowth in memory CD4^{+} T-cells of HIV-infected ART-treated individuals. Memory CD4^{+} T-cells were isolated by MACS from PBMCs of ART-treated PLWH (HIV+ART) individuals (**Supplementary Table S1**; HIV+ART #1–10). **(A)** Shown is the viral outgrowth procedure (VOP) performed as described in the Results and Materials and Methods. **(B)** Shown are integrated HIV-DNA levels (mean ± SD of triplicate wells) in memory CD4^{+} T-cells (10^5 cells/PCR reaction) from each donor *ex vivo*. **(C)** Shown are HIV-p24 levels measured by ELISA in cell-culture supernatants collected at day 3 (1 well/donor), day 6 (2 wells/donor), day 9 (4 wells/donor), day 12 (8 wells/donor) post-culture. At day 12 post-stimulation, cells were harvested and used for intracellular staining with HIV-p24 Abs and subsequent flow cytometry analysis. Shown are **(D)** representative flow cytometry dot plot and **(E)** graphical representation of the percentage of HIV-p24^{+} T-cells (8 wells/individual) in n = 10 HIV+ART individuals. Each symbol represents one experimental replicate well, with a total of 8 wells/individual at day 12.

To determine whether washing/splitting was important for HIV outgrowth, we performed the VOP in the presence or absence of washing and/or splitting in n = 3 HIV+ART individuals (HIV+ART #5, #11, #13; **Supplementary Table S1**). The HIV outgrowth was measured by flow cytometry at day 12 post-culture (**Figures 2A,C**) and by ELISA at days 3, 6, 9, and 12 post-culture (**Figures 2D,E**). Results depicted in **Figure 2C**, as well as **paired ANOVA** and Bonferroni *Post hoc* tests following pairwise paired *t*-test analyses in **Supplementary Table S2**, demonstrate that in the absence of washing/splitting (−/−) viral outgrowth was low/undetectable; cell washing alone (+/−) or splitting alone (−/+) increased the % of HIV-p24$^+$ T-cells in specific donors, without reaching statistical significance when compared to the −/− condition. Noteworthy, a significant increase in HIV outgrowth was observed when cells were both washed and split (+/+) compared to the −/− condition (**Figure 2C** and **Supplementary Table S2**). Similar results were obtained when soluble HIV-p24 levels were measured in cell-culture supernatants, with **linear mixed model** analysis indicating a statistically significant increase in HIV outgrowth in the +/+ versus −/− conditions at both Days 9 and 12 (**Figures 2D,E** and **Supplementary Table S3**). Thus, while splitting and washing alone increased HIV outgrowth in specific donors, optimal viral outgrowth was observed when both washing and splitting were performed. Based on these results, both wash and split were performed in the subsequent experiments.

Reproducibility of the New VOP

Another important issue for this new VOP was to determine its reproducibility. For this, the VOP was performed using memory CD4$^+$ T-cells of HIV+ART individuals (HIV+ART #1, #5, and #7; **Supplementary Table S1**) in two independent experiments. Results in **Supplementary Figure S2** demonstrate that this VOA is reproducible.

ATRA Improves HIV Outgrowth in Memory CD4$^+$ T-Cells

To improve the efficacy of this VOP, memory CD4$^+$ T-cells of HIV+ART individuals were cultured in the presence or in the absence of ATRA, a stimulus demonstrated by our group and others to increase HIV replication either directly by increasing HIV transcription and/or indirectly by rendering neighboring cells highly permissive to infection (Cicala et al., 2009; Monteiro et al., 2011; Li et al., 2016; Gosselin et al., 2017). In a preliminary experiment, the VOP was performed with cells from HIV+ART#5, as described in **Figure 1A**, in the presence of different concentration of ATRA (10, 100, 1,000, and 10,000 nM). HIV-p24 levels were monitored in cell-culture supernatants by ELISA up to 12 days post-stimulation. Results in **Supplementary Figure S3** demonstrate that ATRA significantly improved HIV outgrowth, especially at day 6 post-stimulation, with optimal HIV outgrowth being achieved with ATRA at a concentration of 100 nM.

Further, the VOP was performed in the presence or the absence of 100 nM ATRA in memory CD4$^+$ T-cells from $n = 9$ HIV+ART individuals (HIV+ART #1, #2, #3, #5, #7, #9, #10, #11, and #12; **Supplementary Table S1**). First we observed that ATRA allowed HIV outgrowth detection in cells from individuals where viral outgrowth was low/undetectable in the absence of ATRA, notably ART #3, #7, #9, and #10 (**Figure 3C** and **Supplementary Figure S4**). To determine the effect of ATRA on HIV outgrowth, we used a linear mixed model to compare HIV-p24 levels in supernatants form cell cultures performed in the presence or the absence of ATRA. Results in **Figures 3B,C** and **Supplementary Table S4** demonstrate a statistically significant increase in HIV outgrowth per well at Day 9 (4 wells/donor; Pr (>|z|)= 0.00291) and Day 12 (8 wells per donor; Pr (>|z|)= 0.00857) in the presence of ATRA versus DMSO. Finally, by applying a negative binomial regression model, we observed a statistically significant increase in the number of HIV-p24 positive wells/donor in the presence of ATRA versus DMSO at Day 9 (Pr (>|z|)= 0.0232), with the difference being only marginally significant at Day 12 (Pr (>|z|)= 0.07076) (**Supplementary Table S5**). Together, these results are indicative of an improved HIV outgrowth in the presence of ATRA, both in terms of amplitude of the HIV outgrowth per well and the number of positive wells/donor and time point. Such improvements are important for the accurate quantification of the replication-competent HIV reservoir size.

The ATRA-Based QVOA

To render quantitative the VOP described above, four original replicates of 1×10^6 cells/well (generating 32 splitting replicates at day 12) and six original replicates of 2×10^5 cells/well (generating 48 splitting replicates at day 12) were cultured in 48- and 96-well plates, respectively, in the presence or in the absence of ATRA using a cell-culture protocol illustrated in **Figure 4A**. HIV-p24 quantification by ELISA of all individual splitting replicates allowed the calculation of the IUPM, using the formula established by the group of Dr. Robert Siliciano (https://silicianolab.johnshopkins.edu) (Rosenbloom et al., 2015). An original replicate was considered positive if one or more splitting replicates were positive at two consecutive time points for HIV-p24, as depicted in **Supplementary Figure S5**. Experiments performed with memory CD4$^+$ T-cells from $n = 7$ HIV+ART individuals (**Supplementary Table S1**; HIV+ART #1, #2, #5, #7, #8, #9, and #12) demonstrated a statistically significant increase in the IUPM values when cells were cultured in the presence of ATRA (**Figure 4B** and **Supplementary Figure S5B**), with the IUPM geometric mean increasing from 0.3350 in the absence of ATRA to 0.6591 in the presence of ATRA ($n = 7$; $p = 0.0313$). In conclusion, the ATRA-based QVOA represents a simplified assay that requires a minimum of 5.2×10^6 memory CD4$^+$ T-cells, with the culture of cells in 4–6 replicates of two serial dilutions for 12 days allowing the proper calculation of the number of IUPMs.

Finally, we acknowledge that the HIV-p24 ELISA quantification of supernatants from all individual splitting replicates represents a heavy work load. However, the assay can be further simplified by merging supernatants from "identical" splitting replicates coming from one original well and also by testing only supernatants from days 9 and 12. Thus, instead of testing 150 individual supernatants (10 at day 3, 20 at day 6, 40 wells at day 9, and 80 wells at day 12) per donor, one may test only 20 merged "identical" supernatants (10 wells at day 9 and

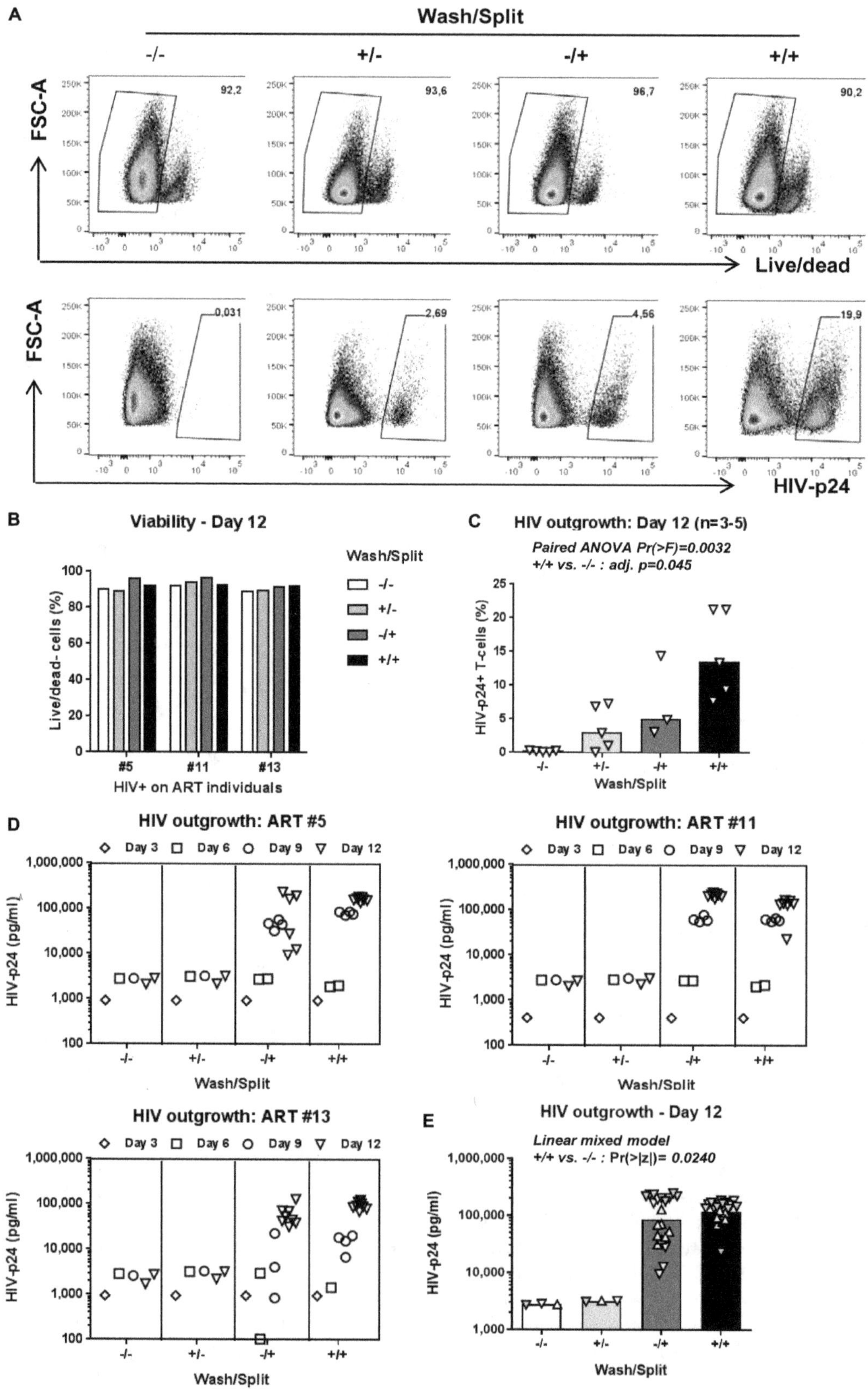

FIGURE 2 | Continued

FIGURE 2 | Optimal cell density in culture is key for HIV outgrowth. The VOP was performed as in **Figure 1A** using memory CD4$^+$ T-cells from $n = 3$–5 HIV-infected ART-treated individuals. To determine the importance of washing at day 3 and splitting at days 3, 6 and 9 post-culture, the VOP was performed in parallel with cells that were washed and split (+/+), only washed (+/−) or split (−/+), and in the absence of (−/−). A viability dye was used to measure cell survival. Intracellular HIV-p24 expression was measured by flow-cytometry at day 12 of culture. Cells from eight wells at day 12 for the conditions with cell splitting (−/+ and +/+) were merged to generated one single value, as for the conditions without cell splitting (−/− and +/−). Shown are results on intracellular HIV-p24 levels and viability from one representative individual (ART #13) at day 12 **(A)**, as well as cell viability **(B)** and the percentage of HIV-p24$^+$ T-cells at day 12 for $n = 3$–5 HIV+ART individuals **(C)**. Bars in **3C** are median values, with symbols for each HIV+ART individual. Paired ANOVA Pr(> F) value and Bonferroni *Post hoc* tests following pairwise paired *t*-tests adjusted (adj.) *p*-values for the + / + versus −/− comparison are indicated on the graph (details in **Supplementary Table S2**). Shown are HIV-p24 levels in cell culture supernatants at days 3, 6, 9, and 12 for three different HIV+ART individuals **(D)**. Bars in **3E** are geometric mean values, with distinct symbols for different wells/donor at Day 12 **(E)**. Linear mixed model Pr(>|z|) values for the +/+ versus −/− comparison are indicated on the graph (details in **Supplementary Table S3**).

10 wells at day 12). This strategy was tested in the laboratory and the IUPM calculation using this simplified strategy generated identical results (data not shown).

DISCUSSION

In this manuscript, we provide new insights into the optimization of the VOP from replication-competent HIV reservoirs by integrating tailored cell-culture strategies, including maintenance of optimal cell density by cell splitting, the preservation of all splitting replicates, as well as supplementing with ATRA, during 12 days in culture. This new VOP was performed with memory CD4$^+$ T-cells from ART-treated PLWH in the absence of feeder/target cells or indicator cell lines. We demonstrate that culturing a minimum of 5.2×10^6 memory CD4$^+$ T-cells in 4 and 6 replicates of two serial dilutions for 12 days allows the calculation of IUPMs, with an efficacy that is significantly increased by ATRA. While this novel simplified ATRA-based QVOA is appropriate for HIV reservoir quantification in small biological samples, it may also serve as a platform to further improving the efficacy of QVOAs by supplementing the culture media with other stimuli that boost HIV reactivation in reservoir cells and facilitate cell-to-cell outgrowth in culture.

This VOP is built based on our expertise in reactivating HIV reservoirs from rare subsets of Th17 cells (Wacleche et al., 2016), a Th cell lineage that require suboptimal TCR triggering for the maintenance of effector functions, as well as culture at optimal cell density for access to nutrients (Kastirr et al., 2015; Mele et al., 2015). The detection of replication-competent HIV reservoirs in this VOP depends on multiple parameters, including the frequency of infected cells (HIV reservoir size), the capacity of reactivated virus to infect new cells (viral fitness), and also on the capacity of neighboring cells to support productive infection (HIV permissiveness). Cell washing at day 3 post-TCR triggering and cell splitting every 3 days significantly improved the efficiency of this VOP. One potential explanation for the importance of washing is that CD4$^+$ T cells, particularly Th1 cells, produce CCR5 ligands (e.g., MIP-1β) that limit cell-to-cell transmission (Casazza et al., 2009; Gosselin et al., 2010; Alvarez et al., 2013). Since Th1 cells are predominant within the pool of CD4$^+$ T-cells (Gosselin et al., 2010), the CCR5 ligands produced upon TCR triggering may limit the detection of viral outgrowth *in vitro*. Another explanation is that cytokines produced by Th1 cells (e.g., IFN-γ) are known to inhibit the transcriptional profile of Th17 cells (Basu et al., 2013; Wacleche et al., 2017), a subset enriched in HIV reservoirs (Gosselin et al., 2017; Planas et al., 2017, 2018; Anderson et al., 2019). Therefore, removal of such soluble factors from cell-culture supernatants remains a plausible explanation for viral outgrowth improvement. An additional improvement was achieved by splitting the cells, indicating that optimal cell density during the culture is critical for VOP, as reported for Th17 survival/function (Kastirr et al., 2015; Mele et al., 2015). The boost in HIV outgrowth by ATRA is explained by its documented capacity to promote HIV replication *via* entry (CCR5 upregulation) and post-entry mechanisms (mTOR activation) (Monteiro et al., 2011; Planas et al., 2017). Noteworthy, retinoic acid (RA) derivatives such as acitretin promote HIV transcription directly (Li et al., 2016), consistent with the presence of RA responsive elements, the DNA binding site of RA receptor alpha, within the HIV LTR (Lee et al., 1994).

Our effort was further focused on finding a strategy to render this ATRA-based VOP quantitative. Our results propose a simple strategy for calculating the IUPMs by culturing cells in multiple original replicates in only two serial dilutions and this for 12 days in culture. The sensitivity of the ATRA-based QVOA could be further improved by including more original replicates in the assay and by culturing the cells for more than 12 days. The positivity in this assay relies on the detection of HIV-p24 by ELISA in cell-culture supernatants. New ultrasensitive single molecule assays (SIMOA) have been recently developed for the detection of HIV-p24, with 1,000-fold superior sensitivity compared to classical HIV-p24 ELISAs (Fan et al., 2015; Kosaka et al., 2017; Passaes et al., 2017); whether SIMOA should be integrated to further optimize ATRA-based QVOAs remains to be determined. Nevertheless, in our ATRA-based QVOA, HIV-p24 levels at days 6–12 post-stimulation were robustly detected in cell-culture supernatants using classical ELISA assays. This new ATRA-based QVOA may be used successfully to quantify HIV reservoirs in small biological samples, but also for fundamental/translational purposes to test the effect of specific drugs acting positively/negatively on HIV transcription (Planas et al., 2017, 2018), a step untargeted by current ART (Barre-Sinoussi et al., 2013; Mousseau et al., 2015b). The IUPM calculation in this ATRA-QVOA can be further simplified by merging supernatants from identical splitting replicates at days 9 and 12 generated from one original well, thus significantly reducing the number of HIV-p24 ELISA wells per donor from 120 to 20. Such a simplification will also allow an increase

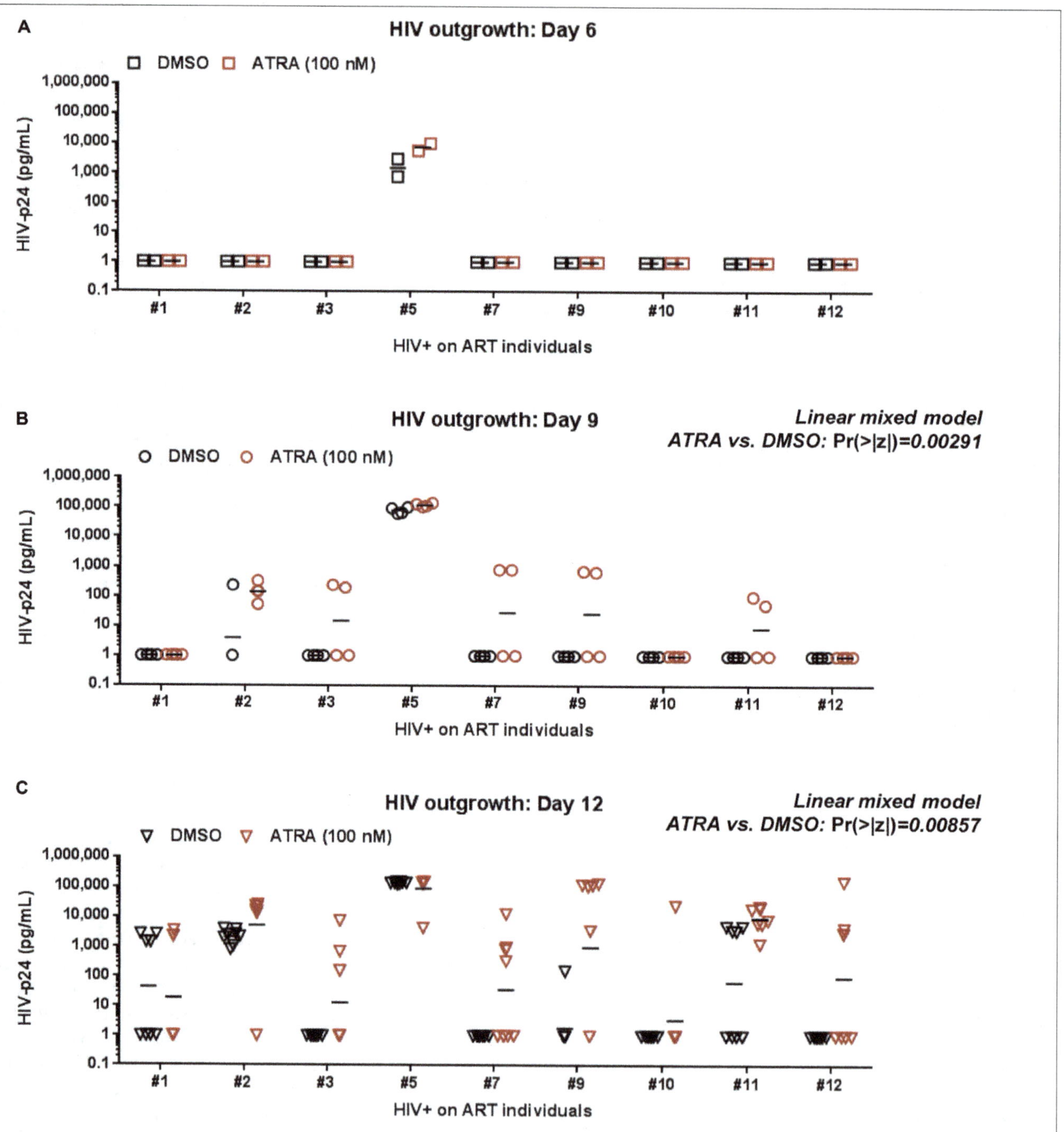

FIGURE 3 | ATRA boosts HIV outgrowth. The VOP was performed with memory CD4$^+$ T-cells of ART-treated PLWH (n = 9 HIV+ART individuals; **Supplementary Table S1**) in the presence (red symbols) or absence (black symbols) of ATRA (100 nM), as described in **Figure 1**. Shown are absolute HIV-p24 levels quantified in cell-culture supernatants collected from splitting replicates at days 6 (2 wells) **(A)**, 9 (4 wells) **(B)**, and 12 (8 wells) **(C)** post-culture. The horizontal black lines indicate the geometric means in **(A–C)**. Linear mixed model Pr (>|z|) values are indicated on the graphs for the comparison ATRA versus DMSO at Day 9 and Day 12 (details in **Supplementary Table S4**).

in the number of original replicates, in an effort to reduce the confidence intervals for IUPM measures that proved to be relatively wide in the current ATRA-based QVOA.

We predict the performance of this ATRA-based QVOA may be further improved by performing the assay on sorted memory CCR6$^+$ T-cells, documented to be enriched in HIV reservoirs (Gosselin et al., 2017; Planas et al., 2017, 2018; Anderson et al., 2019). An ATRA-based QVOA performed with memory CCR6$^+$ T-cells may better orient treatment interruption decisions during

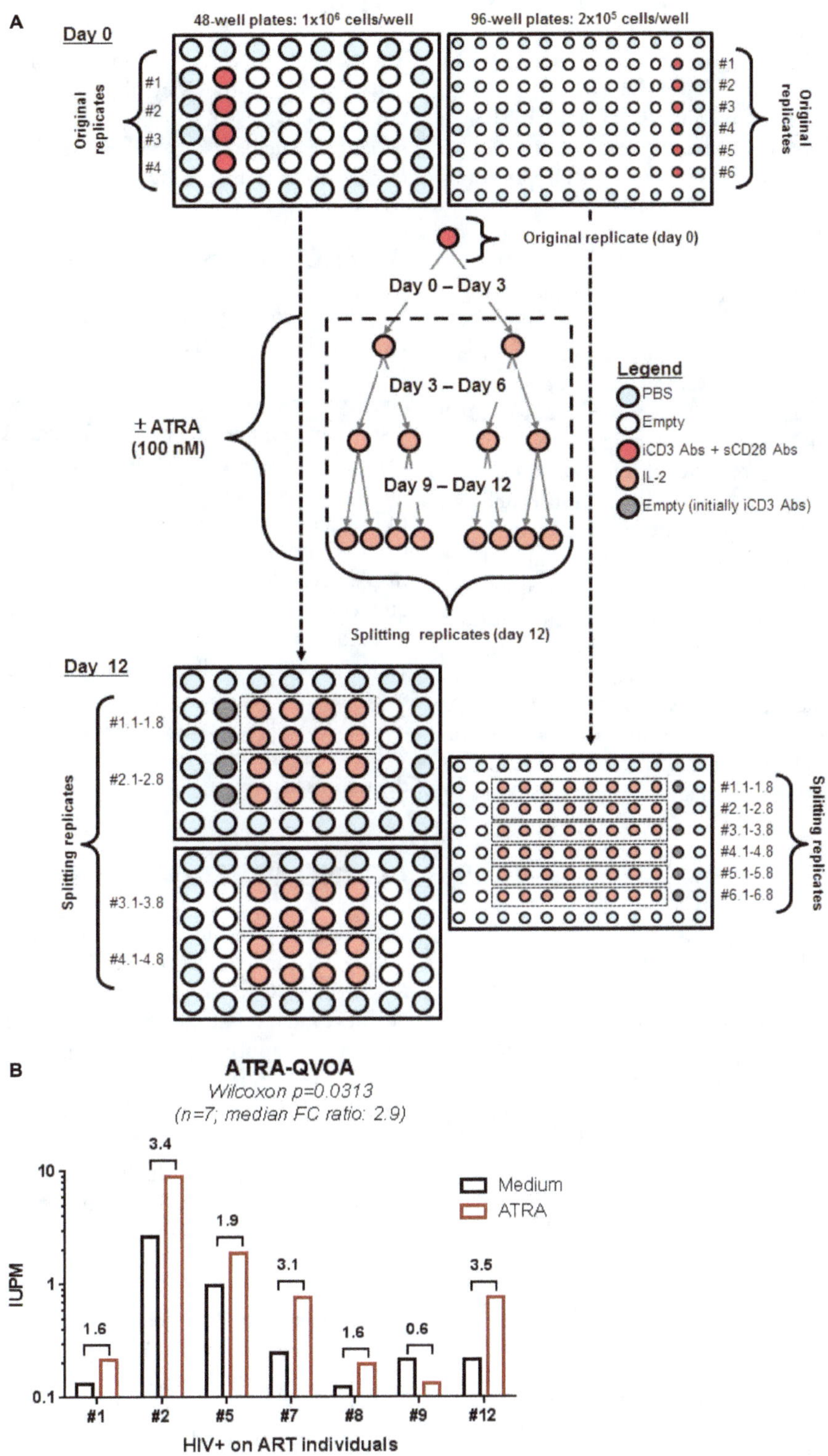

FIGURE 4 | A simplified ATRA-based QVOA. The VOP was performed as described in **Figure 1A** legend, illustrated in **Supplementary Figure S5**, and described in section Materials and Methods using total memory CD4$^+$ T-cells isolated from ART-treated PLWH. **(A)** Briefly, cells were cultured at two cell concentrations, 1×10^6 cells/well in 48-well plates (4 original replicates) and 2×10^5 cells/well in 96 well plates (6 original replicates) and stimulated via CD3/CD28 in the presence or absence of ATRA for 12 days. **(B)** Shown are the IUPM in cells from $n = 7$ HIV+ART PLWH (**Supplementary Table S1**; HIV+ART #1, #2, #5, #7, #8, #9, #12), when the QVOA was performed in the presence and in the absence of ATRA. Fold changes in IUPMs observed in the presence of ATRA versus Medium for each donor cells is annotated on the graph. Wilcoxon matched-pairs signed rank test p-value is indicated on the graph.

HIV cure/remission therapeutic interventions in individuals with low/undetectable viral reservoirs detected in resting, total or memory CD4$^+$ T-cells. Alternatively, the ATRA-based QVOA may be performed on other rare T-cell subsets reported to be enriched in viral reservoirs *in vivo*, such as Tfh (Banga et al., 2016) or PD1$^+$ T-cells (Fromentin et al., 2019), in an effort toward the accurate quantification of intact replication-competent viral reservoirs.

The ATRA-based QVOA we are reporting here may represent an alternative to classical QVOAs that are labor intensive, expensive, and that require several rounds of activation for the accurate estimation of HIV reservoir size (Laird et al., 2013; Soriano-Sarabia et al., 2014; Bruner et al., 2015, 2019; Fun et al., 2017). In this sense, future comparative studies are needed to determine the relative efficacy of these two assays. Noteworthy, a very recent study demonstrated an improved detection of replication-competent HIV reservoirs using a strategy to promote effector memory differentiation thus, emphasizing the importance of appropriate cell activation and culturing conditions for efficient HIV outgrowth quantification (Wonderlich et al., 2019). This new assay called differentiation QVOA (dQVOA) proved to be more efficient compared to the classical QVOA in detecting replication-competent HIV reservoirs (Wonderlich et al., 2019). Future studies are also needed to compare the ATRA-based QVOA and dQVOA in terms of efficacy and simplicity for scalable applications.

CONCLUSION

In conclusion, by combining optimal memory CD4$^+$ T-cell stimulation *via* the TCR and cell density in culture, together with knowledge on the ability of ATRA to promote HIV reactivation and cell-to-cell transmission in culture, we propose a new ATRA-based QVOA that is relatively simple and highly sensitive for the quantification of replication-competent HIV reservoirs in ART-treated PLWH. The fact that viral outgrowth was boosted by ATRA, a key modulator of immunity *via* the imprinting for gut-homing and the modulation of T-cell effector functions (Raverdeau and Mills, 2014; Erkelens and Mebius, 2017), points to its potential use for the optimization of current QVOAs. The existence of other molecular boosters of HIV outgrowth is not excluded and requires future investigations. Such optimizations should also consider current advances in understanding the HIV integration landscape (Hughes and Coffin, 2016) and the unique transcriptional programming of distinct CD4$^+$ T-cell subsets (Ansel et al., 2006; Gaffen et al., 2014; Kallies and Good-Jacobson, 2017) that predominantly carry HIV reservoirs (e.g., Th17 versus Th1) (Sun et al., 2015; Wacleche et al., 2016; Gosselin et al., 2017; Lee et al., 2017; Planas et al., 2017).

ETHICS STATEMENT

The studies involving human participants were reviewed and approved by McGill University Health Centre and the CHUM-Research Centre, Montreal, QC, Canada. The patients/participants provided their written informed consent to participate in this study.

AUTHOR CONTRIBUTIONS

YZ designed experiments, generated results included in **Figures 1–3**, prepared figures, and wrote the manuscript. DP generated results in **Figures 2**, **4**, prepared figures, and participated in manuscript writing. LR generated results in **Figure 4**, prepared figures, and participated in manuscript writing. MM contributed to HIV-DNA PCR quantifications and QVOA set-up. HC performed HIV-p24 ELISA and flow-cytometry quantifications. VW contributed to the initial experimental design. J-PG prepared heat maps. AG performed cell sorting and HIV-DNA PCR quantifications. MF and JP-R insured study participant recruitment, blood cell collection through leukapheresis, and/or access to clinical information. NC contributed with expertise, protocols, and reagents, as well as data analysis for QVOA. PA designed experiments, prepared figures, and wrote the manuscript. All authors revised and approved the manuscript.

ACKNOWLEDGMENTS

We acknowledge the contribution of Dr. Dominique Gauchat (Flow Cytometry Core Facility, CHUM-Research Centre, Montreal, QC, Canada) for expert technical support with flow cytometry analysis and sorting, Mario Legault for help with ethical approvals and informed consents, Josée Girouard, Angie Massicotte, and Maria Fraraccio (McGill University Health Centre-Glen site, Montreal, QC, Canada) for their contribution to blood collection from HIV-infected study participants. We thank Amélie Cattin, and Tomas Wiche Salinas (CRCHUM) for critical reading/revision of the manuscript; as well as Dr. Jonathan Richard and Dr. Andres Finzi (CRCHUM) for recommendations on HIV outgrowth strategies. We also thank Dr. Roger G. Ptak, Dr. Carol Lackman-Smith (Southern Research, Frederick, Maryland, United States of America), and Dr. Deanna A. Kulpa (Department of Pediatrics, Emory University, Atlanta, Georgia, United States of America) for critical reading of the manuscript and expert technical recommendations on QVOA. We also thank Dr. Ali Filali-Mouhim, Research Associate-Senior Bioinformatician at the CHUM Research Center, for professional expertise with statistical analysis. Finally, we acknowledge the key contribution of study participants via their precious gift of biological samples.

REFERENCES

Alvarez, Y., Tuen, M., Shen, G., Nawaz, F., Arthos, J., Wolff, M. J., et al. (2013). Preferential HIV infection of CCR6$^+$ Th17 cells is associated with higher levels of virus receptor expression and lack of CCR5 ligands. *J. Virol.* 87, 10843–10854. doi: 10.1128/JVI.01838-13

Anderson, J. L., Khoury, G., Fromentin, R., Solomon, A., Chomont, N., Sinclair, E., et al. (2019). Human immunodeficiency virus (HIV)-infected CCR6$^+$ rectal CD4$^+$ T cells and HIV persistence on antiretroviral therapy. *J. Infect Dis.* 221, 744-755. doi: 10.1093/infdis/jiz509

Ansel, K. M., Djuretic, I., Tanasa, B., and Rao, A. (2006). Regulation of Th2 differentiation and Il4 locus accessibility. *Annu. Rev. Immunol.* 24, 607–656. doi: 10.1146/annurev.immunol.23.021704.115821

Archin, N. M., Liberty, A. L., Kashuba, A. D., Choudhary, S. K., Kuruc, J. D., Crooks, A. M., et al. (2012). Administration of vorinostat disrupts HIV-1 latency in patients on antiretroviral therapy. *Nature* 487, 482–485.

Archin, N. M., and Margolis, D. M. (2014). Emerging strategies to deplete the HIV reservoir. *Curr. Opin. Infect. Dis.* 27, 29–35. doi: 10.1097/QCO.0000000000000026

Banga, R., Procopio, F. A., Noto, A., Pollakis, G., Cavassini, M., Ohmiti, K., et al. (2016). PD-1$^+$ and follicular helper T cells are responsible for persistent HIV-1 transcription in treated aviremic individuals. *Nat. Med.* 22, 754–761. doi: 10.1038/nm.4113

Barre-Sinoussi, F., Ross, A. L., and Delfraissy, J. F. (2013). Past, present and future: 30 years of HIV research. *Nat. Rev. Microbiol.* 11, 877–883. doi: 10.1038/nrmicro3132

Basu, R., Hatton, R. D., and Weaver, C. T. (2013). The Th17 family: flexibility follows function. *Immunol. Rev.* 252, 89–103. doi: 10.1111/imr.12035

Baxter, A. E., Niessl, J., Fromentin, R., Richard, J., Porichis, F., Charlebois, R., et al. (2016). Single-cell characterization of viral translation-competent reservoirs in HIV-infected individuals. *Cell Host Microbe* 20, 368–380. doi: 10.1016/j.chom.2016.07.015

Baxter, A. E., Niessl, J., Fromentin, R., Richard, J., Porichis, F., Massanella, M., et al. (2017). Multiparametric characterization of rare HIV-infected cells using an RNA-flow FISH technique. *Nat. Protoc.* 12, 2029–2049. doi: 10.1038/nprot.2017.079

Baxter, A. E., O'Doherty, U., and Kaufmann, D. E. (2018). Beyond the replication-competent HIV reservoir: transcription and translation-competent reservoirs. *Retrovirology* 15:18. doi: 10.1186/s12977-018-0392-7

Beliakova-Bethell, N., Hezareh, M., Wong, J. K., Strain, M. C., Lewinski, M. K., Richman, D. D., et al. (2017). Relative efficacy of T cell stimuli as inducers of productive HIV-1 replication in latently infected CD4 lymphocytes from patients on suppressive cART. *Virology* 508, 127–133. doi: 10.1016/j.virol.2017.05.008

Boulassel, M. R., Spurll, G., Rouleau, D., Tremblay, C., Edwardes, M., Sekaly, R. P., et al. (2003). Changes in immunological and virological parameters in HIV-1 infected subjects following leukapheresis. *J. Clin. Apher.* 18, 55–60.

Bounou, S., Leclerc, J. E., and Tremblay, M. J. (2002). Presence of host ICAM-1 in laboratory and clinical strains of human immunodeficiency virus type 1 increases virus infectivity and CD4(+)-T-cell depletion in human lymphoid tissue, a major site of replication in vivo. *J. Virol.* 76, 1004–1014. doi: 10.1128/jvi.76.3.1004-1014.2002

Bruner, K. M., Hosmane, N. N., and Siliciano, R. F. (2015). Towards an HIV-1 cure: measuring the latent reservoir. *Trends Microbiol.* 23, 192–203. doi: 10.1016/j.tim.2015.01.013

Bruner, K. M., Murray, A. J., Pollack, R. A., Soliman, M. G., Laskey, S. B., Capoferri, A. A., et al. (2016). Defective proviruses rapidly accumulate during acute HIV-1 infection. *Nat. Med.* 22, 1043–1049. doi: 10.1038/nm.4156

Bruner, K. M., Wang, Z., Simonetti, F. R., Bender, A. M., Kwon, K. J., Sengupta, S., et al. (2019). A quantitative approach for measuring the reservoir of latent HIV-1 proviruses. *Nature* 566, 120–125. doi: 10.1038/s41586-019-0898-8

Brussel, A., and Sonigo, P. (2003). Analysis of early human immunodeficiency virus type 1 DNA synthesis by use of a new sensitive assay for quantifying integrated provirus. *J. Virol.* 77, 10119–10124.

Bullen, C. K., Laird, G. M., Durand, C. M., Siliciano, J. D., and Siliciano, R. F. (2014). New ex vivo approaches distinguish effective and ineffective single agents for reversing HIV-1 latency in vivo. *Nat. Med.* 20, 425–429. doi: 10.1038/nm.3489

Buzon, M. J., Massanella, M., Llibre, J. M., Esteve, A., Dahl, V., Puertas, M. C., et al. (2010). HIV-1 replication and immune dynamics are affected by raltegravir intensification of HAART-suppressed subjects. *Nat. Med.* 16, 460–465. doi: 10.1038/nm.2111

Buzon, M. J., Sun, H., Li, C., Shaw, A., Seiss, K., Ouyang, Z., et al. (2014). HIV-1 persistence in CD4$^+$ T cells with stem cell-like properties. *Nat. Med.* 20, 139–142. doi: 10.1038/nm.3445

Casazza, J. P., Brenchley, J. M., Hill, B. J., Ayana, R., Ambrozak, D., Roederer, M., et al. (2009). Autocrine production of beta-chemokines protects CMV-Specific CD4 T cells from HIV infection. *PLoS Pathog.* 5:e1000646. doi: 10.1371/journal.ppat.1000646

Chomont, N., Dafonseca, S., Vandergeeten, C., Ancuta, P., and Sekaly, R. P. (2011). Maintenance of CD4$^+$ T-cell memory and HIV persistence: keeping memory, keeping HIV. *Curr. Opin. HIV AIDS* 6, 30–36.

Chomont, N., El-Far, M., Ancuta, P., Trautmann, L., Procopio, F. A., Yassine-Diab, B., et al. (2009). HIV reservoir size and persistence are driven by T cell survival and homeostatic proliferation. *Nat. Med.* 15, 893–900.

Chun, T. W., Moir, S., and Fauci, A. S. (2015). HIV reservoirs as obstacles and opportunities for an HIV cure. *Nat. Immunol.* 16, 584–589. doi: 10.1038/ni.3152

Churchill, M. J., Deeks, S. G., Margolis, D. M., Siliciano, R. F., and Swanstrom, R. (2016). HIV reservoirs: what, where and how to target them. *Nat. Rev. Microbiol.* 14, 55–60. doi: 10.1038/nrmicro.2015.5

Cicala, C., Martinelli, E., McNally, J. P., Goode, D. J., Gopaul, R., Hiatt, J., et al. (2009). The integrin alpha4beta7 forms a complex with cell-surface CD4 and defines a T-cell subset that is highly susceptible to infection by HIV-1. *Proc. Natl. Acad. Sci. U.S.A.* 106, 20877–20882.

Cillo, A. R., Sobolewski, M. D., Bosch, R. J., Fyne, E., Piatak, M. Jr., et al. (2014). Quantification of HIV-1 latency reversal in resting CD4$^+$ T cells from patients on suppressive antiretroviral therapy. *Proc. Natl. Acad. Sci. U.S.A.* 111, 7078–7083. doi: 10.1073/pnas.1402873111

Cohn, L. B., Silva, I. T., Oliveira, T. Y., Rosales, R. A., Parrish, E. H., Learn, G. H., et al. (2015). HIV-1 integration landscape during latent and active infection. *Cell* 160, 420–432. doi: 10.1016/j.cell.2015.01.020

Colby, D. J., Trautmann, L., Pinyakorn, S., Leyre, L., Pagliuzza, A., Kroon, E., et al. (2018). Rapid HIV RNA rebound after antiretroviral treatment interruption in persons durably suppressed in Fiebig I acute HIV infection. *Nat. Med.* 24, 923–926. doi: 10.1038/s41591-018-0026-6

Deeks, S. G., Lewin, S. R., Ross, A. L., Ananworanich, J., Benkirane, M., Cannon, P., et al. (2016). International AIDS society global scientific strategy: towards an HIV cure 2016. *Nat. Med.* 22, 839–850. doi: 10.1038/nm.4108

Eisele, E., and Siliciano, R. F. (2012). Redefining the viral reservoirs that prevent HIV-1 eradication. *Immunity* 37, 377–388.

Eriksson, S., Graf, E. H., Dahl, V., Strain, M. C., Yukl, S. A., Lysenko, E. S., et al. (2013). Comparative analysis of measures of viral reservoirs in HIV-1 eradication studies. *PLoS Pathog.* 9:e1003174. doi: 10.1371/journal.ppat.1003174

Erkelens, M. N., and Mebius, R. E. (2017). Retinoic acid and immune homeostasis: a balancing act. *Trends Immunol.* 38, 168–180. doi: 10.1016/j.it.2016.12.006

Fan, P., Li, X., Su, W., Kong, W., Kong, X., Wang, Z., et al. (2015). Enhanced sensitivity for detection of HIV-1 p24 antigen by a novel nuclease-linked fluorescence oligonucleotide assay. *PLoS ONE* 10:e0125701. doi: 10.1371/journal.pone.0125701

Finzi, D., Hermankova, M., Pierson, T., Carruth, L. M., Buck, C., Chaisson, R. E., et al. (1997). Identification of a reservoir for HIV-1 in patients on highly active antiretroviral therapy. *Science* 278, 1295–1300.

Fromentin, R., DaFonseca, S., Costiniuk, C. T., El-Far, M., Procopio, F. A., Hecht, F. M., et al. (2019). PD-1 blockade potentiates HIV latency reversal ex vivo in CD4(+) T cells from ART-suppressed individuals. *Nat. Commun.* 10:814. doi: 10.1038/s41467-019-08798-7

Fun, A., Mok, H. P., Wills, M. R., and Lever, A. M. (2017). A highly reproducible quantitative viral outgrowth assay for the measurement of the replication-competent latent HIV-1 reservoir. *Sci. Rep.* 7:43231. doi: 10.1038/srep43231

Gaffen, S. L., Jain, R., Garg, A. V., and Cua, D. J. (2014). The IL-23-IL-17 immune axis: from mechanisms to therapeutic testing. *Nat. Rev. Immunol.* 14, 585–600. doi: 10.1038/nri3707

Gianella, S., Anderson, C. M., Richman, D. D., Smith, D. M., and Little, S. J. (2015). No evidence of posttreatment control after early initiation of antiretroviral therapy. *AIDS* 29, 2093–2097. doi: 10.1097/QAD.0000000000000816

Gosselin, A., Monteiro, P., Chomont, N., Diaz-Griffero, F., Said, E. A., Fonseca, S., et al. (2010). Peripheral blood $CCR4^+$ $CCR6^+$ and $CXCR3^+$ $CCR6^+$ $CD4^+$ T cells are highly permissive to HIV-1 infection. *J. Immunol.* 184, 1604–1616.

Gosselin, A., Wiche Salinas, T. R., Planas, D., Wacleche, V. S., Zhang, Y., Fromentin, R., et al. (2017). HIV persists in $CCR6^+CD4^+$ T cells from colon and blood during antiretroviral therapy. *AIDS* 31, 35–48. doi: 10.1097/QAD.0000000000001309

Goulder, P., and Deeks, S. G. (2018). HIV control: is getting there the same as staying there? *PLoS Pathog.* 14:e1007222. doi: 10.1371/journal.ppat.1007222

Henrich, T. J., Hatano, H., Bacon, O., Hogan, L. E., Rutishauser, R., Hill, A., et al. (2017). HIV-1 persistence following extremely early initiation of antiretroviral therapy (ART) during acute HIV-1 infection: an observational study. *PLoS Med.* 14:e1002417. doi: 10.1371/journal.pmed.1002417

Ho, D. D., and Zhang, L. (2000). HIV-1 rebound after anti-retroviral therapy. *Nat. Med.* 6, 736–737. doi: 10.1038/77447

Ho, Y. C., Shan, L., Hosmane, N. N., Wang, J., Laskey, S. B., Rosenbloom, D. I., et al. (2013). Replication-competent noninduced proviruses in the latent reservoir increase barrier to HIV-1 cure. *Cell* 155, 540–551. doi: 10.1016/j.cell.2013.09.020

Hosmane, N. N., Kwon, K. J., Bruner, K. M., Capoferri, A. A., Beg, S., Rosenbloom, D. I., et al. (2017). Proliferation of latently infected $CD4^+$ T cells carrying replication-competent HIV-1: potential role in latent reservoir dynamics. *J. Exp. Med.* 214, 959–972. doi: 10.1084/jem.20170193

Hughes, S. H., and Coffin, J. M. (2016). What integration sites tell us about HIV persistence. *Cell Host Microbe* 19, 588–598. doi: 10.1016/j.chom.2016.04.010

Kallies, A., and Good-Jacobson, K. L. (2017). Transcription factor T-bet orchestrates lineage development and function in the immune system. *Trends Immunol.* 38, 287–297. doi: 10.1016/j.it.2017.02.003

Kastirr, I., Crosti, M., Maglie, S., Paroni, M., Steckel, B., Moro, M., et al. (2015). Signal strength and metabolic requirements control cytokine-induced Th17 differentiation of uncommitted human T cells. *J. Immunol.* 195, 3617–3627. doi: 10.4049/jimmunol.1501016

Kessing, C. F., Nixon, C. C., Li, C., Tsai, P., Takata, H., Mousseau, G., et al. (2017). In vivo suppression of HIV rebound by didehydro-cortistatin A, a "block-and-lock", Strategy for HIV-1 Treatment. *Cell Rep.* 21, 600–611. doi: 10.1016/j.celrep.2017.09.080

Khoury, G., Anderson, J. L., Fromentin, R., Hartogenesis, W., Smith, M. Z., Bacchetti, P., et al. (2016). Persistence of integrated HIV DNA in CXCR3 $^+$ CCR6 $^+$ memory $CD4^+$ T cells in HIV-infected individuals on antiretroviral therapy. *AIDS* 30, 1511–1520. doi: 10.1097/QAD.0000000000001029

Kim, C. J., Rousseau, R., Huibner, S., Kovacs, C., Benko, E., Shahabi, K., et al. (2017). Impact of intensified antiretroviral therapy during early HIV infection on gut immunology and inflammatory blood biomarkers: a randomized controlled trial. *AIDS* 31, 1529–1534. doi: 10.1097/QAD.0000000000001515

Kiselinova, M., De Spiegelaere, W., Buzon, M. J., Malatinkova, E., Lichterfeld, M., and Vandekerckhove, L. (2016). Integrated and total HIV-1 DNA predict ex vivo viral outgrowth. *PLoS Pathog.* 12:e1005472. doi: 10.1371/journal.ppat.1005472

Kosaka, P. M., Pini, V., Calleja, M., and Tamayo, J. (2017). Ultrasensitive detection of HIV-1 p24 antigen by a hybrid nanomechanical-optoplasmonic platform with potential for detecting HIV-1 at first week after infection. *PLoS ONE* 12:e0171899. doi: 10.1371/journal.pone.0171899

Laird, G. M., Eisele, E. E., Rabi, S. A., Lai, J., Chioma, S., Blankson, J. N., et al. (2013). Rapid quantification of the latent reservoir for HIV-1 using a viral outgrowth assay. *PLoS Pathog.* 9:e1003398. doi: 10.1371/journal.ppat.1003398

Laird, G. M., Rosenbloom, D. I., Lai, J., Siliciano, R. F., and Siliciano, J. D. (2016). Measuring the frequency of latent HIV-1 in resting CD4($^+$) T cells using a limiting dilution coculture assay. *Methods Mol. Biol.* 1354, 239–253. doi: 10.1007/978-1-4939-3046-3_16

Lee, G. Q., Orlova-Fink, N., Einkauf, K., Chowdhury, F. Z., Sun, X., Harrington, S., et al. (2017). Clonal expansion of genome-intact HIV-1 in functionally polarized Th1 $CD4^+$ T cells. *J. Clin. Invest.* 127, 2689–2696. doi: 10.1172/JCI93289

Lee, M. O., Hobbs, P. D., Zhang, X. K., Dawson, M. I., and Pfahl, M. (1994). A synthetic retinoid antagonist inhibits the human immunodeficiency virus type 1 promoter. *Proc. Natl. Acad. Sci. U.S.A.* 91, 5632–5636.

Li, P., Kaiser, P., Lampiris, H. W., Kim, P., Yukl, S. A., Havlir, D. V., et al. (2016). Stimulating the RIG-I pathway to kill cells in the latent HIV reservoir following viral reactivation. *Nat. Med.* 22, 807–811. doi: 10.1038/nm.4124

Lorenzi, J. C., Cohen, Y. Z., Cohn, L. B., Kreider, E. F., Barton, J. P., Learn, G. H., et al. (2016). Paired quantitative and qualitative assessment of the replication-competent HIV-1 reservoir and comparison with integrated proviral DNA. *Proc. Natl. Acad. Sci. U.S.A.* 113, E7908–E7916. doi: 10.1073/pnas.1617789113

Margolis, D. M., Garcia, J. V., Hazuda, D. J., and Haynes, B. F. (2016). Latency reversal and viral clearance to cure HIV-1. *Science* 353:aaf6517. doi: 10.1126/science.aaf6517

Martin, A. R., and Siliciano, R. F. (2016). Progress toward HIV eradication: case reports, current efforts, and the challenges associated with cure. *Annu. Rev. Med.* 67, 215–228. doi: 10.1146/annurev-med-011514-023043

Martinelli, E., Tharinger, H., Frank, I., Arthos, J., Piatak, M. Jr., et al. (2011). HSV-2 infection of dendritic cells amplifies a highly susceptible HIV-1 cell target. *PLoS Pathog.* 7:e1002109. doi: 10.1371/journal.ppat.1002109

Massanella, M., and Richman, D. D. (2016). Measuring the latent reservoir in vivo. *J. Clin. Invest.* 126, 464–472. doi: 10.1172/JCI80567

Massanella, M., Yek, C., Lada, S. M., Nakazawa, M., Shefa, N., Huang, K., et al. (2018). Improved assays to measure and characterize the inducible HIV reservoir. *EBioMed.* 36, 113–121. doi: 10.1016/j.ebiom.2018.09.036

Mele, F., Basso, C., Leoni, C., Aschenbrenner, D., Becattini, S., Latorre, D., et al. (2015). ERK phosphorylation and miR-181a expression modulate activation of human memory TH17 cells. *Nat. Commun.* 6:6431. doi: 10.1038/ncomms7431

Miles, B., and Connick, E. (2016). TFH in HIV latency and as sources of replication-competent virus. *Trends Microbiol.* 24, 338–344. doi: 10.1016/j.tim.2016.02.006

Monteiro, P., Gosselin, A., Wacleche, V. S., El-Far, M., Said, E. A., Kared, H., et al. (2011). Memory $CCR6^+CD4^+$ T cells are preferential targets for productive HIV type 1 infection regardless of their expression of integrin beta7. *J. Immunol.* 186, 4618–4630.

Mousseau, G., Kessing, C. F., Fromentin, R., Trautmann, L., Chomont, N., and Valente, S. T. (2015a). The tat inhibitor didehydro-cortistatin A prevents HIV-1 reactivation from latency. *MBio* 6:e00465. doi: 10.1128/mBio.00465-15

Mousseau, G., Mediouni, S., and Valente, S. T. (2015b). Targeting HIV transcription: the quest for a functional cure. *Curr. Top. Microbiol. Immunol.* 389, 121–145. doi: 10.1007/82_2015_435

Pardons, M., Baxter, A. E., Massanella, M., Pagliuzza, A., Fromentin, R., Dufour, C., et al. (2019). Single-cell characterization and quantification of translation-competent viral reservoirs in treated and untreated HIV infection. *PLoS Pathog.* 15:e1007619. doi: 10.1371/journal.ppat.1007619

Passaes, C. P., Bruel, T., Decalf, J., David, A., Angin, M., Monceaux, V., et al. (2017). Ultrasensitive HIV-1 p24 assay detects single infected cells and differences in reservoir induction by latency reversal agents. *J. Virol.* 91, e2296–e2216. doi: 10.1128/JVI.02296-16

Pinzone, M. R., and O'Doherty, U. (2018). Measuring integrated HIV DNA ex vivo and in vitro provides insights about how reservoirs are formed and maintained. *Retrovirology* 15:22. doi: 10.1186/s12977-018-0396-3

Planas, D., Routy, J. P., and Ancuta, P. (2018). New Th17-specific therapeutic strategies for HIV remission. *Curr. Opin. HIV AIDS* 14, 85–92. doi: 10.1097/COH.0000000000000522

Planas, D., Zhang, Y., Monteiro, P., Goulet, J. P., Gosselin, A., Grandvaux, N., et al. (2017). HIV-1 selectively targets gut-homing $CCR6^+CD4^+$ T cells via mTOR-dependent mechanisms. *JCI Insight* 2, e93230. doi: 10.1172/jci.insight.93230

Procopio, F. A., Fromentin, R., Kulpa, D. A., Brehm, J. H., Bebin, A. G., Strain, M. C., et al. (2015). A novel assay to measure the magnitude of the inducible viral reservoir in HIV-infected individuals. *EBioMedicine* 2, 872–881. doi: 10.1016/j.ebiom.2015.06.019

Raverdeau, M., and Mills, K. H. (2014). Modulation of T cell and innate immune responses by retinoic Acid. *J. Immunol.* 192, 2953–2958. doi: 10.4049/jimmunol.1303245

Roederer, M. (2002). Compensation in flow cytometry. *Curr. Protoc. Cytom.* 1:14. doi: 10.1002/0471142956.cy0114s22

Rosenbloom, D. I., Elliott, O., Hill, A. L., Henrich, T. J., Siliciano, J. M., and Siliciano, R. F. (2015). Designing and interpreting limiting dilution assays: general principles and applications to the latent reservoir for human immunodeficiency virus-1. *Open Forum Infect. Dis.* 2:ofv123. doi: 10.1093/ofid/ofv123

Sengupta, S., and Siliciano, R. F. (2018). Targeting the latent reservoir for HIV-1. *Immunity* 48, 872–895. doi: 10.1016/j.immuni.2018.04.030

Siliciano, J. D., and Siliciano, R. F. (2005). Enhanced culture assay for detection and quantitation of latently infected, resting $CD4^+$ T-cells carrying replication-competent virus in HIV-1-infected individuals. *Methods Mol. Biol.* 304, 3–15.

Siliciano, J. D., and Siliciano, R. F. (2018). Assays to measure latency, reservoirs, and reactivation. *Curr. Top. Microbiol. Immunol.* 417, 23–41. doi: 10.1007/82_2017_75

Soriano-Sarabia, N., Bateson, R. E., Dahl, N. P., Crooks, A. M., Kuruc, J. D., Margolis, D. M., et al. (2014). Quantitation of replication-competent HIV-1 in populations of resting $CD4^+$ T cells. *J. Virol.* 88, 14070–14077. doi: 10.1128/JVI.01900-14

Spina, C. A., Anderson, J., Archin, N. M., Bosque, A., Chan, J., Famiglietti, M., et al. (2013). An in-depth comparison of latent HIV-1 reactivation in multiple cell model systems and resting $CD4^+$ T cells from aviremic patients. *PLoS Pathog.* 9:e1003834. doi: 10.1371/journal.ppat.1003834

Sun, H., Kim, D., Li, X., Kiselinova, M., Ouyang, Z., Vandekerckhove, L., et al. (2015). Th1/17 polarization of CD4 T cells supports HIV-1 DNA persistence during antiretroviral therapy. *J. Virol.* 89, 11284–11293. doi: 10.1128/JVI.01595-15

Vandergeeten, C., Fromentin, R., Merlini, E., Lawani, M. B., DaFonseca, S., Bakeman, W., et al. (2014). Cross-clade ultrasensitive PCR-based assays to measure HIV persistence in large-cohort studies. *J. Virol.* 88, 12385–12396. doi: 10.1128/JVI.00609-14

Wacleche, V. S., Goulet, J. P., Gosselin, A., Monteiro, P., Soudeyns, H., Fromentin, R., et al. (2016). New insights into the heterogeneity of Th17 subsets contributing to HIV-1 persistence during antiretroviral therapy. *Retrovirology* 13:59. doi: 10.1186/s12977-016-0293-6

Wacleche, V. S., Landay, A., Routy, J. P., and Ancuta, P. (2017). The Th17 lineage: from barrier surfaces homeostasis to autoimmunity, cancer, and HIV-1 pathogenesis. *Viruses* 9:E303. doi: 10.3390/v9100303

Wang, F. S., Zhang, L., Douek, D., McMichael, A., Xu, X. N., and Lewin, S. R. (2018). Strategies for an HIV cure: progress and challenges. *Nat. Immunol.* 19, 1155–1158. doi: 10.1038/s41590-018-0242-8

Wonderlich, E. R., Subramanian, K., Cox, B., Wiegand, A., Lackman-Smith, C., Bale, M. J., et al. (2019). Effector memory differentiation increases detection of replication-competent HIV-l in resting $CD4^+$ T cells from virally suppressed individuals. *PLoS Pathog.* 15:e1008074. doi: 10.1371/journal.ppat.1008074

Wong, J. K., Hezareh, M., Gunthard, H. F., Havlir, D. V., Ignacio, C. C., Spina, C. A., et al. (1997). Recovery of replication-competent HIV despite prolonged suppression of plasma viremia. *Science* 278, 1291–1295.

9

Quantification of Viral RNA and DNA Positive Cells in Tissues from Simian Immunodeficiency Virus/Simian Human Immunodeficiency Virus Infected Controller and Progressor Rhesus Macaques

Bapi Pahar[1], Dot Kuebler[1], Terri Rasmussen[1], Xiaolei Wang[1], Sudesh K. Srivastav[2], Arpita Das[3] and Ronald S. Veazey[1]*

[1] Division of Comparative Pathology, Tulane National Primate Research Center, Covington, LA, United States, [2] Department of Biostatistics and Bioinformatics, Tulane University, New Orleans, LA, United States, [3] Division of Microbiology, Tulane National Primate Research Center, Covington, LA, United States

***Correspondence:**
Bapi Pahar
bpahar@tulane.edu

Eradication of human immunodeficiency virus 1 (HIV-1) from an infected individual cannot be achieved using current antiretroviral therapy (ART) regimens. Viral reservoirs established in early infection remain unaffected by ART and are able to replenish systemic infection upon treatment interruption. Simian immunodeficiency virus (SIV) infected macaque models are useful for studying HIV pathogenesis, treatments, and persistent viral reservoirs. Here, we used the SIV macaque model to examine and quantify RNA and DNA positive cells in tissues from macaques that control viral replication (controllers) and those that have persistently high plasma viremia (progressors). A positive correlation was detected between tissue RNA+ cells and plasma viral load in both mesenteric lymph node (LN) and spleen. Similarly, a positive correlation also observed between DNA+ cells and plasma viral load in ileum and jejunum. Controllers had a lower frequency of both RNA and DNA+ cells in several tissues compared to progressors. However, DNA+ cells were prevalent in mesenteric LN, inguinal LN, colon, midbrain, and bone marrow tissues in both controller and progressors. Organized lymphoid tissues of LNs, spleen, and intestine were found as the major tissues positive for virus. Viral RNA and DNA positive cells were detected in brain and thymus in macaques with high plasma viremia and SIV-encephalitis. Both T cells and macrophages were shown to be infected in several tissues, indicating vaccines and ART should be specifically designed to protect these cells in organized lymphoid tissues. These results indicate ART should target infected cells in secondary lymphoid organs to reduce both productively and latently infected cells.

Keywords: DNA, HIV, infection, macaque, RNA, SIV, tissue

INTRODUCTION

Human immunodeficiency virus (HIV) continues to be a major dreaded disease, as 37.9 million people are living with HIV/AIDS worldwide[1]. Globally, in 2018 alone, an estimated 1.7 million people became newly infected with HIV and 770,000 people died from AIDS-related illness, emphasizing the need for more effective treatments. Administration of combination antiretroviral therapy (cART) has drastically improved the mortality of HIV infected patients, yet it has little impact on eliminating viral reservoirs or in reducing virus-associated immune activation, which is believed to be primarily responsible for continued viral replication, and the acceleration of cellular senescence and aging in HIV disease (Desai and Landay, 2010). The simian immunodeficiency virus (SIV) non-human primate (NHP) models of AIDS are well established, and have been extremely useful in HIV-1 vaccine development and in advancing the understanding of the pathogenesis of AIDS. HIV and NHP models of SIV infection have shown that persistent latent and active reservoirs are established in tissues within days of infection (Chun et al., 1998; Whitney et al., 2014; Ananworanich et al., 2016; Amedee et al., 2018; Bandera et al., 2019). A recent study demonstrated the presence of SIV in CD4+ T cells and macrophages in ART suppressed SIV infected macaques treated with cART 12 days after infection (Abreu et al., 2019). Resting CD4+ T cells are believed to be the major latent cellular reservoirs for HIV. Further, CD4+ cells with stem-cell like properties, resident memory T cells in cervical mucosa, follicular T cells in germinal centers of organized lymphoid tissues, monocytes/macrophages, dendritic cells, astrocytes, hematopoietic stem cells, and other progenitor cells have all been shown to be reservoirs for HIV (Zhu et al., 2002; Buzon et al., 2014; Fukazawa et al., 2015; Garcia et al., 2017; Zaikos et al., 2018; Bandera et al., 2019; Cantero-Perez et al., 2019). Major HIV tissue reservoir includes lymph node (LN), spleen, gut associate lymphoid tissues, brain, lung, liver, bone marrow, reproductive tissues and adipose tissues (Chun et al., 1997; Blankson et al., 2002; Marcello, 2006; Couturier and Lewis, 2018), thus virus rebounds within days to a few weeks after ART interruption. Cells latently harboring proviral DNA allow the virus to persist indefinitely in tissues, which may eventually be triggered to produce bursts of viral replication during periods of immune activation and in the absence of ART. Further, these latently infected cells are not recognized or eliminated by the cytolytic T cells. The half-life of latently infected cells has been estimated to be 44 months on treatment, suggesting that virus cannot be eliminated within the lifetime of infected individuals (Siliciano et al., 2003; Strain et al., 2003; Crooks et al., 2015; Bruner and Cohn, 2019). Moreover, the rare occurrence of genetically intact provirus (1 in 100,000) in circulating CD4+ T cells (Bruner and Cohn, 2019) and the lack of cellular markers to distinguish HIV-infected and uninfected cells are all major barriers for establishing an effective cure strategy for HIV. A minor population of HIV infected patients known as long term non-progressors (LTNPs) have been shown to naturally control plasma viral loads (pVL) and maintain stable CD4+ T cell counts for years in the absence of ART. However, the mechanism behind this lack of progression to disease remains elusive. Here, we used the NHP-SIV model to compare viral infected cells in macaques that spontaneously control viral replication to those that have persistently high viremia. Although most Indian-origin rhesus macaques (RMs) progress to disease when infected with SIV_{MAC}, a fraction (~20%) of Chinese origin macaques spontaneously control viremia and become LTNP. In these LTNP Chinese macaques, virus has been detected in the large intestine without any significant changes in immune activation when compared to progressors (Ling et al., 2010). Although several lymphoid tissues have been shown to harbor latently infected cells, we hypothesize that differences in the distribution of viral infected cells exist between animals who control viral replication such as LTNP and those that progress to simian AIDS. In this study, we have quantified SIV RNA and DNA positive cells in several tissues from progressing and non-progressing macaques (Chinese and Indian origin) to determine the major infected tissues harboring SIV/SHIV RNA and DNA positive cells.

[1]https://www.who.int/hiv/data/en/

MATERIALS AND METHODS

Ethics Statement

In this study, 32 adult Indian (IND) or Chinese (CHI) RMs (*Macaca mulatta*) were screened and shown to be negative for SIV, HIV-2, type-D retrovirus and simian T-cell leukemia virus 1 infection at the beginning of the study (**Table 1**). All animals were housed and maintained at the Tulane National Primate Research Center (TNPRC) throughout the study. The study was approved by the TNPRC Institutional Animal Care and Use Committee (IACUC) and was conducted within the guidelines of the United States Public Health Service Policy and the *Guide for the Care and Use of Laboratory Animals* (National Research Council, 2011). The TNPRC is fully accredited by the Association for Assessment and Accreditation of Laboratory Animal Care (AAALAC) International. Once infected, animals were housed in Animal Biosafety Level 2 indoor housing with a 12:12-h light/dark cycle, relative humidity of 30–70%, and a temperature of 64–72°F. Water was available *ad libitum* and a standard commercially formulated NHP diet was provided daily and supplemented with fresh fruit and/or forage material no fewer than three times per week as part of the behavioral management program. Animals were housed in stainless steel cages (Allentown, Inc., Allentown, NJ, United States) sized in accordance or in excess of the U.S. Department of Agriculture (USDA) regulations; each cage contained a perch, portable enrichment toy, and a forage board for feeding enrichment. All animal procedures including virus administration, sample collection, and euthanasia were carried out under the direction of TNPRC veterinarians.

Animals and Tissue Sampling

A total of 32 RMs of both sexes between 2.2 and 12.2 years of age were grouped into four groups based on their terminal pVL.

TABLE 1 | List of rhesus macaques examined.

Animal number	Indian/ Chinese[a]	Age at inoculation (year)	Sex[b]	Virus	Days of infection	Dosage ($TCID_{50}$ or vRNA copies)[c]	Route[d]	Terminal plasma viral load (RNA copies/ml)	Cause of death
AL78	CHI	5.2	F	SHIV162P3	204	300	IVAG	<125	Euthanasia
BA69	IND	9.6	F	SHIV162P3	175	300	IVAG	<125	Euthanasia
BA11	IND	10.6	F	SHIV162P3	175	300	IVAG	<125	Euthanasia
BN81	IND	5.9	F	SHIV162P3	520	5000	IR	<125	Intestine Torsion
CR02	CHI	6.2	F	SHIV162P3	129	300	IVAG	699	Euthanasia
BN87	IND	6.7	F	SHIV162P3	175	300	IVAG	2425	Euthanasia
R870	IND	11.3	F	SHIV162P3	175	300	IVAG	181619	Euthanasia
V120	IND	9.7	F	SHIV162P3	175	300	IVAG	916	Euthanasia
GE64	CHI	5.0	F	SHIV162P3	129	500	IVAG	1123	Euthanasia
DE99	IND	4.9	M	$SIV_{MAC}239$	119	100	IV	43244100	Euthanasia due to poor prognosis
DG96	IND	4.7	M	$SIV_{MAC}239$	147	100	IV	12411500	Euthanasia due to poor prognosis
J541	CHI	10.8	F	$SIV_{MAC}239$	556	100	IV	2057775	Colitis
CR83	IND	3.1	F	$SIV_{MAC}239$	616	100	IV	5458	Euthanasia
DD88	IND	2.2	F	$SIV_{MAC}239$	385	100	IV	921755	Euthanasia due to poor prognosis
CA84	IND	4.5	M	$SIV_{MAC}239$	628	100	IV	8285600	AIDS
DD95	IND	2.6	M	$SIV_{MAC}239$	468	100	IV	1819200	Euthanasia due to poor prognosis
V515	CHI	4.2	F	$SIV_{MAC}239$	668	100	IV	183648	*Mycobacterium avium intracellulare*
AL26	CHI	3.1	M	$SIV_{MAC}239$	685	100	IV	949800	Interstitial Pneumonia
P772	CHI	6.5	F	$SIV_{MAC}239$	819	100	IV	2269180	*Pneumocystis carinii* infection
L395	CHI	8.9	F	$SIV_{MAC}239$	1313	100	IV	667	Amyloidosis
V542	CHI	4.1	M	$SIV_{MAC}239$	1845	100	IV	220	Pneumonia
I553	IND	12.2	F	$SIV_{MAC}239$	655	100	IV	1895400	*Pneumocystis carinii* infection
T798	IND	6.3	M	$SIV_{MAC}239$	962	100	IV	85463	*Mycobacterium avium intracellulare*
FA97	CHI	11.8	M	$SIV_{MAC}239$	316	194,981*	IV	3985200	AIDS/CMV infection
BE86	IND	5.9	F	$SIV_{MAC}251$	837	100	IV	76639	*Mycobacterium avium intracellulare*
DG55	IND	3.7	M	$SIV_{MAC}251$	78	100	IR	413577	Euthanasia
CF35	IND	4.2	M	$SIV_{MAC}251$	93	200	IR	2183900	Euthanasia
DB53	IND	4.9	M	$SIV_{MAC}251$	79	200	IR	127999	Euthanasia
DT83	CHI	8.1	F	$SIV_{MAC}251$	456	200	IR	<125	Dehydration
BE64	IND	3.3	F	$SIV_{MAC}251$	752	3,300,000*	IV	265116	Pericarditis
BE65	IND	3.3	M	$SIV_{MAC}251$	1087	3,300,000*	IV	85463	*Mycobacterium avium intracellulare*
CA66	CHI	5.7	M	$SIV_{MAC}251$	746	200	IR	<125	Generalized amyloidosis

[a]IND and CHI denote Indian and Chinese, respectively. [b]F and M denote female and male respectively. [c]All values are expressed as the TCID50, except values denoted by an asterisk (*), which are vRNA copies. $TCID_{50}$ and vRNA represent as tissue culture infectivity dose at 50% and viral RNA respectively. [d]IR, IV, and IVAG denote intrarectal, intravenous, and intravaginal route, respectively. CMV denotes cytomegalovirus.

Animals were infected with either SHIV162P3, or $SIV_{MAC}251$ or $SIV_{MAC}239$ using intravenous (IV), intrarectal (IR) or intravaginal (IVAG) routes as listed in **Table 1**. At necropsy, peripheral blood and tissues including midbrain, mesenteric LN (Mes. LN), inguinal LN (Ing. LN), axillary LN (Ax. LN), spleen, bone marrow, colon, ileum, jejunum, and thymus were collected and processed as both formalin fixed, paraffin embedded tissues and snap frozen in OCT for *in situ* hybridization (ISH) and immunohistochemistry, respectively.

Plasma Viral Load Quantification

Plasma viral load quantification was performed by bDNA signal amplification assay (Siemens Diagnostics, United States) with a lower limit of detection of 125 SIV/SHIV RNA copies/mL of plasma (Pahar et al., 2007, 2016).

SIV RNA *in situ* Hybridization

SIV RNA ISH was performed on tissue sections as described previously (Borda et al., 2004; Wang et al., 2007; Ahsan et al., 2013; Pahar et al., 2017). Formalin-fixed, paraffin-embedded tissue sections were de-paraffinized overnight at 60°C, then dehydrated by xylene washes followed by re-hydration with alcohol and DEPC water. Antigen retrieval was performed by treating tissue slides with steam in 0.01 M citrate buffer pH 6.0 using a conventional microwave. A 60-min pre-hybridization incubation was performed followed by an overnight incubation at 45°C in hybridization buffer with SIV RNA digoxigenin labeled probe comprising essentially the entire SIV genome (Lofstrand Labs Ltd., Gaithersburg, MD, United States). The next day, slides were washed with SSC buffer followed by blocking with protein blocker (Dako, Santa Clara, CA, United States) for 1 h. The slides were further incubated overnight with appropriately diluted anti-digoxigenin alkaline phosphatase antibody (Roche Diagnostics, Indianapolis, IN, United States) in dark humidified chambers at 4°C. On day three, after two washes with post-hybridization buffer, the slides were developed with NBT/BCIP (Roche) substrate. For each run, known positive and negative LN controls sections were included to validate staining. An average of 10–15 fields (200× magnification) were used in each of the slides to quantify SIV RNA positive cells manually using SPOT3 live imaging software (Diagnostic Instruments, Sterling Heights, MI, United States). The sites for all tissue evaluations were selected randomly from each tissue and counted by two different individuals blinded to the samples to avoid bias. The quantification of RNA positive cells was presented as the number of infected cells/mm^2 of tissue.

SIV DNA *in situ* Hybridization

Amplification of the LTR, Gag, and Pol region of the p239SpSp5′ plasmid DNA (NIH AIDS Research and Reference Reagent Program) was performed utilizing 9 primer pairs designed to span the desired regions. The template DNA (50 ng) and 200 nmoL of each primer were added to a PCR mixture tube containing 2.5 U of Taq DNA polymerase, 200 μM each dTP, dCTP, dGTP, 130 μM dATP, 70 μM DIG-UTP (Roche), 10 mM Tris–HCl (pH 8.3), 40 mM KCl, 1.5 mM $MgCl_2$. The volume was adjusted with distilled water to 25 μL. The reaction mixture was subjected to denaturation at 95°C for 1 min followed by 40 cycles of 95°C for 1 min, 60°C for 1 min, and 72°C for 1 min, and then a final extension step of 72°C for 7 min was done. Labeled amplicons varied in length, averaging 670 nucleotides long. ISH was performed as previous described (Wang et al., 2007) using the PCR generated non-radioactive digoxigenin-labeled probe. In brief, slides were deparaffinized in xylene, and rehydrated, followed by antigen retrieval with steam (citrate buffer). The sections were first treated with RNAse followed by incubation at 37°C overnight with the DNA probe, after which the hybridized probe was detected with Anti-DIG-POD followed by NBT/BCIP (Roche) for visualization. The probe was tested on negative control tissue and tissues known to be infected with $SIV_{MAC}239$ and SHIV to determine specificity and efficiency (**Supplementary Figure 1**). Ten fields (200× magnification) were counted from each slide to quantify SIV DNA positive cells manually using SPOT3 live imaging software. The sites for all tissue evaluations were selected randomly from each tissue and counted by two different individuals blinded to the samples to avoid bias as being performed for RNA stained tissues. The quantification of DNA positive cells was presented as the number of infected cells/mm^2 of tissue.

Immunohistochemistry for Detection and Phenotyping of Infected Cells in Tissues

Formalin fixed, paraffin embedded, tissue sections were processed for immunofluorescent staining with one or a combination of primary antibodies as previously described (Wang et al., 2007; Pan et al., 2014; Pahar et al., 2015, 2017). For immunofluorescent staining, tissue sections were stained sequentially for 2–3 colors by first staining with antisense SIV riboprobes. SIV mRNA positive cells were developed by using a 2-hydroxy-3-naphthoic acid-2 phenylanilide phosphate (HNPP) fluorescence detection kit (Roche Diagnostics). SIV RNA stained slides were further stained with any one of the unconjugated primary antibodies (CD3, Ham56, DC-SIGN, or Ki67) sequentially and then incubated with Alexa Fluor 488-conjugated secondary antibodies (1:1000 dilution, Life Technologies, United States) and/or Alexa Fluor 633-conjugated secondary antibodies (1:1000 dilution, Life Technologies) sequentially. After staining, slides were washed, mounted with Prolong® Gold antifade medium (Life Technologies) and scanned for imaging using a TCS SP2 confocal laser scanning microscope (Leica, Germany) equipped with three lasers. ImageJ (version 1.52a; NIH, Bethesda, MD, United States) and Adobe Photoshop CC (20.0.4 release; Adobe, San Jose, CA, United States) was used to assign colors to all four channels collected: HNPP/Fast Red, which fluoresces red when exposed to a 568-nm wavelength laser; Alexa 488 (Life Technologies) fluoresces green; Alexa 633 (Life Technologies) appears blue; and the differential interference contrast (DIC) image is gray scale. Negative control slides were incorporated in each experiment either by omitting the primary antibody or using isotype IgG1 and IgG (H + L) controls (Pan et al., 2012, 2013, 2014; Pahar et al., 2015, 2017). For phenotyping SIV-infected cells, tissues were first processed for SIV RNA ISH and immunohistochemistry for Ham56 (clone Ham56, IgM Kappa; Dako), CD3 (Rabbit anti-human polyclonal; Dako), dendritic cell-specific ICAM-3 grabbing non-integrin (DC-SIGN, clone DCN46, IgG2b kappa; BD Biosciences, San Jose, CA, United States), and Ki67 (clone MIB-1, IgG1 kappa; Dako) by multilabel confocal microscopy as previously described (Pahar et al., 2017).

Graphics and Statistical Analyses

All data was summarized using descriptive statistics including mean, proportions, and standard deviations. Graphical presentation was performed using GraphPad Prism (version 8.1.2. GraphPad Software, United States). The analysis of variance and Chi-square methods were performed to compare the mean and proportional differences data, respectively. A two-sided

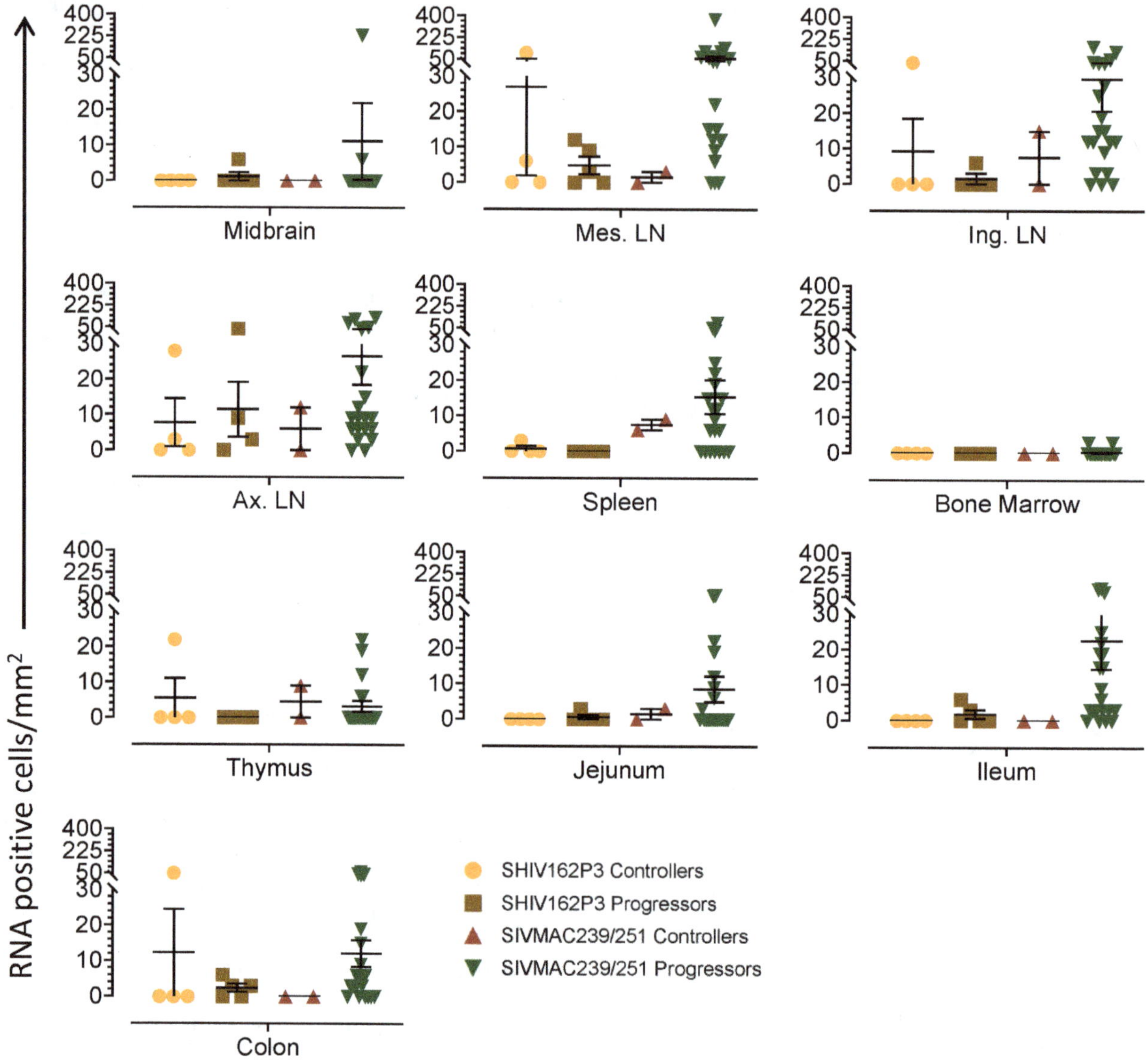

FIGURE 1 | Quantification of RNA positive cells/mm^2 per section in different tissues from animals with different terminal plasma viral loads are shown. Horizontal lines denoted the mean RNA positive cells (±SEM) for each group of animals for the respective tissue.

5% significance level was used throughout. The associations between the frequency of RNA or DNA positive cells in tissues and pVL for both SHIV and SIV controllers and progressors was calculated using the Pearson correlation coefficient method. All data analyses were performed using SAS software (version 9.4 in a Windows environment).

RESULTS

Terminal Plasma Viral Loads in SIV/SHIV Infected Macaques

All RMs were placed into four groups based on their terminal pVL. The first group, SHIV162P3 controllers included four SHIV162P3 infected animals (3 IND and 1 CHI) with undetectable viremia (<125 copies RNA/mL of plasma) (**Table 1**). The second group, SHIV162P3 progressors included five SHIV162P3 infected animals (3 IND and 2 CHI) ranging from 699 copies to 1.8×10^5 copies of RNA/mL of plasma. The third group, $SIV_{MAC}251$ controllers included two $SIV_{MAC}251$ infected CHI RMs (DT83 and CA66) with undetectable plasma viral load (<125 copies RNA/mL of plasma). The ultimate fourth group, $SIV_{MAC}239/251$ progressors included 14 IND and 7 CHI RMs that were infected either with $SIV_{MAC}239$ or $SIV_{MAC}251$ and had detectable plasma viral load ranging from 220 copies to 4.3×10^7 RNA copies/mL of plasma (**Table 1**). No RMs infected with $SIV_{MAC}239$ were found to be controllers based on our criteria in this study. The duration of infection prior to necropsy and tissue collection ranged from 78 days to 1845 days (~5 years) after SIV/SHIV infection. Viremia ranged in SHIV

TABLE 2 | Summary of viral RNA and DNA positive cells in tissues of macaques spontaneously controlling viremia[#].

	Brain		Mes. LN		Ing. LN		Ax. LN		Spleen		Bone marrow		Colon		Ileum		Jejunum		Thymus	
	RNA	**DNA**	**RNA**	**DNA**	**RNA**	**DNA**	**RNA**	**DNA**	**RNA**	**DNA**	**RNA**	**DNA**	**RNA**	**DNA**	**RNA**	**DNA**	**RNA**	**DNA**	**RNA**	**DNA**
AL78	0	0	0	3	0	5	3	0	0	2	0	0	0	0	0	0	0	0	22	0
BA69	0	NE	102	NE	37	NE	28	NE	0	NE	0	NE	49	NE	0	NE	0	NE	0	NE
BA11	0	0	6	11	0	NE	0	NE	3	0	0	0	0	37	0	NE	0	0	0	NE
BN81	0	NE	0	NE	0	0	0	0	0	NE	0	NE	0	NE	0	0	0	NE	0	NE
DT83	0	0	3	1	15	1	12	0	9	0	0	3	0	163	0	0	0	1	1	0
CA66	0	2	0	7	0	14	0	0	6	20	0	0	0	0	0	0	3	3	0	0

[#] *Cells/mm^2, NE indicates tissue was not examined.*

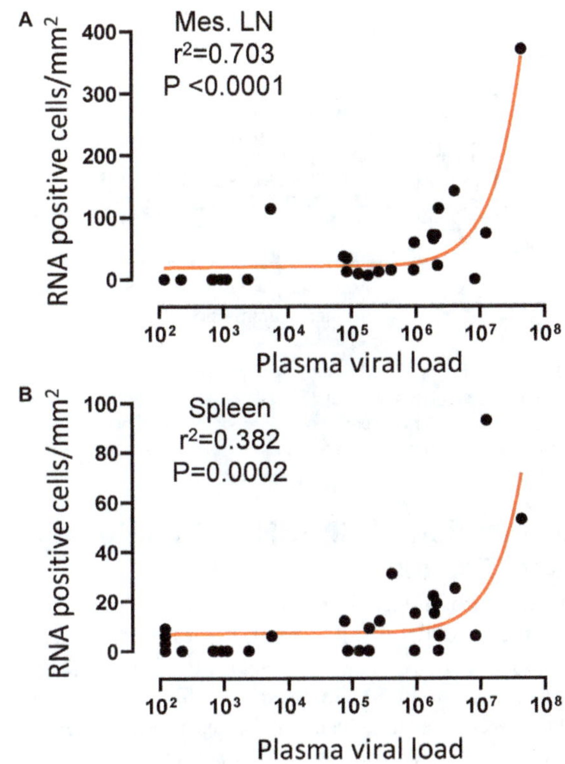

FIGURE 2 | A positive correlation of RNA positive cells and plasma viral RNA copies was shown for both mesenteric lymph node **(A)** and spleen **(B)** tissues. Pearson correlation coefficients analysis of RNA positive cells/mm^2 and plasma viral RNA load (RNA copies/mL of plasma) from all SHIV/SIV controllers and progressors was performed.

infected animals from (<125 copies) to 1.8 × 10^5 RNA copies per mL of plasma at the time of euthanasia irrespective of IVAG or IR challenge (**Table 1**). Four of the SHIV-infected animals that had undetectable pVL (<125 copies) were considered non-progressors, whereas, only one IND macaque (BN81) was categorized as a LTNP having undetectable viremia for over a year. In contrast, 13 out of 15 RMs infected with SIV$_{MAC}$239 had high terminal pVL ranged from 5.5 × 10^3 to 4.3 × 10^7 RNA copies/mL of plasma (**Table 1**). Only two out of 15 RMs infected with SIV$_{MAC}$239 had <1000 copies of plasma RNA copies/mL of plasma at the time of euthanasia, and both were of Chinese origin. Similarly, 6 out of 8 SIV$_{MAC}$251 infected RMs, had high pVL ranging from 7.7 × 10^4 to 2.2 × 10^6 RNA copies/mL of plasma at necropsy. All other RMs that had detectable pVL were considered normal progressors. We did not detect significant differences in terminal pVL between animals infected by different routes of inoculation. The majority of the SIV$_{MAC}$239 infected macaques were euthanized due to AIDS related symptoms or opportunistic infections (**Table 1**). None of the SHIV infected RMs had detectable pathological findings except for one IND macaque (BN81) that was euthanized due to intestinal torsion which was not considered to be associated with the SHIV infection.

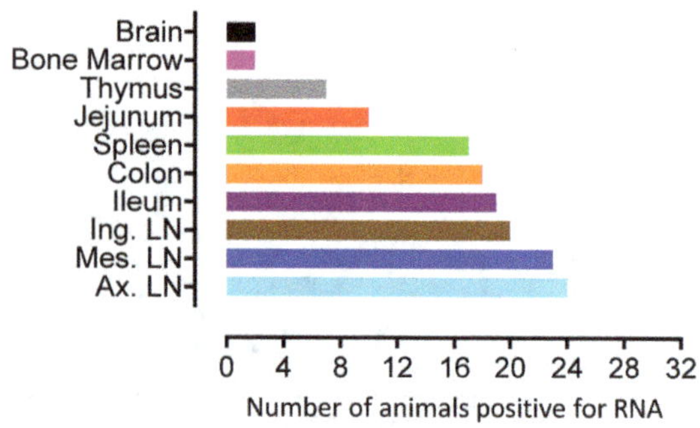

FIGURE 3 | Number of animals with RNA positive cells in each tissue are shown. Ten different tissues in a total of 32 animals were examined. Axillary LN and bone marrow/brain were found to harbor the most, and least number of RNA+ cells, respectively compared to other tissues examined.

Quantification of SIV/SHIV RNA Positive Cells in Tissues

To quantify virus infected cells in animals, we performed ISH staining for viral RNA in different tissues and the frequency was quantified as RNA positive cells/mm^2 of tissue (**Figure 1**). All animals except BN81 (infected with SHIV) had detectable SIV/SHIV RNA positive cells in at least one of the tissues examined. One SHIV progressor (R870) and two SIV progressors (FA97 and J541) had detectable RNA positive cells in midbrain (**Table 1** and **Figure 1**). One IND SHIV controller macaque (BA69) had higher RNA positive cells in mes. LN, ing. LN, ax. LN and colon tissues compared to other SHIV controllers (**Figure 1**). Overall in LTNPs with undetectable pVL, RNA positive cells were still detected in ing. LN, ax. LN, spleen, colon, jejunum and thymus (**Table 2**). Similarly, both the SIV controllers had detectable RNA positive cells in spleen. None of the SHIV/SIV controllers had detectable RNA positive cells in midbrain, bone marrow, and ileum (**Figure 1**). There were no significant differences in numbers of RNA positive cells between controllers and progressors in any of the tissues examined. Total RNA positive cells/mm^2 in some tissues correlated with pVL in all animals. Parametric Pearson correlation coefficient of these independent measures demonstrated a highly significant positive correlation of increased pVL and RNA positive cells in mes. LN ($p < 0.0001$, **Figure 2A**) and spleen ($p = 0.0002$, **Figure 2B**). However, no significant correlation was detected between RNA positive cells in any other tissues (midbrain, ing. LN, ax. LN, bone marrow, thymus, jejunum, ileum and colon) and pVL. We also compared frequencies of tissues that were positive for viral RNA from each animal. Ax. LN was found to be the most frequent infected tissue as 25 out of 32 animals were found positive for viral RNA (**Figure 3**). LNs were the most frequent infected tissues for SIV/SHIV RNA followed by ileum, colon, spleen, jejunum, thymus, midbrain and bone marrow (**Figure 3**).

Quantification of Viral DNA Positive Cells in Tissues

To quantify the DNA positive cells, we performed ISH staining in tissues from 25 animals (**Figure 4**). Cells positive for viral DNA were quantified as DNA positive cells/mm^2 area in tissues as described in methods. All animals except BN81 (infected with SHIV) had detectable DNA positive cells in at least one of the tissues examined. None of the animals with undetectable viremia (<125 copies/mL of plasma) had detectable DNA positive cells in ax. LN, thymus, or ileum, suggesting these may not be the major viral reservoirs for LTNP animals (**Figure 4**). In contrast, mes. LN followed by ing. LN and colon were found to be major source of viral DNA for several macaques with undetectable pVL and LTNPs. All SHIV progressors and 10 out of 14 SIV progressors had detectable DNA positive cells in midbrain suggesting that the frequency of viral DNA is much higher in brain compared to viral RNA copies in those animals. Similarly, 3 out of 5 and 8 out of 14 macaques from SHIV and SIV$_{MAC}$251/239 progressors, respectively were positive for viral DNA in bone marrow (**Figure 4**) which was much higher in frequency than RNA positive cells in that tissue. No significant differences in DNA positive cells were detected between controller and progressor groups in any tissues examined. Total DNA positive cells/mm^2 in each tissue however correlated with pVL for all animals. Parametric Pearson correlation coefficient of these independent measures demonstrated a significant positive correlation with pVL and numbers of DNA positive cells/mm^2 in the ileum ($p = 0.036$, **Figure 5A**) and jejunum ($p = 0.036$, **Figure 5B**). However, no correlation between pVL and tissue DNA positive cells was detected for any other tissue (midbrain, mes. LN, ing. LN, ax. LN, spleen, bone marrow, thymus, or colon). We also quantified the number of animals positive for viral DNA in tissues. Mes. LN was found to be the major infected tissue, where 19 out of 25 animals examined were positive for viral DNA. LNs appeared to be the major infected tissue followed by spleen, midbrain, colon, ileum, bone marrow, jejunum, and thymus. In the sections examined, viral DNA was diffusely distributed throughout the section in several tissues including midbrain (**Figure 6A**, CR02 with pVL 699 RNA copies/mL of plasma), bone marrow (**Figure 6B**, DD88 with pVL 9.2×10^5 RNA copies/mL of plasma), ax. LN (**Figure 6C**, GE64 with pVL 1123 RNA copies/mL of plasma), mes. LN (**Figure 6D**, CR02), ing. LN (**Figure 6E**, DG96 with pVL 1.2×10^7 RNA copies/mL of plasma), jejunum (**Figure 6F**, CA84 with pVL 8.3×10^6 RNA copies/mL of plasma), ileum (**Figure 6G**, DG96) and colon (**Figure 6H**, R870 with pVL 1.8×10^5 RNA copies/mL of plasma).

Quantification of RNA and DNA Positive Cells in Macaques Controlling Viremia

We quantified RNA and DNA positive cells by ISH from the 6 RMs infected with SHIV or SIV$_{MAC}$251 with undetectable viremia (3 IND and 3 CHI, pVL < 125 RNA copies/mL of plasma) in 10 different tissues except BA69, where only RNA was examined, and none of the tissues were examined for viral DNA+ cells (**Figure 7**). Similarly, only selected tissues were used to quantify DNA+ cells in animals BA11 and BN81. In the animals examined, SIV DNA+ cells were diffusely distributed throughout tissues examined, especially in mes. LN (**Figure 7A**, BA11), spleen (**Figure 7B**, CA66), ing. LN (**Figure 7C**, AL78), and

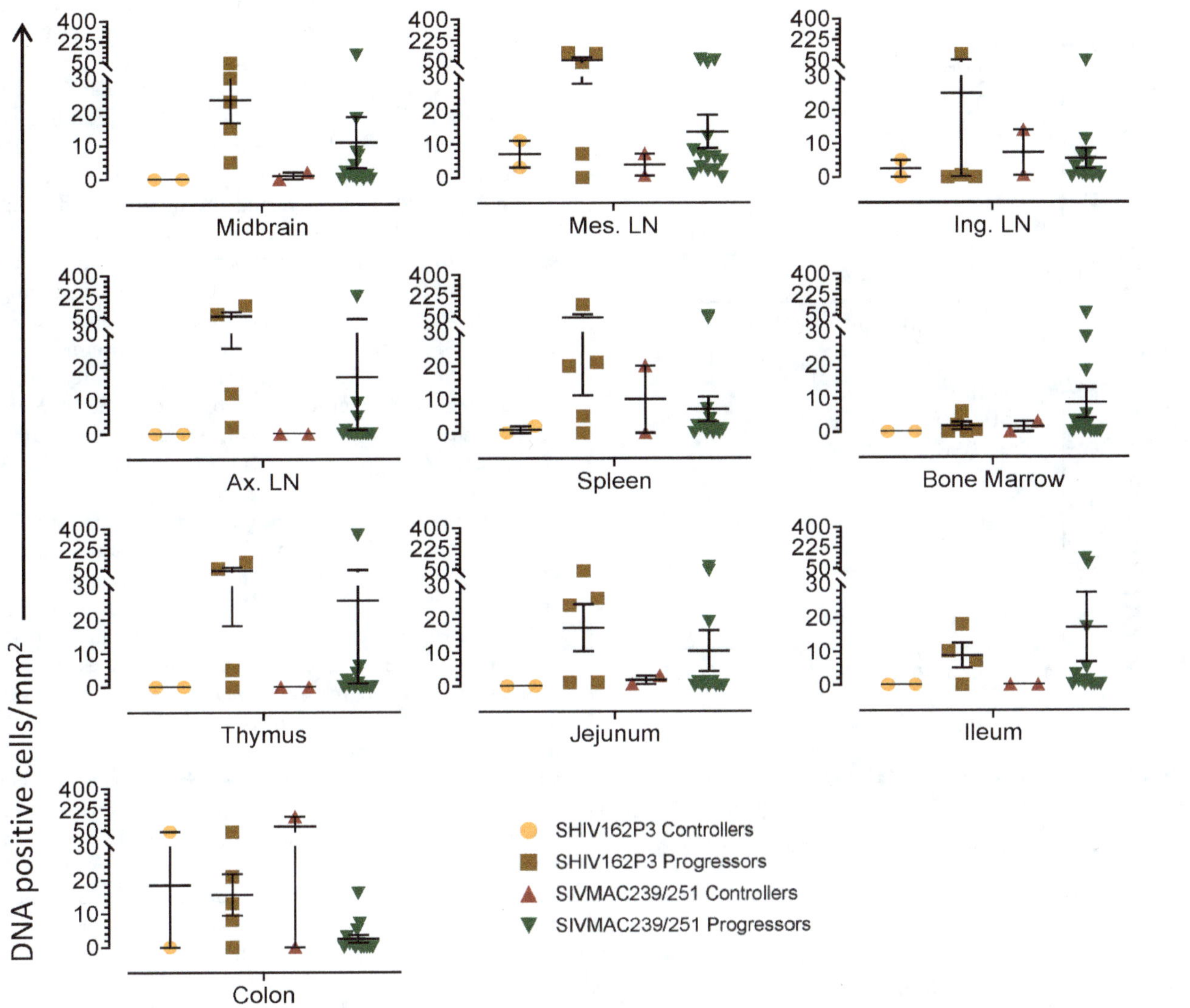

FIGURE 4 | Quantification of DNA positive cells/mm^2 per section in different tissues from animals with different plasma viral loads are shown. Horizontal lines denoted the mean DNA positive cells (±SEM) for each group of animals for the respective tissue.

colon (**Figure 7D**, DT83). RNA positive cells from colon were shown (**Figures 7E,F**, BA69), where some of the RNA positive cells were dividing cells (**Figure 7F**). A summary of the viral reservoirs detected in animals controlling viremia was shown in **Table 2**. One animal (BN81) had no detectable RNA or DNA in the tissues examined, but as noted, only a limited number of tissues were screened for DNA+ cells in this animal.

Phenotyping RNA+ Cells in Tissues

We assessed the phenotype of SIV RNA+ cells in midbrain, thymus, ing. LN, colon, ax. LN, and spleen by multilabel confocal microscopy. As shown in **Figure 8**, T-cells (CD3+), macrophages (HAM56+), and dendritic cells (CD209, DC-SIGN+) were all shown to harbor SIV RNA (**Figure 8**). The midbrain contained multiple multinucleated giant cells infected with SIV surrounded by uninfected macrophages. T cells were the most frequently infected cells but rare DC-SIGN positive cells were occasionally found, mostly in the T-cell zones of LN (**Figure 8C**) and spleen (data not shown). The identification of RNA + HAM56 + DC-SIGN+ cells could either be actively replicating virus infected macrophages that have engulfed virus or virus infected cells (**Figure 8C**). Several HAM56+ cells (macrophages) were detected in the colon lamina propria, however, very few cells colocalized with SIV RNA (data not shown). In thymus SIV infected CD3+ T cells were also detected (**Figure 8B**). The majority of SIV RNA+ cells were found to be non-proliferating (Ki67^{negative}) in this study but several proliferating (Ki67^{positive}) cells were detected in thymus (**Figure 8B**).

Differences in Levels of Infected Cells Between Indian and Chinese Origin Macaques

We quantified RNA and DNA+ cells from twenty IND and twelve CHI RMs for each tissue (**Figure 9**). Overall, higher

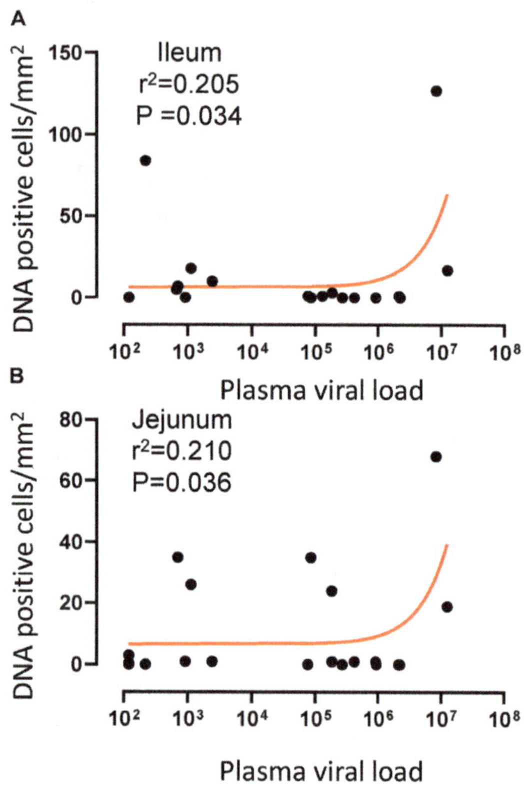

FIGURE 5 | A positive correlation of DNA positive cells and plasma viral RNA copies was shown for both ileum **(A)** and jejunum **(B)** tissues. Pearson correlation coefficients analysis of DNA positive cells/mm^2 and plasma viral RNA load (RNA copies/mL of plasma) from all SHIV/SIV controllers and progressors was performed.

numbers of RNA+ cells were detected in both IND and CHI RMs compared to DNA+ cells in LN tissues. DNA positive cells in brain and bone marrow were detected more frequently in IND compared to CHI macaques, however, the differences were not statistically significant. Similarly, increased DNA+ cells were detected in the thymus of CHI compared to IND macaques, but again the differences were not significant. No significant differences in RNA/DNA+ cells were observed between IND and CHI RMs for the other tissues examined.

DISCUSSION

Combination ART has drastically reduced the mortality rate and improved the life expectancy of HIV infected patients. However, despite years of treatment and years of undetectable plasma viremia in treated patients, cART is still not able to eliminate reservoirs or cure HIV infection. Recent studies with SIV-infected RMs and HIV patients treated with cART showed the presence of both viral RNA and DNA+ cells in several lymphoid tissues indicating long term cART fails to eliminate viral reservoirs in tissues (Estes et al., 2017). Further, most new treatment strategies aimed at reducing viral reservoirs have failed to eliminate actively replicating and latently infected proviruses from tissues (Chun and Fauci, 2012). In addition, cART treated HIV patients also have a higher incidence of age-related diseases than uninfected individuals (Pathai et al., 2014). Interestingly, a small percentage of HIV+ patients spontaneously control pVL below levels of detection, without the administration of cART, although these LTNPs represent less than 1% of the HIV-1 infected population (Blankson, 2010; Mandalia et al., 2012; Imami et al., 2013). Comparing the quantity and distribution of persistent viral reservoirs in tissues from HIV LTNPs compared to HIV progressors may lead to improved treatment and cure strategies. However, recessed tissues, including brain, intestine, bone marrow, etc., are difficult to sample in humans. Thus the SIV infected RM model is the premier model for studying the immunopathogenesis of HIV infection, as well as studying viral reservoir in progressors and LTNPs (Heise et al., 1993; Veazey et al., 1998; Shedlock et al., 2009; Ling et al., 2010; Zaragoza et al., 2011; Pan et al., 2012, 2013, 2014; Pahar et al., 2015).

Here, we showed lower pVL in the majority of RMs infected with SHIV162P3 compared to macaques infected with $SIV_{MAC}251$ or 239, which correlates with lower levels of RNA+ as well as DNA+ levels in SHIV infected animals. However, DNA+ cells persisted, and were prevalent in mes. LN, ing. LN, colon, midbrain and bone marrow tissues in both non-progressors and progressor animals. Mesenteric LN was found to be the major source of viral DNA in macaques with undetectable pVL and LTNPs, which supports previous reports where mes. LN was shown to be the major site of persistent viral reservoir in the presence of cART (North et al., 2010; Horiike et al., 2012; Siddiqui et al., 2019). LNs were found to harbor RNA and DNA+ cells in the majority of the infected animals compared to intestinal tissues. However, only one section of intestinal tissue from each organ was examined, and since the intestinal tract is among the largest organs in the body, single sections may not be representative of the entire tissue reservoir. Organized lymphoid tissues (LN, ileum, colon) are clearly the major tissue for viral RNA and DNA+ cells, likely because virus dissemination is mainly mediated by infected lymphocytes, macrophages and/or dendritic cells that normally re-circulate through organized lymphoid tissues as part of their normal homing process (Moll, 2003). Here, we also show that the large intestine (colon) consistently contains detectable RNA and DNA+ cells, contains more organized lymphoid tissues than the small intestine, and is likely the major persistent viral reservoir in macaques spontaneously controlling viremia in the majority of infected animals, which is also consistent with previous findings of macaques controlling viremia through cART (Van Marle et al., 2007; Ling et al., 2010). A positive correlation between tissue RNA+ cells and plasma viral load in both mes. LN and spleen suggests that these lymphoid tissues may be more exposed to viruses from the gastrointestinal tract compared to other tissues during high SIV/SHIV plasma viral load. Similarly, a positive correlation between DNA+ cells and pVL in ileum and jejunum suggests that perhaps during peak viremia, viral RNA is transcribed to DNA more often in those tissues resulting in larger reservoirs in these tissues compared to other tissues. The presence of RNA+ cells in tissues does not differentiate actively

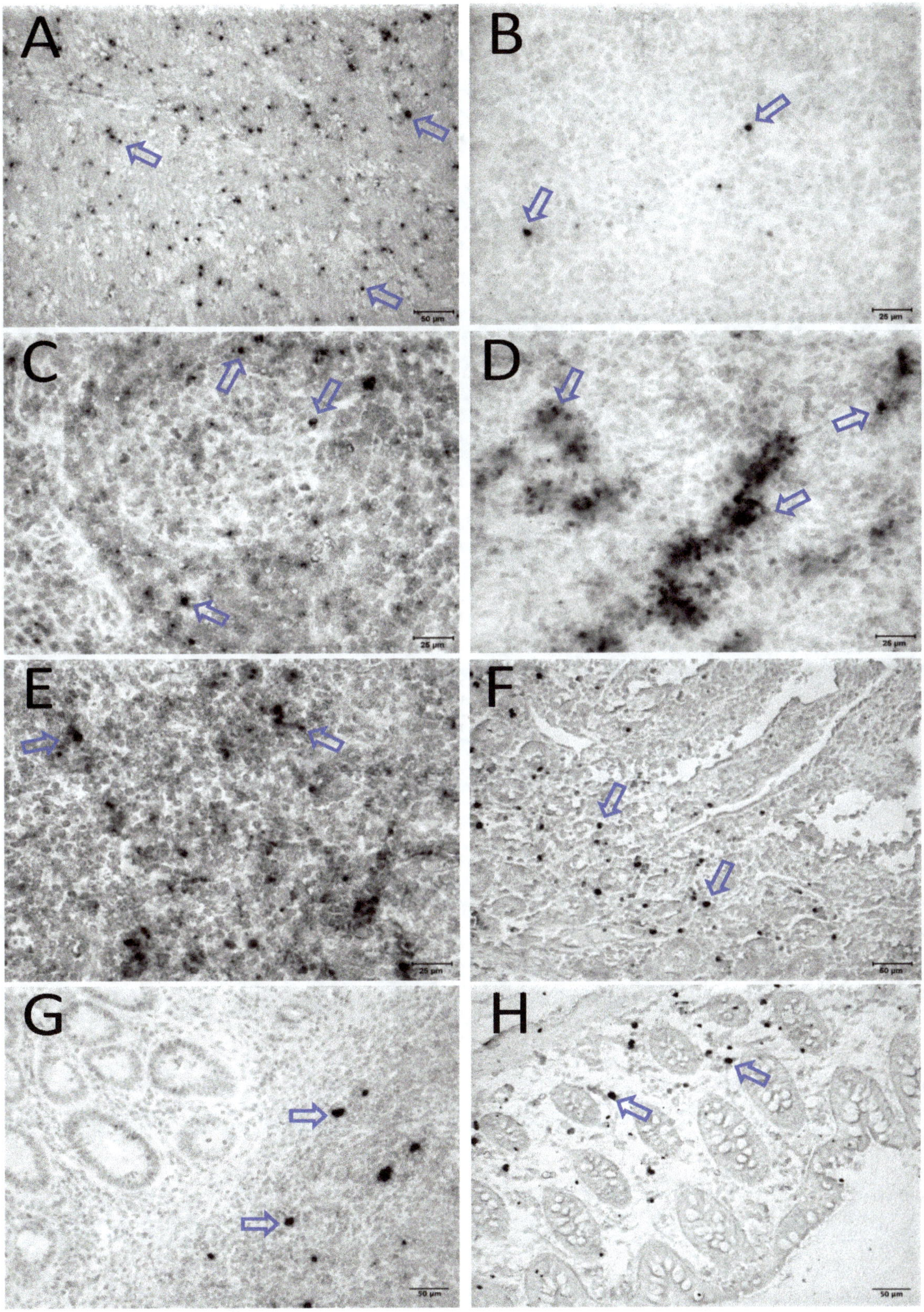

FIGURE 6 | Detection of viral reservoirs in tissues of macaques with high viremia by *in situ* hybridization for viral DNA. SIV DNA positive cells are shown in brown for the brain (CR02, **A**), bone marrow (DD88, **B**), axillary LN (GE64, **C**), mesenteric LN (CR02, **D**), inguinal LN (DG96, **E**), jejunum (CA84, **F**), ileum (DG96, **G**), and colon (R870, **H**). Blue arrows in each figure indicate representative SIV-DNA positive cells.

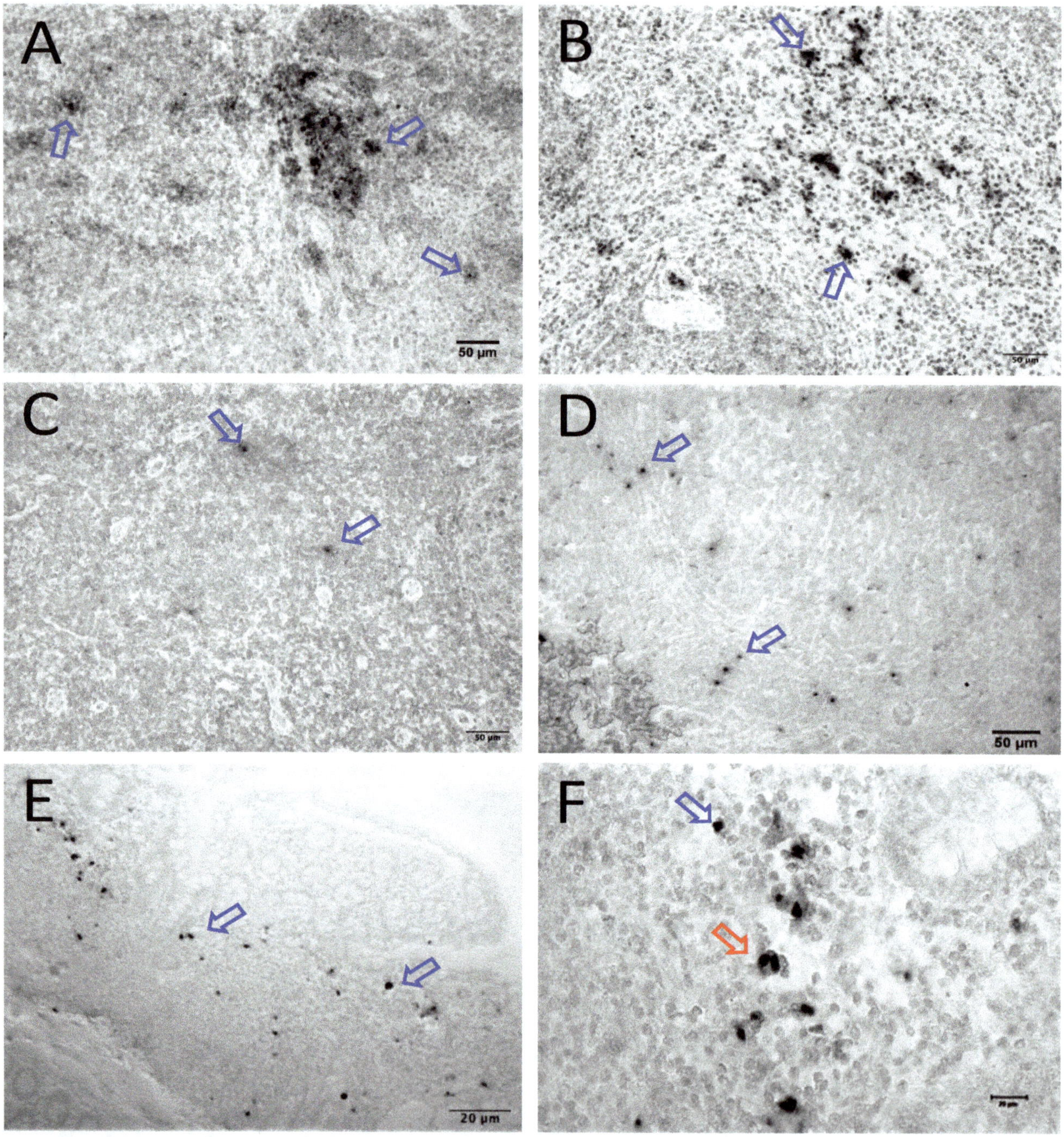

FIGURE 7 | SIV DNA positive cells detected by *in situ* hybridization in LTNP with undetectable viremia are shown in brown for mesenteric LN (BA11, **A**), spleen (CA66, **B**), inguinal LN (AL78, **C**), and colon (DT83, **D**). Similarly, RNA positive cells are shown in brown for colon (BA69, **E,F**) from a LTNP animal with undetectable viremia. All animals had undetectable plasma viral load (<125 copies/ml of plasma) at the time of euthanasia. Blue arrows in each figure indicate representative SIV-DNA/RNA positive cells. Panels **(E,F)** show RNA+ cells in a macaque (BA69), some of which are clearly in the telophase stage of cell division (red arrow). Note, that despite the animals had undetectable plasma viral load, several tissues had productively infected cells as well as DNA positive cells detected at the time of euthanasia.

replicating virus or cells with virus that might have reactivated from latency. Similarly, our assay for DNA+ cells in tissues can not discriminate between cells that harbor latent provirus or replication competent virus.

SIV infected T-cells, HAM56+ macrophages, and DC-SIGN (a marker of dendritic cells) were detected in several tissues, demonstrating that all of these cells contribute to viral persistence and even viral replication which is also in agreement with other

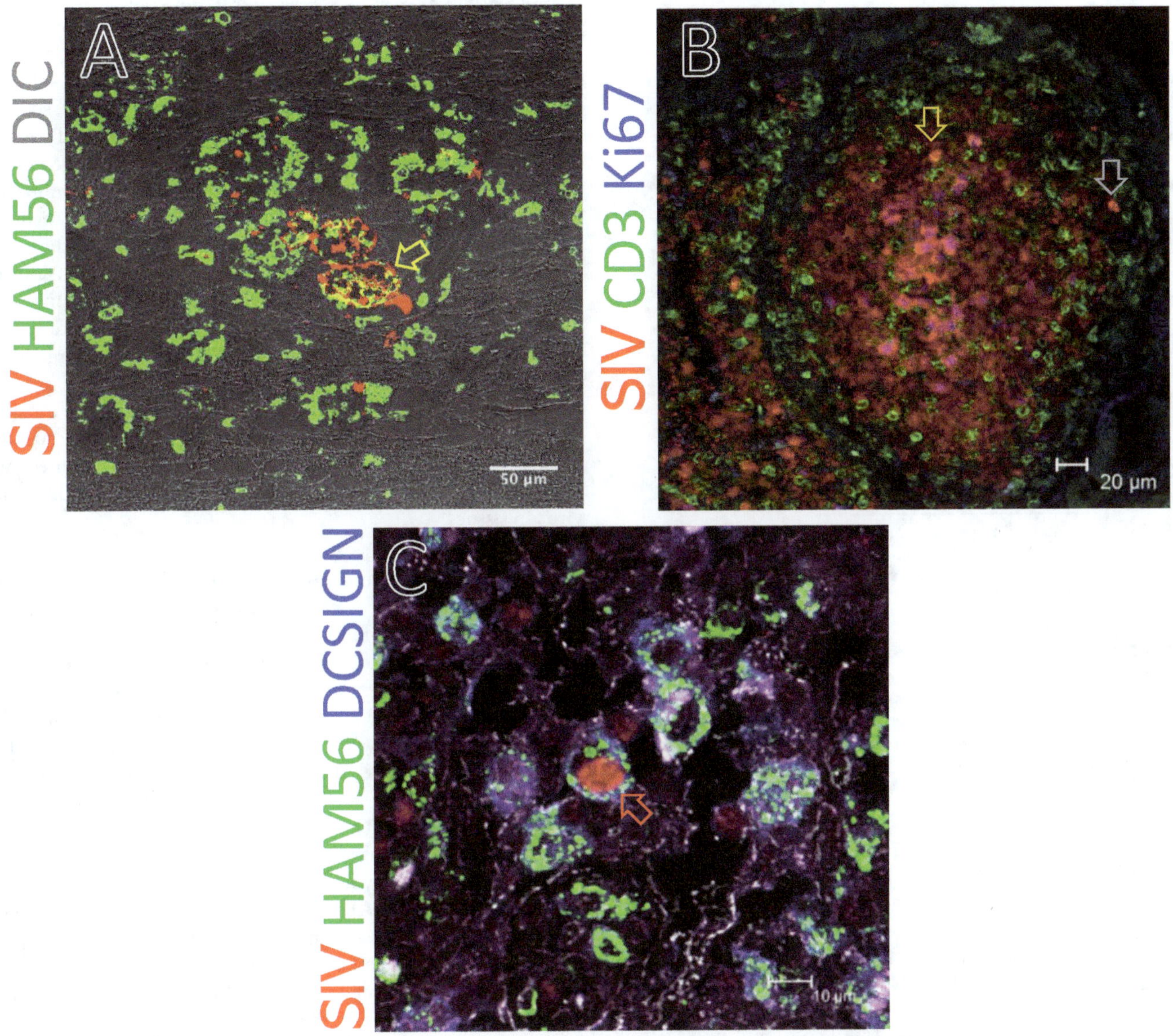

FIGURE 8 | SIV RNA positive cells were detected by *in situ* hybridization and multilabel confocal microscopy in midbrain **(A)**, thymus **(B)**, and inguinal LN **(C)**. Ham56 positive macrophages **(A,C)**, DCSIGN positive dendritic cells **(C)**, and CD3+ T-cells **(B)** are shown in different tissues. Colocalization of Ham56+ and SIV+ cells are shown by yellow arrow. Similarly, distribution of SIV infected cells in proliferating (Ki67^{positive}) and resting (Ki67^{negative}) cells was shown by orange and gray arrow, respectively. Colocalization of Ham56, DC-SIGN and SIV+ cells are shown by red arrow.

reports (Wang et al., 2010; Ribeiro Dos Santos et al., 2011; Soulas et al., 2011; Nowlin et al., 2015; Pahar et al., 2017). Although SIV-infected proliferating cells were frequently detected, the majority of infected cells were Ki67^{negative}, indicating both proliferating and non-proliferating cells serve as source for harboring infection. However, we did detect significant numbers of RNA+ cells that were clearly dividing (**Figure 7E**), lending support to the theory that at least some of the viral reservoir persists through cellular division resulting in clonal expansion of virus (Murray et al., 2016). Several studies have documented that resting memory CD4+ T cells are infected with SIV during acute infection (Zhang et al., 2004; Li et al., 2005). It is believed that SIV infected cells are initially infected when the cells are activated or proliferating, and later convert to resting, non-proliferating cells and remained persistent as latently infected cells in tissues. Notably, bone marrow and brain had the least residual infected cells, especially in animals controlling viremia, indicating those tissues play a minimal role as a source for harboring virus. Other tissues such as reproductive organs, liver, breast tissues, and adipose tissues have been described as potential reservoirs for infection (Svicher et al., 2014; Damouche et al., 2015) but these tissues were not examined in this study.

Both IND and CHI RMs are used for HIV/SIV pathogenesis, therapeutics and vaccine research due to their susceptibility

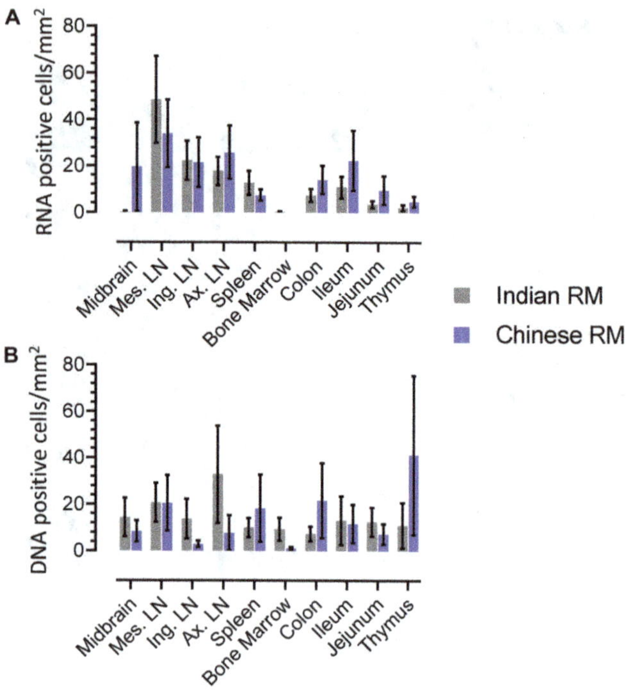

FIGURE 9 | Quantification of RNA **(A)** and DNA **(B)** positive cells in different tissues from Indian and Chinese animals were shown. No statistically significant differences in RNA/DNA+ cells exist between Indian and Chinese animals in each tissue when analyzed using analysis of variance and Chi-square methods. The horizontal bars denoted the mean RNA or DNA positive cells (±SEM) for each group and for the respective tissue.

to SIV/SHIV infection through different routes of inoculation (Joag et al., 1994; Mellors et al., 1996; Smith et al., 1999; Lifson et al., 2001; Ling et al., 2002; Zhou et al., 2013). Although the same genus and species, CHI macaques are more genetically diverse than IND macaques, and some (20–30%) have significantly lower viral set points, generate strong antibody responses, have reduced induction of type I IFN responses, lower levels of immune activation, and reduced mitochondrial antiviral signaling proteins compared to IND RMs, due to still unknown differences in physiological and genetical parameters (Viray et al., 2001; Ling et al., 2002; Doxiadis et al., 2003; Campillo-Gimenez et al., 2010; Zhou et al., 2013; Zhang et al., 2018). However, we did not observe any significant differences in either RNA or DNA positive cells in tissues between these animals, which suggests that despite their differences in levels of control of viremia, or genetic differences, both IND and CHI origin macaques show similar to equal proportions of viral infected cells in tissues, indicating their suitability as animal models for LTNPs and HIV cure strategies. Similarly, we did not observe any significant difference in either RNA or DNA positive cells in tissues when animals were grouped by sex (male or female), viral dose, or route of virus exposure in our study.

Overall, we have shown that non-progressor animals having a lower frequency of both RNA and DNA+ cells in several tissues compared to progressors. In general, organized lymphoid tissues (LNs and colon) were shown to be the major persistent reservoirs for viral RNA and DNA+ cells in animals spontaneously controlling infection. Therefore, ART should be designed to penetrate organized lymphoid tissues so that it can target all tissue-resident infected cells to reduce the burden of both latently and productively infected cells. Notably, RNA+ cells were frequently detected in organized lymphoid tissues of almost every animal, even those spontaneously controlling infection with undetectable pVL. This study has caveats and limitations including the lack of inclusion of reproductive tissues in our tissue list and the sensitivity of the assays. A more sensitive and specific next-generation ISH approach has been developed for the detection of viral RNA and DNA+ cells using RNAscope and DNAscope probes, respectively (Deleage et al., 2016) that can provide more detailed information about the actively replicating and latently infected cells in these tissues but since resources were limited for this study we used our standard ISH techniques for detecting virus in tissues.

In recent years, several approaches have been proposed and tested to eliminate latent viral reservoirs, including lymphocyte ablation by irradiation followed by bone marrow transplantation with CCR5 deletion of stem cells, gene editing technology to disrupt the HIV genome, and "Shock and Kill" strategies to reactivate latent HIV followed by immune clearance by cART (Chun et al., 2015; Elsheikh et al., 2019). So far, these approaches have shown negligible success in clearing latent HIV reservoirs, and failure to generate effective host immune responses. There are several new strategies and compounds under investigation that may either block, or eliminate latent reservoirs from organized lymphoid tissues in combination with ART, especially those designed to block lymphoid homing, or eliminate infected reservoir cells from LNs by enhancing cellular and humoral immune responses in tissues (Riley and Montaner, 2017). Undoubtedly, more studies are needed to understand the mechanism of HIV latency and better tools to identify and eradicate latently infected cells from tissues.

ETHICS STATEMENT

The animal study was reviewed and approved by the Tulane Institutional Animal Care and Use Committee.

AUTHOR CONTRIBUTIONS

BP designed the experiments and wrote the manuscript. DK, AD, and BP performed all the animal experiments. BP, AD, and

RV performed the data analysis. TR helped in making the DNA probe. XW helped with the RNA ISH assay. SS performed the statistical analyses. RV helped in experiment design and writing manuscript. All authors have given approval to the final version of the manuscript.

ACKNOWLEDGMENTS

The authors thank Agegnehu Gettie, Andrew Lackner, Binhua Ling, Carol Coyne, Carys Kenway-Lynch, Cecily Conerly Midkiff, Maury Duplantis, Preston J. Marx, Xavier Alvarez, Wendy Lala Trunch, and all animal care staff of the department of veterinary medicine for their technical assistance and advice.

REFERENCES

Abreu, C. M., Veenhuis, R. T., Avalos, C. R., Graham, S., Queen, S. E., Shirk, E. N., et al. (2019). Infectious Virus Persists in CD4(+) T Cells and Macrophages in Antiretroviral Therapy-Suppressed Simian Immunodeficiency Virus-Infected Macaques. *J. Virol.* 93:e00065-19. doi: 10.1128/JVI.00065-19

Ahsan, M. H., Gill, A. F., Alvarez, X., Lackner, A. A., and Veazey, R. S. (2013). Kinetics of liver macrophages (Kupffer cells) in SIV-infected macaques. *Virology* 446, 77–85. doi: 10.1016/j.virol.2013.07.026

Amedee, A. M., Phillips, B., Jensen, K., Robichaux, S., Lacour, N., Burke, M., et al. (2018). Early Sites of Virus Replication After Oral SIVmac251 Infection of Infant Macaques: Implications for Pathogenesis. *AIDS Res. Hum. Retroviruses* 34, 286–299. doi: 10.1089/AID.2017.0169

Ananworanich, J., Chomont, N., Eller, L. A., Kroon, E., Tovanabutra, S., Bose, M., et al. (2016). HIV DNA Set Point is Rapidly Established in Acute HIV Infection and Dramatically Reduced by Early ART. *EBioMedicine* 11, 68–72. doi: 10.1016/j.ebiom.2016.07.024

Bandera, A., Gori, A., Clerici, M., and Sironi, M. (2019). Phylogenies in ART: HIV reservoirs, HIV latency and drug resistance. *Curr. Opin. Pharmacol.* 48, 24–32. doi: 10.1016/j.coph.2019.03.003

Blankson, J. N. (2010). Effector mechanisms in HIV-1 infected elite controllers: highly active immune responses? *Antiviral. Res.* 85, 295–302. doi: 10.1016/j.antiviral.2009.08.007

Blankson, J. N., Persaud, D., and Siliciano, R. F. (2002). The challenge of viral reservoirs in HIV-1 infection. *Annu. Rev. Med.* 53, 557–593. doi: 10.1146/annurev.med.53.082901.104024

Borda, J. T., Alvarez, X., Kondova, I., Aye, P., Simon, M. A., Desrosiers, R. C., et al. (2004). Cell tropism of simian immunodeficiency virus in culture is not predictive of in vivo tropism or pathogenesis. *Am. J. Pathol.* 165, 2111–2122. doi: 10.1016/s0002-9440(10)63261-0

Bruner, K. M., and Cohn, L. B. (2019). HIV-1 reservoir dynamics in CD4+ T cells. *Curr. Opin. HIV AIDS* 14, 108–114. doi: 10.1097/COH.0000000000000521

Buzon, M. J., Sun, H., Li, C., Shaw, A., Seiss, K., Ouyang, Z., et al. (2014). HIV-1 persistence in CD4+ T cells with stem cell-like properties. *Nat. Med.* 20, 139–142. doi: 10.1038/nm.3445

Campillo-Gimenez, L., Laforge, M., Fay, M., Brussel, A., Cumont, M. C., Monceaux, V., et al. (2010). Nonpathogenesis of simian immunodeficiency virus infection is associated with reduced inflammation and recruitment of plasmacytoid dendritic cells to lymph nodes, not to lack of an interferon type I response, during the acute phase. *J. Virol.* 84, 1838–1846. doi: 10.1128/JVI.01496-09

Cantero-Perez, J., Grau-Exposito, J., Serra-Peinado, C., Rosero, D. A., Luque-Ballesteros, L., Astorga-Gamaza, A., et al. (2019). Resident memory T cells are a cellular reservoir for HIV in the cervical mucosa. *Nat. Commun.* 10:4739. doi: 10.1038/s41467-019-12732-2

Chun, T. W., Engel, D., Berrey, M. M., Shea, T., Corey, L., and Fauci, A. S. (1998). Early establishment of a pool of latently infected, resting CD4(+) T cells during primary HIV-1 infection. *Proc. Natl. Acad. Sci. U.S.A.* 95, 8869–8873. doi: 10.1073/pnas.95.15.8869

Chun, T. W., and Fauci, A. S. (2012). HIV reservoirs: pathogenesis and obstacles to viral eradication and cure. *AIDS* 26, 1261–1268. doi: 10.1097/qad.0b013e328353f3f1

Chun, T. W., Moir, S., and Fauci, A. S. (2015). HIV reservoirs as obstacles and opportunities for an HIV cure. *Nat. Immunol.* 16, 584–589. doi: 10.1038/ni.3152

Chun, T. W., Stuyver, L., Mizell, S. B., Ehler, L. A., Mican, J. A., Baseler, M., et al. (1997). Presence of an inducible HIV-1 latent reservoir during highly active antiretroviral therapy. *Proc. Natl. Acad. Sci. U.S.A.* 94, 13193–13197. doi: 10.1073/pnas.94.24.13193

Couturier, J., and Lewis, D. E. (2018). HIV Persistence in Adipose Tissue Reservoirs. *Curr. HIV/AIDS Rep.* 15, 60–71. doi: 10.1007/s11904-018-0378-z

Crooks, A. M., Bateson, R., Cope, A. B., Dahl, N. P., Griggs, M. K., Kuruc, J. D., et al. (2015). Precise Quantitation of the Latent HIV-1 Reservoir: Implications for Eradication Strategies. *J. Infect. Dis.* 212, 1361–1365. doi: 10.1093/infdis/jiv218

Damouche, A., Lazure, T., Avettand-Fenoel, V., Huot, N., Dejucq-Rainsford, N., Satie, A. P., et al. (2015). Adipose Tissue Is a Neglected Viral Reservoir and an Inflammatory Site during Chronic HIV and SIV Infection. *PLoS Pathog.* 11:e1005153. doi: 10.1371/journal.ppat.1005153

Deleage, C., Wietgrefe, S. W., Del Prete, G., Morcock, D. R., Hao, X. P., Piatak, M., et al. (2016). Defining HIV and SIV Reservoirs in Lymphoid Tissues. *Pathog. Immun.* 1, 68–106.

Desai, S., and Landay, A. (2010). Early immune senescence in HIV disease. *Curr. HIV/AIDS Rep.* 7, 4–10. doi: 10.1007/s11904-009-0038-4

Doxiadis, G. G., Otting, N., De Groot, N. G., De Groot, N., Rouweler, A. J., Noort, R., et al. (2003). Evolutionary stability of MHC class II haplotypes in diverse rhesus macaque populations. *Immunogenetics* 55, 540–551. doi: 10.1007/s00251-003-0590-9

Elsheikh, M. M., Tang, Y., Li, D., and Jiang, G. (2019). Deep latency: A new insight into a functional HIV cure. *EBioMedicine* 45, 624–629. doi: 10.1016/j.ebiom.2019.06.020

Estes, J. D., Kityo, C., Ssali, F., Swainson, L., Makamdop, K. N., Del Prete, G. Q., et al. (2017). Defining total-body AIDS-virus burden with implications for curative strategies. *Nat. Med.* 23, 1271–1276. doi: 10.1038/nm.4411

Fukazawa, Y., Lum, R., Okoye, A. A., Park, H., Matsuda, K., Bae, J. Y., et al. (2015). B cell follicle sanctuary permits persistent productive simian immunodeficiency virus infection in elite controllers. *Nat. Med.* 21, 132–139. doi: 10.1038/nm.3781

Garcia, M., Gorgolas, M., Cabello, A., Estrada, V., Ligos, J. M., Fernandez-Guerrero, M., et al. (2017). Peripheral T follicular helper Cells Make a Difference in HIV Reservoir Size between Elite Controllers and Patients on Successful cART. *Sci. Rep.* 7:16799. doi: 10.1038/s41598-017-17057-y

Heise, C., Vogel, P., Miller, C. J., Halsted, C. H., and Dandekar, S. (1993). Simian immunodeficiency virus infection of the gastrointestinal tract of rhesus macaques. Functional, pathological, and morphological changes. *Am. J. Pathol.* 142, 1759–1771.

Horiike, M., Iwami, S., Kodama, M., Sato, A., Watanabe, Y., Yasui, M., et al. (2012). Lymph nodes harbor viral reservoirs that cause rebound of plasma viremia in SIV-infected macaques upon cessation of combined antiretroviral therapy. *Virology* 423, 107–118. doi: 10.1016/j.virol.2011.11.024

Imami, N., Westrop, S. J., Grageda, N., and Herasimtschuk, A. A. (2013). Long-Term Non-Progression and Broad HIV-1-Specific Proliferative T-Cell Responses. *Front. Immunol.* 4:58. doi: 10.3389/fimmu.2013.00058

Joag, S. V., Stephens, E. B., Adams, R. J., Foresman, L., and Narayan, O. (1994). Pathogenesis of SIVmac infection in Chinese and Indian rhesus macaques: effects of splenectomy on virus burden. *Virology* 200, 436–446. doi: 10.1006/viro.1994.1207

Li, Q., Duan, L., Estes, J. D., Ma, Z. M., Rourke, T., Wang, Y., et al. (2005). Peak SIV replication in resting memory CD4+ T cells depletes gut lamina propria CD4+ T cells. *Nature* 434, 1148–1152. doi: 10.1038/nature03513

Lifson, J. D., Rossio, J. L., Piatak, M Jr, Parks, T., Li, L., Kiser, R., et al. (2001). Role of CD8(+) lymphocytes in control of simian immunodeficiency virus infection and resistance to rechallenge after transient early antiretroviral treatment. *J. Virol.* 75, 10187–10199. doi: 10.1128/jvi.75.21.10187-10199.2001

Ling, B., Mohan, M., Lackner, A. A., Green, L. C., Marx, P. A., Doyle, L. A., et al. (2010). The large intestine as a major reservoir for simian immunodeficiency virus in macaques with long-term, nonprogressing infection. *J. Infect. Dis.* 202, 1846–1854. doi: 10.1086/657413

Ling, B., Veazey, R. S., Luckay, A., Penedo, C., Xu, K., Lifson, J. D., et al. (2002). SIV(mac) pathogenesis in rhesus macaques of Chinese and Indian origin compared with primary HIV infections in humans. *AIDS* 16, 1489–1496. doi: 10.1097/00002030-200207260-00005

Mandalia, S., Westrop, S. J., Beck, E. J., Nelson, M., Gazzard, B. G., and Imami, N. (2012). Are long-term non-progressors very slow progressors? Insights from the Chelsea and Westminster HIV cohort, 1988-2010. *PLoS One* 7:e29844. doi: 10.1371/journal.pone.0029844

Marcello, A. (2006). Latency: the hidden HIV-1 challenge. *Retrovirology* 3:7.

Mellors, J. W., Rinaldo, C. R Jr, Gupta, P., White, R. M., Todd, J. A., and Kingsley, L. A. (1996). Prognosis in HIV-1 infection predicted by the quantity of virus in plasma. *Science* 272, 1167–1170. doi: 10.1126/science.272.5265.1167

Moll, H. (2003). Dendritic cells and host resistance to infection. *Cell. Microbiol.* 5, 493–500. doi: 10.1046/j.1462-5822.2003.00291.x

Murray, A. J., Kwon, K. J., Farber, D. L., and Siliciano, R. F. (2016). The Latent Reservoir for HIV-1: How Immunologic Memory and Clonal Expansion Contribute to HIV-1 Persistence. *J. Immunol.* 197, 407–417. doi: 10.4049/jimmunol.1600343

National Research Council (2011). *Guide For The Care and Use of Laboratory Animals*. 8th Edn, Washington, DC: The National Academies Press.

North, T. W., Higgins, J., Deere, J. D., Hayes, T. L., Villalobos, A., Adamson, L., et al. (2010). Viral sanctuaries during highly active antiretroviral therapy in a nonhuman primate model for AIDS. *J. Virol.* 84, 2913–2922. doi: 10.1128/JVI.02356-09

Nowlin, B. T., Burdo, T. H., Midkiff, C. C., Salemi, M., Alvarez, X., and Williams, K. C. (2015). SIV encephalitis lesions are composed of CD163(+) macrophages present in the central nervous system during early SIV infection and SIV-positive macrophages recruited terminally with AIDS. *Am. J. Pathol.* 185, 1649–1665. doi: 10.1016/j.ajpath.2015.01.033

Pahar, B., Kenway-Lynch, C. S., Marx, P., Srivastav, S. K., Labranche, C., Montefiori, D. C., et al. (2016). Breadth and magnitude of antigen-specific antibody responses in the control of plasma viremia in simian immunodeficiency virus infected macaques. *Virol. J.* 13:200.

Pahar, B., Lala, W., Kuebler, D., and Liu, D. (2017). A significant productive in vivo infection of resting cells with simian immunodeficiency virus in a macaque with AIDS. *J. Med. Primatol.* 46, 59–62. doi: 10.1111/jmp.12252

Pahar, B., Pan, D., Lala, W., Kenway-Lynch, C. S., and Das, A. (2015). Transforming growth factor-beta1 regulated phosphorylated AKT and interferon gamma expressions are associated with epithelial cell survival in rhesus macaque colon explants. *Clin. Immunol.* 158, 8–18. doi: 10.1016/j.clim.2015.03.001

Pahar, B., Wang, X., Dufour, J., Lackner, A. A., and Veazey, R. S. (2007). Virus-specific T cell responses in macaques acutely infected with SHIV(sf162p3). *Virology* 363, 36–47. doi: 10.1016/j.virol.2007.01.010

Pan, D., Das, A., Lala, W., Kenway-Lynch, C. S., Liu, D. X., Veazey, R. S., et al. (2013). Interleukin-10 prevents epithelial cell apoptosis by regulating IFNgamma and TNFalpha expression in rhesus macaque colon explants. *Cytokine* 64, 30–34. doi: 10.1016/j.cyto.2013.06.312

Pan, D., Das, A., Liu, D., Veazey, R. S., and Pahar, B. (2012). Isolation and characterization of intestinal epithelial cells from normal and SIV-infected rhesus macaques. *PLoS One* 7:e30247. doi: 10.1371/journal.pone.0030247

Pan, D., Kenway-Lynch, C. S., Lala, W., Veazey, R. S., Lackner, A. A., Das, A., et al. (2014). Lack of interleukin-10-mediated anti-inflammatory signals and upregulated interferon gamma production are linked to increased intestinal epithelial cell apoptosis in pathogenic simian immunodeficiency virus infection. *J. Virol.* 88, 13015–13028. doi: 10.1128/JVI.01757-14

Pathai, S., Bajillan, H., Landay, A. L., and High, K. P. (2014). Is HIV a model of accelerated or accentuated aging? *J. Gerontol. A Biol. Sci. Med. Sci.* 69, 833–842. doi: 10.1093/gerona/glt168

Ribeiro Dos Santos, P., Rancez, M., Pretet, J. L., Michel-Salzat, A., Messent, V., Bogdanova, A., et al. (2011). Rapid dissemination of SIV follows multisite entry after rectal inoculation. *PLoS One* 6:e19493. doi: 10.1371/journal.pone.0019493

Riley, J. L., and Montaner, L. J. (2017). Cell-Mediated Immunity to Target the Persistent Human Immunodeficiency Virus Reservoir. *J. Infect. Dis.* 215, S160–S171. doi: 10.1093/infdis/jix002

Shedlock, D. J., Silvestri, G., and Weiner, D. B. (2009). Monkeying around with HIV vaccines: using rhesus macaques to define 'gatekeepers' for clinical trials. *Nat. Rev. Immunol.* 9, 717–728. doi: 10.1038/nri2636

Siddiqui, S., Perez, S., Gao, Y., Doyle-Meyers, L., Foley, B. T., Li, Q., et al. (2019). Persistent Viral Reservoirs in Lymphoid Tissues in SIV-Infected Rhesus Macaques of Chinese-Origin on Suppressive Antiretroviral Therapy. *Viruses* 11:105. doi: 10.3390/v11020105

Siliciano, J. D., Kajdas, J., Finzi, D., Quinn, T. C., Chadwick, K., Margolick, J. B., et al. (2003). Long-term follow-up studies confirm the stability of the latent reservoir for HIV-1 in resting CD4+ T cells. *Nat. Med.* 9, 727–728. doi: 10.1038/nm880

Smith, S. M., Holland, B., Russo, C., Dailey, P. J., Marx, P. A., and Connor, R. I. (1999). Retrospective analysis of viral load and SIV antibody responses in rhesus macaques infected with pathogenic SIV: predictive value for disease progression. *AIDS Res. Hum. Retroviruses* 15, 1691–1701. doi: 10.1089/088922299309739

Soulas, C., Conerly, C., Kim, W. K., Burdo, T. H., Alvarez, X., Lackner, A. A., et al. (2011). Recently infiltrating MAC387(+) monocytes/macrophages a third macrophage population involved in SIV and HIV encephalitic lesion formation. *Am. J. Pathol.* 178, 2121–2135. doi: 10.1016/j.ajpath.2011.01.023

Strain, M. C., Gunthard, H. F., Havlir, D. V., Ignacio, C. C., Smith, D. M., Leigh-Brown, A. J., et al. (2003). Heterogeneous clearance rates of long-lived lymphocytes infected with HIV: intrinsic stability predicts lifelong persistence. *Proc. Natl. Acad. Sci. U.S.A.* 100, 4819–4824. doi: 10.1073/pnas.0736332100

Svicher, V., Ceccherini-Silberstein, F., Antinori, A., Aquaro, S., and Perno, C. F. (2014). Understanding HIV compartments and reservoirs. *Curr. HIV/AIDS Rep.* 11, 186–194. doi: 10.1007/s11904-014-0207-y

Van Marle, G., Gill, M. J., Kolodka, D., Mcmanus, L., Grant, T., and Church, D. L. (2007). Compartmentalization of the gut viral reservoir in HIV-1 infected patients. *Retrovirology* 4:87. doi: 10.1186/1742-4690-4-87

Veazey, R. S., Demaria, M., Chalifoux, L. V., Shvetz, D. E., Pauley, D. R., Knight, H. L., et al. (1998). Gastrointestinal tract as a major site of CD4+ T cell depletion and viral replication in SIV infection. *Science* 280, 427–431. doi: 10.1126/science.280.5362.427

Viray, J., Rolfs, B., and Smith, D. G. (2001). Comparison of the frequencies of major histocompatibility (MHC) class-II DQA1 and DQB1 alleles in Indian and Chinese rhesus macaques (*Macaca mulatta*). *Comp. Med.* 51, 555–561.

Wang, X., Rasmussen, T., Pahar, B., Poonia, B., Alvarez, X., Lackner, A. A., et al. (2007). Massive infection and loss of CD4+ T cells occurs in the intestinal tract of neonatal rhesus macaques in acute SIV infection. *Blood* 109, 1174–1181. doi: 10.1182/blood-2006-04-015172

Wang, X., Xu, H., Pahar, B., Alvarez, X., Green, L. C., Dufour, J., et al. (2010). Simian immunodeficiency virus selectively infects proliferating CD4+ T cells in neonatal rhesus macaques. *Blood* 116, 4168–4174. doi: 10.1182/blood-2010-03-273482

Whitney, J. B., Hill, A. L., Sanisetty, S., Penaloza-Macmaster, P., Liu, J., Shetty, M., et al. (2014). Rapid seeding of the viral reservoir prior to SIV viraemia in rhesus monkeys. *Nature* 512, 74–77. doi: 10.1038/nature13594

Zaikos, T. D., Terry, V. H., Sebastian Kettinger, N. T., Lubow, J., Painter, M. M., Virgilio, M. C., et al. (2018). Hematopoietic Stem and Progenitor Cells Are a Distinct HIV Reservoir that Contributes to Persistent Viremia in Suppressed Patients. *Cel.l Rep.* 25, 3759.e9–3773.e9. doi: 10.1016/j.celrep.2018.11.104

Zaragoza, M. M., Sankaran-Walters, S., Canfield, D. R., Hung, J. K., Martinez, E., Ouellette, A. J., et al. (2011). Persistence of gut mucosal innate immune defenses by enteric alpha-defensin expression in the simian immunodeficiency virus model of AIDS. *J. Immunol.* 186, 1589–1597. doi: 10.4049/jimmunol.1002021

Zhang, M., Fu, Z., Chen, J., Zhu, B., Cheng, Y., and Fu, L. (2018). Low level expression of the Mitochondrial Antiviral Signaling protein (MAVS) associated with long-term nonprogression in SIV-infected rhesus macaques. *Virol. J.* 15:159. doi: 10.1186/s12985-018-1069-5

Zhang, Z. Q., Wietgrefe, S. W., Li, Q., Shore, M. D., Duan, L., Reilly, C., et al. (2004). Roles of substrate availability and infection of resting and activated CD4+ T cells in transmission and acute simian immunodeficiency virus infection. *Proc. Natl. Acad. Sci. U.S.A.* 101, 5640–5645. doi: 10.1073/pnas.0308425101

Zhou, Y., Bao, R., Haigwood, N. L., Persidsky, Y., and Ho, W. Z. (2013). SIV infection of rhesus macaques of Chinese origin: a suitable model for HIV infection in humans. *Retrovirology* 10:89. doi: 10.1186/1742-4690-10-89

Zhu, T., Muthui, D., Holte, S., Nickle, D., Feng, F., Brodie, S., et al. (2002). Evidence for human immunodeficiency virus type 1 replication in vivo in CD14(+) monocytes and its potential role as a source of virus in patients on highly active antiretroviral therapy. *J. Virol.* 76, 707–716. doi: 10.1128/jvi.76.2.707-716.2002

10

Targeting Cellular and Tissue HIV Reservoirs with Toll-Like Receptor Agonists

Amanda B. Macedo [1], *Camille L. Novis* [2] *and Alberto Bosque* [1*]

[1] *Department of Microbiology, Immunology and Tropical Medicine, George Washington University, Washington, DC, United States,* [2] *Department of Pathology, Division of Microbiology and Immunology, The University of Utah, Salt Lake City, UT, United States*

Correspondence:
Alberto Bosque
abosque@gwu.edu

The elimination of both cellular and tissue latent reservoirs is a challenge toward a successful HIV cure. "Shock and Kill" are among the therapeutic strategies that have been more extensively studied to target these reservoirs. These strategies are aimed toward the reactivation of the latent reservoir using a latency-reversal agent (LRA) with the subsequent killing of the reactivated cell either by the cytotoxic arm of the immune system, including NK and CD8 T cells, or by viral cytopathic mechanisms. Numerous LRAs are currently being investigated *in vitro*, *ex vivo* as well as *in vivo* for their ability to reactivate and reduce latent reservoirs. Among those, several toll-like receptor (TLR) agonists have been shown to reactivate latent HIV. In humans, there are 10 TLRs that recognize different pathogen-associated molecular patterns. TLRs are present in several cell types, including CD4 T cells, the cell compartment that harbors the majority of the latent reservoir. Besides their ability to reactivate latent HIV, TLR agonists also increase immune activation and promote an antiviral response. These combined properties make TLR agonists unique among the different LRAs characterized to date. Additionally, some of these agonists have shown promise toward finding an HIV cure in animal models. When in combination with broadly neutralizing antibodies, TLR-7 agonists have shown to impact the SIV latent reservoir and delay viral rebound. Moreover, there are FDA-approved TLR agonists that are currently being investigated for cancer therapy and other diseases. All these has prompted clinical trials using TLR agonists either alone or in combination toward HIV eradication approaches. In this review, we provide an extensive characterization of the state-of-the-art of the use of TLR agonists toward HIV eradication strategies and the mechanism behind how TLR agonists target both cellular and tissue HIV reservoirs.

Keywords: HIV, toll-like receptors, latency-reversal agents, shock and kill, reservoirs

INTRODUCTION

HIV infection is still one of the highest causes of mortality and morbidity worldwide. The introduction of anti-retroviral therapy (ART) in 1996 decreased the mortality due to HIV infection and transformed the disease from deadly to chronic. Cure is still not attainable due to a small reservoir of infected cells that harbor the virus in a latent form and become unrecognizable by the immune system and current therapies (1–5). Several strategies have been proposed to eliminate this latent reservoir (6). Among these strategies, the "shock and kill" approach rely on the notion that a pharmacological agent that reactivates the latent virus or latency-reversing agent (LRA) in the presence of ART will reduce the latent reservoir and could be followed by two potential outcomes. "Shock and kill" strategies can lead to complete viral eradication. In this case, the final goal is to eliminate all latent viruses. In a way, these strategies will try to echo the Berlin or the London patient, whom underwent remission due to bone marrow transplants and became undetectable for viral reservoirs (7, 8). Another outcome could be that a reduction of the latent reservoir due to the "shock and kill" strategy may be sufficient to allow the immune system control viral replication in the absence of ART (9–12). This has been termed "functional cure" and it is exemplified with the VISCONTI study. In this study, a subset of HIV-infected individuals who started ART early were able to control viremia in the absence of ART (termed Post-Treatment Controllers or PTCs) (11, 12). The authors of this study found a strong association between a low HIV reservoir in blood with the ability of the immune system to control viremia after ART treatment interruption (11).

As of today, several LRAs have been developed and some have reached clinical trials. The first generation LRAs that reached human testing include Valproic Acid (13–18), SAHA (19–21), Romidepsin (22), Panobinostat (23), Bryostatin-1 (24), and Disulfiram (25, 26). However, these LRAs have resulted in limited to no clinical effect on the size of the latent reservoir (27–29). Some potential explanations for the failure of these LRAs are the following. First, the lack of or low reactivation of latent viruses with these LRAs *in vivo*. Second, the reduced killing of reactivated cells either by the low frequency or compartmentalization of HIV-specific cells on patients under ART, immune exhaustion or the presence of defective proviruses that divert the immune response from the reactivated cells carrying replication competent virus. Third, a survival advantage of latently infected cells (30–36). To that end, strategies that can efficiently reactivate latent HIV *in vivo* and also enhance immune responses against HIV may overcome these obstacles encountered by the current cure efforts.

Recently, a second generation of LRAs targeting toll-like receptors (TLRs) have reached clinical trials. TLRs are pathogen-recognition receptors (PRRs) capable of sensing small molecular motifs conserved within microbes (37, 38). In addition to their ability to reactivate latent HIV, TLR agonists also increase immune activation and promote antiviral responses (39–44). These combined properties make TLR agonists unique among the LRAs characterized to date.

In 1891, William Coley demonstrated how several bacterial components could be used to treat cancer patients (45). Since then, several TLR ligands are being investigated and in clinical trials to enhance immunity for their use in treatment of cancer (46), viral infection (47), and bacterial infection (48). Several reviews have previously focused in the development and use of TLR agonists for cancer and other diseases (49–51). Here, we provide a comprehensive literature review specifically focused on the development of TLR agonists as LRAs and their potential use of these agonists for HIV eradication purposes.

TOLL-LIKE RECEPTORS

TLRs and Their Ligands

TLRs are transmembrane PRRs that recognize a plethora of molecules present in virus, bacteria, fungi or protozoa such as lipids, proteins, nucleic acids, and carbohydrates (52, 53). PRRs are germline-encoded receptors which function as first line of detection of pathogenic infections and recognize conserved molecular structures called pathogen-associated molecular patterns (PAMPs) (54). PRRs can also recognize soluble molecules released during cell death or damage. These structures are called damage-associated molecular patterns (DAMPs) (55, 56). In humans, there are 10 TLRs that differ both in their location within the cell as well as their cognate PAMP (**Figure 1**). TLR-1, 2, 4, 5, 6, and 10 are localized on the surface of the cells and recognize PAMPs present at the exterior of bacteria, fungi, and protozoa. On the other hand, TLR-3, 7, 8, and 9 are localized within endosomal structures and recognize nucleic acids derived from bacteria and viruses (53, 57). TLRs recognize their cognate ligand through either homodimers or heterodimers and are expressed in cells of the innate and adaptive immune system (such as dendritic cells, macrophages, granulocytes, T cells, B cells, NK cells, and mast cells) as well as epithelial and endothelial cells [reviewed in (37)].

TLRs in the Plasma Membrane

TLR-2 has a broader spectrum of ligand recognition than other TLRs due to its ability to dimerize with other receptors (58, 59). TLR-2 can recognize diacylated lipopeptides in the surface of gram-positive bacteria in conjunction with TLR-6 (60, 61). Whereas, TLR-2 can recognize triacylated lipopeptides present in gram-negative bacteria together with TLR-1 (62). TLR-2 has been shown to also induce signaling as a homodimer when recognizing lipoarabidomannan of *Mycobacterium smegmatis* (LAM-MS) and polysaccharide A of *Bacteroides fragilis* (PSA) (63, 64). Finally, TLR-2 can complex to the c-type lectin Dectin-1 to recognize zymosan, a β-glucan present in yeast cell wall (65). TLR-4 recognizes lipopolysaccharide (LPS), the principal component of gram-negative bacteria, and its truncated versions lipooligosaccharide and lipid A (66). CD14 and MD-2 are also needed for proper TLR-4 signaling (67, 68). TLR-5 recognizes flagellin, the main component of bacterial flagella (69). Lastly, TLR-10 has been an orphan receptor for a long time with no clearly defined ligand (70). TLR-10 has been shown to be involved in triacylated lipopeptides recognition by TLR-2 (71, 72). Recently, TLR-10 has been shown to sense gp41 and other HIV proteins in conjunction with TLR-1 and TLR-2 (73).

TLRs in the Endosomal Membrane

Several TLRs are present in endosomes, lysosomes and endolysosomes (74). TLR-3 recognizes double-stranded RNA (dsRNA) generated during viral infections while TLR-7 and TLR-8 both recognize single stranded RNA (ssRNA) (75, 76). Finally, TLR-9 can recognize unmethylated double-stranded DNA derived from both bacteria and viruses (77).

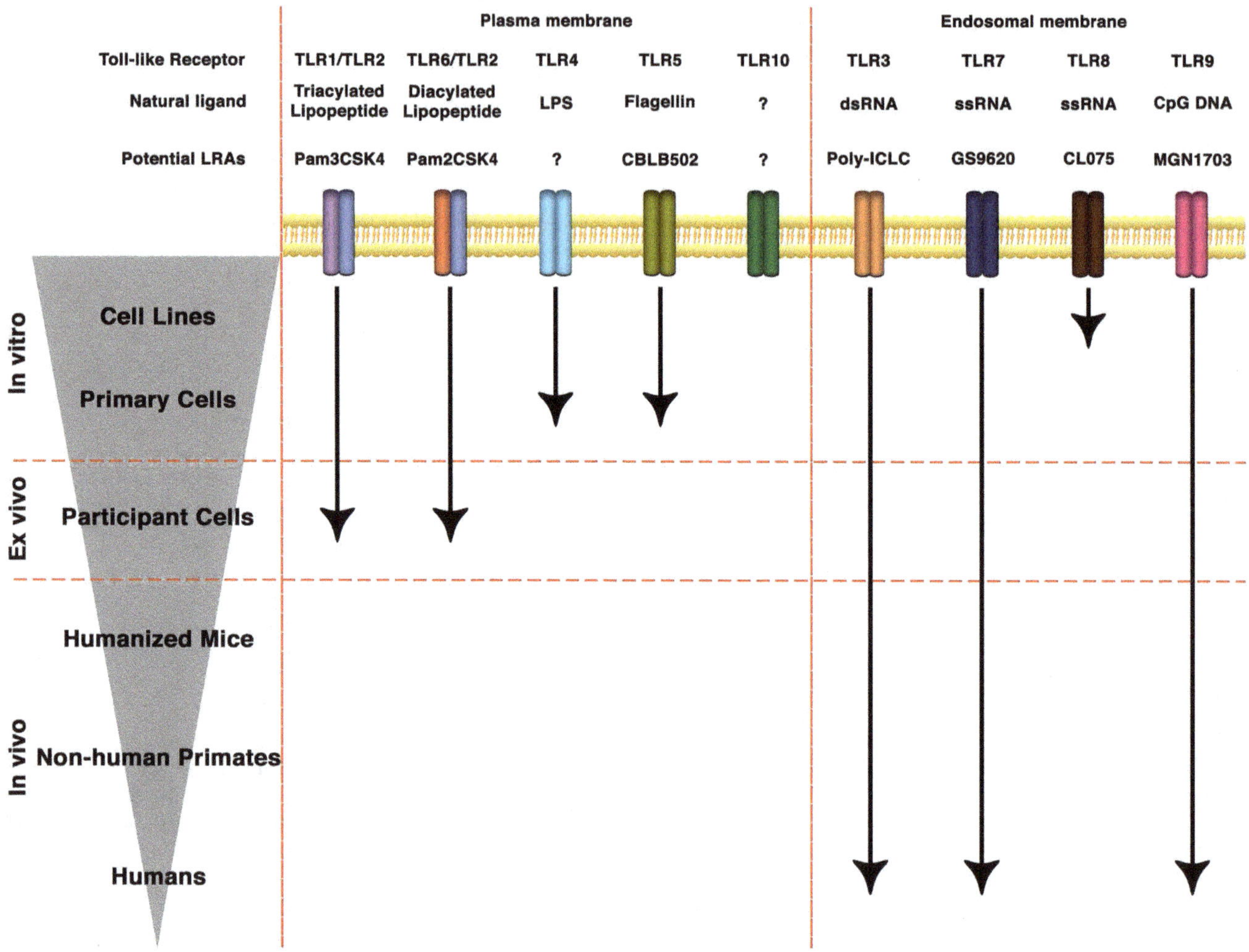

FIGURE 1 | State of the art of TLRs as LRAs for HIV eradication. TLRs can be expressed either in the plasma membrane or in endosomal membranes. They recognize molecular patterns such as lipids, proteins, nucleic acids and carbohydrates present in bacteria, protozoa, viruses or fungi. Based on the structure of the natural ligands, several synthetic derivatives and small molecules have been developed to specifically target different TLRs. Several of them are being investigated toward HIV cure strategies in cell lines, animal models or clinical trials.

Synthetic Ligands

Due to their immunostimulatory properties, the discovery of small molecules that can "mimic" a TLR response is an area of active research. Over the past years, several small molecules have been developed to specifically target TLRs and are being investigated for the treatment of bacterial and viral infections, for cancer immunotherapy and to optimize vaccine efficacy [reviewed in (50, 78, 79)].

Synthetic lipopeptides have been the gold standard TLR-2 ligands. Pam2CSK4 is a synthetic diacylated lipopeptide that engages TLR-2/TLR-6 heterodimers or TLR-2 homodimers (60, 80). Pam3CSK4 is a synthetic triacylated lipopeptide that engages TLR-2/TLR-1 heterodimers (62, 81). Mono-acyl lipopeptides are the minimal structure required for TLR-2 activity (82). Guan and colleagues identified a series of compounds with a similar core structure consisting of 3-carboxylbenzothiophene linked via a carbonothioyl amino bridge to an anilino group (83). Further structure-activity relationship (SAR) studies have yielded an optimized novel compound termed CU-T12-9 (84). This compound has shown higher efficacy than the original compound and shows a specificity toward TLR-2/TLR-1 heterodimers over TLR-2/TLR-6 heterodimers (84). Using structure-based virtual screening of over 10.5 million compounds, Chen and colleagues identified ethyl 2-(4-methylpiperazine-1-carboxamido)-5,6-dihydro-4H-cyclopenta[b]thiophene-3-carboxylate (SMU127) as a specific TLR-2/TLR-1 heterodimer ligand (85). Recently, the same group has developed 2-(1-(2-(Methylamino)-5-nitrophenyl)-1H-imidazol-4-yl)-5-(trifluoromethyl)phenol (SMU-Z1) as a specific TLR-2/TLR-1 heterodimer ligand (86). Finally, a screening in PMA-differentiated THP-1 cell line of nearly 100,000 compounds identified diprovocims as inducers of TLR-2 and TLR-1 receptor dimerization and activation in the low pM range (87).

The main synthetic ligand used for TLR-3 is polyinosinic-polycytidylic acid [poly(I:C)]. Poly(I:C) mimics dsRNA and it is formed of a strand of inosine poly(I) homopolymer annealed to a strand of cytidine poly(C) homopolymer. The antiviral and antitumoral activities of Poly(I:C) were described in the 1960's but it was not characterized as a TLR-3 agonist until the early 2000's (75). Other derivatives of Poly(I:C) have been developed such as a combination of polyinosinic-polycytidylic acid and poly-L-lysine (Poly-ICLC/Hiltonol®), or the introduction of uridine in the Poly(I:C) strand (poly(I:C$_{12}$U)/rintatolimod/Ampligen®), or Polyadenylic–polyuridylic acid [poly(A:U)] (88–90).

Monophosphoryl lipid A (MPL) is a detoxified form of the TLR4 agonist LPS from *Salmonella minnesota* that retains immunostimulatory properties but lacks the toxic effects of LPS (91). RC599 is a synthetic mimetic of MPL derived from aminoalkyl glucosaminide 4-phosphate (92). Both, MPL and RC599 have been shown to be efficient adjuvants and promote CD4 T cell responses (93). MPL has been used in a number of complex adjuvants included in human vaccines (Supervax®, Cervarix, Melacine®, Stimuvax) [reviewed in (94)]. Other lipid A mimetics (AS04, GLA-SE, GSK1795091, and OM-174) have been developed as vaccine adjuvants and are in licensed vaccines or in Phase I or II clinical trials as anticancer therapeutics [reviewed in (95)].

The polypeptide CBLB502 (Entolimod) derived from Flagellin is a potent TLR-5 ligand under extensive investigation as vaccine adjuvant, cancer and ischemia (96–99).

Imiquimod is an imidazoquinoline amine analog to guanosine that specifically activates TLR-7 (100). Several other agonists derived of imidazoquinoline have been developed that target TLR-7 such as Gardiquimod™ and PF-04878691 [also known as 852A or 3M-001) (101, 102)], or to target TLR-7 and TLR-8 simultaneously such as CL075, CL097, or Resiquimod (also known as R-848) (103–105). In addition, guanosine analogs such as Loxoribine have been generated as specific TLR-7 ligands (106). ANA975 and ANA773, also guanosine analogs, are prodrugs derived of the TLR-7 agonist isatoribine (107, 108). CL264 and SM360320 are derivatives of 9-benzyl-8 hydroxyadenine that have been shown to stimulate TLR-7

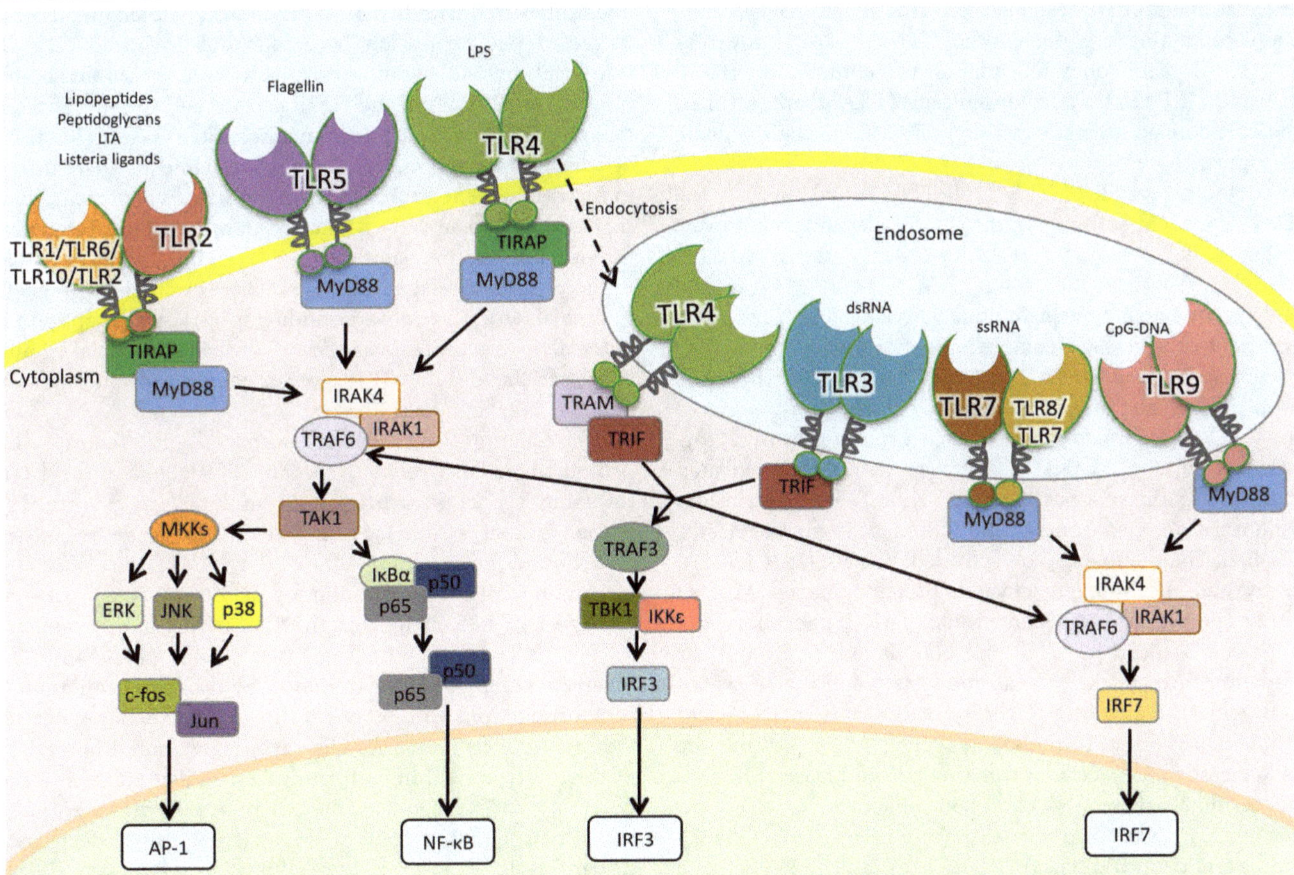

FIGURE 2 | Toll-like receptors signaling pathways. TLRs are the sentinels of host defense. The homodimers TLR5, TLR4, and TLR2 and the heterodimers TLR2-TLR1, TLR2-TLR6, and TLR2-TLR10 bind to their specific ligand at the cell surface, whereas TLR3, TLR7, TLR7-TLR8, and TLR9 localize to the endosomes, where they interact to their ligands. TLR4 following microbial detection is endocytosed into the endosome. When TLRs are activated by interaction with their ligands, adaptor molecules are recruited to stimulate downstream signaling pathways including NF- κB, AP1, and IRFs.

(109, 110). Finally, GS-9620 (Vesatolimod) and its close analog GS-986 are also a 9-benzyl-8 hydroxyadenine derivatives that targets TLR-7 with higher activity than CL264 (41, 42, 111).

All the synthetic TLR-9 ligands generated to date are derived from CpG oligodeoxynucleotides (CpG ODNs). CpGs ODNs can be classified into three classes (A, B, or C) that differ in their structure as well as their immunostimulatory properties (112, 113). Among others, CpG ODNs include CPG10101, IMO-2125, SD-101, CpG7909 (ProMune), MGN1703 (Lefitolimod) (114–118).

Finally, a series of synthetic TLR ligands that covalently link two or more TLR ligands are under investigation. These multi-TLR ligands have been designed to enhance immune responses through the synergistic activation of two or more TLRs with different downstream pathways (42, 119).

TLR Signaling Pathway

TLRs are type I transmembrane glycoproteins composed of a leucine-rich-repeat (LRR) motifs on the extracellular or endosomal domain that mediates ligand recognition and the Toll/IL-1R (TIR) in the cytoplasmic domain responsible for signaling (120). The signaling cascades following TLR activation involves multiple steps. Adaptor proteins such as myeloid differentiation primary-response protein 88 (MyD88), TIR-domain containing adaptor protein (TIRAP, also known as MAL), TIR-domain containing adaptor protein inducing IFN-β (TRIF) and TRIF-related adaptor molecule (TRAM) are recruited to the TIR domain after interaction of PAMPs to their cognate TLR (**Figure 2**).

With the exception of TLR-3, all TLRs signal through the MyD88-dependent pathway. In the MyD88-dependent pathway, TLR-2 and TLR-4 require TIRAP in order to recruit MyD88 to start signal transduction while TLR-5, TLR-7, TLR-8, and TLR-9 initiate signaling using uniquely MyD88 (121, 122). After recruitment of MyD88, a complex is formed with interleukin-1 receptor-associated kinase-1 (IRAK1) and IRAK4. IRAK1 is phosphorylated and associates with TNF receptor-associated factor 6 (TRAF6), which activates transforming growth factor-β-activated kinase 1 (TAK1), also known as mitogen-activated protein kinase kinase kinase 7 (MAP3K7). TAK1 activates, by phosphorylation, two routes; the IκB kinase—nuclear factor kappa-light-chain-enhancer of activated B cells (IKK-NF-κB) pathway and the mitogen-activated protein kinases (MAPK) pathway (**Figure 2**). In the first route, TAK-1 phosphorylates I-kappa-B-α/β (IκBα/β). This phosphorylation leads to their degradation through the proteasome system and the release of NF-κB, which translocates to the nucleus, binds to DNA and initiates transcription. In the second route, TAK1 activates the MAPK members extracellular signal-regulated kinase (ERK), c-Jun N-terminal kinase (JNK) and p38, which lead to activation of the nuclear factor activator protein-1 (AP-1) (57, 123). In plasmocytoid dendritic cells (pDCs), TLR-7, and TLR-9 activate MyD88 signaling that leads to the phosphorylation and activation of the transcription factor interferon regulatory factor 7 (IRF7), which regulates the expression of IFN-α (124).

In the MyD88-independent pathway, TRIF is recruited to TLR-3 to initiate signaling (125). Besides TLR-3, TLR-4 can be endocytosed and signal through TRIF using the adaptor molecule TRAM (126, 127). TRAF6 and TRAF3 are recruited to TRIF. While TRAF6 engages IKK and MAPK, leading to the activation of NF-κB, AP-1, and IRF7; TRAF3 recruits TBK1/IKK-ε complex that activates IRF3 culminating in IFN-β expression (**Figure 2**) (128, 129).

TOLL-LIKE RECEPTOR AGONISTS AS LATENCY-REVERSING AGENTS

In vitro Studies

The importance of TLRs in the physiopathology of HIV was first postulated after observations on increased plasma viral loads seen in HIV-infected individuals exposed to vaccination regimens, suffering of opportunistic bacterial infections or sexually transmitted diseases, or had translocation of microbial products from the gut (130–138). Early studies have shown that PAMPs and their corresponding microorganisms transactivate the HIV long-terminal repeat (LTR) promoter. For example, it was described that purified protein derivative (PPD) of *Mycobacterium tuberculosis* increased viral mRNA expression in HIV infected monocytes (139). Furthermore, monocytic cell lines stimulated with live *M. tuberculosis* or lipomannan (LAM) increased p24 expression by 3-fold and enhanced HIV LTR transcription (140). Additionally, it has been shown that both *M. tuberculosis* PPD from the H37Ra strain and the mycobacterial major cell wall component mannosylated LAM (ManLAM) activated transcription of HIV in the T cell line Jurkat. ManLAM-induced HIV gene expression was mediated via protein kinases that culminated in NF-κB nuclear translocation. Mutations in the NF-κB binding sites in the HIV LTR abolished PDD-induced HIV expression (141, 142). These findings suggested that microbial products could be inducing HIV transcription. The latter discovery of TLRs as sensors of these microbial products suggested the idea that TLR agonists could reactivate latent HIV and could be potential LRAs.

Subsequently increasing number of reports have demonstrated the role of specific TLR agonists as latency reversing agents *in vitro*. Equils and colleagues transfected human dermal endothelial cells with an LTR luciferase construct and showed that stimulation of TLR-4 with LPS leads to NF-κB activation and transactivation of HIV-LTR (143). However, the effect of LPS in the reactivation of the HIV promoter in T cells has been disputed by other groups (144–146). These divergent results could be explained by the use of contaminated LPS formulations with other PAMPs, like bacterial lipopeptides. Other possible reasons for the discrepancy could be variation in the cell type used in each study, since different cells respond differently to TLR agonists, the cell culture environment, which component could escalate or impair an agonists effect, and/or disparities in TLR-4 binding affinity to LPS from different bacteria. Recently, LPS has been shown to reactivate latent HIV in macrophages isolated from the urethra of patients under ART (147).

The TLR-9 agonist CpG ODNs has been shown to activate HIV replication in the chronically infected human cell lines

U1 and ACH2 in an NF-κB dependent manner (148, 149). Furthermore, DNA from *F. nucleatum* increased HIV promoter activity through TLR-9 signaling in the THP89GFP cell line (144). Recently, the TLR9 MGN1703 has been shown to induced HIV RNA release in peripheral blood mononuclear cells (PBMCs) from aviremic HIV-infected donors on antiretroviral therapy (ART) (150).

Mycobacteria have been shown to induce HIV transcription in a TLR-2 dependent manner. Bhat et al. observed that the *M. tuberculosis* and *M. smegmatis* proline-proline-glutamic acid protein Rv1168c (PPE17) interacts with TLR-2 resulting in activation of NF-κB and HIV transactivation in the human monocytic cell line THP1 (151). Our group has shown that the TLR-2 agonists Pam2CSK4 and Pam3CSK4 have latency reversal activity in CD4 T cells from aviremic HIV-infected participants and in a primary T_{CM} cell model of latency (42, 146, 152). Finally, the component of the *M. tuberculosis* membrane phosphatidylinositol mannoside 6 (PIM6) as well as whole bacteria in co-culture reactivated HIV in a primary T_{CM} cell model of latency. As for previous studies with *M. tuberculosis,* viral reactivation was dependent on TLR-2 (153).

R-848, a TLR-7/-8 agonist, induced p24 expression in the latently infected monocytic cell lines U1 and OM10 (154). Furthermore, a combination of the PKC agonist and LRA prostratin with a TLR-8 agonist 3M-002 was tested in a coculture of latently infected cells (J-Lat) and monocyte-derived dendritic cells (MDDCs). The combination of protratin and 3M-002 resulted in greater reactivation of HIV latency in J-Lat than each compounds alone. This synergistic interaction was dependent on TNF-α and on MDDC-T cell interactions (155).

Flagellin, the structural protein in bacterial flagella and a TLR5 agonist, has been shown to reactivate latent HIV in J-Lat, a transformed cell line latently infected with HIV derived of Jurkat (146, 156, 157). Thibault and colleagues also shown activity of flagellin in central memory T cells previously infected with a VSV-G pseudotyped NL43. However, resting CD4 T cells from aviremic patients, when challenged with flagellin, failed to elicit detectable levels of viral gene expression (157).

The TLR-3 agonist Poly(I:C) has been shown to reactivate latent HIV via NF-κB and JNK in the monocytic cell line U38 that contains a stably integrated and silent copy of the HIV LTR promoter linked to the chloramphenicol acetyltransferase (CAT) gene (158).

The selective TLR-7 agonist GS-9620 induced extracellular HIV RNA release in the supernatants of PBMCs isolated from HIV-infected participants on ART but not in purified CD4 T cells (159). In this study, Tsai and colleagues attributed this viral reactivation to type I IFN produced by pDCs. Therefore, this last finding suggests two complementary mechanisms of latency reversal mediated by TLR agonists. One that requires a subset of immune cells to be activated with the TLR agonist and these cells release soluble factors with latency reversal activity. And a second mechanism in which the TLR agonists have a direct effect on latently infected CD4T cells. Based on this idea, we have recently characterized the mechanisms of viral reactivation mediated by the TLR-2 agonist Pam2CSK4 and the TLR-7 agonist GS-9620 and compared with that of synthetic dual TLR-2 and TLR-7 agonists (dual TLR-2/7 agonists). We found that TLR-2 and TLR-7 agonists reactivate latency by two distinct and complementary mechanisms. TLR-2 agonists reactivate HIV by directly inducing NF-κB activation in memory CD4 T cells, while TLR7 agonists induced the secretion of soluble factors that can reactivate latent HIV in CD4 T cells. Our results suggests that TNF-α but not type-I IFN secreted by monocytes and plasmacytoid dendritic cells (pDCs) promotes viral reactivation in CD4 T cells (42).

TLR agonists have also shown to reactivate latent HIV in other cell subsets besides CD4 T cells and monocytes/macrophages. Poly (I:C) and bacterial ribosomal RNA induced HIV reactivation through TLR-3 in a latency model using immortalized human primary microglia with simian virus-40 (SV40) large T antigen and human telomerase reverse transcriptase (160). Furthermore, stimulation with TLR-2, TLR-4, or TLR-9 agonists induced HIV replication in a primary latency model using human progenitor mast cells (161).

In vivo Studies: From Small Animals to Clinical Trials

Mouse models have been a tool to study the role of TLR agonists on the pathogenesis of HIV. Initial studies were done using a transgenic mouse model that contains intact copies of HIV proviral DNA (162). Infection of these animals with *Mycobacterium avium* or *Toxoplasma gondii* increased viral production in monocytes/macrophages (163, 164). Using *ex vivo* spleens from these transgenic mice, Equils and colleagues demonstrated that ligands for TLR-2 (soluble Mycobacterium tuberculosis factor or STF), TLR-4 (LPS), and TLR-9 (CpG) increased viral production and that combination of LPS with either STF or CpG increased viral production in an additive manner (165). Furthermore, Bafica and colleagues crossed this HIV transgenic mouse with either a TLR-2-deficient or a control mouse to investigate the role of TLR-2 in the activation of HIV expression. Culture filtrate proteins, phosphatidyl-inositol mannoside from *M. tuberculosis* and the synthetic lipopeptdide Pam3CSK4 induced p24 expression in spleen cells from HIV transgenic mouse expressing TLR-2 but not the TLR-2 deficient mice (166).

Several studies have specifically looked at the effects of TLR agonists on the latent reservoir *in vivo* (**Table 1**). A study using a humanized mice model of HIV latency demonstrated that the TLR-3 agonists poly(I:C) can reactivate latent HIV *in vivo* (167). In this study, the co-administration of poly(I:C) with a vaccination regimen including recombinant anti-human CD40 antibody fused to 5 HIV peptide regions (αCD40.HIV5pep) reduced the levels of cell-associated HIV DNA and delayed 1 week viral rebound after ART interruption in these animals (167). The selective TLR-7 small-molecule agonist GS-9620 has demonstrated antiviral activity in animal models of hepatitis B virus, good safety profiles and has progressed to clinical testing (171–173). As such, TLR-7 agonists have also been tested as LRAs in SIV-infected rhesus macaques. So far, there has been 4 different studies on the administration of GS-9620 or its analog GS-986 in infected macaques under suppressive ART.

TABLE 1 | Summary of *in vivo* studies using TLR ligands as LRAs.

	Administration	Study arms	Specie	Viral blips	Effects on reservoir	References
Poly I:C (TLR3)	Two doses 2.5 weeks apart, half IP half IM	PBS Poly I:C αCD40.HIV5pep/ Poly I:C	NRG hu-mice	Yes (US/7)	Reduction on cell-associated DNA in lymphoid tissue (4/4) Delayed rebound (αCD40.HIV5pep/Poly I:C 1 week)	(167)
Poly-ICLC (TLR3)	Two consecutively daily doses, SC	Randomize (3:1) vs placebo	Human	0/12	Reduction on cell-associated DNA (0/12)	(168)
GS-986 (TLR7)	Ten doses two weeks apart, OG	Sham Ad26/MVA GS-986 GS-986/Ad26/MVA	Rhesus macaque	Sham (0/9) Ad26/MVA (0/9) GS-986 (0/9) GS-986/Ad26/MVA (1/9)	Reduction on cell-associated DNA in lymph nodes week 70 (Sham 1/9, Ad26/MVA 1/9, GS-986 4/8; GS-986/Ad26/MVA 6/8) Reduction on cell-associated DNA in PBMCs week 70 (Sham 3/9, Ad26/MVA 9/9, GS-986 4/8; GS-986/Ad26/MVA 6/8) Virologic control (Sham 0/9, Ad26/MVA 0/9, GS-986 0/8, GS-986/Ad26/MVA 3/8)	(39)
GS-9620 (TLR7)	Ten doses two weeks apart, OG	Sham PGT121 GS-9620 GS-9620/PGT121	Rhesus macaque	Sham (0/11) PGT121 (0/11) GS-9620 (0/11) GS-9620/ PGT121 (0/11)	Reduction of viral DNA in lymph nodes week 120 (Sham 4/11, PGT121 7/11, GS-9620 3/11, GS-9620/PGT121 11/11) Virologic control (Sham 0/11, PGT121 3/11, GS-9620 1/11, GS-9620/PGT121 5/11)	(40)
GS-986 (TLR7)	Dose scalation 2 weeks apart, OG	Sham GS-986	Rhesus macaque	Sham (0/3) GS-986 (4/4)	Reduction of viral DNA in memory CD4 T cells from PBMCs (3/4), LNMCs (4/4) and GMMCs (4/4)	(41)
GS-9620 (TLR7)	Ten doses 2 weeks apart, OG	Sham GS-9620 0.05 mg/kg GS-9620 0.1 mg/kg GS-9620 0.15 mg/kg	Rhesus macaque	Sham (0/3) GS-9620 0.05 mg/kg (3/3) GS-9620 0.1 mg/kg (3/3) GS-9620 0.15 mg/kg (3/3)	Reduction of viral DNA in memory CD4 T cells from PBMCs (Sham 2/2, GS-9620 0.05 mg/kg 3/3, GS-9620 0.1 mg/kg 3/3, GS-9620 0.15 mg/kg 3/3) Reduction of viral DNA in memory CD4 T cells from LNMCs (Sham 1/2, GS-9620 0.05 mg/kg 1/3, GS-9620 0.1 mg/kg 2/3, GS-9620 0.15 mg/kg 1/3) Reduction of viral DNA in memory CD4 T cells from GMMCs (Sham 0/2, GS-9620 0.05 mg/kg 2/3, GS-9620 0.1 mg/kg 3/3, GS-9620 0.15 mg/kg 3/3) Virologic control (Sham 0/2, GS-9620 0.05 mg/kg 0/3, GS-9620 0.1 mg/kg 1/3, GS-9620 0.15 mg/kg 1/3)	(41)
GS-9620 (TLR7)	First course of twelve doses 2 weeks apart, OG Second course of five dose 2 weeks apart, OG	Sham GS-9620	Rhesus macaque	Sham (0/2) GS-9620 (0/4)	No effects in viral HIV DNA	(169)
GS-9620 (TLR7)	Tablet(s) administered orally once every 2 weeks	Randomized, blinded, placebo-controlled dose-escalation study	Human	Completed trial	Completed trial	NCT02858401

(*Continued*)

TABLE 1 | Continued

	Administration	Study arms	Specie	Viral blips	Effects on reservoir	References
GS-9620 (TLR7)	Up to 10 doses administered as four 2 mg tablets orally every 14 days	Randomized, Double-Blind, Placebo-controlled Study	Human	Ongoing trial	Ongoing trial	NCT03060447
CpG-ODN 7909 (TLR9)	Immunized with double the standard dose of PCV7 (Prevnar®, Wyeth) at 0 and 3 months and with one single dose of PPV-23 (Pneumo Novum®, Sanofi-Pasteur MSD)	Placebo CpG-ODN 7909	Human	ND	Decrease in viral HIV DNA in PBMCs in CpG-ODN 7909 group relative to placebo control	(170)
MGN1703 (TLR9)	Eight doses twice weekly for 4 week, SC	Single-arm, open-label study	Human	6/15	No effects in viral HIV DNA in CD4 T cells	(43)
MGN1703 (TLR9)	Forty-eight doses twice weekly for 24 week, SC	Single-arm, open-label study	Human	ND	No effects in viral HIV DNA in CD4 T cells No changes in CA US HIV RNA in CD4 T cells No changes in IUPM	(44)

IP, intraperitoneally; IM, intramuscularly; SC, subcutaneously; OG, oral gavage; NRG mice, NOD.Cg-Rag1^{tm1Mom}Il2rg^{tm1Wjl}/SzJ mice; US, Unspecified; ND, Non-determined; CA US, cell-associated unspliced; IUPM, infectious units per million.

The first study combined the therapeutic vaccine Ad26/MVA (recombinant adenovirus serotype 26 (Ad26) prime, modified vaccinia Ankara (MVA) boost) with GS-986. They found that this combination resulted in decreased levels of viral DNA in lymph nodes and peripheral blood, and improved virologic control and delayed viral rebound following discontinuation of antiretroviral therapy (39). In another study from the same group, GS-9620 was combined with the V3 glycan-dependent bNAb PGT121 in rhesus monkeys during ART (40). This combination delayed viral rebound after ART discontinuation. Interestingly, 5 out of 11 monkeys did not show viral rebound even after CD8-depletion or adoptive transfer of PBMCs and LNMCs into naïve monkeys (40). In a third study, repeated administration of GS-9620 or its analog G-986 to SIVmac251-infected rhesus macaques under ART was associated with transient plasma viremia that peaked 24 to 48 h after dosing (41). Furthermore, TLR-7 agonists induced a reduction in cell-associated SIV DNA in sorted memory CD4 T cells obtained from peripheral blood, gastrointestinal mucosa and lymph nodes (41). Finally, a recent study also evaluated the effects of repeated doses of the TLR7 agonist GS-9620 in SIV-infected rhesus macaques receiving ART (169). The rhesus macaques that received GS-9620 during ART presented with immunologic effects due to the TLR-7 agonist, such as upregulation of IFN-stimulated genes in both blood and tissues, an increase in different plasma cytokines such as IFN-α and IL-1RA, and changes in CD8, NK and macrophage activation. In contrast with the study from Lim and colleagues, GS-9620 did not result in a measurable increase in plasma viremia or changes in viral RNA–to–viral DNA ratio in PBMCs or tissues, nor decreases in viral DNA in PBMC or tissues (169). Several differences can account for the discrepancies in these two studies. First, ART was initiated at different times after initial infection (65 vs. 13 days). Second, GS-9620 was administrated at different times post-ART initiation (60 vs. 75 weeks). Third, the SIV strain used in each study were different (SIVmac251 vs. SIVmac239X). Forth, the route of inoculation was also different (intrarectally vs. intravenously). All of these differences could lead to variations in the formation of viral reservoirs and their sensitivity to TLR-7 agonists. Further studies are warranted to fully understand the discrepancies of these two studies.

TLR agonists have also reached clinical testing in ART-suppressed participants (**Table 1**). The TLR-9 agonist CpG-ODN 7909, a class B CpG ODN, was administered as adjuvant in HIV-infected individuals (174). Interestingly, those participants receiving the TLR9 agonist as adjuvant in the immunization protocol had some decrease in the HIV proviral reservoir compared the control group (170). This led to the idea of using TLR-9 agonists to reduce the latent reservoir. As such, two different clinical trials aimed toward HIV eradication have been done using the TLR-9 ligand MGN1703. In the first clinical trial, a single-arm, open-label study in which 15 (13 male, 2 female) virologically suppressed HIV infected individuals on ART received 60 mg MGN1703 subcutaneously twice weekly for 4 weeks (43). In this study, they characterized pDC, NK, and T-cell activation using flow cytometry on baseline and after 4 weeks of treatment. Additionally, HIV transcription was quantified by measuring plasma HIV RNA. MGN1703 treatment increased the activation of pDCs, upregulated levels of cytokines, and enhanced activation of cytotoxic NK cells and effector $CD8^+$ T cells. Furthermore, treatment with MGN1703 induced plasma HIV RNA blips up to >1,500 copies/mL in 6 of 15 participants (43). From this trial, biopsies from sigmoid colon were collected from 11 participants. Increased in solely type-1 interferon response but not a broad inflammatory response was observed in intestinal mononuclear cells. Interestingly, increased transcription of either *TLR9* or *IFNAR1* before MGN1703 administration was associated with improved efficacy in eliminating HIV DNA-containing cells in the intestine during the course of treatment (175). In the second clinical trial, the same group enrolled HIV-infected individuals on ART for an exploratory, single-arm clinical trial that tested the safety and immune enhancement effects of 24-weeks of MGN1703 (60 mg 2 weekly) therapy (44). A total of twelve individuals completed the treatment phase and nine underwent analytical treatment interruption (ATI). MGN1703 led to potent T-cell activation and increased HIV-specific T-cell responses, however there were no changes in CD4 T cells containing viral DNA nor differences in the time to rebound after ATI. In this study, a single patient was able to control viremia for 150 days after ATI. This participant had strong HIV-specific cellular and antibody-mediated immune responses, however as the study did not contain a placebo arm, the delayed viral rebound cannot exclusively be associated to MGN1703 treatment (44). The TLR-3 agonist Poly-ICLC (Hiltonol®) has also been tested in a randomized, placebo-controlled, double-blinded trial in ART-suppressed participants (168). In this study, participants received two daily doses of Poly-ICLC subcutaneously. Both, Poly-ICLC and placebo control were observed for adverse events, immune activation, and viral replication. As for other TLR agonists, Poly-ICLC administration lead to transient innate immune stimulation without generalized immune activation. While no effects of Poly-ICLC in reversing HIV latency or on the size of the viral reservoirs were observed; Poly-ICLC was reported safe and well-tolerated (168). Finally, the TLR7 agonist GS-9620 is currently being evaluated in clinical trials in HIV infected controllers (NCT03060447) and in those on suppressive ART (NCT02858401). These studies will provide information regarding safety and biological activity, including their impact on viral reservoirs, in HIV-infected patients.

MODULATION OF HIV-HOST IMMUNE RESPONSES BY TLR STIMULATION

Besides their potential ability to reactivate latent HIV, TLR agonists have been shown to have immunostimulatory and antiviral properties to modulate anti-HIV immune responses.

The TLR-2 agonist Pam3CSK4 has been shown to prime latently-infected CD4 T cells for CD8 T cell recognition (176). We have characterized that TLR-2 and dual TLR-2/7 agonists, besides reactivating latent HIV, they can activate NK cells and induce IL-22. We demonstrated a protective role for IL-22 in both cell-free and cell-to-cell HIV infection of CD4 T cells (42). Whether TLR-2 agonists enhance the ability of NK cells to kill HIV-infected cells has not been demonstrated yet. Furthermore, the dual TLR-2/7 agonist PamadiFectin has been shown to enhance humoral responses in a mouse model immunized with p24 coupled to nanoparticles (119).

The TLR-3 agonist poly(I:C) enhanced the generation of HIV-specific T cell responses in BALB/c mice and in humanize mouse vaccination models (167, 177). *In vitro*, the TLR-7 agonist GS-9620 has been shown to both inhibit HIV replication in an IFN-α-mediated mechanism as well as enhance the anti-HIV activity of CD8 T and NK cells (159, 178). The TLR-7/8 agonist 3M-012, an analog of R-848, has been given as vaccine adjuvant in combination with HIV Gag antigen to non-human primates. The addition of 3M-012 to the Gag vaccine substantially enhanced Gag-specific T helper 1 and CD8 T cell responses compared to animals given the Gag protein alone (179). Furthermore, TLR-7/-8 activation through ssRNA or R-848 interfered with HIV replication cycle in lymphocyte cultures (154). In addition, The TLR-7/8 agonists 3M-002 and R-848 were able to promote HIV control *in vitro* in HIV-infected PBMCs through the activation of CD8 T cells and NK cells (180).

A randomized controlled vaccine trial conducted with 95 HIV-infected subjects investigated the impact of TLR-9 agonist as an adjuvant for pneumococcal vaccine. The trial showed that the TLR-9 agonist, CpG-ODN 7909, enhanced vaccine immunogenicity in the experimental group compared with the control group (174). *Post-hoc* analyses of the vaccine trial confirmed that patients that received TLR-9 ligand as adjuvant expressed more CD107a and macrophage inflammatory protein 1β (MIP1β) markers in CD8 T cells. The increase in these markers was associated with a reduction in HIV proviral load (170). Furthermore, the TLR-9 agonist CpG-ODN 2216 has been shown to activate NK cells in a pDC-mediated mechanism and enhance NK lysis of autologous HIV-infected CD4 T cells (181). In addition, TLR ligands such as Imiquimod (TLR-7), R-848 (TLR-7/8), CpG ODN (TLR-9), and Poly(I:C) (TLR-3) have been also shown to enhance the generation of HIV-specific CD8 T cells *in vitro* (182).

CONCLUDING REMARKS

The use of TLR ligands as LRAs has shown promising results in efforts toward HIV eradication either alone or in combination with other therapeutic strategies because of their ability to reactivate latent HIV, to enhance immune responses and promote antiviral responses. Several TLR agonists are under investigation both in pre-clinical models of HIV latency as well as in clinical trials (**Figure 1**). These preclinical and clinical studies have shown a wide variety of response even in studies using the same TLR agonists (**Table 1**). Why such differences are currently unknown. Based on these studies, we can speculate several factors that may be influencing the response to TLR agonists including the time of ART initiation, the length of ART treatment, the cellular composition of the latent reservoir, or the strain of SIV or HIV. There are also other factors that may influence the activity of these agonists that will need to be considered in future cure strategies. First, TLRs contain polymorphisms that influence their activity (183, 184). How these polymorphisms affect the efficacy of different TLR ligands in HIV eradication approaches has not been characterized. Second, it is well-known that biological sex influences the responses of certain TLRs, in particular TLR-7 (185, 186). The *in vivo* evaluation of GS-9620 or other TLR-7 agonists will need to take this into account. As research progresses, emphasis also needs to be done in understanding whether these TLR agonists can reach all the different tissue compartments where HIV may hide, including lymph nodes, intestinal mucosal, and brain [reviewed in (187–191)]. Furthermore, HIV has been shown to reside latent in other cell types besides CD4 T cell (147, 192). As such, it is possible that a single TLR agonist may not be sufficient to reactivate all latent virus present in different cellular compartments as the expression of TLRs differs among different cell subsets. Additional research is warranted to fully understand which TLR agonists reactivate latent HIV in each cell compartment. Also, it will be important to address whether reactivation is due to a direct targeting of the TLR in the reservoir cell or whether other soluble factors secreted by other cells are required for efficient viral reactivation. The mechanisms involved in HIV latency are complex and involve a plethora of cellular factors as well as epigenetic mechanisms (193). As such, TLR agonists may need to be combined with other LRAs with different mechanisms of action to efficiently reactivate all latent viruses. Finally, recent studies using animal models suggest the use of additional strategies, such as bNAbs, might be required to generate meaningful remission. Therefore, it is important to continue the investigation of TLR agonists as potential adjuvants for novel HIV cure strategies.

AUTHOR CONTRIBUTIONS

AM, CN, and AB contributed to the conception of the review and wrote the first draft of the manuscript. All authors contributed to manuscript revision, read, and approved the submitted version.

REFERENCES

Chun TW, Stuyver L, Mizell SB, Ehler LA, Mican JA, Baseler M, et al. Presence of an inducible HIV-1 latent reservoir during highly active antiretroviral therapy. *Proc Natl Acad Sci USA.* (1997) 94:13193–7. doi:10.1073/pnas.94.24.13193

Finzi D, Hermankova M, Pierson T, Carruth LM, Buck C, Chaisson RE, et al. Identification of a reservoir for HIV-1 in patients on highly active antiretroviral therapy. *Science.* (1997) 278:1295–300. doi:10.1126/science.278.5341.1295

Wong JK, Hezareh M, Gunthard HF, Havlir DV, Ignacio CC, Spina CA, et al. Recovery of replication-competent HIV despite prolonged suppression of plasma viremia. *Science.* (1997) 278:1291–5. doi:10.1126/science.278.5341.1291

Brenchley JM, Hill BJ, Ambrozak DR, Price DA, Guenaga FJ, Casazza JP, et al. T-cell subsets that harbor human immunodeficiency virus (HIV) *in vivo*: implications for HIV pathogenesis. *J Virol.* (2004) 78:1160–8. doi: 10.1128/JVI.78.3.1160-1168.2004

Chomont N, El-Far M, Ancuta P, Trautmann L, Procopio FA, Yassine- Diab B, et al. HIV reservoir size and persistence are driven by T cell survival and homeostatic proliferation. *Nat Med.* (2009) 15:893–900. doi:10.1038/nm.1972

Barouch DH, Deeks SG. Immunologic strategies for HIV-1 remission and eradication. *Science.* (2014) 345:169–74. doi: 10.1126/science.1255512

Gupta RK, Abdul-Jawad S, McCoy LE, Mok HP, Peppa D, Salgado M, et al. HIV-1 remission following CCR5Delta32/Delta32 haematopoietic stem-cell transplantation. *Nature.* (2019) 568:244–8. doi: 10.1038/s41586-019-1027-4

Hutter G, Nowak D, Mossner M, Ganepola S, Mussig A, Allers K, et al. Long- term control of HIV by CCR5 Delta32/Delta32 stem-cell transplantation. *N Engl J Med.* (2009) 360:692–8. doi: 10.1056/NEJMoa0802905

Cheret A, Bacchus-Souffan C, Avettand-Fenoel V, Melard A, Nembot G, Blanc C, et al. Combined ART started during acute HIV infection protects central memory CD4+ T cells and can induce remission. *J Antimicrob Chemother.* (2015) 70:2108–20. doi: 10.1093/jac/dkv084

Hocqueloux L, Prazuck T, Avettand-Fenoel V, Lafeuillade A, Cardon B, Viard JP, et al. Long-term immunovirologic control following antiretroviral therapy interruption in patients treated at the time of primary HIV-1 infection. *AIDS.* (2010) 24:1598–601. doi: 10.1097/QAD.0b013e32833b61ba

Saez-Cirion A, Bacchus C, Hocqueloux L, Avettand-Fenoel V, Girault I, Lecuroux C, et al. Post-treatment HIV-1 controllers with a long-term virological remission after the interruption of early initiated antiretroviral therapy ANRS VISCONTI Study. *PLoS Pathog.* (2013) 9:e1003211. doi:10.1371/journal.ppat.1003211

Samri A, Bacchus-Souffan C, Hocqueloux L, Avettand-Fenoel V, Descours B, Theodorou I, et al. Polyfunctional HIV-specific T cells in Post-Treatment Controllers. *AIDS.* (2016) 30:2299–302. doi:10.1097/QAD.0000000000001195

Archin NM, Cheema M, Parker D, Wiegand A, Bosch RJ, Coffin JM, et al. Antiretroviral intensification and valproic acid lack sustained effect on residual HIV-1 viremia or resting CD4+ cell infection. *PLoS ONE.* (2010) 5:e9390. doi: 10.1371/journal.pone.0009390

Archin NM, Eron JJ, Palmer S, Hartmann-Duff A, Martinson JA, Wiegand A, et al. Valproic acid without intensified antiviral therapy has limited impact on persistent HIV infection of resting CD4+ T cells. *AIDS.* (2008) 22:1131–5. doi: 10.1097/QAD.0b013e3282fd6df4

Lehrman G, Hogue IB, Palmer S, Jennings C, Spina CA, Wiegand A, et al. Depletion of latent HIV-1 infection *in vivo*: a proof-of-concept study. *Lancet.* (2005) 366:549–55. doi: 10.1016/S0140-6736(05)67098-5

Routy JP, Tremblay CL, Angel JB, Trottier B, Rouleau D, Baril JG, et al. Valproic acid in association with highly active antiretroviral therapy for reducing systemic HIV-1 reservoirs: results from a multicentre randomized clinical study. *HIV Med.* (2012) 13:291–6. doi:10.1111/j.1468-1293.2011.00975.x

Sagot-Lerolle N, Lamine A, Chaix ML, Boufassa F, Aboulker JP, Costagliola D, et al. Prolonged valproic acid treatment does not reduce the size of latent HIV reservoir. *AIDS.* (2008) 22:1125–9. doi:10.1097/QAD.0b013e3282fd6ddc

Siliciano JD, Lai J, Callender M, Pitt E, Zhang H, Margolick JB, et al. Stability of the latent reservoir for HIV-1 in patients receiving valproic acid. *J Infect Dis.* (2007) 195:833–6. doi: 10.1086/511823

Archin NM, Bateson R, Tripathy MK, Crooks AM, Yang KH, Dahl NP, et al. HIV-1 expression within resting CD4+ T cells after multiple doses of vorinostat. *J Infect Dis.* (2014) 210:728–35. doi: 10.1093/infdis/jiu155

Archin NM, Liberty AL, Kashuba AD, Choudhary SK, Kuruc JD, Crooks AM, et al. Administration of vorinostat disrupts HIV-1 latency in patients on antiretroviral therapy. *Nature.* (2012) 487:482–5. doi: 10.1038/nature11286

Elliott JH, Wightman F, Solomon A, Ghneim K, Ahlers J, Cameron MJ, et al. Activation of HIV transcription with short-course vorinostat in HIV- infected patients on suppressive antiretroviral therapy. *PLoS Pathog.* (2014) 10:e1004473. doi: 10.1371/journal.ppat.1004473

Sogaard OS, Graversen ME, Leth S, Olesen R, Brinkmann CR, Nissen SK, et al. The depsipeptide romidepsin reverses HIV-1 latency *in vivo*. *PLoS Pathog.* (2015) 11:e1005142. doi: 10.1371/journal.ppat.10 05142

Rasmussen TA, Tolstrup M, Brinkmann CR, Olesen R, Erikstrup C, Solomon A, et al. Panobinostat, a histone deacetylase inhibitor, for latent-virus reactivation in HIV-infected patients on suppressive antiretroviral therapy: a phase 1/2, single group, clinical trial. *Lancet HIV.* (2014) 1:e13–21. doi: 10.1016/S2352-3018(14)70014-1

Gutierrez C, Serrano-Villar S, Madrid-Elena N, Perez-Elias MJ, Martin ME, Barbas C, et al. Bryostatin-1 for latent virus reactivation in HIV- infected patients on antiretroviral therapy. *AIDS.* (2016) 30:1385–92. doi: 10.1097/QAD.0000000000001064

Elliott JH, McMahon JH, Chang CC, Lee SA, Hartogensis W, Bumpus N, et al. Short-term administration of disulfiram for reversal of latent HIV infection: a phase 2 dose-escalation study. *Lancet HIV.* (2015) 2:e520–529. doi:10.1016/S2352-3018(15)00226-X

Spivak AM, Andrade A, Eisele E, Hoh R, Bacchetti P, Bumpus NN, et al. A pilot study assessing the safety and latency-reversing activity of disulfiram in HIV-1-infected adults on antiretroviral therapy. *Clin Infect Dis.* (2014) 58:883–90. doi: 10.1093/cid/cit813

Rasmussen TA, Schmeltz Sogaard O, Brinkmann C, Wightman F, Lewin SR, Melchjorsen J, et al. Comparison of HDAC inhibitors in clinical development: effect on HIV production in latently infected cells and T-cell activation. *Hum Vaccin Immunother.* (2013) 9:993–1001. doi:10.4161/hv.23800

Spivak AM, Planelles V. HIV-1 eradication: early trials (and Tribulations). *Trends Mol Med.* (2016) 22:10–27. doi: 10.1016/j.molmed.2015.11.004

Van Lint C, Bouchat S, Marcello A. HIV-1 transcription and latency: an update. *Retrovirology.* (2013) 10:67. doi: 10.1186/1742-4690-10-67

Day CL, Kaufmann DE, Kiepiela P, Brown JA, Moodley ES, Reddy S, et al. PD-1 expression on HIV-specific T cells is associated with T-cell exhaustion and disease progression. *Nature.* (2006) 443:350–4. doi: 10.1038/nature05115

Ho YC, Shan L, Hosmane NN, Wang J, Laskey SB, Rosenbloom DI, et al. Replication-competent noninduced proviruses in the latent reservoir increase barrier to HIV-1 cure. *Cell.* (2013) 155:540–51. doi:10.1016/j.cell.2013.09.020

Huang SH, Ren Y, Thomas AS, Chan D, Mueller S, Ward AR, et al. Latent HIV reservoirs exhibit inherent resistance to elimination by CD8+ T cells. *J Clin Invest.* (2018) 128:876–89. doi: 10.1172/JCI97555

Kuo HH, Ahmad R, Lee GQ, Gao C, Chen HR, Ouyang Z, et al. Anti-apoptotic Protein BIRC5 Maintains Survival of HIV- 1-Infected CD4(+) T Cells. *Immunity.* (2018) 48:1183–94.e1185. doi:10.1016/j.immuni.2018.04.004

Pollack RA, Jones RB, Pertea M, Bruner KM, Martin AR, Thomas AS, et al. Defective HIV-1 proviruses are expressed and can be recognized by cytotoxic T lymphocytes, which shape the proviral landscape. *Cell Host Microbe.* (2017) 21:494–506.e494. doi: 10.1016/j.chom.2017.03.008

Shan L, Deng K, Shroff NS, Durand CM, Rabi SA, Yang HC, et al. Stimulation of HIV-1-specific cytolytic T lymphocytes facilitates elimination of latent viral reservoir after virus reactivation. *Immunity.* (2012) 36:491– 501. doi: 10.1016/j.immuni.2012.01.014

Trautmann L, Janbazian L, Chomont N, Said EA, Gimmig S, Bessette B, et al. Upregulation of PD-1 expression on HIV-specific CD8+ T cells leads to reversible immune dysfunction. *Nat Med.* (2006) 12:1198–202. doi: 10.1038/nm1482

Hopkins PA, Sriskandan S. Mammalian Toll-like receptors: to immunity and beyond. *Clin Exp Immunol.* (2005) 140:395–407. doi:10.1111/j.1365-2249.2005.02801.x

Janeway CA Jr, Medzhitov R. Innate immune recognition. *Annu Rev Immunol.* (2002) 20:197–216. doi: 10.1146/annurev.immunol. 20.083001.084359

Borducchi EN, Cabral C, Stephenson KE, Liu J, Abbink P, Ng'ang'a D, et al. Ad26/MVA therapeutic vaccination with TLR7 stimulation in SIV-infected rhesus monkeys. *Nature.* (2016) 540:284–7. doi: 10.1038/nature20583

Borducchi EN, Liu J, Nkolola JP, Cadena AM, Yu WH, Fischinger S, et al. Antibody and TLR7 agonist delay viral rebound in SHIV-infected monkeys. *Nature.* (2018) 563:360–4. doi: 10.1038/s41586-018-0600-6

Lim SY, Osuna CE, Hraber PT, Hesselgesser J, Gerold JM, Barnes TL, et al. TLR7 agonists induce transient viremia and reduce the viral reservoir in SIV-infected rhesus macaques on antiretroviral therapy. *Sci Transl Med.* (2018) 10:aao4521. doi: 10.1126/scitranslmed.aao4521

Macedo AB, Novis CL, De Assis CM, Sorensen ES, Moszczynski P, Huang SH, et al. Dual TLR2 and TLR7 agonists as HIV latency-reversing agents. *JCI Insight.* (2018) 3:e122673. doi: 10.1172/jci.insight.122673

Vibholm L, Schleimann MH, Hojen JF, Benfield T, Offersen R, Rasmussen K, et al. Short-course toll-like receptor 9 agonist treatment impacts innate immunity and plasma viremia in individuals with human immunodeficiency virus infection. *Clin Infect Dis.* (2017) 64:1686–95. doi: 10.1093/cid/cix201

Vibholm LK, Konrad CV, Schleimann MH, Frattari G, Winckelmann A, Klastrup V, et al. Effects of 24 Week toll-like receptor 9 agonist treatment in HIV-1+ individuals: a single-arm, phase 1B/2A trial. *AIDS.* (2019) 33:1315– 25. doi: 10.1097/QAD.0000000000002213

Coley WB. II. Contribution to the Knowledge of Sarcoma. *Ann Surg.* (1891) 14:199–220. doi: 10.1097/00000658-189112000-00015

Vacchelli E, Eggermont A, Sautes-Fridman C, Galon J, Zitvogel L, Kroemer G, et al. Trial Watch: toll-like receptor agonists for cancer therapy. *Oncoimmunology.* (2013) 2:e25238. doi: 10.4161/onci.25238

Horscroft NJ, Pryde DC, Bright H. Antiviral applications of Toll- like receptor agonists. *J Antimicrob Chemother.* (2012) 67:789–801. doi: 10.1093/jac/dkr588

Hancock RE, Nijnik A, Philpott DJ. Modulating immunity as a therapy for bacterial infections. *Nat Rev Microbiol.* (2012) 10:243–54. doi: 10.1038/nrmicro2745

Galluzzi L, Vacchelli E, Eggermont A, Fridman WH, Galon J, Sautes-Fridman C, et al. Trial Watch: experimental Toll-like receptor agonists for cancer therapy. *Oncoimmunology.* (2012) 1:699–716. doi: 10.4161/onci.20696

Savva A, Roger T. Targeting toll-like receptors: promising therapeutic strategies for the management of sepsis-associated pathology and infectious diseases. *Front Immunol.* (2013) 4:387. doi: 10.3389/fimmu.2013.00387

Vacchelli E, Galluzzi L, Eggermont A, Fridman WH, Galon J, Sautes-Fridman C, et al. Trial watch: FDA-approved Toll-like receptor agonists for cancer therapy. *Oncoimmunology.* (2012) 1:894–907. doi: 10.4161/onci.20931

Kawai T, Akira S. The role of pattern-recognition receptors in innate immunity: update on Toll-like receptors. *Nat Immunol.* (2010) 11:373–84. doi: 10.1038/ni.1863

Kumar H, Kawai T, Akira S. Pathogen recognition by the innate immune system. *Int Rev Immunol.* (2011) 30:16–34. doi: 10.3109/08830 185.2010.529976

Schnare M, Holt AC, Takeda K, Akira S, Medzhitov R. Recognition of CpG DNA is mediated by signaling pathways dependent on the adaptor protein MyD88. *Curr Biol.* (2000) 10:1139–42. doi: 10.1016/S0960-9822(00)00700-4

Bianchi ME. DAMPs, PAMPs and alarmins: all we need to know about danger. *J Leukoc Biol.* (2007) 81:1–5. doi: 10.1189/jlb.0306164

Venereau E, Ceriotti C, Bianchi ME. DAMPs from cell death to new life. *Front Immunol.* (2015) 6:422. doi: 10.3389/fimmu.2015.00422

Akira S, Uematsu S, Takeuchi O. Pathogen recognition and innate immunity. *Cell.* (2006) 124:783–801. doi: 10.1016/j.cell.2006.02.015

Akira S, Takeda K. Toll-like receptor signalling. *Nat Rev.* (2004) 4:499–511. doi: 10.1038/nri1391

Ozinsky A, Underhill DM, Fontenot JD, Hajjar AM, Smith KD, Wilson CB, et al. The repertoire for pattern recognition of pathogens by the innate immune system is defined by cooperation between toll-like receptors. *Proc Natl Acad Sci USA.* (2000) 97:13766–71. doi: 10.1073/pnas.250476497

Kang JY, Nan X, Jin MS, Youn SJ, Ryu YH, Mah S, et al. Recognition of lipopeptide patterns by Toll-like receptor 2-Toll-like receptor 6 heterodimer. *Immunity.* (2009) 31:873–84. doi: 10.1016/j.immuni.2009.09.018

Takeuchi O, Kawai T, Muhlradt PF, Morr M, Radolf JD, Zychlinsky A, et al. Discrimination of bacterial lipoproteins by Toll-like receptor 6. *Int Immunol.* (2001) 13:933–40. doi: 10.1093/intimm/13.7.933

Jin MS, Kim SE, Heo JY, Lee ME, Kim HM, Paik SG, et al. Crystal structure of the TLR1-TLR2 heterodimer induced by binding of a tri-acylated lipopeptide. *Cell.* (2007) 130:1071–82. doi: 10.1016/j.cell.2007.09.008

Means TK, Lien E, Yoshimura A, Wang S, Golenbock DT, Fenton MJ. The CD14 ligands lipoarabinomannan and lipopolysaccharide differ in their requirement for Toll-like receptors. *J Immunol.* (1999) 163:6748–55.

Round JL, Lee SM, Li J, Tran G, Jabri B, Chatila TA, et al. The Toll- like receptor 2 pathway establishes colonization by a commensal of the human microbiota. *Science.* (2011) 332:974–7. doi: 10.1126/science. 1206095

Gantner BN, Simmons RM, Canavera SJ, Akira S, Underhill DM. Collaborative induction of inflammatory responses by dectin-1 and Toll-like receptor 2. *J Exp Med.* (2003) 197:1107–17. doi: 10.1084/jem.20021787

Poltorak A, He X, Smirnova I, Liu MY, Van Huffel C, Du X, et al. Defective LPS signaling in C3H/HeJ and C57BL/10ScCr mice: mutations in Tlr4 gene. *Science.* (1998) 282:2085–8. doi: 10.1126/science.282.5396.2085

Chow JC, Young DW, Golenbock DT, Christ WJ, Gusovsky F. Toll-like receptor-4 mediates lipopolysaccharide-induced signal transduction. *J Biol Chem.* (1999) 274:10689–92. doi: 10.1074/jbc.274.16. 10689

Shimazu R, Akashi S, Ogata H, Nagai Y, Fukudome K, Miyake K, et al. MD-2, a molecule that confers lipopolysaccharide responsiveness on Toll- like receptor 4. *J Exp Med.* (1999) 189:1777–82. doi: 10.1084/jem.189. 11.1777

Hayashi F, Smith KD, Ozinsky A, Hawn TR, Yi EC, Goodlett DR, et al. The innate immune response to bacterial flagellin is mediated by Toll-like receptor 5. *Nature.* (2001) 410:1099–103. doi: 10.1038/35074106

Chuang T, Ulevitch RJ. Identification of hTLR10: a novel human Toll-like receptor preferentially expressed in immune cells. *Biochim Biophys Acta.* (2001) 1518:157–61. doi: 10.1016/S0167-4781(00)00289-X

Guan Y, Ranoa DR, Jiang S, Mutha SK, Li X, Baudry J, et al. Human TLRs 10 and 1 share common mechanisms of innate immune sensing but not signaling. *J Immunol.* (2010) 184:5094–103. doi: 10.4049/jimmunol.0901888

Oosting M, Cheng SC, Bolscher JM, Vestering-Stenger R, Plantinga TS, Verschueren IC, et al. Human TLR10 is an anti-inflammatory pattern-recognition receptor. *Proc Natl Acad Sci USA.* (2014) 111:E4478–84. doi: 10.1073/pnas.1410293111

Henrick BM, Yao XD, Zahoor MA, Abimiku A, Osawe S, Rosenthal KL. TLR10 senses HIV-1 proteins and significantly enhances HIV-1 infection. *Front Immunol.* (2019) 10:482. doi: 10.3389/fimmu.2019.00482

Akira S, Takeda K, Kaisho T. Toll-like receptors: critical proteins linking innate and acquired immunity. *Nat Immunol.* (2001) 2:675–80. doi: 10.1038/90609

Alexopoulou L, Holt AC, Medzhitov R, Flavell RA. Recognition of double-stranded RNA and activation of NF-kappaB by Toll-like receptor 3. *Nature.* (2001) 413:732–8. doi: 10.1038/35099560

Heil F, Hemmi H, Hochrein H, Ampenberger F, Kirschning C, Akira S, et al. Species-specific recognition of single-stranded RNA via toll-like receptor 7 and 8. *Science.* (2004) 303:1526–9. doi: 10.1126/science.1093620

Hemmi H, Takeuchi O, Kawai T, Kaisho T, Sato S, Sanjo H, et al. A Toll-like receptor recognizes bacterial DNA. *Nature.* (2000) 408:740–5. doi: 10.1038/35047123

Ho NI, Huis In 't Veld LGM, Raaijmakers TK, Adema GJ. Adjuvants enhancing cross-presentation by dendritic cells: the key to more effective vaccines? *Front Immunol.* (2018) 9:2874. doi: 10.3389/fimmu.2018.02874

Smith M, Garcia-Martinez E, Pitter MR, Fucikova J, Spisek R, Zitvogel L, et al. Trial Watch: toll-like receptor agonists in cancer immunotherapy. *Oncoimmunology.* (2018) 7:e1526250. doi: 10.1080/2162402X.2018.1526250

Buwitt-Beckmann U, Heine H, Wiesmuller KH, Jung G, Brock R, Akira S, et al. Toll-like receptor 6-independent signaling by diacylated lipopeptides. *Eur J Immunol.* (2005) 35:282–9. doi: 10.1002/eji.200424955

Redecke V, Hacker H, Datta SK, Fermin A, Pitha PM, Broide DH, et al. Cutting edge: activation of Toll-like receptor 2 induces a Th2 immune response and promotes experimental asthma. *J Immunol.* (2004) 172:2739– 43. doi: 10.4049/jimmunol.172.5.2739

Agnihotri G, Crall BM, Lewis TC, Day TP, Balakrishna R, Warshakoon HJ, et al. Structure-activity relationships in toll-like receptor 2-agonists leading to simplified monoacyl lipopeptides. *J Med Chem.* (2011) 54:8148–60. doi: 10.1021/jm201071e

Guan Y, Omueti-Ayoade K, Mutha SK, Hergenrother PJ, Tapping RI. Identification of novel synthetic toll-like receptor 2 agonists by high throughput screening. *J Biol Chem.* (2010) 285:23755–62. doi: 10.1074/jbc.M110.116046

Cheng K, Gao M, Godfroy JI, Brown PN, Kastelowitz N, Yin H. Specific activation of the TLR1-TLR2 heterodimer by small-molecule agonists. *Sci Adv.* (2015) 1:e1400139. doi: 10.1126/sciadv.1400139

Chen Z, Cen X, Yang J, Tang X, Cui K, Cheng K. Structure-based discovery of a specific TLR1-TLR2 small molecule agonist from the ZINC drug library database. *Chem Commun.* (2018) 54:11411–4. doi: 10.1039/C8CC06618C

Cen X, Zhu G, Yang J, Yang J, Guo J, Jin J, et al. TLR1/2 specific small-molecule agonist suppresses leukemia cancer cell growth by stimulating cytotoxic T lymphocytes. *Adv Sci.* (2019) 6:1802042. doi: 10.1002/advs.201802042

Morin MD, Wang Y, Jones BT, Mifune Y, Su L, Shi H, et al. Diprovocims: a new and exceptionally potent class of toll-like receptor agonists. *J Am Chem Soc.* (2018) 140:14440–54. doi: 10.1021/jacs.8b09223

Lepe-Zuniga JL, Rotbein J, Gutterman JU. Production of interferon- alpha induced by dsRNA in human peripheral blood mononuclear cell cultures: role of priming by dsRNA-induced interferons-gamma and -beta. *J Interferon Res.* (1989) 9:445–56. doi: 10.1089/jir.1989.9.445

Wang L, Smith D, Bot S, Dellamary L, Bloom A, Bot A. Noncoding RNA danger motifs bridge innate and adaptive immunity and are potent adjuvants for vaccination. *J Clin Invest.* (2002) 110:1175–84. doi: 10.1172/JCI0215536

Zhu X, Nishimura F, Sasaki K, Fujita M, Dusak JE, Eguchi J, et al. Toll like receptor-3 ligand poly-ICLC promotes the efficacy of peripheral vaccinations with tumor antigen-derived peptide epitopes in murine CNS tumor models. *J Transl Med.* (2007) 5:10. doi: 10.1186/1479-5876-5-10

Ulrich JT, Myers KR. Monophosphoryl lipid A as an adjuvant. Past experiences and new directions. *Pharm Biotechnol.* (1995) 6:495–524. doi: 10.1007/978-1-4615-1823-5_21

Johnson DA, Sowell CG, Johnson CL, Livesay MT, Keegan DS, Rhodes MJ, et al. Synthesis and biological evaluation of a new class of vaccine adjuvants: aminoalkyl glucosaminide 4-phosphates (AGPs). *Bioorg Med Chem Lett.* (1999) 9:2273–8. doi: 10.1016/S0960-894X(99)00374-1

Thompson BS, Chilton PM, Ward JR, Evans JT, Mitchell TC. The low- toxicity versions of LPS, MPL adjuvant and RC529, are efficient adjuvants for CD4+ T cells. *J Leukoc Biol.* (2005) 78:1273–80. doi: 10.1189/jlb.0305172

Toussi DN, Massari P. Immune adjuvant effect of molecularly- defined toll-like receptor ligands. *Vaccines.* (2014) 2:323–53. doi: 10.3390/vaccines2020323

Zaffaroni L, Peri F. Recent advances on Toll-like receptor 4 modulation: new therapeutic perspectives. *Future Med Chem.* (2018) 10:461–76. doi: 10.4155/fmc-2017-0172

Burdelya LG, Krivokrysenko VI, Tallant TC, Strom E, Gleiberman AS, Gupta D, et al. An agonist of toll-like receptor 5 has radioprotective activity in mouse and primate models. *Science.* (2008) 320:226–30. doi: 10.1126/science.1154986

Fukuzawa N, Petro M, Baldwin WM III, Gudkov AV, Fairchild RL. A TLR5 agonist inhibits acute renal ischemic failure. *J Immunol.* (2011) 187:3831–9. doi: 10.4049/jimmunol.1003238

Mizel SB, Bates JT. Flagellin as an adjuvant: cellular mechanisms and potential. *J Immunol.* (2010) 185:5677–82. doi: 10.4049/jimmunol.1002156

Yoon SI, Kurnasov O, Natarajan V, Hong M, Gudkov AV, Osterman AL, et al. Structural basis of TLR5-flagellin recognition and signaling. *Science.* (2012) 335:859–64. doi: 10.1126/science.1215584

Lee J, Chuang TH, Redecke V, She L, Pitha PM, Carson DA, et al. Molecular basis for the immunostimulatory activity of guanine nucleoside analogs: activation of Toll-like receptor 7. *Proc Natl Acad Sci USA.* (2003) 100:6646– 51. doi: 10.1073/pnas.0631696100

Gorden KB, Gorski KS, Gibson SJ, Kedl RM, Kieper WC, Qiu X, et al. Synthetic TLR agonists reveal functional differences between human TLR7 and TLR8. *J Immunol.* (2005) 174:1259–68. doi: 10.4049/jimmunol.174.3.1259

Kalali BN, Kollisch G, Mages J, Muller T, Bauer S, Wagner H, et al. Double-stranded RNA induces an antiviral defense status in epidermal keratinocytes through TLR3-, PKR-, and MDA5/RIG-I-mediated differential signaling. *J Immunol.* (2008) 181:2694–704. doi: 10.4049/jimmunol. 181.4.2694

Ahonen CL, Gibson SJ, Smith RM, Pederson LK, Lindh JM, Tomai MA, et al. Dendritic cell maturation and subsequent enhanced T-cell stimulation induced with the novel synthetic immune response modifier R-848. *Cell Immunol.* (1999) 197:62–72. doi: 10.1006/cimm.1999.1555

Petricevic B, Wessner B, Sachet M, Vrbanec D, Spittler A, Bergmann M. CL097, a TLR7/8 ligand, inhibits TLR-4–dependent activation of IRAK-M and BCL-3 expression. *Shock.* (2009) 32:484–90. doi:10.1097/SHK.0b013e3181a5ac8a

Spranger S, Javorovic M, Burdek M, Wilde S, Mosetter B, Tippmer S, et al. Generation of Th1-polarizing dendritic cells using the TLR7/8 agonist CL075. *J Immunol.* (2010) 185:738–47. doi: 10.4049/jimmunol.1000060

Pope BL, Chourmouzis E, Sigindere J, Capetola RJ, Lau CY. *In vivo* enhancement of murine natural killer cell activity by 7-allyl-8- oxoguanosine (loxoribine). *Int J Immunopharmacol.* (1992) 14:1375–82. doi:10.1016/0192-0561(92)90008-9

Bergmann JF, de Bruijne J, Hotho DM, de Knegt RJ, Boonstra A, Weegink CJ, et al. Randomised clinical trial: anti-viral activity of ANA773, an oral inducer of endogenous interferons acting via TLR7, in chronic HCV. *Aliment Pharmacol Ther.* (2011) 34:443–53. doi: 10.1111/j.1365-2036.2011.04745.x

Xiang AX, Webber SE, Kerr BM, Rueden EJ, Lennox JR, Haley GJ, et al. Discovery of ANA975: an oral prodrug of the TLR-7 agonist isatoribine. *Nucleosides Nucleotides Nucleic Acids.* (2007) 26:635–40. doi:10.1080/15257770701490472

Hayashi T, Gray CS, Chan M, Tawatao RI, Ronacher L, McGargill MA, et al. Prevention of autoimmune disease by induction of tolerance to Toll-like receptor 7. *Proc Natl Acad Sci USA.* (2009) 106:2764–9. doi: 10.1073/pnas.0813037106

Hilbert T, Steinhagen F, Weisheit C, Baumgarten G, Hoeft A, Klaschik S. Synergistic stimulation with different TLR7 ligands modulates gene expression patterns in the human plasmacytoid dendritic cell line CAL-1. *Mediators Inflamm.* (2015) 2015:948540. doi: 10.1155/2015/948540

Rebbapragada I, Birkus G, Perry J, Xing W, Kwon H, Pflanz S. Molecular determinants of GS-9620-dependent TLR7 activation. *PLoS ONE.* (2016) 11:e0146835. doi: 10.1371/journal.pone.0146835

Liu Y, Luo X, Yang C, Yu S, Xu H. Three CpG oligodeoxynucleotide classes differentially enhance antigen-specific humoral and cellular immune responses in mice. *Vaccine.* (2011) 29:5778–84. doi:10.1016/j.vaccine.2011.05.087

Vollmer J, Weeratna R, Payette P, Jurk M, Schetter C, Laucht M, et al. Characterization of three CpG oligodeoxynucleotide classes with distinct immunostimulatory activities. *Eur J Immunol.* (2004) 34:251–62. doi:10.1002/eji.200324032

Agrawal S, Kandimalla ER. Synthetic agonists of Toll-like receptors 7, 8 and 9. *Biochem Soc Trans.* (2007) 35:1461–7. doi: 10.1042/BST0351461

Paul S. Technology evaluation: CpG-7909, Coley. *Curr Opin Mol Ther.* (2003) 5:553–9.

Vicari AP, Schmalbach T, Lekstrom-Himes J, Morris ML, Al-Adhami MJ, Laframboise C, et al. Safety, pharmacokinetics and immune effects in normal volunteers of CPG 10101 (ACTILON), an investigational synthetic toll-like receptor 9 agonist. *Antivir Ther.* (2007) 12:741–51.

Wang S, Campos J, Gallotta M, Gong M, Crain C, Naik E, et al. Intratumoral injection of a CpG oligonucleotide reverts resistance to PD-1 blockade by expanding multifunctional CD8+ T cells. *Proc Natl Acad Sc USA.* (2016) 113:E7240–9. doi: 10.1073/pnas.1608555113

Wittig B, Schmidt M, Scheithauer W, Schmoll HJ. MGN1703, an immunomodulator and toll-like receptor 9 (TLR-9) agonist: from bench to bedside. *Crit Rev Oncol Hematol.* (2015) 94:31–44. doi:10.1016/j.critrevonc.2014.12.002

Gutjahr A, Papagno L, Nicoli F, Lamoureux A, Vernejoul F, Lioux T, et al. Cutting edge: a Dual TLR2 and TLR7 ligand induces highly potent humoral and cell-mediated immune responses. *J Immunol.* (2017) 198:4205– 9. doi: 10.4049/jimmunol.1602131

Yamamoto M, Takeda K, Akira S. TIR domain-containing adaptors define the specificity of TLR signaling. *Mol Immunol.* (2004) 40:861–8. doi:10.1016/j.molimm.2003.10.006

Verstak B, Nagpal K, Bottomley SP, Golenbock DT, Hertzog PJ, Mansell MyD88 adapter-like (Mal)/TIRAP interaction with TRAF6 is critical for TLR2- and TLR4-mediated NF-kappaB proinflammatory responses. *J Biol Chem.* (2009) 284:24192–203. doi: 10.1074/jbc.M109.023044

Yamamoto M, Sato S, Hemmi H, Sanjo H, Uematsu S, Kaisho T, et al. Essential role for TIRAP in activation of the signalling cascade shared by TLR2 and TLR4. *Nature.* (2002) 420:324–9. doi: 10.1038/nature01182

Kawasaki T, Kawai T. Toll-like receptor signaling pathways. *Front Immunol.* (2014) 5:461. doi: 10.3389/fimmu.2014.00461

Ning S, Pagano JS, Barber GN. IRF7: activation, regulation, modification and function. *Genes Immun.* (2011) 12:399–414. doi: 10.1038/gene.2011.21

Yamamoto M, Sato S, Hemmi H, Hoshino K, Kaisho T, Sanjo H, et al. Role of adaptor TRIF in the MyD88-independent toll-like receptor signaling pathway. *Science.* (2003) 301:640–3. doi: 10.1126/science.1087262

Kagan JC, Su T, Horng T, Chow A, Akira S, Medzhitov R. TRAM couples endocytosis of Toll-like receptor 4 to the induction of interferon-beta. *Nat Immunol.* (2008) 9:361–8. doi: 10.1038/ni1569

Yamamoto M, Sato S, Hemmi H, Uematsu S, Hoshino K, Kaisho T, et al. TRAM is specifically involved in the Toll-like receptor 4-mediated MyD88-independent signaling pathway. *Nat Immunol.* (2003) 4:1144–50. doi: 10.1038/ni986

Hacker H, Redecke V, Blagoev B, Kratchmarova I, Hsu LC, Wang GG, et al. Specificity in Toll-like receptor signalling through distinct effector functions of TRAF3 and TRAF6. *Nature.* (2006) 439:204–7. doi: 10.1038/nature04369

Xie P. TRAF molecules in cell signaling and in human diseases. *J Mol Signal.* (2013) 8:7. doi: 10.1186/1750-2187-8-7

Bentwich Z, Maartens G, Torten D, Lal AA, Lal RB. Concurrent infections and HIV pathogenesis. *AIDS.* (2000) 14:2071–81. doi: 10.1097/00002030-200009290-00002

Brichacek B, Swindells S, Janoff EN, Pirruccello S, Stevenson M. Increased plasma human immunodeficiency virus type 1 burden following antigenic challenge with pneumococcal vaccine. *J Infect Dis.* (1996) 174:1191–9. doi: 10.1093/infdis/174.6.1191

Donovan RM, Bush CE, Markowitz NP, Baxa DM, Saravolatz LD. Changes in virus load markers during AIDS-associated opportunistic diseases in human immunodeficiency virus-infected persons. *J Infect Dis.* (1996) 174:401–3. doi: 10.1093/infdis/174.2.401

Goletti D, Weissman D, Jackson RW, Graham NM, Vlahov D, Klein RS, et al. Effect of Mycobacterium tuberculosis on HIV replication. Role of immune activation. *J Immunol.* (1996) 157:1271–8.

Mole L, Ripich S, Margolis D, Holodniy M. The impact of active herpes simplex virus infection on human immunodeficiency virus load. *J Infect Dis.* (1997) 176:766–70. doi: 10.1086/517297

O'Brien WA, Grovit-Ferbas K, Namazi A, Ovcak-Derzic S, Wang HJ, Park J, et al. Human immunodeficiency virus-type 1 replication can be increased in peripheral blood of seropositive patients after influenza vaccination. *Blood.* (1995) 86:1082–9.

Stanley SK, Ostrowski MA, Justement JS, Gantt K, Hedayati S, Mannix M, et al. Effect of immunization with a common recall antigen on viral expression in patients infected with human immunodeficiency virus type 1. *N Engl J Med.* (1996) 334:1222–30. doi: 10.1056/NEJM199605093341903

Staprans SI, Hamilton BL, Follansbee SE, Elbeik T, Barbosa P, Grant RM, et al. Activation of virus replication after vaccination of HIV-1-infected individuals. *J Exp Med.* (1995) 182:1727–37. doi: 10.1084/jem.182.6.1727

Sulkowski MS, Chaisson RE, Karp CL, Moore RD, Margolick JB, Quinn TC. The effect of acute infectious illnesses on plasma human immunodeficiency virus (HIV) type 1 load and the expression of serologic markers of immune activation among HIV-infected adults. *J Infect Dis.* (1998) 178:1642–8. doi:10.1086/314491

Toossi Z, Xia L, Wu M, Salvekar A. Transcriptional activation of HIV by Mycobacterium tuberculosis in human monocytes. *Clin Exp Immunol.* (1999) 117:324–30. doi: 10.1046/j.1365-2249.1999.00952.x

Zhang Y, Nakata K, Weiden M, Rom WN. Mycobacterium tuberculosis enhances human immunodeficiency virus-1 replication by transcriptional activation at the long terminal repeat. *J Clin Invest.* (1995) 95:2324–31. doi: 10.1172/JCI117924

Bernier R, Barbeau B, Olivier M, Tremblay MJ. Mycobacterium tuberculosis mannose-capped lipoarabinomannan can induce NF-kappaB-dependent activation of human immunodeficiency virus type 1 long terminal repeat in T cells. *J Gen Virol.* (1998) 79:1353–61. doi: 10.1099/0022-1317-79-6-1353

Lederman MM, Georges DL, Kusner DJ, Mudido P, Giam CZ, Toossi Z.

Mycobacterium tuberculosis and its purified protein derivative activate expression of the human immunodeficiency virus. *J Acquir Immune Defic Syndr.* (1994) 7:727–33.

Equils O, Faure E, Thomas L, Bulut Y, Trushin S, Arditi M. Bacterial lipopolysaccharide activates HIV long terminal repeat through Toll-like receptor 4. *J Immunol.* (2001) 166:2342–7. doi: 10.4049/jimmunol.166.4.2342

Gonzalez OA, Li M, Ebersole JL, Huang CB. HIV-1 reactivation induced by the periodontal pathogens *Fusobacterium nucleatum* and *Porphyromonas gingivalis* involves Toll-like receptor 2 [corrected] and 9 activation in monocytes/macrophages. *Clin Vaccine Immunol.* (2010) 17:1417–27. doi: 10.1128/CVI.00009-10

Nordone SK, Ignacio GA, Su L, Sempowski GD, Golenbock DT, Li L, et al. Failure of TLR4-driven NF-kappa B activation to stimulate virus replication in models of HIV type 1 activation. *AIDS Res Hum Retroviruses.* (2007) 23:1387–95. doi: 10.1089/aid.2007.0033

Novis CL, Archin NM, Buzon MJ, Verdin E, Round JL, Lichterfeld M, et al. Reactivation of latent HIV-1 in central memory CD4(+) T cells through TLR-1/2 stimulation. *Retrovirology.* (2013) 10:119. doi:10.1186/1742-4690-10-119

Ganor Y, Real F, Sennepin A, Dutertre CA, Prevedel L, Xu L, et al. HIV-1 reservoirs in urethral macrophages of patients under suppressive antiretroviral therapy. *Nat Microbiol.* (2019) 4:633–44. doi:10.1038/s41564-018-0335-z

Scheller C, Ullrich A, Lamla S, Dittmer U, Rethwilm A, Koutsilieri E. Dual activity of phosphorothioate CpG oligodeoxynucleotides on HIV: reactivation of latent provirus and inhibition of productive infection in human T cells. *Ann N Y Acad Sci.* (2006) 1091:540–7. doi:10.1196/annals.1378.095

Scheller C, Ullrich A, McPherson K, Hefele B, Knoferle J, Lamla S, et al. CpG oligodeoxynucleotides activate HIV replication in latently infected human T cells. *J Biol Chem.* (2004) 279:21897–902. doi: 10.1074/jbc.M311609200

Offersen R, Nissen SK, Rasmussen TA, Ostergaard L, Denton PW, Sogaard OS, et al. A novel toll-like receptor 9 agonist, MGN1703, enhances HIV-1 transcription and NK cell-mediated inhibition of HIV-1-infected autologous CD4+ T cells. *J Virol.* (2016) 90:4441–53. doi: 10.1128/JVI.00222-16

Bhat KH, Chaitanya CK, Parveen N, Varman R, Ghosh S, Mukhopadhyay S. Proline-proline-glutamic acid (PPE) protein Rv1168c of Mycobacterium tuberculosis augments transcription from HIV-1 long terminal repeat promoter. *J Biol Chem.* (2012) 287:16930–46. doi: 10.1074/jbc.M111.327825

Macedo AB, Resop RS, Martins LJ, Szaniawski MA, Sorensen ES, Spivak AM, et al. Influence of biological sex, age and HIV status in an *in vitro* primary cell model of HIV latency using a CXCR4 tropic virus. *AIDS Res Hum Retroviruses.* (2018) 34:769–77. doi: 10.1089/aid.2018.0098

Larson EC, Novis CL, Martins LJ, Macedo AB, Kimball KE, Bosque A, et al. *Mycobacterium tuberculosis* reactivates latent HIV-1 in T cells *in vitro*. *PLoS ONE.* (2017) 12:e0185162. doi: 10.1371/journal.pone.0185162

Schlaepfer E, Audige A, Joller H, Speck RF. TLR7/8 triggering exerts opposing effects in acute versus latent HIV infection. *J Immunol.* (2006) 176:2888–95. doi: 10.4049/jimmunol.176.5.2888

Rochat MA, Schlaepfer E, Speck RF. Promising role of toll-like receptor 8 agonist in concert with prostratin for activation of silent HIV. *J Virol.* (2017) 91:e02084-16. doi: 10.1128/JVI.02084-16

Jordan A, Bisgrove D, Verdin E. HIV reproducibly establishes a latent infection after acute infection of T cells *in vitro*. *EMBO J.* (2003) 22:1868–77. doi:10.1093/emboj/cdg188

Thibault S, Imbeault M, Tardif MR, Tremblay MJ. TLR5 stimulation is sufficient to trigger reactivation of latent HIV-1 provirus in T lymphoid cells and activate virus gene expression in central memory CD4+ T cells. *Virology.* (2009) 389:20–5. doi: 10.1016/j.virol.2009.04.019

Bhargavan B, Woollard SM, Kanmogne GD. Toll-like receptor-3 mediates HIV-1 transactivation via NFkappaB and JNK pathways and histone acetylation, but prolonged activation suppresses Tat and HIV-1 replication. *Cell Signal.* (2016) 28:7–22. doi: 10.1016/j.cellsig.2015.11.005

Tsai A, Irrinki A, Kaur J, Cihlar T, Kukolj G, Sloan DD, et al. Toll-like receptor 7 agonist GS-9620 induces HIV expression and HIV-specific immunity in cells from HIV-infected individuals on suppressive antiretroviral therapy. *J Virol.* (2017) 91:e02166-16. doi: 10.1128/JVI.02166-16

Alvarez-Carbonell D, Garcia-Mesa Y, Milne S, Das B, Dobrowolski C, Rojas R, et al. Toll-like receptor 3 activation selectively reverses HIV latency in microglial cells. *Retrovirology.* (2017) 14:9. doi: 10.1186/s12977-017-0335-8

Sundstrom JB, Little DM, Villinger F, Ellis JE, Ansari AA. Signaling through Toll-like receptors triggers HIV-1 replication in latently infected mast cells. *J Immunol.* (2004) 172:4391–401. doi: 10.4049/jimmunol.172.7.4391

Leonard JM, Abramczuk JW, Pezen DS, Rutledge R, Belcher JH, Hakim F, et al. Development of disease and virus recovery in transgenic mice containing HIV proviral DNA. *Science.* (1988) 242:1665–70. doi: 10.1126/science.3201255

Doherty TM, Chougnet C, Schito M, Patterson BK, Fox C, Shearer GM, et al. Infection of HIV-1 transgenic mice with Mycobacterium avium induces the expression of infectious virus selectively from a Mac-1-positive host cell population. *J Immunol.* (1999) 163:1506–15.

Gazzinelli RT, Sher A, Cheever A, Gerstberger S, Martin MA, Dickie P. Infection of human immunodeficiency virus 1 transgenic mice with *Toxoplasma gondii* stimulates proviral transcription in macrophages *in vivo*. *J Exp Med.* (1996) 183:1645–55. doi: 10.1084/jem.183.4.1645

Equils O, Schito ML, Karahashi H, Madak Z, Yarali A, Michelsen KS, et al. Toll-like receptor 2 (TLR2) and TLR9 signaling results in HIV-long terminal repeat trans-activation and HIV replication in HIV-1 transgenic mouse spleen cells: implications of simultaneous activation of TLRs on HIV replication. *J Immunol.* (2003) 170:5159–64. doi:10.4049/jimmunol.170.10.5159

Bafica A, Scanga CA, Schito ML, Hieny S, Sher A. Cutting edge: *in vivo* induction of integrated HIV-1 expression by mycobacteria is critically dependent on Toll-like receptor 2. *J Immunol.* (2003) 171:1123–7. doi:10.4049/jimmunol.171.3.1123

Cheng L, Wang Q, Li G, Banga R, Ma J, Yu H, et al. TLR3 agonist and CD40-targeting vaccination induces immune responses and reduces HIV-1 reservoirs. *J Clin Invest.* (2018) 128:4387–96. doi: 10.1172/JCI99005

Saxena M, Sabado RL, La Mar M, Mohri H, Salazar AM, Dong H, et al. Poly-ICLC, a TLR3 agonist, induces transient innate immune responses in patients with treated HIV-infection: a randomized double-blinded placebo controlled trial. *Front Immunol.* (2019) 10:725. doi: 10.3389/fimmu.2019.00725

Del Prete GQ, Alvord WG, Li Y, Deleage C, Nag M, Oswald K, et al. TLR7 agonist administration to SIV-infected macaques receiving early initiated cART does not induce plasma viremia. *JCI Insight.* (2019) 4:127717. doi: 10.1172/jci.insight.127717

Winckelmann AA, Munk-Petersen LV, Rasmussen TA, Melchjorsen J, Hjelholt TJ, Montefiori D, et al. Administration of a Toll-like receptor 9 agonist decreases the proviral reservoir in virologically suppressed HIV-infected patients. *PLoS ONE.* (2013) 8:e62074. doi:10.1371/journal.pone.0062074

Lanford RE, Guerra B, Chavez D, Giavedoni L, Hodara VL, Brasky KM, et al. GS-9620, an oral agonist of Toll-like receptor-7, induces prolonged suppression of hepatitis B virus in chronically infected chimpanzees. *Gastroenterology.* (2013) 144:1508–17, 1517.e1501–10. doi:10.1053/j.gastro.2013.02.003

Lopatin U, Wolfgang G, Tumas D, Frey CR, Ohmstede C, Hesselgesser J, et al. Safety, pharmacokinetics and pharmacodynamics of GS-9620, an oral Toll-like receptor 7 agonist. *Antivir Ther.* (2013) 18:409–18. doi: 10.3851/IMP2548

Menne S, Tumas DB, Liu KH, Thampi L, AlDeghaither D, Baldwin BH, et al. Sustained efficacy and seroconversion with the Toll-like receptor 7 agonist GS-9620 in the Woodchuck model of chronic hepatitis B. *J Hepatol.* (2015) 62:1237–45. doi: 10.1016/j.jhep.2014.12.026

Sogaard OS, Schonheyder HC, Bukh AR, Harboe ZB, Rasmussen TA, Ostergaard L, et al. Pneumococcal conjugate vaccination in persons with HIV: the effect of highly active antiretroviral therapy. *AIDS.* (2010) 24:1315–22. doi: 10.1097/QAD.0b013e328339fe0b

Krarup AR, Abdel-Mohsen M, Schleimann MH, Vibholm L, Engen PA, Dige A, et al. The TLR9 agonist MGN1703 triggers a potent type I interferon response in the sigmoid colon. *Mucosal Immunol.* (2018) 11:449–61. doi: 10.1038/mi.2017.59

Jones RB, Mueller S, O'Connor R, Rimpel K, Sloan DD, Karel D, et al. A subset of latency-reversing agents expose HIV-infected resting CD4+ T-cells to recognition by cytotoxic T-lymphocytes. *PLoS Pathog.* (2016) 12:e1005545. doi: 10.1371/journal.ppat.1005545

Fujimoto C, Nakagawa Y, Ohara K, Takahashi H. Polyriboinosinic polyribocytidylic acid [poly(I:C)]/TLR3 signaling allows class I processing of exogenous protein and induction of HIV-specific CD8+ cytotoxic T lymphocytes. *Int Immunol.* (2004) 16:55–63. doi: 10.1093/intimm/dxh025

Bam RA, Hansen D, Irrinki A, Mulato A, Jones GS, Hesselgesser J, et al. TLR7 agonist GS-9620 is a potent inhibitor of acute HIV-1 infection in human peripheral blood mononuclear cells. *Antimicrob Agents Chemother.* (2017) 61:e01369-16. doi: 10.1128/AAC. 01369-16

Wille-Reece U, Wu CY, Flynn BJ, Kedl RM, Seder RA. Immunization with HIV-1 Gag protein conjugated to a TLR7/8 agonist results in the generation of HIV-1 Gag-specific Th1 and CD8+ T cell responses. *J Immunol.* (2005) 174:7676–83. doi: 10.4049/jimmunol.174.12.7676

Schlaepfer E, Speck RF. Anti-HIV activity mediated by natural killer and CD8+ cells after toll-like receptor 7/8 triggering. *PLoS ONE.* (2008) 3:e1999. doi: 10.1371/journal.pone.0001999

Tomescu C, Chehimi J, Maino VC, Montaner LJ. NK cell lysis of HIV-1- infected autologous CD4 primary T cells: requirement for IFN-mediated NK activation by plasmacytoid dendritic cells. *J Immunol.* (2007) 179:2097–104. doi: 10.4049/jimmunol.179.4.2097

Lore K, Betts MR, Brenchley JM, Kuruppu J, Khojasteh S, Perfetto S, et al. Toll-like receptor ligands modulate dendritic cells to augment cytomegalovirus- and HIV-1-specific T cell responses. *J Immunol.* (2003) 171:4320–8. doi: 10.4049/jimmunol.171.8.4320

Mukherjee S, Huda S, Sinha Babu SP. Toll-like receptor polymorphism in host immune response to infectious diseases: a review. *Scand J Immunol.* (2019) 90:e12771. doi: 10.1111/sji.12771

Skevaki C, Pararas M, Kostelidou K, Tsakris A, Routsias JG. Single nucleotide polymorphisms of Toll-like receptors and susceptibility to infectious diseases. *Clin Exp Immunol.* (2015) 180:165–77. doi: 10.1111/cei. 12578

Laffont S, Rouquie N, Azar P, Seillet C, Plumas J, Aspord C, et al. X- Chromosome complement and estrogen receptor signaling independently contribute to the enhanced TLR7-mediated IFN-alpha production of plasmacytoid dendritic cells from women. *J Immunol.* (2014) 193:5444–52. doi: 10.4049/jimmunol.1303400

Meier A, Chang JJ, Chan ES, Pollard RB, Sidhu HK, Kulkarni S, et al. Sex differences in the Toll-like receptor-mediated response of plasmacytoid dendritic cells to HIV-1. *Nat Med.* (2009) 15:955–9. doi: 10.1038/ nm.2004

Belmonte L, Olmos M, Fanin A, Parodi C, Bare P, Concetti H, et al. The intestinal mucosa as a reservoir of HIV-1 infection after successful HAART. *AIDS.* (2007) 21:2106–8. doi: 10.1097/QAD.0b013e3282efb74b

Lamers SL, Rose R, Maidji E, Agsalda-Garcia M, Nolan DJ, Fogel GB, et al. HIV DNA is frequently present within pathologic tissues evaluated at autopsy from combined antiretroviral therapy-treated patients with undetectable viral loads. *J Virol.* (2016) 90:8968–83. doi: 10.1128/JVI.00674-16

Licht A, Alter G. A Drug-Free Zone–Lymph Nodes as a Safe Haven for HIV. *Cell Host Microbe.* (2016) 19:275–6. doi: 10.1016/j.chom.2016.02.018

Rose R, Nolan DJ, Maidji E, Stoddart CA, Singer EJ, Lamers SL, et al. Eradication of HIV from tissue reservoirs: challenges for the cure. *AIDS Res Hum Retroviruses.* (2018) 34:3–8. doi: 10.1089/aid.2017.0072

Yukl SA, Shergill AK, Ho T, Killian M, Girling V, Epling L, et al. The distribution of HIV DNA and RNA in cell subsets differs in gut and blood of HIV-positive patients on ART: implications for viral persistence. *J Infect Dis.* (2013) 208:1212–20. doi: 10.1093/infdis/jit308

McNamara LA, Ganesh JA, Collins KL. Latent HIV-1 infection occurs in multiple subsets of hematopoietic progenitor cells and is reversed by NF-kappaB activation. *J Virol.* (2012) 86:9337–50. doi: 10.1128/JVI.00 895-12

Khoury G, Darcis G, Lee MY, Bouchat S, Van Driessche B, Purcell DFJ, et al. The molecular biology of HIV latency. *Adv Exp Med Biol.* (2018) 1075:187–212. doi: 10.1007/978-981-13-0484-2_8

11

Microglial Cells: The Main HIV-1 Reservoir in the Brain

Clementine Wallet[1], Marco De Rovere[1], Jeanne Van Assche[1], Fadoua Daouad[1], Stéphane De Wit[2], Virginie Gautier[3], Patrick W. G. Mallon[3], Alessandro Marcello[4], Carine Van Lint[5], Olivier Rohr[1] and Christian Schwartz[1*†]*

[1] Université de Strasbourg, EA7292, FMTS, IUT Louis Pasteur, Schiltigheim, France, [2] Division of Infectious Diseases, Saint-Pierre University Hospital, Université Libre de Bruxelles (ULB), Brussels, Belgium, [3] UCD Centre for Experimental Pathogen Host Research (CEPHR), School of Medicine, University College Dublin, Dublin, Ireland, [4] Laboratory of Molecular Virology, International Centre for Genetic Engineering and Biotechnology (ICGEB), Trieste, Italy, [5] Service of Molecular Virology, Department of Molecular Biology (DBM), Université Libre de Bruxelles (ULB), Gosselies, Belgium

***Correspondence:**
Olivier Rohr
olivier.rohr@unistra.fr
Christian Schwartz
schwartz.christian@unistra.fr

†Lead contact

Despite efficient combination of the antiretroviral therapy (cART), which significantly decreased mortality and morbidity of HIV-1 infection, a definitive HIV cure has not been achieved. Hidden HIV-1 in cellular and anatomic reservoirs is the major hurdle toward a functional cure. Microglial cells, the Central Nervous system (CNS) resident macrophages, are one of the major cellular reservoirs of latent HIV-1. These cells are believed to be involved in the emergence of drugs resistance and reseeding peripheral tissues. Moreover, these long-life reservoirs are also involved in the development of HIV-1-associated neurocognitive diseases (HAND). Clearing these infected cells from the brain is therefore crucial to achieve a cure. However, many characteristics of microglial cells and the CNS hinder the eradication of these brain reservoirs. Better understandings of the specific molecular mechanisms of HIV-1 latency in microglial cells should help to design new molecules and new strategies preventing HAND and achieving HIV cure. Moreover, new strategies are needed to circumvent the limitations associated to anatomical sanctuaries with barriers such as the blood brain barrier (BBB) that reduce the access of drugs.

Keywords: HIV-1, Ctip2, microglial cells, reservoirs, latency, brain

INTRODUCTION

Since the introduction of the combination antiretroviral therapy (cART) in 1996 the fatal evolution of the HIV-1 infection has stopped and became a chronic disease. However, despite continual efforts definitive cure has not been achieved. This is mainly due to the lack of efficient vaccination and to the existence of viral reservoirs. Indeed, as soon as the treatment is interrupted, a viral rebound is observed within a couple of weeks and viremia is comparable to the one encountered before the introduction of cART (Davey et al., 1999; García et al., 1999; Mata et al., 2005). Moreover, with ultrasensitive methods, we can still notice a residual viremia in patients under cART (Dornadula et al., 1999; Bouchat et al., 2016). The main reservoirs are the resting CD4+ T cells but we have now enough evidence which argues for the existence of many other cell reservoirs such as hematopoietic stem cells, dendritic cells, microglial cells and cells from the monocyte-macrophage lineage (reviewed in Marcello, 2006; García et al., 2018; Sung and Margolis, 2018).

In addition, some of these reservoirs are found in sanctuaries such as the genital tract, the adipose tissue, the bone marrow and the brain. Targeting the infected cells in these reservoirs is even more difficult (Sadowski and Hashemi, 2019). The brain for instance constitutes a typical anatomical site, which has poor drug penetration and reduced immune surveillance due to the blood brain barrier (BBB). As a consequence, the genetical information exchange of the virus confined in the brain and other compartments such as the blood is poor (Canestri et al., 2010; Dahl et al., 2014). The measureable pool of latently infected, resting CD4+ T cells does not account fully for the early rebounding plasma HIV-1. It has been shown that the rebounding HIV-1 was genetically different suggesting that these viruses came from other cell reservoirs (Chun et al., 2000). In addition, the result of recent phylogenetic studies is in favor of other physiological observations suggesting that HIV-1 production in the brain is associated with the emergence of virus resistance (Smit et al., 2004; Strain et al., 2005) and with HIV-1 associated neurocognitive disease (HAND) (Salemi et al., 2005; Lamers et al., 2010). Up to 50% of patients under cART with undetectable virus in the blood suffer of less severe forms of HAND (Eggers et al., 2017). The pathogenesis of HAND is not fully understood but appears to be multifactorial: drug neurotoxicity of the cART, HIV replication in the central nervous system (CNS) from quiescent/latent infected cells, CNS inflammation and co-infection with other viruses such as hepatitis C virus (reviewed in Sutherland and Brew, 2018). Indeed production of newly synthesized viral protein such as Tat or gp120 from infected cells might lead to direct neural injury (reviewed in Rao et al., 2014). Recent reports described new mechanisms for HIV-1 Tat-mediated microglial inflammation which involves a novel miRNA-34a- NOD-like receptor C5 (NLRC5)-NFκB signaling axis or activation of the methyl CpG binding protein 2 (MEPC2)-STAT3 axis (Periyasamy et al., 2018, 2019). Activation by Tat of the microglial nucleotide-binding domain leucin-rich repeat and pyrin-containing receptor 3 (NLRP3) inflammasome also lead to the occurrence of neuroinflammation (Chivero et al., 2017). Indirect impact on the integrity of neurons is also observed during sustained chronic inflammation induced by secreting perivascular macrophages or microglial cells (reviewed in Eggers et al., 2017). Following activation these immune cells release neurotoxic host factors such as pro-inflammatory cytokines (TNFα, IFNα, IL6, IL8, IL1β) (Nolting et al., 2012; Zhou et al., 2016; Abassi et al., 2017) and chemokines (CCL2 and CCL5) (Woods et al., 2006; Zhou et al., 2016). All together these indirect evidences strongly support the existence of cellular reservoirs in the CNS. At least, three different types of infected cells have been described in the CNS referred as a compartment (Bednar et al., 2015): astrocytes, cells from the monocyte lineage (Wong et al., 2019) and microglial cells (Joseph et al., 2015). These putative true reservoirs are established very early during HIV-1 infection (within 3 to 5 days following infection) (Koenig et al., 1986; Whitney et al., 2014). It is well-documented that infection of the CNS results from transmigration of infected CD4+ cells (reviewed in Williams et al., 2012) and of infected monocytes across the BBB (Williams et al., 2012). However, these infected cells entering the CNS do not constitute an HIV reservoir since they have a very short half-life. Instead they will be the source of the infection of three long lived cell types: astrocytes, perivascular macrophages and microglial cells. Whether or not these cells constitute true cell reservoirs is still debated (Gray et al., 2014; Al-Harti et al., 2018; Vanhamel et al., 2019). Criteria for a cell reservoir are the followings: (i) presence of HIV-1 DNA integrated in the host genome of long lived cells, (ii) existence of mechanisms which allow the virus to persist for long period in latent cells which include mechanisms allowing establishment and maintenance of a latent infection and (iii) formation of replication-competent particles following activation of the reservoirs (Eisele and Siliciano, 2012). Two criteria of a true latency reservoir have been described in these cells: the presence of HIV-1 integrated DNA in long lived cells and the existence of mechanisms which allow the virus to persist for long period in latent cells (Blankson et al., 2002). On the other hand, it cannot be explored whether these cells can produce replication-competent viruses in human due to ethical and technical problems.

The astrocyte is the most abundant infected cell type in the CNS with up to 10–20% having HIV-1 DNA in the cell genome (Churchill et al., 2009). However a recent study using sensitive methods detected HIV-1 in brain macrophages and microglial cells but not in astrocytes (Ko et al., 2019). Moreover, the infection appears to be non-productive. Thus they might not constitute a true viral reservoir for HIV-1 (Gorry et al., 2003). On the contrary there is evidence that both macrophages and microglial cells are susceptible to HIV-1 infection and support productive infection (reviewed in Joseph et al., 2015). As already mentioned, the productive infection in these later cells in the CNS has been associated with HAND in humans and in animal models such as the macaques. Therefore, both macrophages and microglial cells can be considered as true reservoirs in the brain. However, their relative importance is not the same due to their differences in size and constitution in the brain. The macrophages are bone marrow-derived with a half-life of months and they do not undergo cell division (Koppensteiner et al., 2012). They are repopulated from monocytes crossing the BBB. Under a very efficient cART or by using therapeutic strategies preventing the specific subset of infected monocytes to cross the BBB we might expect in the future to drastically decrease this reservoir in the brain. The microglial cells originate from erythromyeloid progenitors in the yolk sac during embryogenesis and colonize the forming CNS (Kierdorf et al., 2013). They constitute therefore the main resident cells of the brain which can serve as brain macrophages. Due to their long half-life of years they constitute a very stable population (Réu et al., 2017). In addition unlike macrophages they can undergo cell division enabling HIV-1 to persist in the brain (Lawson et al., 1992). Moreover, a recent report suggests that microglial cells are highly susceptible to HIV-1 infection (Cenker et al., 2017). Altogether, the microglial cells might constitute one of the main HIV-1 reservoir in the brain.

In the review we will first present microglial cells and discuss why they might be the main HIV-1 cell reservoirs in the cART era. We suggest that microglial cells should be the main target in the brain in order to achieve cure. As a prerequisite it is needed to decipher the molecular mechanisms of the establishment and the maintenance of HIV-1 latency in these cells. In further section, we will discuss the therapeutic implications of these mechanisms followed by the discussion of the challenges facing when targeting microglial cells and how to circumvent these limitations.

MICROGLIAL CELLS, A KEY PLAYER DURING THE COURSE OF HIV-1 INFECTION

The Biology of Microglial Cells

Microglial cells constitute the CNS resident innate immune cells (Bilimoria and Stevens, 2015). They are the most abundant mono nuclear macrophages which are found in the totality of the brain parenchyma. These cells appear very early during embryogenesis and derive from early myeloid precursors in the embryogenic yolk sac (Gomez Perdiguero et al., 2015; Sheng et al., 2015). Microglial cells colonize the entire brain parenchyma before the formation of the BBB and subsist by slow cell division during life (Gomez Perdiguero et al., 2015). The median rate of human microglial cell renewal is around 30% per year. In a recent report, it was estimated that microglial cells are on average 4.2 years old and most of the cells in the population regenerates throughout life (Réu et al., 2017). Contrary to the other potentially infected cells in the brain this slow cell division allows the persistence of HIV-1 in the brain throughout the life of the patient. Both resting and activated microglial cells are ramified cells with multiple branches and processes which contact neurons, astrocytes and blood vessels (reviewed in Sominsky et al., 2018). Resting cells are transformed to activated macrophage like state when sensing a change in their microenvironment (reviewed in Colonna and Butovsky, 2017). They are also very mobile and rapidly reach the site of brain damage. When activated, these cells release many cytokines, chemokines and other neurotoxic proteins. These secretory factors might contribute to the pathological neuroinflammation observed in HAND (Hong and Banks, 2015). Many other diseases have been associated with pathological neuroinflammation and are described elsewhere (Salter and Stevens, 2017). Microglial cells express numerous pattern-recognition receptors (PRRs) such as TLR1/2, TLR3, and TLR4 (reviewed in Colonna and Butovsky, 2017). Many other immune receptors are also expressed in microglial cells including CD4+, chemokine receptors, receptors which regulate the activation of microglial cells such as Triggering Receptor Expressed on Myeloid cell 2 (TREM2). These receptors might serve as a marker of inflammation during the course of HIV-1 infection (Gisslén et al., 2019). Many receptors for pro-inflammatory factors (TNFα, IL1β, IL10) and anti-inflammatory factors (IFNα/β) are also expressed (Lee et al., 2002). Interestingly, released anti-inflammatory factors transfer signals to the cell interior via a specific receptor complex to generate an antiviral response (Taniguchi and Takaoka, 2002). An exhaustive review of the wide range of immune receptors is described elsewhere (Colonna and Butovsky, 2017). Apart its function in immune surveillance to eliminate the microbes, microglial cells can also eliminate dead cells, redundant synapses, protein aggregates such as amyloid plaques (reviewed in Colonna and Butovsky, 2017; Salter and Stevens, 2017; Sominsky et al., 2018). These cells are involved in several functions of the CNS, including neurogenesis, the control of synaptic density and connectivity and the regulation of synaptic plasticity through the release of many cytokines such as Brain-Derived Neurotrophic Factor (BNDF). Of note HIV-1 Tat protein can inhibit BNDF by up regulating the microRNA mir-34a (Santerre et al., 2019). Microglial cells can also engulf neurotransmitters released in excess and therefore prevent excitotoxicity and participate in the cross talk between microglial cells and astrocytes. Due to their multifunction, any dysfunction in microglia cells will lead to many diverse diseases including brain aging or neurodegenerative diseases such as Alzheimer disease, Parkinson disease and amyotrophic lateral sclerosis. They are also central players in the occurrence of pathological neuroinflammation observed in patients under cART. HAND is thought to be related to excessive secretion of cytokines and chemokines (Yadav and Collman, 2009; Burdo et al., 2013; Eggers et al., 2017). In a recent study the gene expression profile in microglial cells from infected patients under cART with or without HIV encephalitis (HIVE) has been investigated which showed differential expression of several classes of genes compared to non-infected patients. 64% of the genes were effected in HIVE positive patients and 24% in HIVE negative patients (Ginsberg et al., 2018). This report strongly suggests that neuroinflammation, which leads to neurodegenerative diseases such as HAND, is associated with microglial impairment. Neuroimaging such as positron emission tomography (PET) has shown that neuroinflammation develops even under effective cART (Tavazzi et al., 2014; Vera et al., 2016). This approach has highlighted the importance of microglial activation in HIV+ patients under efficient cART with or without any cognitive impairments. PET also allows to follow the level of microglial activation by targeting translocator protein (TSPO) (Sinharay and Hammoud, 2019). Indeed, upregulation of TSPO during microglial activation is related to the degree of neuroinflammation (Venneti et al., 2004). Activation of microglial cells will further lead to the progression of neurodegenerative diseases by impacting the BBB (reviewed in da Fonseca et al., 2014; Osipova et al., 2018). Indeed microglial cells activation modulates tight junctions of endothelial cells of the BBB (Sumi et al., 2010). Of note, inhibition of microglial activation by minocycline is associated with preservation of BBB integrity *in vitro* and with reduced disruption of the BBB *in vivo* (Yenari et al., 2006; Sheng et al., 2018).

In conclusion, microglial cells fulfill several criteria of a brain reservoir. Most importantly they can subsist for a very long time in the brain and they can colonize the brain parenchyma. Contrary to other potential reservoirs in the brain, these cells divide slowly expanding the viral reservoirs in the brain and thus allowing virus persistence and reseeding of the blood. They are also involved in many functions including immune surveillance. As a consequence, any dysfunction of these cells might explain the occurrence of HAND.

Evidence Supporting That Microglial Cells Are Susceptible to HIV-1 Infection and They Contribute to the Formation of a Cell Reservoir in the Brain

It is believed that microglial cell infection arises from transmigration of infected monocytes occurring very early in the course of infection. Recently, a specific subset of infected monocytes which preferentially cross the BBB, the HIV+ CD14+ CD16+ monocytes, has been characterized (Veenstra et al., 2017). These cells express abundantly junctional proteins such as Junctional Adhesion Molecule-A (JAM-A) and Activated Leukocyte Cell Adhesion Molecule (ALCAM) and chemokine receptors CCR2 which help these cells to cross the BBB. In turn these infected monocytes may infect microglial cells. Alternatively, but still debated, infected CD4+ T cells migrating into the brain might be ingested by microglial cells (Murooka et al., 2012). Although it has not been clearly demonstrated, this later mechanism could be more efficient to spread the virus than exposure to the free virus (Baxter et al., 2014). Whatever the mechanism of infection, it appears that brain microglial cells are permissive to HIV-1 infection. This is despite high level of the restriction factor SAM domain and HD domain 1 (SAMHD1) (Rodrigues et al., 2017). The absence of restriction by SAMDH1 is due to its phosphorylation by the cyclin kinase 1 (CDK1) which is induced in microglial cells that cycle between G0 to G1 state (Cribier et al., 2013; Mlcochova et al., 2017). There is now evidence supporting that microglial cells are infected by HIV-1 both *in vitro* and *in vivo* (reviewed in Joseph et al., 2015). Previous studies from autopsy have identified HIV-1 DNA, RNA and protein in microglial cells (Cosenza et al., 2002; Churchill et al., 2006). However, it was pointed out that these patients died from severe form of HAND. A recent study confirmed that microglial cells are infected in patients whose viral level is suppressed but died from an HIV-1 unrelated outcome (Ko et al., 2019). In this study the authors used a unique cohort from the National Neuro AIDS Tissue Consortium (NTTC) which comprised 16 patients on cART with well-documented, sustained control of HIV-1. They used highly specific technology to detect and quantify both HIV-1 DNA and RNAs at the cellular level. Very interestingly they showed that both perivascular macrophages and microglial cells but not astrocytes harbored HIV-1 DNA. In 6 out 16 cases they also found HIV-1 RNA in these cells when HIV-1 RNA was undetectable in the cerebro Spinal Fluid (CSF) and in the blood. This result strongly argues in favor that virus production can take place in the CNS. Other studies have also shown that microglial cells are susceptible to infection *in vitro*. Several *in vitro* models of human microglial cells susceptible of infection have been developed (Janabi et al., 1995; Nagai et al., 2001; Garcia-Mesa et al., 2017; Rawat and Spector, 2017; Dello Russo et al., 2018). Some models for latency have been derived from these previous models and constitute valuable tools to study the mechanism of infection and the molecular mechanisms underlying the establishment and maintenance of HIV-1 latency in microglial cells (Garcia-Mesa et al., 2017; Alvarez-Carbonell et al., 2019). Evidence that the virus was detected in the CSF in patients under effective cART who had otherwise undetectable plasma HIV-1 also argues in favor for the production of HIV-1 in the brain (Edén et al., 2010, 2016; Ferretti et al., 2015). In addition, phylogenetic analyses also suggest an important compartmentalization of HIV-1 in the CSF even early in infection (Salemi and Rife, 2016; Bavaro et al., 2019).

Finally, infection of microglial cells is clearly demonstrated in animal models such as the macaque and the humanized mouse (reviewed in Kumar et al., 2016; Marsden and Zack, 2017; Gama et al., 2018; Abreu et al., 2019). In these models HIV-1 DNA, RNA and protein were detected in the brain. Importantly, studies on these models showed that the viral reservoir is established very early at 3 days post infection (Whitney et al., 2014). More interestingly, there is evidence that microglial cells can be latently infected (Avalos et al., 2017; Gama et al., 2017). A macaque model has recently been designed and a mechanism for the establishment of HIV-1 transcription suggested (Barber et al., 2006). In this model, microglial cells can be reactivated in response to cytokine stimulation (Qin et al., 2015; Xu et al., 2017). Interestingly, in a cell model developed in Karn's laboratory, the glucocorticoid receptor and the toll-like receptor 3 appeared to be crucial receptors for HIV-1 activation (Alvarez-Carbonell et al., 2017, 2019). In brain autopsies from patients whose infection was controlled HIV-1 DNAs in microglial cells and macrophages were also detected (Thompson et al., 2011; Desplats et al., 2013). Humanized mouse models were generated in which microglial cells were infected by HIV-1 *in vivo* (Asahchop et al., 2017; Llewellyn et al., 2018; Mathews et al., 2019; Su et al., 2019). These models will allow us to study the pathophysiology of microglial cell activation and to develop strategies aiming to reduce the pool of these reservoirs.

Altogether, there are now numerous evidence supporting that microglial cells constitute a major cellular reservoir in the brain. Perivascular macrophages might also be considered as a cellular reservoir but not a true lifelong existing one. Moreover, we might expect to reduce drastically this pool by intensifying cART or by preventing the transmigration of infected monocytes into the brain. Concerning astrocytes it is still debated whether they constitute a true reservoir (Al-Harti et al., 2018; Ko et al., 2019).

Thus, a complete understanding of the molecular mechanisms underlying establishment and persistence of HIV-1 latency in microglial cells is needed in order to design original strategies aiming to target these reservoirs.

ESTABLISHMENT AND PERSISTENCE OF HIV-1 LATENCY IN MICROGLIAL CELLS

Infection and the constitution of a microglial cell reservoir might occur very early in the evolution of HIV-1 infection (Whitney et al., 2014). Some features of the microglial cells allow for the persistence of HIV-1 in the brain. When infected they are far more resistant to cytopathic effects and on the contrary of CD4+ T cells they are non-lytic. In addition, these cells are resistant to apoptosis. The mechanism of apoptosis resistance to HIV-1 deserves considerable attention since it helps to design alternative strategies based on the increase of apoptosis susceptibility

(Kumar et al., 2014). Indeed, strategies aiming to reactivate HIV-1 from infected cells should consider the problem of resistance to apoptosis since the reinforced therapy might not be efficient against the newly productive but non-apoptotic cells. Finally, the antiretroviral drug efficiency is drastically reduced in anatomical and pharmacological sanctuaries such as the brain where microglial cells are mostly found and thus contributing also to viral persistence (Asahchop et al., 2017; Honeycutt et al., 2017).

Two forms of latency have been described which explain HIV-1 persistence in microglial cells. Latency which occurs before the integration of the HIV-1 genome into the host is called pre-integration latency. This form of latency has been frequently observed in CD4+ T cells and in cells of the monocyte-macrophage lineage (discussed in Le Douce et al., 2010). In the latter cells, pre-integration latency might constitute a viral defense mechanism which could lead to the establishment and persistence of HIV-1 infection (Cara and Klotman, 2006; Hansen et al., 2016). This type of latency has not been described in microglia yet. We call post integration latency when HIV-1 genome has been incorporated into the host DNA genome. The integrated HIV-1 provirus can then be in an active-replication state enabling strong transcription of the HIV-1 promoter or in an inactive-state with a marked repression of HIV-1 transcription (Pai and Weinberger, 2017; Cao et al., 2018). In CD4+ T cells, latency is a very rare event with 1 to 10^6-10^7 cells being latently infected (Weinberger and Weinberger, 2013). This rare event has not yet been described but might occur in the other reservoirs infected with HIV-1. Mechanisms involved in CD4+ T cell latency are well-described (Khoury et al., 2018). The strength of the HIV Tat positive feedback loop regulates principally the viral fate selection (**Figure 1**) (Pai and Weinberger, 2017). In other word, there is stochasticity in HIV-1 transcription which explains that each single cell differs in many parameters (stage of cell cycle, level of expression of transcriptional activators/repressors, metabolic state…). Any mechanism reducing the level of HIV-1 Tat expression under a threshold level might therefore facilitate the establishment of latency (Karn, 2011). Integration of the viral genome into repressive heterochromatin environment (Jordan et al., 2001), transcriptional interference (Han et al., 2008), the lack of host transcriptional activators (Le Douce et al., 2010; Churchill et al., 2015), the presence of host transcriptional repressors (Le Douce et al., 2010; Churchill et al., 2015) or the influence of viral miRNA on the chromatin environment (Wang et al., 2009) are thought to favor the establishment of HIV-1 latency since all these mechanisms significantly decrease the strength of the Tat positive feedback. Of note, the mechanism involving viral miRNAs is however controversial and deserves further studies (Balasubramaniam et al., 2018). Additionally, post-transcriptional mechanisms regulating reactivation from latency have also been proposed (Sarracino et al., 2018). On the other hand, in microglial cells host transcription factors that facilitate the establishment of latency have been described. Intriguingly, it was observed that a new CNS strain of the virus has evolved with specific promoters (the 5' long terminal repeat or 5′ LTR) probably due to the compartmentalization of the virus in the brain (Churchill et al., 2015; Gray et al., 2016). Moreover, in contrast to other reservoirs, the NF-κB and the core region including Sp1 sites are sufficient for HIV-1 transcription in microglial cells (Rohr et al., 2003b). In particular, Sp1 proteins allow the anchorage of many transcriptional activators such as NF-IL6 also referred as liver-enriched transcriptional activator protein (LAP), CREB and Coup-Tf (**Figure 1**). Unlike CD4+ T cells which express only Sp1, microglial cells express both Sp1 and Sp3 which operate as transcriptional repressors. In addition, we and others have shown that in macrophages and microglial cells, a truncated form of NF-IL6, liver-enriched transcriptional inhibitory protein (LIP) and/or C-EBPγ is expressed and acts as repressor by competing with the transcriptional activator NF-IL6 (Schwartz et al., 2000) and (Tesmer and Bina, 1996). Noteworthy, this latter mechanism explains HIV-1 latency in microglial cells of a macaque model (Barber et al., 2006). Epigenetic regulation is also involved in the establishment of latency. Coup-TF interacting protein 2 (CTIP2 also known as BCL11b) is a key factor in promoting the formation of heterochromatin, the compact-inactive form of the promoter, in microglial cells. Indeed, CTIP2, apart its crucial role in establishing latency, is also involved in the persistence of latency by preventing HIV-1 reactivation, and in the generation of a cell microenvironment favorable to the establishment of HIV-1 latency. In addition, CTIP2 is described as an anti-apoptotic protein (Kamimura et al., 2007) and thus might also be involved in the apoptosis resistance in microglial cells (Le Douce et al., 2010; Kumar et al., 2014). Interestingly a new mechanism to prevent apoptosis in infected macrophage/microglia cells which survived the infection and became latently infected has been described (Castellano et al., 2017). They notably showed that apoptosis is blocked at a very early step and that the pro-apoptotic protein BIM which accumulate into mitochondria might serve as a new bio-marker of latently-infected macrophage/microglia cells *in vivo*.

CTIP2 is a Zinc finger transcription regulator which has been implicated in many functions required during development and in adult animal (reviewed in Le Douce et al., 2014). Germline disruption of CTIP2 is mortal stressing its importance during development. In fact, the essential role of CTIP2 in T cell development, odontogenesis, skin development and neuronal development are now well-documented (Le Douce et al., 2014). It was shown that CTIP2 is a transcriptional regulator binding directly on a promoter specific sequence (Avram et al., 2002) or binding indirectly to other promoter-bound transcription factors such as Sp1 (Avram et al., 2000).

CTIP2 is involved in the establishment of HIV-1 latency by favoring the formation of heterochromatin in the vicinity of the viral promoter. It serves as a platform anchoring a chromatin modifying complex (Marban et al., 2007). Indeed, our work showed that in the presence of CTIP2 histone deacetylases HDAC1, HDAC2, and histone methyltransferase (HMT) SUV39H1are simultaneously recruited on the viral promoter which generates the H3K9me3 epigenetic mark (trimetylation of H3K9) (**Figure 2**). This work was the first to demonstrate the recruitment of HMT at the latent HIV-1 promoter. It paved the way for reactivation strategies that use a combination of molecules targeting multiple enzymatic activities. Furthermore, we characterized a new factor working in synergy with CTIP2 i.e., the lysine specific demethylase 1

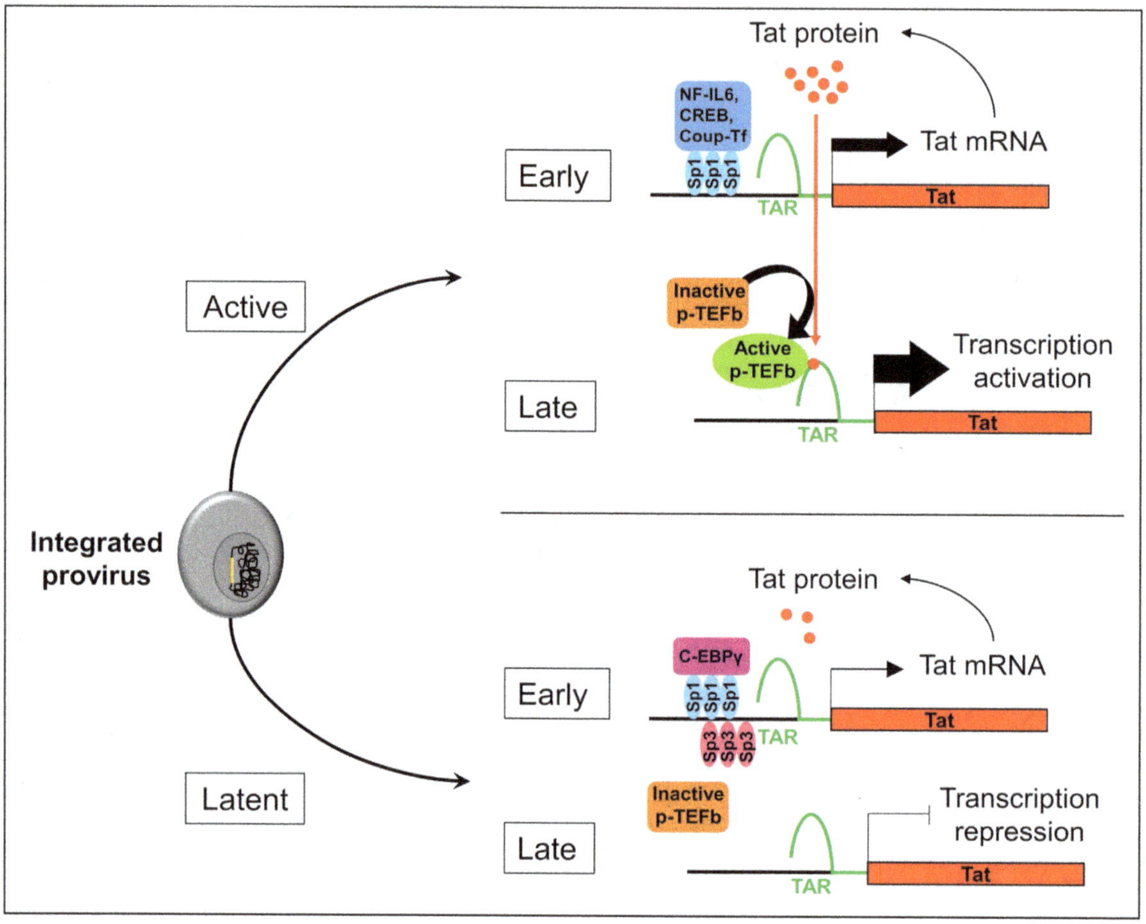

FIGURE 1 | Stochasticity of transcription in microglial cells. The provirus (in yellow) integration in the genome of the microglial host cell (in gray) leads to two possible fates of the cell: active or latent. In active cells, Sp1 allows the anchorage of transcriptional activators like NF-IL6, CREB, and Coup-Tf. It enhances Nf-κB activity and allows the transcription of the viral transactivator Tat in the early phase of transcription. Then, Tat promotes the recruitment of active p-TEFb elongation complex at TAR regions. This recruitment allows viral RNA elongation and transcription activation during the late phase. It results a Tat production which promotes a Tat positive feedback loop and enables a strong transcription of the HIV-1 promoter. In the early phase in latently infected microglial cells, Sp3 act as a transcriptional repressor. In addition, C-EBPγ competes with the transcriptional activator NF-IL6. These repressors reduce Tat expression, p-TEFb recruitment, and viral RNA elongation during the late phase of transcription. If Tat production is under a threshold level, transcription is inhibited and the virus is inactive.

(LSD1), which we showed to be a key factor in the molecular mechanisms of establishment of HIV-1 latency (Le Douce et al., 2012). In particular we established that LSD1 inhibits HIV-1 transcription and viral expression by recruiting hSet1 and WDR5 on the HIV-1 promoter, two members of the hCOMPASS complex, which induce H3K4me3 epigenetic mark (trimetylation of H3K4) (**Figure 2**). The association of H3K4me3 and H3K9me3 epigenetic marks might represent a new level of eukaryotic gene regulation. It was suggested that gene repression linked to H3K4me3 prevents the expression of cryptic promoters (Pinskaya and Morillon, 2009). This is supported by the findings that HIV-1 better integrates in active genes and thus can be considered as a cryptic gene (Wang et al., 2007).

Recently, we showed that CTIP2 is in another complex, which is able to counteract HIV-1 reactivation. In the initial report it was suggested that CTIP2 represses, the Tat-dependent late phase of HIV-1 transcription (Rohr et al., 2003a). Later experiments showed that an inactive form of the elongation factor pTEFb is recovered in a complex containing the non-coding 7SK snRNA and the proteins CTIP2 and HEXIM1 are attached to viral and cellular gene promoters in the absence of the HIV-1 factor Tat (Cherrier et al., 2013). pTEFb is a dimer comprising a regulatory subunit CyclinT1 and a catalytic subunit CDK9. CDK9 is a kinase which phosphorylates the Ser2 residue of the carboxyl terminal end of the RNA polymerase II and the negative transcriptional elongation factors NELF and DSIF. We showed that in this complex CTIP2 significantly inhibited CDK9 kinase activity thus inhibiting pTEFb function (Cherrier et al., 2013). In a following paper, we showed that the cellular protein High Mobility Group AT-hook 1 (HMGA1), which also belongs to the 7SK snRNA complex, recruited the inactive CTIP2/pTEFb complex onto the HIV-1 and cellular target promoters thus regulating their gene expressions (Eilebrecht et al., 2014). HMGA1 has been previously shown to interact with

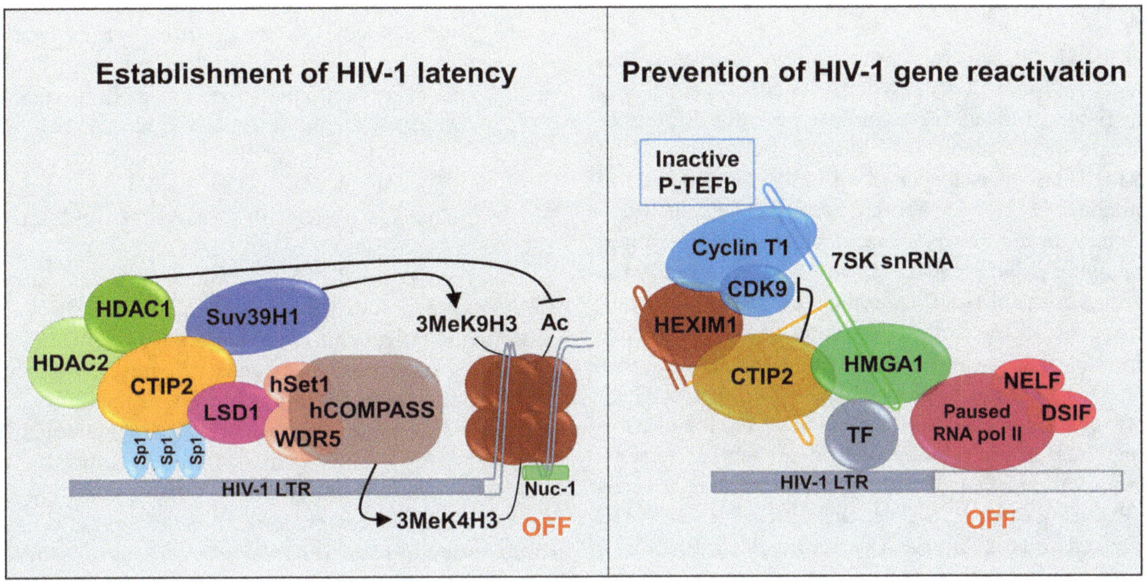

FIGURE 2 | Establishment and persistence of HIV-1 latency in microglial cells: CTIP2 as a central actor. **(Left)** CTIP2 is involved in the establishment of HIV-1 latency by recruiting a chromatin modifying complex at the viral promoter (HIV-1 LTR). CTIP2 is anchored at Sp1 sites on the viral promoter and act as a scaffolding for the recruitment of several chromatin modifying proteins. They perform epigenetic modifications of histones of the nucleosome located at the promoter. CTIP2 recruits simultaneously HDAC2, HDAC1 and the HMT Suv39H1. HDAC1 deacetylate histones while Suv39H1 generates the trimethylation of H3K9 (H3K9me3). In addition, LSD1 promotes the trimethylation of H3K4 by the hCOMPASS methyltransferase complex through hSet1 and WDR5 recruitment. These two epigenetic marks are sufficient to promote chromatin compaction (heterochromatin) and inhibit transcription. **(Right)** CTIP2 prevents transcription restart by sequestrating the elongation factor pTEF-B in an inactive complex. 7SK snRNA complex is recruited at promoter via HMGA1 by interaction with transcription factors (TF). HMGA1 then recruits CTIP2 associated with the inactive form of PTEF-B (Cyclin T1 and CDK9) and HEXIM1, on the 7SK snRNA. Transcription is inhibited at two levels. First, CTIP2 inhibits the kinase activity of CDK9, a pTEF-B subunit which prevent RNA pol II activation by inhibiting the phosphorylation of RNA pol II and the two subunits NELF and DSIF. Second, the persistence of inactive pTEF-B at the promoter prevents any recruitment of active pTEF-B.

TAR to modulate Tat-dependent HIV transcription (Eilebrecht et al., 2013). It seems that HMGA1 is critical for the repressive function of CTIP2. We propose a model in which HMGA1 facilitates the recruitment of CTIP2-inactivated P-TEFb onto cellular and viral gene promoters (**Figure 2**).

As suggested above, CTIP2 has an important role in the regulation of the expression of many infected cells genes. Microarray analysis of a microglial cell line knocked down for CTIP2 showed up or down regulation of several genes (Cherrier et al., 2013). Among them the cellular cyclin-dependent kinase inhibitor CDKN1A/p21^{waf} was up regulated. When recruited to the p21 promoter, CTIP2 represses p21 gene transcription with the same mechanism described for the HIV-1 promoter (Cherrier et al., 2009). The p21 gene repression may favor HIV-1 latency since activation of p21 gene stimulates viral expression in macrophages (Vazquez et al., 2005). In addition, CTIP2 counteracts HIV-1 Vpr which is required for p21 expression. Interestingly we recently showed that HIV-1 Vpr mediates the depletion of the cellular repressor CTIP2 to counteract viral gene silencing (Forouzanfar et al., 2019). Altogether our findings strongly support the findings that CTIP2 generates a cellular environment which is favorable for HIV-1 latency. Furthermore, our results support that CTIP2 is a major actor involved in HIV-1 latency in microglial cells. In agreement with our findings, CTIP2 colocalized with the microglial marker Ionized calcium binding adaptor molecule 1 (Iba1) in latently infected patients but not in HIV encephalitis (HIVE) patients (Desplats et al., 2013). Moreover, the levels of CTIP2 and markers of heterochromatin such as HDACs and heterochromatin 1 (HP1) were increased in microglial cells from HIV-1 positive latent cases. This work and others suggested that CTIP2 can be used as an HIV brain latency biomarker (Cysique et al., 2019).

Recently we have identified and characterized a new cellular factor i.e., Hypermethylated in Cancer 1 (HIC1). This factor regulates together with CTIP2 and HMGA1 cellular and HIV-1 gene transcriptions (Le Douce et al., 2016). However, the repressive activity of the complex requires the deacetylase activity of Sirtuin 1 (SIRT1) in microglial cells. We showed that HIC1 interacted and cooperated with HMGA1 and modulated Tat dependent HIV-1 transcription. However, intriguingly it occurs in the presence of Tat but it is independent of the elongation factor PTEFb. The need for HMGA1 to interact with HIC1 to repress the Tat dependent HIV-1 transcription might suggest a new role for HMGA1 in this process (discussed in Le Douce et al., 2016). Our findings support the idea that the TAR element serves as a HIC-1 reservoir to promote HIC-1/Tat interaction.

We are far from elucidating all the molecular mechanisms which underlie HIV-1 latency in microglial cells. Further investigation in this field is needed in order to identify new potential targets in HIV-1 therapy.

TARGETING THE MICROGLIAL CELLS

Targeting all the HIV-1 reservoirs including the microglial cells in the brain is important in order to achieve either a sterilizing or a functional cure. Indeed, these cells are potential sources of HIV-1 reseeding in the blood. In addition, production of the virus in these cells has been associated with HIV-1 resistance and the development of HAND. However, targeting these cells which are located in anatomic and pharmacologic sanctuaries might be very challenging (Marban et al., 2016). Most importantly the access of drugs used in cART is limited by the blood brain barrier. Poor access of the drugs contributes to the persistence of HIV-1 in microglial cells (Cosenza et al., 2002). Another limitation is the existence of a residual neuroinflammation which is responsible for the occurrence of HAND in up to 50% of HIV-1 infected patients. A main concern is to prevent deleterious neuroinflammation associated with infected microglial cells (Rock and Peterson, 2006). To date, three strategies are used to target infected microglial cells (Veenhuis et al., 2019): (i) the Shock and Kill strategy, (ii) the Block and Lock strategy, and (iii) gene therapy. We will discuss in the following section the principles of these three approaches and outline their limitations. Finally, we briefly discuss how these limitations can be circumvented and how to rationalize treatments aiming the eradication or reduction of the pool of latently infected microglial cells.

Strategies to Struggle Latently-Infected Microglial Cells

The Shock and Kill Strategy

The Shock and Kill strategy is based on the reactivation of the latent virus. In this strategy the intensification of cART aims to clear the reservoirs either by the cytopathic effect of the reactivated virus or by the immune system via the actions of cytotoxic T cells (CTLs) (Schwartz et al., 2017). Latency reversing agents (LRAs) used in the reactivation target identified and characterized cellular factors involved in HIV-1 latency (**Figure 3**). Many LRAs are now used *ex vivo* and in clinical trials. However, the main targets are circulating CD4+ T cells and not the microglial cells (Kumar et al., 2015; Spivak and Planelles, 2018). There are currently 160 compounds used as LRAs which belong to two main families or to a third one which includes uncommon drugs with unique or unknown mechanisms (e.g., disulfiram and ixazomid) (Abner and Jordan, 2019). Screening of new LRAs is still a field of intensive research (Richard et al., 2018).

One family of LRAs targets epigenetic mechanisms that occur in latency (Darcis et al., 2016). This class comprises HDAC inhibitors (HDACi) such as Valproic acid, Vorinostat, panobinostat, and romidepsin; Histone methyl transferases inhibitors (HMTi) such as chaetocin and BIX 01294; and DNA methylation inhibitors such as 5-AzadC.

In the second family T cell activating agents are listed. These drugs induce the expression of positive cellular factors and/or their release from inactive complex (Jiang and Dandekar, 2015; Rice, 2016). Prostratin, bryostatin, and ingenol B by activating the PKC pathway release NF-KB and pTEFb from inactive complexes and increase pTEFb expression (Sung and Rice, 2006; Fujinaga et al., 2012; Pandeló José et al., 2014) which leads to HIV-1 reactivation (Darcis et al., 2015). Bromodomain inhibitors such as JQ1 and others are able to release pTEFb from the BRD4-pTEFb complex (Bartholomeeusen et al., 2012; Li et al., 2013; Darcis et al., 2015). Many other compounds including TLR agonists, TNFα, cytokines, and antibodies are also used as LRAs. A comprehensive review of these compounds are described elsewhere (Abner and Jordan, 2019).

However, these drugs used alone failed to fully reactivate HIV-1 expression *ex vivo* (Cary et al., 2016; Darcis et al., 2016). This might reflect the multi factorial mechanisms involved in promoting latency and the stochastic nature of latency (Sengupta and Siliciano, 2018). Another important inability of LRAs relies in their lack of specificity and to the heterogeneity of the reservoirs (Ait-Ammar et al., submitted). Indeed, the LRAs are mainly used in clinical assays to target circulating CD4+ cells but not the other reservoirs such as microglial cells. Therefore, combination of LRAs is now used to circumvent these problems. We expect synergistic effect which improves the efficiency of reactivation and reduces toxicity because of the lower doses used. Moreover, a recent report demonstrated the importance of the timing of the LRA combination treatment in the reactivation of HIV (Bouchat et al., 2016).

Reactivation of reservoirs should be followed by the elimination of the virus (Kim et al., 2018). There is now evidence that eradication of latently-infected reservoirs in patients involves humoral and cell mediated immune responses (Schwartz et al., 2017). Humoral immune response plays an important role in controlling HIV infection (reviewed in Ferrari et al., 2017). Over the past years, a new class of antibodies, called broadly neutralizing antibodies, have been shown to neutralize a wide range of HIV strains (Halper-Stromberg and Nussenzweig, 2016). Preclinical studies in which SHIVs infected macaque monkeys and HIV-1 infected humanized mice were treated by antibodies gave promising results (Halper-Stromberg and Nussenzweig, 2016). The efficacy of the treatment was even enhanced when various broadly neutralizing antibodies in combination was applied (Bruel et al., 2016) or when using multi-specific engineered antibodies like bi and tri-specific antibodies (Ferrari et al., 2016; Sun et al., 2016). Numerous strategies were proposed to enhance cell-mediated immune responses, e.g., CD8+ T cell or natural killer cell activities (Scully and Alter, 2016; Trautmann, 2016). Some methods aim to redirect HIV-specific cell mediated immune responses (Patel et al., 2016). In one strategy, redirected T cells recognizing a range of HIV antigens are expanded *ex vivo*. In another strategy genetically modified lentiviruses expressing artificial T cell receptors (TCRs) or chimeric antigen receptors (CARs) are used in the treatment (Patel et al., 2016). Increasing the specificity and the affinity of the epitopes of the receptors to achieve wider HIV epitope recognition is also realistic (Patel et al., 2016). The possibility to increase HIV-specific CD8+ T cell responses with heterocyclic peptides is currently tested. It is assumed that these peptides stimulate deeper the cell-mediated immune responses than native epitopes (Buhrman et al., 2013).

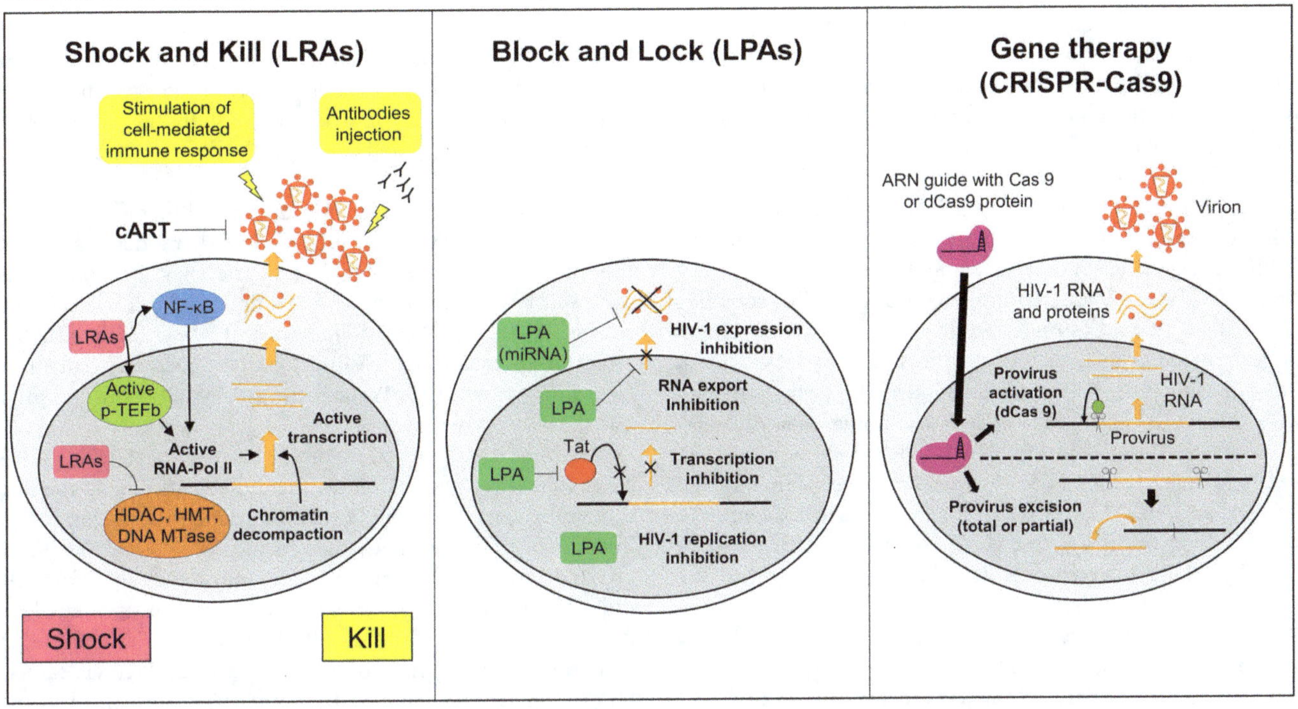

FIGURE 3 | Strategies to struggle latently-infected microglial cells. The shock and kill: the strategy is based on the reactivation of virus expression, in order to eliminate reservoirs and to target latently-infected cells. Latency reversing agents (LRAs) are investigated to reactivate transcription for the "shock." A first family of LRAs are HDAC, HMT, or DNA Mtases inhibitors and target epigenetic mechanisms. These LRAs induce chromatin decompaction and promote virus transcription. Another family of LRAs induce the expression of positive cellular factors (e.g., NF-κB and pTEFB) and/or their recruitment under their active form. These LRAs promote ARN pol II recruitment and favor transcription. The cART is maintained during this phase to clear reservoir without virus propagation in other cells. The "kill" can be enhanced by stimulation of the cell-mediated immune response or by using neutralizing antibodies and/or engineered antibodies. The block and lock: this strategy relates on the induction of a state of deep-latency which prevents any HIV-1 transcription. Several latency-promoting agents (LPAs) are investigated. They inhibit various step of virus expression like replication, transcription by Tat inhibition and RNA export. One promising LPA is a miRNA which inhibit virus expression. The gene therapy (CRISPR-Cas9): this strategy is based on the use of molecular scissors to excise total, or more reasonably, partial sequence of the provirus. Another strategy would be to use deficient Cas9 (dCas9) to carry reactivators or repressors of HIV-1 expression.

An original approach took advantage of the importance of co-stimulatory and co-inhibitory molecules involved in the regulation of T-cell responses (Sharpe and Abbas, 2006). Indeed, treatment by specific antibodies targeting the co-inhibitory molecule PD-1 is thought to reduce the size of the latently-infected reservoir and help to recover CD8+ T cell function from collapse. Finally, therapeutic vaccines might help CTLs to target HIV-1 infected cells derived from latent reservoirs (Deng et al., 2015).

The Block and Lock Strategy

An alternative approach to achieve long term control over HIV-1 infection without the need of cART is to induce a long lasting inhibition of HIV-1 gene expression (**Figure 3**) (Darcis et al., 2017). The molecules used to induce this process are called latency-promoting agents (LPAs). LPAs are expected to suppress the HIV-1 gene expression by inducing a deep latency state (the block) and thus preventing HIV-1 gene transcription (the lock) (Elsheikh et al., 2019). The first LPA identified from a marine sponge is a chemical derivative of corticostatin i.e., Didehydro-corticostatin (dCA). It inhibits Tat activity by preventing Tat-TAR interaction (Mousseau et al., 2015). To date many other LPAs have also been described (reviewed in Castro-Gonzalez et al., 2018). One of them, the ABX464, an inhibitor of Rev which is involved in the RNA export blocks HIV-1 replication *in vitro* as well as in animal models (Campos et al., 2015). Cellular mi RNAs are also potential molecules to be used in the Block and Lock strategy. It has been known for a long time that miRNAs are important modulator of HIV-1 latency (Huang et al., 2007). Screening and computational analysis have allowed the characterization of many miRNAs which impact HIV-1 transcription. One such promising miRNA, i.e., miRNA29a, which inhibits the virus transcription in Jurkat cells should be investigated for its effects in microglial cells (Hariharan et al., 2005). It is suggested that inducing miRNA29a expression in these cells could lead to suppression of HIV-1 gene expression.

The Gene Therapy

Gene therapy has been widely considered as a tool to combat HIV-1. It relies on nuclease-mediated gene editing tools such as the zinc fingers nuclease (ZFN1), the transcription activator-like effector nucleases (TALEN) and the CRISPR/Cas9 technologies (Panfil et al., 2018; Wang et al., 2018). Various gene therapies have been launched since the sterilizing cure of the Berlin patient

(Allers et al., 2011). This patient received transplantation of hematopoietic stem cells from a donor who was homozygous for the CCR5-delta32 mutation (ΔCCR5) conferring resistance to HIV infection. Recently a second patient who shared similar medical contexts, the London patient, was also cured from HIV-1 infection (Gupta R. K. et al., 2019). From this example, the idea to build HIV-1 resistant cells has arisen (Barmania and Pepper, 2013). Clinical trials using ZFN targeting CCR5 are ongoing and deserve attention (Mehta et al., 2017). However, The CRISPR/Cas9 gene editing has become the tool of choice, since ZFN and TALEN are costly and time consuming. This tool uses a guided RNA and a Cas9 nuclease that excise DNA sequences of target specific cellular factors such as CCR5 or HIV-1 DNA thus eliminating the HIV-1 provirus (**Figure 3**). The first targeted DNA sequence by the CRISPR/Cas9 technology was the NF-KB binding site located in the HIV-1 LTR (Ebina et al., 2013). Since then, many other HIV-1 sequences have been targeted (Xiao et al., 2019). This technology may serve to redesign the gene expression of cells such as CTLs so that they target more specifically HIV-1 infected cells. It is believed that by this way the antiviral immunity system could be more efficiently boosted against HIV-1 infected cells and activated reservoirs producing new virions (Mehta et al., 2017). We might even use a variation of the CRISPR/Cas9 technology to reactivate latently infected cells or to induce deep latency (Wang et al., 2018). For this purpose, a defective Cas9 (dCas9) protein is fused to activators to reactivate latently-infected cells (**Figure 3**) or to repressors to suppress HIV-1 expression (Wang et al., 2018). *In vitro* trials suggested a potential application of CRISPR/dCas9 in the reactivation of latent HIV (Zhang et al., 2015). These trials showed reactivation of HIV expression in CD4+ T cells and in microglial cell lines (Cary and Peterlin, 2016). Interestingly, CRISPR/dCas9 when associated with HDAC inhibitors and PKC activators reactivated HIV in a synergistic manner (Limsirichai et al., 2016).

Limitations and Challenges When Targeting Brain Microglial Cells

The current therapeutic strategies have limited efficacy to achieve cure. Their limitations comes from (i) the intrinsic nature of the strategy, (ii) the nature of the cells targeted, or (iii) the attributes of the virus to escape antiviral responses. Regarding microglial cells their specific cell properties and their location in anatomical and pharmacological sanctuaries make them difficult to target. In consequence, the presence of the BBB drastically reduces drug access to currently used drugs in cART (Asahchop et al., 2017). New antiviral drugs with improved CNS penetrance have been introduced in the last years (Veenhuis et al., 2019). However, some showed important side effects. For example, a new integrase inhibitor which showed important CNS uptake (Letendre et al., 2014) was neurotoxic showing severe neuropsychiatric effects (Scheper et al., 2018). Various technics improving delivery of drugs in the CNS and in the CNS-cell types are currently explored. Mechanisms underlying weak drug penetrance are mainly related to differential expression of efflux transporter and to multidrug resistance proteins (Valcour et al., 2011; da Fonseca et al., 2014). Several invasive and non-invasive methods for drug delivery are currently explored including modulation of brain barrier, ultrasound based BBB opening, endogenous transporter, nanoparticles, liposomes, dendrimers... (reviewed in Barnabas, 2019). Original route of drug delivery to the CNS are also explored such as drug delivery from the nose to the brain (Gupta S. et al., 2019).

We should also consider immune-based therapeutics to clear reservoirs activated by the LRAs. Animal models have shown the importance of the CTLs and neutralizing antibodies raised against HIV-1 in immune activation and clearing infected reservoirs in the CNS. Therefore it deserves considerable attention to ensure the feasibility of the Shock and Kill strategy (Brockman et al., 2015; Trautmann, 2016; Subra and Trautmann, 2019).

An important limitation of the use of the Shock and Kill strategy is that reactivation of microglial cells during the Shock therapy leads to neuroinflammation, since the release of pro-inflammatory factors and some viral proteins such as Tat and gp120 during the shock therapy are neurotoxic. Therefore, LRAs induced reactivation of reservoirs has to be associated with drugs preventing the adverse effects of neuroinflammation. One way to prevent inflammation is to improve cART via targeting HIV-1 transcription and/or by inhibiting RNA export in order to counteract the effects of the pro-inflammatory cytokines and to prevent synthesis of viral proteins (Schwartz et al., 2017). Molecules which have anti-inflammatory effects such as curcurmin are also investigated in microglial inflammatory responses (Chen et al., 2018). A new drug formulation using lipid nano-carrier and administration by intra nasal route are currently investigated (Vaz et al., 2017). Remarkably, many drugs targeting the NF-κB pathway (G1V001), the protein Tat (dCA, triptolides...) and rev (ABX4641) induce a deep latency and are thought to be used in the Block and Lock strategy as an alternative to the Shock and Kill strategy. We might use both strategies in a sequential time schedule. First, the Shock and Kill strategy which reactivates and decreases the pool of reservoirs. Followed by application of drugs exploiting the Block and Lock strategy, which suppresses transcription in persisting reservoirs and induces deep latency. Although, it is still an emerging field of research the Block and Lock strategy appears to be more than just an alternative to other strategies. Interestingly, less adverse effects with drugs targeting viral proteins are awaited. We believe that combination of the Block and Lock strategy with the Shock and Kill might allow the reduction of all HIV-1 reservoirs, including the microglial cell reservoir to a level, which does not need any further treatment to achieve a functional cure.

Gene therapy compared to a pharmacological approach such as the Shock and Kill strategy is still in its infancy but appears to be very promising. A recent review compares the advantages and weaknesses of these two approaches i.e., the pharmacological vs. CRISPR/Cas9-based shock strategies (Darcis et al., 2018). Gene therapy, in the same way as pharmacological approaches, does not resolve the problem of drug penetrance in the CNS where microglial cells are located. Indeed, currently used adeno-viruses in *in vitro* essays induce severe inflammation

(Chew et al., 2016). Moreover, another important limitation of gene editing was discovered; HIV-1 can escape CRISPR/cas9 mediated suppression. Indeed, following an initial attempt to establish proof of concept of the use of gene editing targeting specifically HIV-1 (Kaminski et al., 2016), it soon appeared that the virus was able to subvert the DNA repair machinery to evolve quickly into CRISPR/Cas9 resistant strains (Liang et al., 2016; Wang G. et al., 2016; Wang Z. et al., 2016; Yoder and Bundschuh, 2016). On the other hand combination of guided RNAs targeting different HIV-1 specific sequences may drastically reduce the occurrence of HIV-1 escape (Wang et al., 2018). A major off-target of this gene editing tool is the increase of undesirable gene mutations and chromosomal translocations (Yee, 2016). Efforts in reducing these off-target effects are required in order to improve this elegant and attractive approach. For example, bioinformatics could help to select the correct guided RNAs that avoid unexpected DNA cleavage (Zhu et al., 2017). Another limitation of the use of gene editing technology is that it has been mainly tested *in vitro* and mainly in CD4+ T cells. Experiments conducted *ex vivo* showed that redirected immune cells reached only a tiny fraction of the HIV-1 reservoirs. Therefore, this technology does not make possible to drastically reduce the number of infected cells, which is required to achieve functional cure (Wang et al., 2018).

Rationalization of these strategies is required to optimize either of these strategies to target microglial cells. Since we cannot make brain biopsies due to ethical concerns, it is critical to design these strategies and test their feasibility in adequate animal models. Indeed, the efficacy and the pharmacokinetic and pharmacodynamic characteristics of drugs are tested only in preclinical studies. Non-human primates (NHP) and humanized mice are currently the best-suited animal models to study either strategies. However, there are many ways to evaluate the efficiency of a therapy and to evaluate HIV infection in the brain. The search of specific biomarkers for latently infected microglial cells may lead to the development of original strategies, which specifically target brain reservoirs. One such specific marker of the CD4+ T cell reservoir, CD32a, has been described (Descours et al., 2017), although its specificity is debated (Badia et al., 2018). Much research has been focused on finding new specific biomarkers for brain reservoirs, nonetheless their use will be very challenging. Indeed, it will be difficult to target brain reservoirs *ex vivo*, even though it is technically possible for blood cells, and very difficult to target them *in vivo* due to their paucity and localization in the entire brain parenchyma. For example, the invasive techniques used to evaluate the evolution of biomarkers in the CSF such as neopterin, CTIP2, TREM2, and NFL after a treatment cannot be performed too frequently (Jessen Krut et al., 2014). Non-invasive methods such as neuroimaging are therefore needed for brain evaluation (discussed in Garrido and Margolis, 2015). Comprehensive neuropsychological testing is also required to detect subclinical deficits (Haddow et al., 2013). It will be essential to evaluate the efficiency of each strategy that target microglial cells. For this purpose, highly sensitive methods have been developed such as the single copy assay (SCA) which allows the detection of HIV RNA in the CSF from infected patients on cART or from elite controllers whose HIV RNA level was initially undetectable in the plasma and the CSF (Dahl et al., 2013).

CONCLUSION

HIV cure is theoretically possible but not yet feasible with current approaches. Complete cure demands targeting not only the CD4+ T cells reservoirs but also all the other potential reservoirs located in sanctuaries with low drug penetrance. This is particularly true for the microglial cells in the CNS which is considered as the main reservoir for HIV. Indeed, due to their properties (slow turn over, long half-life...), these cells are thought to persist lifelong. Other true reservoirs such as macrophages may be eliminated by intensifying cART and/or by targeting HIV infected monocytes which is the source of infection. Other reservoirs such as astrocytes or the newly identified pericytes (Bertrand et al., 2019) may constitute true reservoirs, but these are still debated and deserve far more investigations. Currently, three strategies are considered, which allow functional cure: two pharmacological approaches including the shock and kill strategy and the alternative block and lock strategy and the CRISPR/cas9 based technology, which is a gene editing tool based strategy. However, the Shock and Kill strategy is not suitable to eliminate reservoirs like microglial cells, since the reactivation of microglial cell reservoirs leads to neuroinflammation, which is the origin of HAND. The search for potential epigenetic regulators that control microglial cells are therefore needed. The most investigated epigenetic regulators are the long non-coding RNAs (Qu et al., 2019) and the mi RNAs (reviewed in Cheray and Joseph, 2018). However, due to the stochasticity of HIV-1 transcription the Shock and Kill strategy does not allow reactivation of all latently infected microglial cells. Alternative strategies are therefore considered. The Block and Lock strategy has the advantage that the risk of inflammation in the brain is drastically reduced. More importantly, this strategy since it targets transcription and/or RNA export might be used following the Shock and Kill strategy. The combination of strategies should lead to the decrease of the pool of the microglial reservoir. It may also induce deep latency in reservoirs that are not reactivated by LRAs. The gene editing tool, such as the CRISPR/Cas9 technology, because it operates on specific sequences is also very promising. Still in its infancy, this elegant approach can target either cellular factors, which are involved in HIV-1 resistance, or viral factors. This technology can be used either to reactivate the virus or to excise and eliminate the provirus from its host genome. However, several challenges have to be overcome such as *in vivo* delivery in the brain and long-term toxicity before its use in the clinic and thus needs far more investigations. An original way to deliver CRISPR/cas9 guided RNA across the BBB has been developed recently and hold promises (Kaushik et al., 2019). Notably, it was shown that this non-invasive method which uses magnetically guided delivery of RNAs inhibits latent infection of microglial cells and cross the BBB in *in vitro* models.

In conclusion, targeting microglial cells is crucial but might be very challenging. We have to keep in mind that these cells are resistant to the cytopathic effects of the virus and resistant to apoptosis. Thus strategies aiming to induce apoptosis in infected microglial cells have to be developed (Le Douce et al., 2010). It appears that the cellular factor CTIP2 (Bcl11b) has a pivotal role in the establishment and persistence of HIV latency, in the genesis of a favorable environment for HIV latency and in the resistance to apoptosis (Le Douce et al., 2014). CTIP2 silencing by RNA interference has been proposed in cancer since downregulation of CTIP2 leads to apoptosis in malignant cells but not in normal mature cells (Grabarczyk et al., 2007; Huang et al., 2007). We might also design drugs targeting CTIP2 interacting proteins specifically involved in HIV-1 latency and apoptosis resistance. Moreover, establishing a protein interaction network focused on CTIP2 interactions in microglial cells will allow the identification and characterization of new actors involved in HIV-1 latency and apoptosis resistance.

AUTHOR CONTRIBUTIONS

CS and OR wrote the review. CW designed the figures and wrote the legends. CW, MD, JV, FD, SD, VG, PM, AM, and CV participated in the writing of the review.

ACKNOWLEDGMENTS

We are grateful to Andrea Janossy for a careful and critical reading of the manuscript.

REFERENCES

Abassi, M., Morawski, B. M., Nakigozi, G., Nakasujja, N., Kong, X., Meya, D. B., et al. (2017). Cerebrospinal fluid biomarkers and HIV-associated neurocognitive disorders in HIV-infected individuals in Rakai, Uganda. *J. Neurovirol.* 23, 369–375. doi: 10.1007/s13365-016-0505-9

Abner, E., and Jordan, A. (2019). HIV "shock and kill" therapy: in need of revision. *Antiviral Res.* 166, 19–34. doi: 10.1016/j.antiviral.2019.03.008

Abreu, C., Shirk, E. N., Queen, S. E., Mankowski, J. L., Gama, L., and Clements, J. E. (2019). A quantitative approach to SIV functional latency in brain macrophages. *J. Neuroimmune Pharmacol.* 14, 23–32. doi: 10.1007/s11481-018-9803-8

Al-Harti, L., Joseph, J., and Nath, A. (2018). Astrocytes as an HIV CNS reservoir: highlights and reflections of an NIMH-sponsored symposium. *J. Neurovirol.* 24, 665–669. doi: 10.1007/s13365-018-0691-8

Allers, K., Hutter, G., Hofmann, J., Loddenkemper, C., Rieger, K., Thiel, E., et al. (2011). Evidence for the cure of HIV infection by CCR5 32/ 32 stem cell transplantation. *Blood* 117, 2791–2799. doi: 10.1182/blood-2010-09-309591

Alvarez-Carbonell, D., Garcia-Mesa, Y., Milne, S., Das, B., Dobrowolski, C., Rojas, R., et al. (2017). Toll-like receptor 3 activation selectively reverses HIV latency in microglial cells. *Retrovirology* 14:9. doi: 10.1186/s12977-017-0335-8

Alvarez-Carbonell, D., Ye, F., Ramanath,N., Dobrowolski, C., and Karn, J. (2019). The glucocorticoid receptor is a critical regulator of HIV latency in human microglial cells. *J. Neuroimmune Pharmacol.* 14, 94–109. doi: 10.1007/s11481-018-9798-1

Asahchop, E. L., Meziane, O., Mamik, M. K., Chan, W. F., Branton, W. G., Resch, L., et al. (2017). Reduced antiretroviral drug efficacy and concentration in HIV-infected microglia contributes to viral persistence in brain. *Retrovirology* 14:47. doi: 10.1186/s12977-017-0370-5

Avalos, C. R., Abreu, C. M., Queen, S. E., Li, M., Price, S., Shirk, E. N., et al. (2017). Brain macrophages in simian immunodeficiency virus-infected, antiretroviral-suppressed macaques: a functional latent reservoir. *MBio* 8:e01186-17. doi: 10.1128/mBio.01186-17

Avram, D., Fields, A., Pretty On Top, K., Nevrivy, D. J., Ishmael, J. E., and Leid, M. (2000). Isolation of a novel family of C(2)H(2) zinc finger proteins implicated in transcriptional repression mediated by chicken ovalbumin upstream promoter transcription factor (COUP-TF) orphan nuclear receptors. *J. Biol. Chem.* 275, 10315–10322. doi: 10.1074/jbc.275.14.10315

Avram, D., Fields, A., Senawong, T., Topark-Ngarm, A., and Leid, M. (2002). COUP-TF (chicken ovalbumin upstream promoter transcription factor)-interacting protein 1 (CTIP1) is a sequence-specific DNA binding protein. *Biochem. J.* 368, 555–563. doi: 10.1042/bj200 20496

Badia, R., Ballana, E., Castellví, M., García-Vidal, E., Pujantell, M., Clotet, B., et al. (2018). CD32 expression is associated to T-cell activation and is not a marker of the HIV-1 reservoir. *Nat. Commun.* 9:2739. doi: 10.1038/s41467-01 8-05157-w

Balasubramaniam, M., Pandhare, J., and Dash, C. (2018). Are microRNAs important players in HIV-1 infection? An update. *Viruses* 10:E110. doi: 10.3390/v10030110

Barber, S. A., Gama, L., Dudaronek, J. M., Voelker, T., Tarwater, P. M., and Clements, J. E. (2006). Mechanism for the establishment of transcriptional HIV latency in the brain in a simian immunodeficiency virus–macaque model. *J. Infect. Dis.* 193, 963–970. doi: 10.1086/500983

Barmania, F., and Pepper, M. S. (2013). C-C chemokine receptor type five (CCR5): an emerging target for the control of HIV infection. *Appl. Transl. Genomics* 2, 3–16. doi: 10.1016/j.atg.2013.05.004

Barnabas, W. (2019). Drug targeting strategies into the brain for treating neurological diseases. *J. Neurosci. Methods* 311, 133–146. doi: 10.1016/j.jneumeth.2018.10.015

Bartholomeeusen, K., Xiang, Y., Fujinaga, K., and Peterlin, B. M. (2012). Bromodomain and Extra-terminal (BET) bromodomain inhibition activate transcription via transient release of positive transcription elongation factor b (P-TEFb) from 7SK small nuclear ribonucleoprotein. *J. Biol. Chem.* 287, 36609–36616. doi: 10.1074/jbc.M112.410746

Bavaro, D. F., Calamo, A., Lepore, L., Fabrizio, C., Saracino, A., Angarano, G., et al. (2019). Cerebrospinal fluid compartmentalization of HIV-1 and correlation with plasma viral load and blood–brain barrier damage. *Infection* 47, 441–446. doi: 10.1007/s15010-019-01268-8

Baxter, A. E., Russell, R. A., Duncan, C. J. A., Moore, M. D., Willberg, C. B., Pablos, J. L., et al. (2014). Macrophage infection via selective capture of HIV-1-infected $CD4^+$ T cells. *Cell Host Microbe* 16, 711–721. doi: 10.1016/j.chom.2014.10.010

Bednar, M. M., Sturdevant, C. B., Tompkins, L. A., Arrildt, K. T., Dukhovlinova, E., Kincer, L. P., et al. (2015). Compartmentalization, viral evolution, and viral latency of HIV in the CNS. *Curr. HIV/AIDS Rep.* 12, 262–271. doi: 10.1007/s11904-015-0265-9

Bertrand, L., Cho, H. J., and Toborek, M. (2019). Blood–brain barrier pericytes as a target for HIV-1 infection. *Brain* 142, 502–511. doi: 10.1093/brain/awy339

Bilimoria, P. M., and Stevens, B. (2015). Microglia function during brain development: new insights from animal models. *Brain Res.* 1617, 7–17. doi: 10.1016/j.brainres.2014.11.032

Blankson, J. N., Persaud, D., and Siliciano, R. F. (2002). The challenge of viral reservoirs in HIV-1 infection. *Annu. Rev. Med.* 53, 557–593. doi: 10.1146/annurev.med.53.082901.104024

Bouchat, S., Delacourt,N., Kula, A., Darcis, G., Van Driessche, B., Corazza, F., et al. (2016). Sequential treatment with 5-aza-2'-deoxycytidine and deacetylase inhibitors reactivates HIV-1. *EMBO Mol. Med.* 8, 117–138. doi: 10.15252/emmm.201505557

Brockman, M. A., Jones, R. B., and Brumme, Z. L. (2015). Challenges and opportunities for T-cell-mediated strategies to eliminate HIV reservoirs. *Front. Immunol.* 6:506. doi: 10.3389/fimmu.2015.00506

Bruel, T., Guivel-Benhassine, F., Amraoui, S., Malbec, M., Richard, L., Bourdic, K., et al. (2016). Elimination of HIV-1-infected cells by broadly neutralizing antibodies. *Nat. Commun.* 7:10844. doi: 10.1038/ncomms10844

Buhrman, J. D., Jordan, K. R., Munson, D. J., Moore, B. L., Kappler, J. W., and Slansky, J. E. (2013). Improving antigenic peptide vaccines for cancer immunotherapy using a dominant tumor-specific T cell receptor. *J. Biol. Chem.* 288, 33213–33225. doi: 10.1074/jbc.M113.509554

Burdo, T. H., Lackner, A., and Williams, K. C. (2013). Monocyte/macrophages and their role in HIV neuropathogenesis. *Immunol. Rev.* 254, 102–113. doi: 10.1111/imr.12068

Campos, N., Myburgh, R., Garcel, A., Vautrin, A., Lapasset, L., Nadal, E. S., et al. (2015). Long lasting control of viral rebound with a new drug ABX464 targeting Rev – mediated viral RNA biogenesis. *Retrovirology* 12:30. doi: 10.1186/s12977-015-0159-3

Canestri, A., Lescure, F., Jaureguiberry, S., Moulignier, A., Amiel, C., Marcelin, A. G., et al. (2010). Discordance between cerebral spinal fluid and plasma HIV replication in patients with neurological symptoms who are receiving suppressive antiretroviral therapy. *Clin. Infect. Dis.* 50, 773–778. doi: 10.1086/650538

Cao, Y., Lei, X., Ribeiro, R. M., Perelson, A. S., and Liang, J. (2018). Probabilistic control of HIV latency and transactivation by the Tat gene circuit. *Proc. Natl. Acad. Sci. U S A.* 115, 12453–12458. doi: 10.1073/pnas.1811195115

Cara, A., and Klotman, M. E. (2006). Retroviral E-DNA: persistence and gene expression in nondividing immune cells. *J. Leukoc. Biol.* 80, 1013–1017. doi: 10.1189/jlb.0306151

Cary, D. C., Fujinaga, K., and Peterlin, B. M. (2016). Molecular mechanisms of HIV latency. *J. Clin. Invest.* 126, 448–454. doi: 10.1172/JCI80565

Cary, D. C., and Peterlin, B. M. (2016). Targeting the latent reservoir to achieve functional HIV cure. *F1000Res* 5:F1000. doi: 10.12688/f1000research.8109.1

Castellano, P., Prevedel, L., and Eugenin, E. A. (2017). HIV-infected macrophages and microglia that survive acute infection become viral reservoirs by a mechanism involving Bim. *Sci. Rep.* 7:12866. doi: 10.1038/s41598-017-12758-w

Castro-Gonzalez, S., Colomer-Lluch, M., and Serra-Moreno, R. (2018). Barriers for HIV cure: the latent reservoir. *AIDS Res. Hum. Retroviruses* 34, 739–759. doi: 10.1089/aid.2018.0118

Cenker, J. J., Stultz, R. D., and McDonald, D. (2017). Brain Microglial cells are highly susceptible to HIV-1 infection and spread. *AIDS Res. Hum. Retroviruses* 33, 1155–1165. doi: 10.1089/aid.2017.0004

Chen, G., Liu, S., Pan, R., Li, G., Tang, H., Jiang, M., et al. (2018). Curcumin attenuates gp120-induced microglial inflammation by inhibiting autophagy via the PI3K pathway. *Cell. Mol. Neurobiol.* 38, 1465–1477. doi: 10.1007/s10571-018-0616-3

Cheray, M., and Joseph, B. (2018). Epigenetics control microglia plasticity. *Front. Cell. Neurosci.* 12:243. doi: 10.3389/fncel.2018.00243

Cherrier, T., Le Douce, V., Eilebrecht, S., Riclet, R., Marban, C., Dequiedt, F., et al. (2013). CTIP2 is a negative regulator of P-TEFb. *Proc. Natl. Acad. Sci. U.S.A.* 110, 12655–12660. doi: 10.1073/pnas.1220136110

Cherrier, T., Suzanne, S., Redel, L., Calao, M., Marban, C., Samah, B., et al. (2009). p21WAF1 gene promoter is epigenetically silenced by CTIP2 and SUV39H1. *Oncogene* 28, 3380–3389. doi: 10.1038/onc.2009.193

Chew, W. L., Tabebordbar, M., Cheng, J. K. W., Mali, P., Wu, E. Y., Ng, A. H. M., et al. (2016). A multifunctional AAV-CRISPR-Cas9 and its host response. *Nat. Methods* 13, 868–874. doi: 10.1038/nmeth.3993

Chivero, E. T., Guo, M.-L., Periyasamy, P., Liao, K., Callen, S. E., and Buch, S. (2017). HIV-1 Tat primes and activates microglial NLRP3 inflammasome-mediated neuroinflammation. *J. Neurosci.* 37, 3599–3609. doi: 10.1523/JNEUROSCI.3045-16.2017

Chun, T. W., Davey, R. T., Ostrowski, M., Shawn Justement, J., Engel, D., Mullins, J. I., et al. (2000). Relationship between pre-existing viral reservoirs and the re-emergence of plasma viremia after discontinuation of highly active anti-retroviral therapy. *Nat. Med.* 6, 757–761. doi: 10.1038/77481

Churchill, M. J., Cowley, D. J., Wesselingh, S. L., Gorry, P. R., and Gray, L. R. (2015). HIV-1 transcriptional regulation in the central nervous system and implications for HIV cure research. *J. Neurovirol.* 21, 290–300. doi: 10.1007/s13365-014-0271-5

Churchill, M. J., Gorry, P. R., Cowley, D., Lal, L., Sonza, S., Purcell, D. F., et al. (2006). Use of laser capture microdissection to detect integrated HIV-1 DNA in macrophages and astrocytes from autopsy brain tissues. *J. Neurovirol.* 12, 146–152. doi: 10.1080/13550280600748946

Churchill, M. J., Wesselingh, S. L., Cowley, D., Pardo, C. A., McArthur, J. C., Brew, B. J., et al. (2009). Extensive astrocyte infection is prominent in human immunodeficiency virus-associated dementia. *Ann. Neurol.* 66, 253–258. doi: 10.1002/ana.21697

Colonna, M., and Butovsky, O. (2017). Microglia function in the central nervous system during health and neurodegeneration. *Annu. Rev. Immunol.* 35, 441–468. doi: 10.1146/annurev-immunol-051116-052358

Cosenza, M. A., Zhao, M.-L., Si, Q., and Lee, S. C. (2002). Human brain parenchymal microglia express CD14 and CD45 and are productively infected by HIV-1 in HIV-1 encephalitis. *Brain Pathol.* 12, 442–455. doi: 10.1111/j.1750-3639.2002.tb00461.x

Cribier, A., Descours, B., Valadão, A. L. C., Laguette,N., and Benkirane, M. (2013). Phosphorylation of SAMHD1 by Cyclin A2/CDK1 regulates its restriction activity toward HIV-1. *Cell Rep.* 3, 1036–1043. doi: 10.1016/j.celrep.2013.03.017

Cysique, L. A., Jugé, L., Lennon, M. J., Gates, T. M., Jones, S. P., Lovelace, M. D., et al. (2019). HIV brain latency as measured by CSF BcL11b relates to disrupted brain cellular energy in virally suppressed HIV infection. *AIDS* 33, 433–441. doi: 10.1097/QAD.0000000000002076

da Fonseca, A. C. C., Matias, D., Garcia, C., Amaral, R., Geraldo, L. H., Freitas, C., et al. (2014). The impact of microglial activation on blood-brain barrier in brain diseases. *Front. Cell. Neurosci.* 8:362. doi: 10.3389/fncel.2014.00362

Dahl, V., Gisslen, M., Hagberg, L., Peterson, J., Shao, W., Spudich, S., et al. (2014). An example of genetically distinct HIV type 1 variants in cerebrospinal fluid and plasma during suppressive therapy. *J. Infect. Dis.* 209, 1618–1622. doi: 10.1093/infdis/jit805

Dahl, V., Peterson, J., Spudich, S., Lee, E., Shacklett, B. L., Price, R. W., et al. (2013). Single-copy assay quantification of HIV-1 RNA in paired cerebrospinal fluid and plasma samples from elite controllers. *AIDS* 27, 1145–1149. doi: 10.1097/QAD.0b013e32835cf235

Darcis, G., Das, A., and Berkhout, B. (2018). Tackling HIV persistence: pharmacological versus CRISPR-based shock strategies. *Viruses* 10:157. doi: 10.3390/v10040157

Darcis, G., Kula, A., Bouchat, S., Fujinaga, K., Corazza, F., Ait-Ammar, A., et al. (2015). An in-depth comparison of latency-reversing agent combinations in various *in vitro* and *ex vivo* HIV-1 latency models identified bryostatin-1+JQ1 and ingenol-B+JQ1 to potently reactivate viral gene expression. *PLoS Pathog.* 11:e1005063. doi: 10.1371/journal.ppat.1005063

Darcis, G., Van Driessche, B., and Van Lint, C. (2016). Preclinical shock strategies to reactivate latent HIV-1: an update. *Curr. Opin. HIV AIDS* 11, 388–393. doi: 10.1097/COH.0000000000000288

Darcis, G., Van Driessche, B., and Van Lint, C. (2017). HIV latency: should we shock or lock? *Trends Immunol.* 38, 217–228. doi: 10.1016/j.it.2016.12.003

Davey, R. T., Bhat, N., Yoder, C., Chun, T. W., Metcalf, J. A., Dewar, R., et al. (1999). HIV-1 and T cell dynamics after interruption of highly active antiretroviral therapy (HAART) in patients with a history of sustained viral suppression. *Proc. Natl. Acad. Sci. U.S.A.* 96, 15109–15114. doi: 10.1073/pnas.96.26.15109

Dello Russo, C., Cappoli, N., Coletta, I., Mezzogori, D., Paciello, F., Pozzoli, G., et al. (2018). The human microglial HMC3 cell line: where do we stand? A systematic literature review. *J. Neuroinflammation* 15:259. doi: 10.1186/s12974-018-1288-0

Deng, K., Pertea, M., Rongvaux, A., Wang, L., Durand, C. M., Ghiaur, G., et al.

(2015). Broad CTL response is required to clear latent HIV-1 due to dominance of escape mutations. *Nature* 517, 381–385. doi: 10.1038/nature14053

Descours, B., Petitjean, G., López-Zaragoza, J.-L., Bruel, T., Raffel, R., Psomas, C., et al. (2017). CD32a is a marker of a CD4 T-cell HIV reservoir harbouring replication-competent proviruses. *Nature* 543, 564–567. doi: 10.1038/nature21710

Desplats, P., Dumaop, W., Smith, D., Adame, A., Everall, I., Letendre, S., et al. (2013). Molecular and pathologic insights from latent HIV-1 infection in the human brain. *Neurology* 80, 1415–1423. doi: 10.1212/WNL.0b013e31828c2e9e

Dornadula, G., Zhang, H., VanUitert, B., Stern, J., Livornese, L., Ingerman, M. J., et al. (1999). Residual HIV-1 RNA in blood plasma of patients taking suppressive highly active antiretroviral therapy. *JAMA* 282, 1627–1632. doi: 10.1001/jama.282.17.1627

Ebina, H., Misawa,N., Kanemura, Y., and Koyanagi, Y. (2013). Harnessing the CRISPR/Cas9 system to disrupt latent HIV-1 provirus. *Sci. Rep.* 3:2510. doi: 10.1038/srep02510

Edén, A., Fuchs, D., Hagberg, L., Nilsson, S., Spudich, S., Svennerholm, B., et al. (2010). HIV-1 viral escape in cerebrospinal fluid of subjects on suppressive antiretroviral treatment. *J. Infect. Dis.* 202, 1819–1825. doi: 10.1086/657342

Edén, A., Nilsson, S., Hagberg, L., Fuchs, D., Zetterberg, H., Svennerholm, B., et al. (2016). Asymptomatic cerebrospinal fluid HIV-1 viral blips and viral escape during antiretroviral therapy: a longitudinal study. *J. Infect. Dis.* 214, 1822–1825. doi: 10.1093/infdis/jiw454

Eggers, C., Arendt, G., Hahn, K., Husstedt, I. W., Maschke, M., Neuen-Jacob, E., et al. (2017). HIV-1-associated neurocognitive disorder: epidemiology, pathogenesis, diagnosis, and treatment. *J. Neurol.* 264, 1715–1727. doi: 10.1007/s00415-017-8503-2

Eilebrecht, S., Le Douce, V., Riclet, R., Targat, B., Hallay, H., Van Driessche, B., et al. (2014). HMGA1 recruits CTIP2-repressed P-TEFb to the HIV-1 and cellular target promoters. *Nucleic Acids Res.* 42, 4962–4971. doi: 10.1093/nar/gku168

Eilebrecht, S., Wilhelm, E., Benecke, B.-J., Bell, B., and Benecke, A. G. (2013). HMGA1 directly interacts with TAR to modulate basal and Tat-dependent HIV transcription. *RNA Biol.* 10, 436–444. doi: 10.4161/rna.23686

Eisele, E., and Siliciano, R. F. (2012). Redefining the viral reservoirs that prevent HIV-1 eradication. *Immunity* 37, 377–388. doi: 10.1016/j.immuni.2012.08.010

Elsheikh, M. M., Tang, Y., Li, D., and Jiang, G. (2019). Deep latency: a new insight into a functional HIV cure. *EBioMedicine* 45, 624–629. doi: 10.1016/j.ebiom.2019.06.020

Ferrari, G., Haynes, B. F., Koenig, S., Nordstrom, J. L., Margolis, D. M., and Tomaras, G. D. (2016). Envelope-specific antibodies and antibody-derived molecules for treating and curing HIV infection. *Nat. Rev. Drug Discov.* 15, 823–834. doi: 10.1038/nrd.2016.173

Ferrari, G., Pollara, J., Tomaras, G. D., and Haynes, B. F. (2017). Humoral and innate antiviral immunity as tools to clear persistent HIV infection. *J. Infect. Dis.* 215, S152–S159. doi: 10.1093/infdis/jiw555

Ferretti, F., Gisslen, M., Cinque, P., and Price, R. W. (2015). Cerebrospinal fluid HIV escape from antiretroviral therapy. *Curr. HIV/AIDS Rep.* 12, 280–288. doi: 10.1007/s11904-015-0267-7

Forouzanfar, F., Ali, S., Wallet, C., Ducloy, C., El Mekdad, H., and El Maassarani, M., et al. (2019). HIV-1 Vpr mediates the depletion of the cellular repressor CTIP2 to counteract viral gene silencing. *Sci. Rep.* 9:13154. doi: 10.1038/s41598-019-48689-x

Fujinaga, K., Barboric, M., Li, Q., Luo, Z., Price, D. H., and Peterlin, B. M. (2012). PKC phosphorylates HEXIM1 and regulates P-TEFb activity. *Nucleic Acids Res.* 40, 9160–9170. doi: 10.1093/nar/gks682

Gama, L., Abreu, C., Shirk, E. N., Queen, S. E., Beck, S. E., Metcalf Pate, K. A., et al. (2018). SIV latency in macrophages in the CNS. *Curr. Top. Microbiol. Immunol.* 417, 111–130. doi: 10.1007/82_2018_89

Gama, L., Abreu, C. M., Shirk, E. N., Price, S. L., Li, M., Laird, G. M., et al. (2017). Reactivation of simian immunodeficiency virus reservoirs in the brain of virally suppressed macaques. *AIDS* 31, 5–14. doi: 10.1097/QAD.0000000000001267

García, F., Plana, M., Vidal, C., Cruceta, A., O'Brien, W. A., Pantaleo, G., et al. (1999). Dynamics of viral load rebound and immunological changes after stopping effective antiretroviral therapy. *AIDS* 13, F79–F86. doi: 10.1097/00002030-199907300-00002

García, M., Buzón, M. J., Benito, J. M., and Rallón,N. (2018). Peering into the HIV reservoir. *Rev. Med. Virol.* 28:e1981. doi: 10.1002/rmv.1981

Garcia-Mesa, Y., Jay, T. R., Checkley, M. A., Luttge, B., Dobrowolski, C., Valadkhan, S., et al. (2017). Immortalization of primary microglia: a new platform to study HIV regulation in the central nervous system. *J. Neurovirol.* 23, 47–66. doi: 10.1007/s13365-016-0499-3

Garrido, C., and Margolis, D. M. (2015). Translational challenges in targeting latent HIV infection and the CNS reservoir problem. *J. Neurovirol.* 21, 222–226. doi: 10.1007/s13365-014-0269-z

Ginsberg, S. D., Alldred, M. J., Gunnam, S. M., Schiroli, C., Lee, S. H., Morgello, S., et al. (2018). Expression profiling suggests microglial impairment in human immunodeficiency virus neuropathogenesis. *Ann. Neurol.* 83, 406–417. doi: 10.1002/ana.25160

Gisslén, M., Heslegrave, A., Veleva, E., Yilmaz, A., Andersson, L.-M., Hagberg, L., et al. (2019). CSF concentrations of soluble TREM2 as a marker of microglial activation in HIV-1 infection. *Neurol. Neuroimmunol. Neuroinflamm.* 6:e512. doi: 10.1212/NXI.0000000000000512

Gomez Perdiguero, E., Klapproth, K., Schulz, C., Busch, K., Azzoni, E., Crozet, L., et al. (2015). Tissue-resident macrophages originate from yolk-sac-derived erythro-myeloid progenitors. *Nature* 518, 547–551. doi: 10.1038/nature13989

Gorry, P. R., Ong, C., Thorpe, J., Bannwarth, S., Thompson, K. A., Gatignol, A., et al. (2003). Astrocyte infection by HIV-1: mechanisms of restricted virus replication, and role in the pathogenesis of HIV-1-associated dementia. *Curr. HIV Res.* 1, 463–473. doi: 10.2174/1570162033485122

Grabarczyk, P., Przybylski, G. K., Depke, M., Völker, U., Bahr, J., Assmus, K., et al. (2007). Inhibition of BCL11B expression leads to apoptosis of malignant but not normal mature T cells. *Oncogene* 26, 3797–3810. doi: 10.1038/sj.onc.1210152

Gray, L. R., Cowley, D., Welsh, C., Lu, H. K., Brew, B. J., Lewin, S. R., et al. (2016). CNS-specific regulatory elements in brain-derived HIV-1 strains affect responses to latency-reversing agents with implications for cure strategies. *Mol. Psychiatry* 21, 574–584. doi: 10.1038/mp.2015.111

Gray, L. R., Roche, M., Flynn, J. K., Wesselingh, S. L., Gorry, P. R., and Churchill, M. J. (2014). Is the central nervous system a reservoir of HIV-1? *Curr. Opin. HIV AIDS* 9, 552–558. doi: 10.1097/COH.0000000000000108

Gupta, R. K., Abdul-Jawad, S., McCoy, L. E., Mok, H. P., Peppa, D., Salgado, M., et al. (2019). HIV-1 remission following CCR5Δ32/Δ32 haematopoietic stem-cell transplantation. *Nature* 568, 244–248. doi: 10.1038/s41586-019-1027-4

Gupta, S., Kesarla, R., and Omri, A. (2019). Approaches for CNS delivery of drugs – nose to brain targeting of antiretroviral agents as a potential attempt for complete elimination of major reservoir site of HIV to aid AIDS treatment. *Expert Opin. Drug Deliv.* 16, 287–300. doi: 10.1080/17425247.2019.1583206

Haddow, L. J., Floyd, S., Copas, A., and Gilson, R. J. C. (2013). A systematic review of the screening accuracy of the HIV dementia scale and international HIV dementia scale. *PLoS ONE* 8:e61826. doi: 10.1371/journal.pone.0061826

Halper-Stromberg, A., and Nussenzweig, M. C. (2016). Towards HIV-1 remission: potential roles for broadly neutralizing antibodies. *J. Clin. Invest.* 126, 415–423. doi: 10.1172/JCI80561

Han, Y., Lin, Y. B., An, W., Xu, J., Yang, H.-C., O'Connell, K., et al. (2008). Orientation-dependent regulation of integrated HIV-1 expression by host gene transcriptional readthrough. *Cell Host Microbe* 4, 134–146. doi: 10.1016/j.chom.2008.06.008

Hansen, E. C., Ransom, M., Hesselberth, J. R., Hosmane, N. N., Capoferri, A. A., Bruner, K. M., et al. (2016). Diverse fates of uracilated HIV-1 DNA during infection of myeloid lineage cells. *Elife* 5:e18447. doi: 10.7554/eLife.18447

Hariharan, M., Scaria, V., Pillai, B., and Brahmachari, S. K. (2005). Targets for human encoded microRNAs in HIV genes. *Biochem. Biophys. Res. Commun.* 337, 1214–1218. doi: 10.1016/j.bbrc.2005.09.183

Honeycutt, J. B., Thayer, W. O., Baker, C. E., Ribeiro, R. M., Lada, S. M., Cao, Y., et al. (2017). HIV persistence in tissue macrophages of humanized myeloid-only mice during antiretroviral therapy. *Nat. Med.* 23, 638–643. doi: 10.1038/nm.4319

Hong, S., and Banks, W. A. (2015). Role of the immune system in HIV-associated neuroinflammation and neurocognitive implications. *Brain. Behav. Immun.* 45, 1–12. doi: 10.1016/j.bbi.2014.10.008

Huang, J., Wang, F., Argyris, E., Chen, K., Liang, Z., Tian, H., et al. (2007). Cellular microRNAs contribute to HIV-1 latency in resting primary CD4+ T lymphocytes. *Nat. Med.* 13, 1241–1247. doi: 10.1038/nm1639

Janabi,N., Peudenier, S., Héron, B., Ng, K. H., and Tardieu, M. (1995). Establishment of human microglial cell lines after transfection of primary cultures of embryonic microglial cells with the SV40 large T antigen. *Neurosci. Lett.* 195, 105–108. doi: 10.1016/0304-3940(94)11792-H

Jessen Krut, J., Mellberg, T., Price, R. W., Hagberg, L., Fuchs, D., Rosengren, L., et al. (2014). Biomarker evidence of axonal injury in neuroasymptomatic HIV-1 patients. *PLoS ONE* 9:e88591. doi: 10.1371/journal.pone.0088591

Jiang, G., and Dandekar, S. (2015). Targeting NF-κB signaling with protein kinase C agonists as an emerging strategy for combating HIV latency. *AIDS Res. Hum. Retroviruses* 31, 4–12. doi: 10.1089/aid.2014.0199

Jordan, A., Defechereux, P., and Verdin, E. (2001). The site of HIV-1 integration in the human genome determines basal transcriptional activity and response to Tat transactivation. *EMBO J.* 20, 1726–1738. doi: 10.1093/emboj/20.7.1726

Joseph, S. B., Arrildt, K. T., Sturdevant, C. B., and Swanstrom, R. (2015). HIV-1 target cells in the CNS. *J. Neurovirol.* 21, 276–289. doi: 10.1007/s13365-014-0287-x

Kamimura, K., Mishima, Y., Obata, M., Endo, T., Aoyagi, Y., and Kominami, R. (2007). Lack of Bcl11b tumor suppressor results in vulnerability to DNA replication stress and damages. *Oncogene* 26, 5840–5850. doi: 10.1038/sj.onc.1210388

Kaminski, R., Bella, R., Yin, C., Otte, J., Ferrante, P., Gendelman, H. E., et al. (2016). Excision of HIV-1 DNA by gene editing: a proof-of-concept *in vivo* study. *Gene Ther.* 23, 690–695. doi: 10.1038/gt.2016.41

Karn, J. (2011). The molecular biology of HIV latency: breaking and restoring the Tat-dependent transcriptional circuit. *Curr. Opin. HIV AIDS* 6, 4–11. doi: 10.1097/COH.0b013e328340ffbb

Kaushik, A., Yndart, A., Atluri, V., Tiwari, S., Tomitaka, A., Gupta, P., et al. (2019). Magnetically guided non-invasive CRISPR-Cas9/gRNA delivery across blood-brain barrier to eradicate latent HIV-1 infection. *Sci. Rep.* 9:3928. doi: 10.1038/s41598-019-40222-4

Khoury, G., Darcis, G., Lee, M. Y., Bouchat, S., Van Driessche, B., Purcell, D. F. J., et al. (2018). The molecular biology of HIV latency. *Adv. Exp. Med. Biol.* 1075, 187–212. doi: 10.1007/978-981-13-0484-2_8

Kierdorf, K., Erny, D., Goldmann, T., Sander, V., Schulz, C., Perdiguero, E. G., et al. (2013). Microglia emerge from erythromyeloid precursors via Pu.1- and Irf8-dependent pathways. *Nat. Neurosci.* 16, 273–280. doi: 10.1038/nn.3318

Kim, Y., Anderson, J. L., and Lewin, S. R. (2018). Getting the "Kill" into "Shock and Kill": strategies to eliminate latent HIV. *Cell Host Microbe* 23, 14–26. doi: 10.1016/j.chom.2017.12.004

Ko, A., Kang, G., Hattler, J. B., Galadima, H. I., Zhang, J., Li, Q., et al. (2019). Macrophages but not astrocytes harbor HIV DNA in the brains of HIV-1-infected aviremic individuals on suppressive antiretroviral therapy. *J. Neuroimmune Pharmacol.* 14, 110–119. doi: 10.1007/s11481-018-9809-2

Koenig, S., Gendelman, H. E., Orenstein, J. M., Dal Canto, M. C., Pezeshkpour, G. H., Yungbluth, M., et al. (1986). Detection of AIDS virus in macrophages in brain tissue from AIDS patients with encephalopathy. *Science* 233, 1089–1093. doi: 10.1126/science.3016903

Koppensteiner, H., Brack-Werner, R., and Schindler, M. (2012). Macrophages and their relevance in human immunodeficiency virus type I infection. *Retrovirology* 9:82. doi: 10.1186/1742-4690-9-82

Kumar, A., Abbas, W., and Herbein, G. (2014). HIV-1 latency in monocytes/macrophages. *Viruses* 6, 1837–1860. doi: 10.3390/v6041837

Kumar, A., Darcis, G., Van Lint, C., and Herbein, G. (2015). Epigenetic control of HIV-1 post integration latency: implications for therapy. *Clin. Epigenetics* 7:103. doi: 10.1186/s13148-015-0137-6

Kumar, N., Chahroudi, A., and Silvestri, G. (2016). Animal models to achieve an HIV cure. *Curr. Opin. HIV AIDS* 11, 432–441. doi: 10.1097/COH.0000000000000290

Lamers, S. L., Salemi, M., Galligan, D. C., Morris, A., Gray, R., Fogel, G., et al. (2010). Human immunodeficiency virus-1 evolutionary patterns associated with pathogenic processes in the brain. *J. Neurovirol.* 16, 230–241. doi: 10.3109/13550281003735709

Lawson, L. J., Perry, V. H., and Gordon, S. (1992). Turnover of resident microglia in the normal adult mouse brain. *Neuroscience* 48, 405–415. doi: 10.1016/0306-4522(92)90500-2

Le Douce, V., Cherrier, T., Riclet, R., Rohr, O., and Schwartz, C. (2014). The many lives of CTIP2: from AIDS to cancer and cardiac hypertrophy. *J. Cell. Physiol.* 229, 533–537. doi: 10.1002/jcp.24490

Le Douce, V., Colin, L., Redel, L., Cherrier, T., Herbein, G., Aunis, D., et al. (2012). LSD1 cooperates with CTIP2 to promote HIV-1 transcriptional silencing. *Nucleic Acids Res.* 40, 1904–1915. doi: 10.1093/nar/gkr857

Le Douce, V., Forouzanfar, F., Eilebrecht, S., Van Driessche, B., Ait-Ammar, A., Verdikt, R., et al. (2016). HIC1 controls cellular- and HIV-1- gene transcription via interactions with CTIP2 and HMGA1. *Sci. Rep.* 6:34920. doi: 10.1038/srep34920

Le Douce, V., Herbein, G., Rohr, O., and Schwartz, C. (2010). Molecular mechanisms of HIV-1 persistence in the monocyte-macrophage lineage. *Retrovirology* 7:32. doi: 10.1186/1742-4690-7-32

Lee, Y. B., Nagai, A., and Kim, S. U. (2002). Cytokines, chemokines, and cytokine receptors in human microglia. *J. Neurosci. Res.* 69, 94–103. doi: 10.1002/jnr.10253

Letendre, S. L., Mills, A. M., Tashima, K. T., Thomas, D. A., Min, S. S., Chen, S., et al. (2014). ING116070: a study of the pharmacokinetics and antiviral activity of dolutegravir in cerebrospinal fluid in HIV-1-infected, antiretroviral therapy-naive subjects. *Clin. Infect. Dis.* 59, 1032–1037. doi: 10.1093/cid/ciu477

Li, Z., Guo, J., Wu, Y., and Zhou, Q. (2013). The BET bromodomain inhibitor JQ1 activates HIV latency through antagonizing Brd4 inhibition of Tat-transactivation. *Nucleic Acids Res.* 41, 277–287. doi: 10.1093/nar/gks976

Liang, C., Wainberg, M. A., Das, A. T., and Berkhout, B. (2016). CRISPR/Cas9: a double-edged sword when used to combat HIV infection. *Retrovirology* 13:37. doi: 10.1186/s12977-016-0270-0

Limsirichai, P., Gaj, T., and Schaffer, D. V. (2016). CRISPR-mediated activation of latent HIV-1 expression. *Mol. Ther.* 24, 499–507. doi: 10.1038/mt.2015.213

Llewellyn, G. N., Alvarez-Carbonell, D., Chateau, M., Karn, J., and Cannon, P. M. (2018). HIV-1 infection of microglial cells in a reconstituted humanized mouse model and identification of compounds that selectively reverse HIV latency. *J. Neurovirol.* 24, 192–203. doi: 10.1007/s13365-017-0604-2

Marban, C., Forouzanfar, F., Ait-Ammar, A., Fahmi, F., El Mekdad, H., Daouad, F., et al. (2016). Targeting the brain reservoirs: toward an HIV Cure. *Front. Immunol.* 7:397. doi: 10.3389/fimmu.2016.00397

Marban, C., Suzanne, S., Dequiedt, F., de Walque, S., Redel, L., Van Lint, C., et al. (2007). Recruitment of chromatin-modifying enzymes by CTIP2 promotes HIV-1 transcriptional silencing. *EMBO J.* 26, 412–423. doi: 10.1038/sj.emboj.7601516

Marcello, A. (2006). Latency: the hidden HIV-1 challenge. *Retrovirology* 3:7. doi: 10.1186/1742-4690-3-7

Marsden, M. D., and Zack, J. A. (2017). Humanized mouse models for human immunodeficiency virus infection. *Annu. Rev. Virol.* 4, 393–412. doi: 10.1146/annurev-virology-101416-041703

Mata, R. C., Viciana, P., de Alarcón, A., López-Cortés, L. F., Gómez-Vera, J., Trastoy, M., et al. (2005). Discontinuation of antiretroviral therapy in patients with chronic HIV infection: clinical, virologic, and immunologic consequences. *AIDS Patient Care STDS* 19, 550–562. doi: 10.1089/apc.2005.19.550

Mathews, S., Branch Woods, A., Katano, I., Makarov, E., Thomas, M. B., Gendelman, H. E., et al. (2019). Human Interleukin-34 facilitates microglia-like cell differentiation and persistent HIV-1 infection in humanized mice. *Mol. Neurodegener.* 14:12. doi: 10.1186/s13024-019-0311-y

Mehta, V., Chandramohan, D., and Agarwal, S. (2017). Genetic modulation therapy through stem cell transplantation for human immunodeficiency virus 1 infection. *Cureus* 9:e1093. doi: 10.7759/cureus.1093

Mlcochova, P., Sutherland, K. A., Watters, S. A., Bertoli, C., de Bruin, R. A., Rehwinkel, J., et al. (2017). A G1-like state allows HIV-1 to bypass SAMHD1 restriction in macrophages. *EMBO J.* 36, 604–616. doi: 10.15252/embj.201696025

Mousseau, G., Kessing, C. F., Fromentin, R., Trautmann, L., Chomont,N., and Valente, S.T. (2015). The Tat inhibitor didehydro-cortistatin A prevents HIV-1 reactivation from latency. *MBio* 6:e00465. doi: 10.1128/mBio.00465-15

Murooka, T. T., Deruaz, M., Marangoni, F., Vrbanac, V. D., Seung, E., von Andrian, U. H., et al. (2012). HIV-infected T cells are migratory vehicles for viral dissemination. *Nature* 490, 283–287. doi: 10.1038/nature11398

Nagai, A., Nakagawa, E., Hatori, K., Choi, H. B., McLarnon, J. G., Lee, M. A., et al. (2001). Generation and characterization of immortalized human microglial cell lines: expression of cytokines and chemokines. *Neurobiol. Dis.* 8, 1057–1068. doi: 10.1006/nbdi.2001.0437

Nolting, T., Lindecke, A., Hartung, H.-P., Koutsilieri, E., Maschke, M., Husstedt, I.-W., et al. (2012). Cytokine levels in CSF and neuropsychological performance in HIV patients. *J. Neurovirol.* 18, 157–161. doi: 10.1007/s13365-012-0091-4

Osipova, E. D., Semyachkina-Glushkovskaya, O. V., Morgun, A. V., Pisareva, N. V., Malinovskaya, N. A., Boitsova, E. B., et al. (2018). Gliotransmitters and cytokines in the control of blood-brain barrier permeability. *Rev. Neurosci.* 29, 567–591. doi: 10.1515/revneuro-2017-0092

Pai, A., and Weinberger, L. S. (2017). Fate-regulating circuits in viruses: from discovery to new therapy targets. *Annu. Rev. Virol.* 4, 469–490. doi: 10.1146/annurev-virology-110615-035606

Pandeló José, D., Bartholomeeusen, K., da Cunha, R. D., Abreu, C. M., Glinski, J., and da Costa, T. B. F., et al. (2014). Reactivation of latent HIV-1 by new semi-synthetic ingenol esters. *Virology* 462–463, 328–339. doi: 10.1016/j.virol.2014.05.033

Panfil, A. R., London, J. A., Green, P. L., and Yoder, K. E. (2018). CRISPR/Cas9 genome editing to disable the latent HIV-1 provirus. *Front. Microbiol.* 9:3107. doi: 10.3389/fmicb.2018.03107

Patel, S., Jones, R. B., Nixon, D. F., and Bollard, C. M. (2016). T-cell therapies for HIV: preclinical successes and current clinical strategies. *Cytotherapy* 18, 931–942. doi: 10.1016/j.jcyt.2016.04.007

Periyasamy, P., Thangaraj, A., Bendi, V. S., and Buch, S. (2019). HIV-1 Tat-mediated microglial inflammation involves a novel miRNA-34a-NLRC5-NFκB signaling axis. *Brain. Behav. Immun.* 80, 227–237. doi: 10.1016/j.bbi.2019.03.011

Periyasamy, P., Thangaraj, A., Guo, M.-L., Hu, G., Callen, S., and Buch, S. (2018). Epigenetic promoter DNA methylation of miR-124 promotes HIV-1 Tat-mediated microglial activation via MECP2-STAT3 Axis. *J. Neurosci.* 38, 5367–5383. doi: 10.1523/JNEUROSCI.3474-17.2018

Pinskaya, M., and Morillon, A. (2009). Histone H3 lysine 4 di-methylation: a novel mark for transcriptional fidelity? *Epigenetics* 4, 302–306. doi: 10.4161/epi.4.5.9369

Qin, Y., Sun, X., Shao, X., Cheng, C., Feng, J., Sun, W., et al. (2015). Macrophage-microglia networks drive M1 microglia polarization after mycobacterium infection. *Inflammation* 38, 1609–1616. doi: 10.1007/s10753-015-0136-y

Qu, D., Sun, W.-W., Li, L., Ma, L., Sun, L., Jin, X., et al. (2019). Long noncoding RNA MALAT1 releases epigenetic silencing of HIV-1 replication by displacing the polycomb repressive complex 2 from binding to the LTR promoter. *Nucleic Acids Res.* 47, 3013–3027. doi: 10.1093/nar/gkz117

Rao, V. R., Ruiz, A. P., and Prasad, V. R. (2014). Viral and cellular factors underlying neuropathogenesis in HIV associated neurocognitive disorders (HAND). *AIDS Res. Ther.* 11:13. doi: 10.1186/1742-6405-11-13

Rawat, P., and Spector, S. A. (2017). Development and characterization of a human microglia cell model of HIV-1 infection. *J. Neurovirol.* 23, 33–46. doi: 10.1007/s13365-016-0472-1

Réu, P., Khosravi, A., Bernard, S., Mold, J. E., Salehpour, M., Alkass, K., et al. (2017). The lifespan and turnover of microglia in the human brain. *Cell Rep.* 20, 779–784. doi: 10.1016/j.celrep.2017.07.004

Rice, A. P. (2016). Cyclin-dependent kinases as therapeutic targets for HIV-1 infection. *Expert Opin. Ther. Targets* 20, 1453–1461. doi: 10.1080/14728222.2016.1254619

Richard, K., Williams, D. E., de Silva, E. D., Brockman, M. A., Brumme, Z. L., Andersen, R. J., et al. (2018). Identification of novel HIV-1 latency-reversing agents from a library of marine natural products. *Viruses* 10:348. doi: 10.3390/v10070348

Rock, R. B., and Peterson, P. K. (2006). Microglia as a pharmacological target in infectious and inflammatory diseases of the brain. *J. Neuroimmune Pharmacol.* 1, 117–126. doi: 10.1007/s11481-006-9012-8

Rodrigues, V., Ruffin,N., San-Roman, M., and Benaroch, P. (2017). Myeloid cell interaction with HIV: a complex relationship. *Front. Immunol.* 8:1698. doi: 10.3389/fimmu.2017.01698

Rohr, O., Lecestre, D., Chasserot-Golaz, S., Marban, C., Avram, D., Aunis, D., et al. (2003a). Recruitment of Tat to heterochromatin protein HP1 via interaction with CTIP2 inhibits human immunodeficiency virus type 1 replication in microglial cells. *J. Virol.* 77, 5415–5427. doi: 10.1128/JVI.77.9.5415-5427.2003

Rohr, O., Marban, C., Aunis, D., and Schaeffer, E. (2003b). Regulation of HIV-1 gene transcription: from lymphocytes to microglial cells. *J. Leukoc. Biol.* 74, 736–749. doi: 10.1189/jlb.0403180

Sadowski, I., and Hashemi, F. B. (2019). Strategies to eradicate HIV from infected patients: elimination of latent provirus reservoirs. *Cell. Mol. Life Sci.* 76, 3583–3600. doi: 10.1007/s00018-019-03156-8

Salemi, M., Lamers, S. L., Yu, S., de Oliveira, T., Fitch, W. M., and McGrath, M. S. (2005). Phylodynamic analysis of human immunodeficiency virus type 1 in distinct brain compartments provides a model for the neuropathogenesis of AIDS. *J. Virol.* 79, 11343–11352. doi: 10.1128/JVI.79.17.11343-11352.2005

Salemi, M., and Rife, B. (2016). Phylogenetics and phyloanatomy of HIV/SIV intra-host compartments and reservoirs: the key role of the central nervous system. *Curr. HIV Res.* 14, 110–120. doi: 10.2174/1570162X13666151029102413

Salter, M. W., and Stevens, B. (2017). Microglia emerge as central players in brain disease. *Nat. Med.* 23, 1018–1027. doi: 10.1038/nm.4397

Santerre, M., Bagashev, A., Gorecki, L., Lysek, K. Z., Wang, Y., Shrestha, J., et al. (2019). HIV-1 Tat protein promotes neuronal dysregulation by inhibiting E2F transcription factor 3 (E2F3). *J. Biol. Chem.* 294, 3618–3633. doi: 10.1074/jbc.RA118.003744

Sarracino, A., Gharu, L., Kula, A., Pasternak, A. O., Avettand-Fenoel, V., Rouzioux, C., et al. (2018). Posttranscriptional regulation of HIV-1 gene expression during replication and reactivation from latency by nuclear matrix protein MATR3. *MBio* 9:e02158-18. doi: 10.1128/mBio.02158-18

Scheper, H., van Holten,N., Hovens, J., and de Boer, M. (2018). Severe depression as a neuropsychiatric side effect induced by dolutegravir. *HIV Med.* 19, e58–e59. doi: 10.1111/hiv.12538

Schwartz, C., Bouchat, S., Marban, C., Gautier, V., Van Lint, C., Rohr, O., et al. (2017). On the way to find a cure: purging latent HIV-1 reservoirs. *Biochem. Pharmacol.* 146, 10–22. doi: 10.1016/j.bcp.2017.07.001

Schwartz, C., Catez, P., Rohr, O., Lecestre, D., Aunis, D., and Schaeffer, E. (2000). Functional interactions between C/EBP, Sp1, and COUP-TF regulate human immunodeficiency virus type 1 gene transcription in human brain cells. *J. Virol.* 74, 65–73. doi: 10.1128/JVI.74.1.65-73.2000

Scully, E., and Alter, G. (2016). NK cells in HIV disease. *Curr. HIV/AIDS Rep.* 13, 85–94. doi: 10.1007/s11904-016-0310-3

Sengupta, S., and Siliciano, R. F. (2018). Targeting the Latent Reservoir for HIV-1. *Immunity* 48, 872–895. doi: 10.1016/j.immuni.2018.04.030

Sharpe, A. H., and Abbas, A. K. (2006). T-cell costimulation–biology, therapeutic potential, and challenges. *N. Engl. J. Med.* 355, 973–975. doi: 10.1056/NEJMp068087

Sheng, J., Ruedl, C., and Karjalainen, K. (2015). Most tissue-resident macrophages except microglia are derived from fetal hematopoietic stem cells. *Immunity* 43, 382–393. doi: 10.1016/j.immuni.2015.07.016

Sheng, Z., Liu, Y., Li, H., Zheng, W., Xia, B., Zhang, X., et al. (2018). Efficacy of minocycline in acute ischemic stroke: a systematic review and meta-analysis of rodent and clinical studies. *Front. Neurol.* 9:1103. doi: 10.3389/fneur.2018.01103

Sinharay, S., and Hammoud, D. A. (2019). Brain PET imaging: value for understanding the pathophysiology of HIV-Associated Neurocognitive Disorder (HAND). *Curr. HIV/AIDS Rep.* 16, 66–75. doi: 10.1007/s11904-019-00419-8

Smit, T. K., Brew, B. J., Tourtellotte, W., Morgello, S., Gelman, B. B., and Saksena,N.K. (2004). Independent evolution of Human Immunodeficiency Virus (HIV) drug resistance mutations in diverse areas of the brain in HIV-infected patients, with and without dementia, on antiretroviral treatment. *J. Virol.* 78, 10133–10148. doi: 10.1128/JVI.78.18.10133-10148.2004

Sominsky, L., De Luca, S., and Spencer, S. J. (2018). Microglia: key players in neurodevelopment and neuronal plasticity. *Int. J. Biochem. Cell Biol.* 94, 56–60. doi: 10.1016/j.biocel.2017.11.012

Spivak, A. M., and Planelles, V. (2018). Novel latency reversal agents for HIV-1 cure. *Annu. Rev. Med.* 69, 421–436. doi: 10.1146/annurev-med-052716-031710

Strain, M. C., Letendre, S., Pillai, S. K., Russell, T., Ignacio, C. C., Gunthard, H. F., et al. (2005). Genetic composition of human immunodeficiency virus type 1 in cerebrospinal fluid and blood without treatment and during failing antiretroviral therapy. *J. Virol.* 79, 1772–1788. doi: 10.1128/JVI.79.3.1772-1788.2005

Su, H., Cheng, Y., Sravanam, S., Mathews, S., Gorantla, S., Poluektova, L. Y., et al. (2019). Immune activations and viral tissue compartmentalization during progressive HIV-1 infection of humanized mice. *Front. Immunol.* 10:340. doi: 10.3389/fimmu.2019.00340

Subra, C., and Trautmann, L. (2019). Role of T lymphocytes in HIV neuropathogenesis. *Curr. HIV/AIDS Rep.* 16, 236–243. doi: 10.1007/s11904-019-00445-6

Sumi, N., Nishioku, T., Takata, F., Matsumoto, J., Watanabe, T., Shuto, H., et al. (2010). Lipopolysaccharide-activated microglia induce dysfunction of the blood–brain barrier in rat microvascular endothelial cells co-cultured with microglia. *Cell. Mol. Neurobiol.* 30, 247–253. doi: 10.1007/s10571-009-9446-7

Sun, M., Li, Y., Zheng, H., and Shao, Y. (2016). Recent progress toward engineering HIV-1-specific neutralizing monoclonal antibodies. *Front. Immunol.* 7:391. doi: 10.3389/fimmu.2016.00391

Sung, J. M., and Margolis, D. M. (2018). HIV persistence on antiretroviral therapy and barriers to a cure. *Adv. Exp. Med. Biol.* 1075, 165–185. doi: 10.1007/978-981-13-0484-2_7

Sung, T.-L., and Rice, A. P. (2006). Effects of prostratin on Cyclin T1/P-TEFb function and the gene expression profile in primary resting CD4$^+$ T cells. *Retrovirology* 3:66. doi: 10.1186/1742-4690-3-66

Sutherland, E. J., and Brew, B. J. (2018). Human immunodeficiency virus and the nervous system. *Neurol. Clin.* 36, 751–765. doi: 10.1016/j.ncl.2018.07.002

Taniguchi, T., and Takaoka, A. (2002). The interferon-alpha/beta system in antiviral responses: a multimodal machinery of gene regulation by the IRF family of transcription factors. *Curr. Opin. Immunol.* 14, 111–116. doi: 10.1016/S0952-7915(01)00305-3

Tavazzi, E., Morrison, D., Sullivan, P., Morgello, S., and Fischer, T. (2014). Brain inflammation is a common feature of HIV-infected patients without HIV encephalitis or productive brain infection. *Curr. HIV Res.* 12, 97–110. doi: 10.2174/1570162X12666140526114956

Tesmer, V. M., and Bina, M. (1996). Regulation of HIV-1 gene expression by NF-IL6. *J. Mol. Biol.* 262, 327–335. doi: 10.1006/jmbi.1996.0516

Thompson, K. A., Cherry, C. L., Bell, J. E., and McLean, C. A. (2011). Brain cell reservoirs of latent virus in presymptomatic HIV-infected individuals. *Am. J. Pathol.* 179, 1623–1629. doi: 10.1016/j.ajpath.2011.06.039

Trautmann, L. (2016). Kill. *Curr. Opin. HIV AIDS* 11, 409–416. doi: 10.1097/COH.0000000000000286

Valcour, V., Paul, R., Chiao, S., Wendelken, L. A., and Miller, B. (2011). Screening for cognitive impairment in human immunodeficiency virus. *Clin. Infect. Dis.* 53, 836–842. doi: 10.1093/cid/cir524

Vanhamel, J., Bruggemans, A., and Debyser, Z. (2019). Establishment of latent HIV-1 reservoirs: what do we really know? *J. Virus Erad.* 5, 3–9.

Vaz, G. R., Hädrich, G., Bidone, J., Rodrigues, J. L., Falkembach, M. C., Putaux, J.-L., et al. (2017). Development of nasal lipid nanocarriers containing curcumin for brain targeting. *J. Alzheimers. Dis.* 59, 961–974. doi: 10.3233/JAD-160355

Vazquez, N., Greenwell-Wild, T., Marinos, N. J., Swaim, W. D., Nares, S., Ott, D. E., et al. (2005). Human immunodeficiency virus type 1-induced macrophage gene expression includes the p21 gene, a target for viral regulation. *J. Virol.* 79, 4479–4491. doi: 10.1128/JVI.79.7.4479-4491.2005

Veenhuis, R. T., Clements, J. E., and Gama, L. (2019). HIV eradication strategies: implications for the central nervous system. *Curr. HIV/AIDS Rep.* 16, 96–104. doi: 10.1007/s11904-019-00428-7

Veenstra, M., León-Rivera, R., Li, M., Gama, L., Clements, J. E., and Berman, J. W. (2017). Mechanisms of CNS viral seeding by HIV$^+$ CD14$^+$ CD16$^+$ monocytes: establishment and reseeding of viral reservoirs contributing to HIV-associated neurocognitive disorders. *MBio* 8:e01280-17. doi: 10.1128/mBio.01280-17

Venneti, S., Lopresti, B. J., Wang, G., Bissel, S. J., Mathis, C. A., Meltzer, C. C., et al. (2004). PET imaging of brain macrophages using the peripheral benzodiazepine receptor in a macaque model of neuroAIDS. *J. Clin. Invest.* 113, 981–989. doi: 10.1172/JCI20227

Vera, J. H., Guo, Q., Cole, J. H., Boasso, A., Greathead, L., Kelleher, P., et al. (2016). Neuroinflammation in treated HIV-positive individuals: a TSPO PET study. *Neurology* 86, 1425–1432. doi: 10.1212/WNL.0000000000002485

Wang, G., Zhao,N., Berkhout, B., and Das, A.T. (2016). CRISPR-Cas9 can inhibit HIV-1 replication but NHEJ repair facilitates virus escape. *Mol. Ther.* 24, 522–526. doi: 10.1038/mt.2016.24

Wang, G., Zhao,N., Berkhout, B., and Das, A.T. (2018). CRISPR-Cas based antiviral strategies against HIV-1. *Virus Res.* 244, 321–332. doi: 10.1016/j.virusres.2017.07.020

Wang, G. P., Ciuffi, A., Leipzig, J., Berry, C. C., and Bushman, F. D. (2007). HIV integration site selection: analysis by massively parallel pyrosequencing reveals association with epigenetic modifications. *Genome Res.* 17, 1186–1194. doi: 10.1101/gr.6286907

Wang, X., Ye, L., Hou, W., Zhou, Y., Wang, Y.-J., Metzger, D. S., et al. (2009). Cellular microRNA expression correlates with susceptibility of monocytes/macrophages to HIV-1 infection. *Blood* 113, 671–674. doi: 10.1182/blood-2008-09-175000

Wang, Z., Pan, Q., Gendron, P., Zhu, W., Guo, F., Cen, S., et al. (2016). CRISPR/Cas9-derived mutations both inhibit HIV-1 replication and accelerate viral escape. *Cell Rep.* 15, 481–489. doi: 10.1016/j.celrep.2016.03.042

Weinberger, A. D., and Weinberger, L. S. (2013). Stochastic fate selection in HIV-infected patients. *Cell* 155, 497–499. doi: 10.1016/j.cell.2013.09.039

Whitney, J. B., Hill, A. L., Sanisetty, S., Penaloza-MacMaster, P., Liu, J., Shetty, M., et al. (2014). Rapid seeding of the viral reservoir prior to SIV viraemia in rhesus monkeys. *Nature* 512, 74–77. doi: 10.1038/nature13594

Williams, D. W., Eugenin, E. A., Calderon, T. M., and Berman, J. W. (2012). Monocyte maturation, HIV susceptibility, and transmigration across the blood brain barrier are critical in HIV neuropathogenesis. *J. Leukoc. Biol.* 91, 401–415. doi: 10.1189/jlb.0811394

Wong, M. E., Jaworowski, A., and Hearps, A. C. (2019). The HIV reservoir in monocytes and macrophages. *Front. Immunol.* 10:1435. doi: 10.3389/fimmu.2019.01435

Woods, S. P., Morgan, E. E., Marquie-Beck, J., Carey, C. L., and Grant, I., Letendre, S. L., et al. (2006). Markers of macrophage activation and axonal injury are associated with prospective memory in HIV-1 disease. *Cogn. Behav. Neurol.* 19, 217–221. doi: 10.1097/01.wnn.0000213916.10514.57

Xiao, Q., Guo, D., and Chen, S. (2019). Application of CRISPR/Cas9-based gene editing in HIV-1/AIDS therapy. *Front. Cell. Infect. Microbiol.* 9:69. doi: 10.3389/fcimb.2019.00069

Xu, H., Wang, Z., Li, J., Wu, H., Peng, Y., Fan, L., et al. (2017). The polarization states of microglia in TBI: a new paradigm for pharmacological intervention. *Neural Plast.* 2017, 1–11. doi: 10.1155/2017/5405104

Yadav, A., and Collman, R. G. (2009). CNS inflammation and macrophage/microglial biology associated with HIV-1 infection. *J. Neuroimmune Pharmacol.* 4, 430–447. doi: 10.1007/s11481-009-9174-2

Yee, J.-K. (2016). Off-target effects of engineered nucleases. *FEBS J.* 283, 3239–3248. doi: 10.1111/febs.13760

Yenari, M. A., Xu, L., Tang, X. N., Qiao, Y., and Giffard, R. G. (2006). Microglia potentiate damage to blood-brain barrier constituents: improvement by minocycline *in vivo* and *in vitro*. *Stroke* 37, 1087–1093. doi: 10.1161/01.STR.0000206281.77178.ac

Yoder, K. E., and Bundschuh, R. (2016). Host double strand break repair generates HIV-1 strains resistant to CRISPR/Cas9. *Sci. Rep.* 6:29530. doi: 10.1038/srep29530

Zhang, Y., Yin, C., Zhang, T., Li, F., Yang, W., Kaminski, R., et al. (2015). CRISPR/gRNA-directed synergistic activation mediator (SAM) induces specific, persistent and robust reactivation of the HIV-1 latent reservoirs. *Sci. Rep.* 5:16277. doi: 10.1038/srep16277

Zhou, Y., Tang, H., and Xiong, H. (2016). Chemokine CCL2 enhances NMDA receptor-mediated excitatory postsynaptic current in rat hippocampal slices-a potential mechanism for HIV-1-associated neuropathy? *J. Neuroimmune Pharmacol.* 11, 306–315. doi: 10.1007/s11481-016-9660-2

Zhu, L. J., Lawrence, M., Gupta, A., Pagès, H., Kucukural, A., Garber, M., et al. (2017). GUIDEseq: a bioconductor package to analyze GUIDE-Seq datasets for CRISPR-Cas nucleases. *BMC Genomics* 18:379. doi: 10.1186/s12864-017-3746-y

12

The Quest for Cellular Markers of HIV Reservoirs: Any Color You Like

Gilles Darcis[1,2]*, *Ben Berkhout*[1] *and Alexander O. Pasternak*[1]*

[1] *Laboratory of Experimental Virology, Department of Medical Microbiology, Amsterdam UMC, University of Amsterdam, Amsterdam, Netherlands,* [2] *Infectious Diseases Department, Liège University Hospital, Liège, Belgium*

***Correspondence:**
Gilles Darcis
gdarcis@chuliege.be
Alexander O. Pasternak
a.o.pasternak@amc.uva.nl

Combination antiretroviral therapy (ART) suppresses human immunodeficiency virus (HIV) replication and improves immune function, but is unable to eradicate the virus. Therefore, development of an HIV cure has become one of the main priorities of the HIV research field. The main obstacle for an HIV cure is the formation of latent viral reservoirs, where the virus is able to "hide" despite decades of therapy, just to reignite active replication once therapy is stopped. Revealing HIV hiding places is thus central to HIV cure research, but the absence of markers of these reservoir cells greatly complicates the search for a cure. Identification of one or several marker(s) of latently infected cells would represent a significant step forward toward a better description of the cell types involved and improved understanding of HIV latency. Moreover, it could provide a "handle" for selective therapeutic targeting of the reservoirs. A number of cellular markers of HIV reservoir have recently been proposed, including immune checkpoint molecules, CD2, and CD30. CD32a is perhaps the most promising of HIV reservoir markers as it is reported to be associated with a very prominent enrichment in HIV DNA, although this finding has been challenged. In this review, we provide an update on the current knowledge about HIV reservoir markers. We specifically highlight studies that characterized markers of persistently infected cells in the lymphoid tissues.

Keywords: HIV, biomarker, viral reservoirs, HIV latent reservoir, HIV persistence

INTRODUCTION

Antiretroviral therapy (ART) allows the clinical management of the vast majority of human immunodeficiency virus (HIV) infected individuals, resulting in the prevention of AIDS and in the drastic reduction of the virus transmission risk. Unfortunately, ART is not curative. Interruption of therapy almost invariably leads to a quick viral rebound to pre-ART levels (1–6). Moreover, chronic immune activation and inflammation despite ART contribute to the excessive risk of non-AIDS events in ART-treated individuals (7). The etiology of persistent immune activation in the context of successful ART is considered multifactorial and involves microbial translocation, co-infections, metabolic disorders, regulatory T cell (Treg) deficiency, and decreased thymic function (8–11).

Presence of latent HIV reservoirs forms the major obstacle to an HIV cure. There is currently no consensus definition of the viral reservoirs due to their heterogeneous and dynamic nature. Viral reservoirs are commonly defined as cell types or anatomical sites that support the long-term persistence of replication-competent virus (12–14). This definition limits the HIV reservoirs to proviruses capable of triggering viral rebound after ART interruption (15). However, there is evidence that some defective proviruses that cannot reignite infection may still elicit immune activation through the production of viral proteins or novel antigens and thus participate in residual

HIV pathogenesis (16–19). The eradication of this fraction of the HIV reservoir should therefore also be considered in the context of a durable cure. This concept led to extension of the HIV reservoir definition to all infected cells (20–22).

The definition of the HIV latent reservoir was initially restricted to transcriptionally silent proviruses (12). However, HIV post-integration latency is a multifactorial phenomenon controlled by mechanisms that operate not only at the transcriptional but also posttranscriptional levels (e.g., splicing and nuclear export of HIV RNA, translation, viral particle assembly, and maturation) (23, 24). These multiple blocks to virus production (25, 26) explain why subsets of latently infected cells in individuals on long-term ART can express HIV RNA and proteins (27–29). Such latently infected but transcription-competent cells have been defined as active HIV reservoirs (30–32). HIV latency has thus to be seen as a continuum with blocks to productive infection at different stages of the viral replication cycle in different populations of latently infected cells (33, 34). It has therefore been suggested to avoid the word "latent" when describing these cellular HIV reservoirs (22), and the term "leaky latency" has been proposed (Conference on Retroviruses and Opportunistic Infections 2015). However, it might be more practical to use a wider definition of HIV latency, integrating all the transcriptional and post-transcriptional blocks to virus production (34). Interestingly, those blocks are not "frozen" but can evolve over time. For instance, DNA methylation of the HIV promoter progressively increases during ART, possibly strengthening HIV latency (35). HIV reservoir expression also leads to clearance of infected cells due to immune surveillance or viral cytotoxicity, as suggested by a recent longitudinal HIV sequencing study (36). Prolonged ART is consequently associated with enrichment for proviral sequences that exhibit multiple features of deeper latency, such as positioning of the provirus in intergenic regions, in opposite orientation to host genes, and in either proximity to or increased distance from host transcription start sites and accessible chromatin (37).

In summary, a complex interplay of viral and host factors is continuously reshaping the HIV reservoirs. Moreover, this likely varies in different tissues, which are characterized by different anatomic properties and enriched for specific CD4$^+$ T-cell subsets. It is therefore not surprising that mechanisms underlying HIV latency might differ between the peripheral blood and the tissues, as recently proposed (38). Viral and host markers of HIV reservoirs have been the focus of two recent reviews (39, 40). Here, we provide an update on some recent developments in the quest to distinguish the HIV reservoir cells from the plethora of cells in blood and tissues of an infected individual.

HETEROGENEOUS NATURE OF HIV RESERVOIRS

Understanding the cell types and anatomical sites that harbor latent HIV proviruses is essential for the design of therapeutic strategies to eradicate HIV from an infected individual. The developmental profile of a memory T cell has been increasingly well conceptualized, and is currently best characterized as a linear program during which highly immature, long-lasting memory T cells progressively transition toward more mature, differentiated and short-lived effector-memory cells (41, 42). HIV can persist in stem cell-like memory (T_{SCM}), central (T_{CM}), transitional (T_{TM}), and effector (T_{EM}) memory CD4$^+$ T cells, in addition to naïve (T_N) CD4$^+$ T cells (43–47). Although the frequency of HIV-infected cells is lower in T_N compared to T_{CM}, Zerbato et al. demonstrated that T_N harbor a large inducible reservoir of replication-competent HIV, suggesting that T_N cells may constitute an important HIV reservoir (48). Confirming these results, Venanzi Rullo et al. recently reported a large proportion of intact proviruses in T_N from two ART-treated subjects (49). Hiener et al. showed that, among memory CD4$^+$ T cells, T_{EM} contain the larger proportion of intact HIV genomes (50). These studies indicate that the advent of improved culture- or PCR-based assays to measure the different reservoirs does seriously challenge the dogma that resting CD4$^+$ memory T cells constitute the main HIV reservoir.

T cells can also be categorized according to functional properties, defined by specific antimicrobial properties or distinctive cytokine secretion patterns. Th1, Th2, Th17, Th9, regulatory T cell (Treg), and follicular T helper cell (Tfh) T-cell subpopulations have been identified based on functional polarization (42). Functionally polarized CD4$^+$ T cells can support HIV persistence by distinct mechanisms related to their discrete functional profiles. Functional commitment toward a Th1 profile is possible during all stages of memory CD4$^+$ T-cell development including the most immature and most durable subpopulations (51). Interestingly, proliferation of HIV-infected Th1 cells can play a crucial role in HIV persistence by maintaining the number of cells that harbor intact, replication-competent HIV (52). Recent evidence also highlights the contribution of long-lived Th17 cells to HIV persistence during ART, particularly in the gut (53). Th1/17 cells have been understood as a long-lasting subpopulation that may be somewhat more mature than Th17 cells, but retain the developmental program of long-lasting precursor cells for effector lymphocytes (54). CD4$^+$ T cells enriched for Th1/17 polarization harbor high levels of HIV DNA in ART treated individuals and contribute disproportionately to the viral reservoirs that remain stable over many years of ART (45, 55).

Besides the gut and the lymph nodes (LN) that constitute major anatomical sites for HIV persistence, multiple other tissues and organs harbor HIV provirus in ART-suppressed individuals (56). Besides T cells, other cell types such as monocytes, astrocytes and tissue resident macrophages (splenic, alveolar, and microglia) may potentially serve as stable viral reservoirs in the tissues (20, 57–63). Given the difficulties in accessing tissue biopsies from humans, animal models such as humanized mouse models or SIV-infected non-human primate (NHP) models have been very helpful for examining HIV dynamics. These models have been used to show the persistence of HIV reservoirs in various tissues of HIV- or SIV-suppressed animals, with new tools allowing for demonstrating the intactness of these reservoirs (64–66).

Altogether, these studies highlight the highly heterogeneous nature of HIV reservoirs and underline the urgent need for identification of marker(s) of latently infected cells. Such markers could provide a "handle" to further dissect the complex and dynamic nature of the reservoirs and might even enable their selective targeting for eradication (67, 68). So far, no cellular marker has been discovered that is capable of identifying all HIV reservoirs. However, several HIV reservoir markers have recently been proposed and their further characterization could represent a significant step toward a better understanding of the HIV reservoirs.

IMMUNE CHECKPOINT MOLECULES

In chronic viral infections, high antigenic loads constantly stimulate T cells, resulting in progressive loss of function termed T-cell exhaustion (69, 70). During this period, T cells demonstrate increased expression of some inhibitory receptors, known as immune checkpoint molecules (ICs), which increase the threshold for activation, leading to suppressed immune responses. Such ICs include programmed cell death-1 (PD-1), cytotoxic T-lymphocyte-associated protein 4 (CTLA-4), lymphocyte activation gene 3 (LAG-3), T cell immunoglobulin, and ITIM domain (TIGIT), T cell immunoglobulin and mucin 3 (TIM-3), CD160, and 2B4 (CD244). Fromentin et al. showed that expression of PD-1, LAG-3, and TIGIT in $CD4^+$ T cells was positively associated with the frequency of cells harboring integrated HIV DNA (71). More importantly, they observed that cells expressing these markers were enriched for HIV infection in several memory $CD4^+$ T-cell subsets during ART. The majority of inducible HIV proviruses were found in memory $CD4^+$ T cells that expressed at least one of these markers (71). More recently, the same group demonstrated a modest enrichment for HIV capsid (CA-p24)-producing cells (5.4-fold) in ART-suppressed individuals-derived cells displaying a $CD45RA^-$, $\alpha4\beta1^+$, $TIGIT^+$ phenotype (72). In line with these studies, Fromentin et al. recently reported that *ex vivo* HIV reactivation from latency is enhanced by a PD-1 blockade in $CD4^+$ T cells from ART-suppressed individuals (73), although another group could not demonstrate such effect (74). In addition, Hurst et al. found that the expression of ICs measured prior to ART predicts time to viral rebound following ART interruption, confirming that T-cell exhaustion markers can identify latently infected cells with a higher tendency to viral transcription (75).

LN $PD\text{-}1^+$/Tfh cells, as well as their circulating counterpart in peripheral blood ($CXCR3^+CD4^+$), represent a major cellular location for persistent virus in untreated and treated HIV-infected individuals, as demonstrated by the Perreau group (76–78). Notably, Tfh are localized to the germinal centers within the LN B-cell follicles, which are an immunologically privileged site with restricted CTL function (79). This may explain why $PD\text{-}1^+$/Tfh cells are enriched in replication-competent HIV as compared to any other PD-1 negative memory $CD4^+$ T-cell population isolated from blood or LN (77). However, intracellular concentrations of a number of antiretroviral drugs have been shown to be reduced in LN compared to peripheral blood (80–82), providing another possible reason for the persistence of infectious virus in the LNs. Interestingly, McGary et al. reported that $CTLA\text{-}4^+PD\text{-}1^-$ memory $CD4^+$ T cells significantly contribute to SIV persistence in ART-treated rhesus macaques (83). $CTLA\text{-}4^+PD\text{-}1^-$ memory $CD4^+$ T cells, a subset comprised predominantly of Tregs, were shown to be enriched for SIV DNA in several tissues and to contain replication-competent and infectious virus. In contrast to $PD\text{-}1^+$/Tfh cells, SIV-enriched $CTLA\text{-}4^+PD\text{-}1^-$ Treg cells localized outside the LN B-cell follicle. Moreover, in HIV-infected individuals on ART, $CTLA\text{-}4^+PD\text{-}1^-$ memory $CD4^+$ T cells harboring HIV DNA also persisted outside the B-cell follicle and contributed to the long-term latent viral reservoir (83).

Better definition of the parameters that dictate exhaustion is promoting the development of methods that prevent functionally inferior responses or "revitalize" them (84). IC inhibitors are already currently used to treat malignancies. This treatment would work for HIV infection in two ways: through boosting HIV-specific $CD8^+$ T-cell effector function and through reactivating HIV expression from latency (85, 86). However, the case reports and clinical trials investigating the use of IC blockers have produced conflicting results (87, 88). Toxicity also appears as an important concern (89).

CD2, CD30, AND CD20

Using an *in vitro* primary $CD4^+$ T-cell model for HIV post-integration latency (90), Iglesias-Ussel et al. studied the expression profile of latently infected $CD4^+$ T cells (91). Among the markers identified in this study, CD2 was selected for further analysis. Resting memory $CD4^+$ $CD2^{high}$ T cells harbored higher HIV DNA copy numbers compared with the other cell subsets, although the fold enrichment was limited (5.7-fold). Iglesias-Ussel et al. further showed that $CD4^+$ $CD2^{high}$ T cells could be stimulated to express high levels of HIV RNA, although no evidence was provided that infectious viruses could be produced (91). In contrast to the other markers described in this review and for which some tissue data is available, the relevance of CD2 still has to be confirmed in lymphoid tissues.

CD30 is expressed in Hodgkin and other aggressive lymphomas and on a small fraction of lymphocytes in healthy individuals (92). CD30 expression can be triggered by infections with several viruses, including human T-cell lymphotropic virus and Epstein-Barr virus (92). It is known for more than 20 years that triggering CD30 may play an important role in both HIV replication and HIV-infected $CD4^+$ T-cell death (93). More recently, Hogan et al. demonstrated that $CD30^+CD4^+$ T cells were significantly enriched for cell-associated HIV RNA but not for HIV DNA in several individuals regardless of ART use (94). CD30 expression and HIV transcriptional activity co-localized in gut-associated lymphoid tissue from ART-treated or ART-naïve individuals. Following *ex vivo* culture of peripheral blood cells in the presence of brentuximab vedotin, an anti-CD30 antibody-drug conjugate, they observed a significant reduction in total HIV DNA. These data suggested that CD30 may be a relevant HIV therapeutic target as it is not expressed on a vast majority of cells (93). Subsequently, the same group studied the impact of 3 doses of brentuximab vedotin therapy for Hodgkin lymphoma on HIV persistence and immune phenotype in an individual on long-term ART (95). An encouraging but transient reduction of $CD4^+$ T cells expressing CD30 was observed, accompanied by reductions in $CD4^+$ T-cell–associated HIV RNA, low-level plasma viremia, and to lesser extent HIV DNA levels (95). The reason for the lack of a sustained effect of brentuximab vedotin on CD30-expressing T cells is currently unknown.

Very recently, Serra-Peinado et al. reported a higher percentage of HIV RNA^+ cells among cells expressing CD20 (96). CD20 is a known B-cell surface marker but is dimly expressed on a small subpopulation of $CD4^+$ T cells. Although the contribution of $CD20^{dim}CD4^+$ T cells to the total pool of HIV RNA^+ cells was modest (median of 18.6% in ART-treated and 25.0% in viremic HIV-infected individuals), *ex vivo* treatment of primary peripheral blood mononuclear cells (PBMCs) from ART-suppressed individuals with the anti-CD20 monoclonal antibody Rituximab appeared to reduce the pool of HIV RNA^+ cells when combined with latency-reversing agents (96). Further studies are needed to elucidate whether Rituximab treatment is also capable of reducing the total or intact HIV DNA reservoir.

CD32a

CD32a, also known as Fc gamma receptor IIa (FcγIIa), is the low-affinity receptor for the immunoglobulin G Fc fragment that is highly expressed on myeloid cells and expressed on a small subset of T cells (97, 98). CD32a was recently proposed by Descours et al. as a marker of HIV reservoir cells (99). Notably, CD32 has already been identified by an earlier study among several surface markers overexpressed in latently infected vs. uninfected $CD4^+$ T cells in a primary $CD4^+$ T-cell model for HIV latency (91). In contrast to all the markers described above that are associated with very limited HIV DNA enrichment, an extremely high (~1,000-fold) enrichment in HIV DNA was observed by Descours et al. in $CD4^+$ T cells with high CD32a expression as compared to $CD32^-CD4^+$ T cells (99). They also demonstrated an enrichment for replication-competent proviruses in these cells, although not to a higher degree than the enrichment for total HIV DNA. If confirmed, these findings would represent a milestone in the efforts to develop a cure for HIV infection. However, a number of subsequent reports questioned whether CD32a would be a *bona fide* marker of the HIV latent reservoir (100–105), which decreased the initial enthusiasm. Some studies observed limited enrichment for HIV DNA in $CD32^+$ cells in some participants but not in others (101, 102). Other reports could not demonstrate any enrichment for total HIV DNA or for replication-competent proviruses in $CD32^+$ cells (100, 103–105).

The key for this controversy likely resides in the technical difficulty to obtain a sufficiently pure population of *bona fide* $CD32^+CD4^+$ T cells. The frequency of $CD32^+$ cells among antigen-presenting cells (APCs) is much higher than among $CD4^+$ T cells. Therefore, even if the residual APC contamination of $CD4^+$ T cells is low in general, APCs will be disproportionally overrepresented in the $CD32^+$ fraction, as reported by several groups (101, 103) and also observed in our initial attempts to purify $CD32^+CD4^+$ cells (**Figure 1A**) (106). The excess of residual non-T cells in the sorted $CD32^+$ fraction can easily obscure the enrichment for HIV DNA in $CD32^+CD4^+$ cells. Alternatively, certain cell sorting strategies and/or settings might result in the isolation of T-B cell doublets or conjugates instead of *bona fide* $CD32^+CD4^+$ T cells, as reported by two groups (105, 107). Because another CD32 isoform, CD32b, is highly expressed on the surface of B cells, and consequently on T-B cell doublets or conjugates, the latter cells may be preferentially recognized during FACS sorting for $CD32^+CD4^+$ cells as most anti-CD32 antibodies do not discriminate between the CD32a and CD32b isoforms. The extracellular domains of these two proteins are very similar, and no CD32a-specific antibody is available yet. Depending on the sorting settings and/or antibody titers, *bona fide* $CD32^+CD4^+$ T cells, which likely express less CD32 molecules per cell than T-B cell doublets/conjugates, might be missed, unless specific efforts are made to thoroughly deplete the $CD32^+$ non-T cells.

To overcome these problems, we performed two consecutive rounds of $CD4^+$ T-cell negative selection by magnetic cell sorting before we started with $CD32^+$ cell isolation. This sequential cell purification strategy could efficiently deplete the vast majority of contaminating non-T cells, including any T-B cell doublets, which allowed us to obtain a purified population of $CD32^+CD4^+$ cells (**Figure 1B**) (106). Remarkably, we demonstrated a progressive increase in HIV DNA enrichment in $CD32^+CD4^+$ cells with further purification of these cells, and in the purified population we measured a very prominent enrichment for HIV DNA (average, 292-fold) (106), confirming the results of Descours et al. (99). Interestingly, several groups found that the majority of peripheral blood $CD32^+CD4^+$ T cells express the activation marker HLA-DR (100–102, 106, 108, 109). Although it has been shown previously that HIV can establish latent infection in activated $CD4^+$ T cells (110, 111) and that the peripheral blood HIV DNA load is higher in activated compared to resting cells in ART-treated individuals (112), the existence of latently infected CD4+ cells that are activated, and therefore relatively short-lived, suggests continuous replenishment of this component of the reservoir by cellular proliferation (113). At present, however, high HLA-DR expression on $CD32^+CD4^+$ cells should be interpreted with caution, as it cannot be ruled out that the HLA-DR signal may partly originate from the non-T cells within the contaminating $CD32^+$ T-non-T cell doublets or conjugates, as recently demonstrated by Thornhill et al. (107).

Persistence of $CD32^+$ cells has also been studied in tissues. Abdel-Mohsen et al. showed that a high percentage of HIV-expressing cells localized within the B-cell follicle co-express CD32a, whereas CD32a single-positive cells were rarely observed (100). These RNA *in situ* hybridization (ISH) experiments showing the co-expression of CD32a RNA and HIV RNA in lymphoid tissue support the notion that CD32a is associated with transcriptionally active tissue reservoirs. Similar results were recently obtained by Vásquez et al. in the gut tissue (114). By using ISH-based methods, they demonstrated co-expression of HIV and CD32a mRNA, with most of the $CD3^+CD32^+$

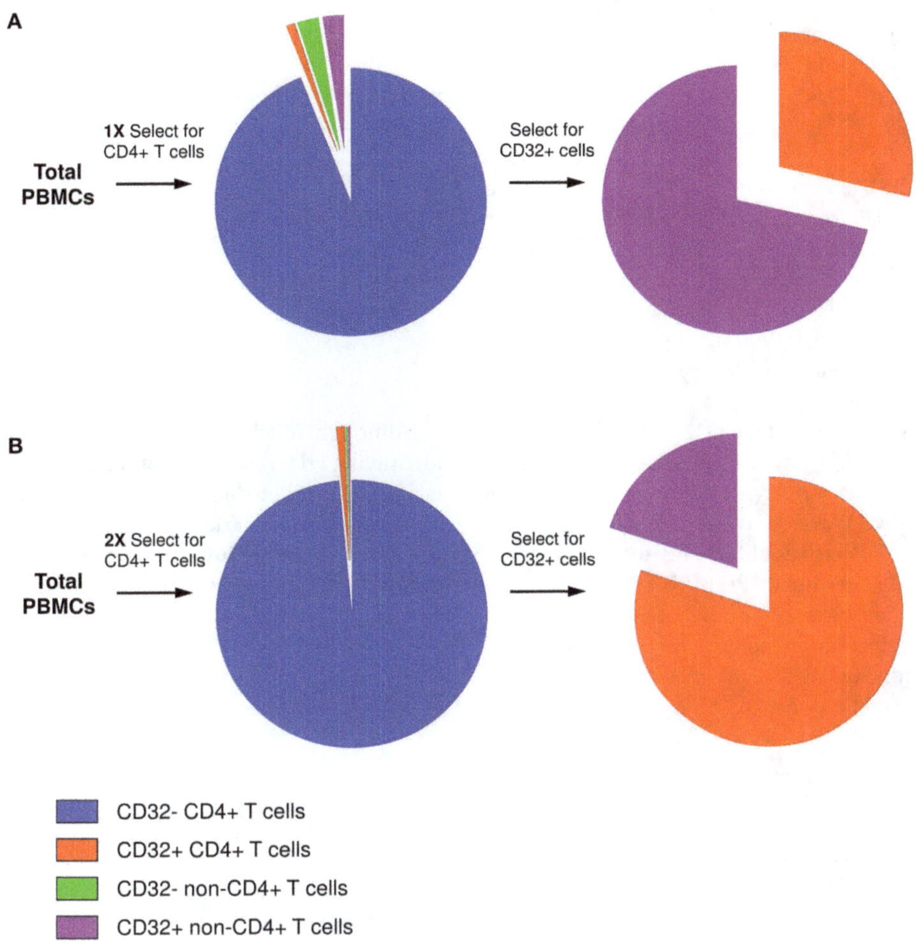

FIGURE 1 | Presence of residual non-CD4$^+$ T cells in the CD32$^+$ cell fraction. **(A)** After one round of selection for CD4$^+$ T cells, although the residual non-CD4$^+$ T-cell contamination is low in general, the percentage of CD32$^+$ cells among non-T cells is much higher than among CD4$^+$ T cells. Therefore, after selection for CD32-expressing cells, the majority of CD32$^+$ cells will be non-T cells. **(B)** Two consecutive rounds of CD4$^+$ T-cell selection result in much purer CD4$^+$ T-cell population, and the majority of CD4$^+$ T cells is maintained even in the CD32$^+$ fraction.

cells in the gut co-expressing HIV RNA. Moreover, Thornhill et al. recently found that the T cells within the CD32$^+$ T-B cell doublets in the gut and tonsil tissues of ART-treated individuals were associated with a Tfh phenotype (107). As Tfh cells have been previously shown to harbor high levels of HIV RNA and infectious virus in LN (77), this may provide a clue why CD32$^+$ cells are associated with HIV transcription in tissues.

Two groups studied co-expression of CD32a and other HIV reservoir markers in tissues. Noto et al. analyzed HIV transcription in LN memory CD4$^+$ T-cell populations sorted for CD32a and PD-1 expression (108). The CD32$^+$ and PD-1$^+$ CD4$^+$ T-cell populations overlapped to a large extent and CD32$^+$PD-1$^+$ cells were significantly enriched for HIV RNA compared to CD32$^-$PD-1$^-$, CD32$^+$PD-1$^-$, and CD32$^-$PD-1$^+$ cells. In the LNs, CD32$^+$ and PD-1$^+$ CD4$^+$ T cells expressed high levels of the HIV co-receptors CCR5 and CXCR4, potentially making these cells a preferential target for HIV infection, as well as higher levels of activation markers, which can explain why these cells are characterized by a high level of HIV transcription (108). Hogan et al. sorted rectal biopsy cells for the expression of CD32a and CD30 (94). The highest HIV RNA and DNA levels from rectal tissue-derived cells were measured in cells co-expressing CD30 and CD32. These two studies demonstrate that different HIV reservoir markers can be co-expressed on CD4$^+$ T cells, raising the possibility that there is some overlap in the reservoirs identified by these markers.

Taken together, these studies suggest an association between CD32a expression and active HIV transcription in tissues. In contrast, in peripheral blood we found no enrichment for cell-associated HIV RNA in CD32$^+$CD4$^+$ cells, and significantly reduced HIV RNA/DNA ratios were measured in these cells compared to CD32$^-$CD4$^+$ cells (106), indicating that HIV is transcriptionally silent in most of the infected peripheral blood CD32$^+$ cells and suggesting that CD32a indeed marks latently infected cells. These seemingly discrepant results might suggest differences in the underlying mechanisms of persistence of

HIV-infected CD32^{+} cells between blood and tissues. Residual HIV replication in tissue compartments can be quite prominent due to poor antiretroviral drug penetration (80–82, 115, 116) and CD32a expression in CD4^{+} T cells is induced upon *in vitro* HIV infection (29, 99, 100, 102). Therefore, in tissues, CD32a could mark cells that were recently infected despite ART. Alternatively, CD32a expression may be up-regulated upon re-activation of HIV transcription in long-lived latently infected cells in tissues, although the reverse association between HIV transcription and CD32a expression in peripheral blood makes this possibility less likely. To study the association between CD32a expression and HIV transcription in tissues, it will also be important to determine the relative contribution of CD32b^{+} T-B cell doublets vs. *bona fide* CD32a^{+}CD4^{+} T cells to the total pool of tissue CD32^{+} T cells, and to which extent these two cell types are associated with active HIV transcription vs. viral latency. Interestingly, Thornhill et al. observed a positive correlation between the frequency of Tfh cells in CD32^{+} T-B cell doublets and total HIV DNA in the rectum (but not terminal ileum or PBMC) (107), suggesting that these doublets might be associated with a higher level of HIV infection in some sites. As B cells are capable of transmission of infectious HIV to T cells via CD21-complement interactions or DC-SIGN-mediated virion capture (117, 118), some of the observed T-B cell doublets can even be involved in residual B-to-T-cell HIV trans-infection in tissues.

Despite the considerable interest triggered by the Descours study (99), many questions with regard to the CD32a-HIV link are still open. Mechanisms of CD32a expression in HIV-infected cells remain to be investigated, as well as the role of CD32a in HIV reservoir formation and/or persistence. Notably, the contribution of CD32^{+} CD4^{+} T cells to the HIV reservoirs seems to be highly variable from one HIV-infected individual to the other, both in peripheral blood and in tissues (94, 99, 100, 106). This may restrict the efficiency of CD32a therapeutic targeting for HIV reservoir eradication in some individuals. In general, targeting of CD32a alone is not a feasible option because this would deplete the majority of an individual's myeloid immune cells. However, advanced targeting strategies (e.g., bi- and tri-specific antibodies) can be used to guarantee high specificity of CD32^{+}CD4^{+} cell targeting. Targeting downstream CD32a signaling in CD4^{+} T cells could also be a feasible alternative.

CONCLUSIONS

The identification of a marker of latently infected cells has long been considered the "Holy Grail" of HIV cure programs (67). Several CD4^{+} T-cell subsets have been shown to harbor important HIV reservoirs, including resting memory CD4^{+} T cells. However, this picture is getting more complex every day as numerous other cell types were found to contribute to the HIV reservoirs. Activated T cells, naïve T cells, Tregs, Tfh, and their circulating counterpart, but also tissue macrophages, appear as major sites of HIV persistence.

Although much progress has been made in recent years in identifying HIV reservoir markers, no single cell surface molecule is currently able to mark all HIV-infected cells. However, some of the putative markers, including CD32a, CD30, and ICs, will likely play an important role in future studies aimed at understanding and eradicating the HIV reservoirs. Although a significant overlap was found in the expression of different HIV reservoir markers, targeting several markers at the same time in a "multicolor" approach may significantly increase the proportion of the reservoir that is eradicated.

AUTHOR CONTRIBUTIONS

AP, GD, and BB wrote the manuscript. AP made the figure. All authors approved the final manuscript.

ACKNOWLEDGMENTS

We are thankful to Jeroen den Dunnen and Rogier Sanders for helpful discussions. GD is post-doctorate clinical master specialist for the National Fund for Scientific Research (FNRS). The content is solely the responsibility of the authors and does not necessarily represent the official views of the National Institutes of Health. We thank the Rotary Foundation and the Fonds Léon Fredericq.

REFERENCES

Chun TW, Carruth L, Finzi D, Shen X, DiGiuseppe JA, Taylor H, et al. Quantification of latent tissue reservoirs and total body viral load in HIV-1 infection. *Nature.* (1997) 387:183–8. doi: 10.1038/387183a0

Chun TW, Finzi D, Margolick J, Chadwick K, Schwartz D, Siliciano RF. *In vivo* fate of HIV-1-infected T cells: quantitative analysis of the transition to stable latency. *Nat Med.* (1995) 1:1284–90. doi: 10.1038/nm1295-1284

Finzi D, Blankson J, Siliciano JD, Margolick JB, Chadwick K, Pierson T, et al. Latent infection of CD4+ T cells provides a mechanism for lifelong persistence of HIV-1, even in patients on effective combination therapy. *Nat Med.* (1999) 5:512–7. doi: 10.1038/8394

Siliciano JD, Kajdas J, Finzi D, Quinn TC, Chadwick K, Margolick JB, et al. Long-term follow-up studies confirm the stability of the latent reservoir for HIV-1 in resting CD4+ T cells. *Nat Med.* (2003) 9:727–8. doi: 10.1038/nm880

Chun TW, Davey RT Jr, Ostrowski M, Shawn Justement J, Engel D, Mullins JI, et al. Relationship between pre-existing viral reservoirs and the re- emergence of plasma viremia after discontinuation of highly active anti- retroviral therapy. *Nat Med.* (2000) 6:757–61. doi: 10.1038/77481

Davey RT Jr, Bhat N, Yoder C, Chun TW, Metcalf JA, Dewar R, et al. HIV-1 and T cell dynamics after interruption of highly active antiretroviral therapy (HAART) in patients with a history of sustained viral suppression. *Proc Natl Acad Sci USA.* (1999) 96:15109–14. doi: 10.1073/pnas.96.26.15109

Deeks SG, Tracy R, Douek DC. Systemic effects of inflammation on health during chronic HIV infection. *Immunity.* (2013) 39:633–45. doi: 10.1016/j.immuni.2013.10.001

Paiardini M, Muller-Trutwin M. HIV-associated chronic immune activation. *Immunol Rev.* (2013) 254:78–101. doi: 10.1111/imr.12079

Klatt NR, Chomont N, Douek DC, Deeks SG. Immune activation and HIV persistence: implications for curative approaches to HIV infection. *Immunol Rev.* (2013) 254:326–42. doi: 10.1111/imr.12065

Douek DC. Immune activation, HIV persistence, and the cure. *Top Antivir Med.* (2013) 21:128–32.

De Voeght A, Martens H, Renard C, Vaira D, Debruche M, Simonet J, et al. Exploring the link between innate immune activation and thymic function by measuring sCD14 and TRECs in HIV patients living in Belgium. *PLoS ONE.* (2017) 12:e0185761. doi: 10.1371/journal.pone.0185761

Darcis G, Van Driessche B, Van Lint C. HIV latency: should we shock or lock? *Trends Immunol.* (2017) 38:217–28. doi: 10.1016/j.it.2016.12.003

Pasternak AO, Berkhout B. HIV reservoir: finding the right needles in a needlestack. *Cell Host Microbe.* (2016) 20:280–2. doi: 10.1016/j.chom.2016.08.011

Eisele E, Siliciano RF. Redefining the viral reservoirs that prevent HIV-1 eradication. *Immunity.* (2012) 37:377–88. doi: 10.1016/j.immuni.2012.08.010

Bruner KM, Hosmane NN, Siliciano RF. Towards an HIV-1 cure: measuring the latent reservoir. *Trends Microbiol.* (2015) 23:192–203. doi: 10.1016/j.tim.2015.01.013

Imamichi H, Dewar RL, Adelsberger JW, Rehm CA, O'Doherty U, Paxinos EE, et al. Defective HIV-1 proviruses produce novel protein-coding RNA species in HIV-infected patients on combination antiretroviral therapy. *Proc Natl Acad Sci USA.* (2016) 113:8783–8. doi: 10.1073/pnas.1609057113

Pollack RA, Jones RB, Pertea M, Bruner KM, Martin AR, Thomas AS, et al. Defective HIV-1 proviruses are expressed and can be recognized by cytotoxic T lymphocytes, which shape the proviral landscape. *Cell Host Microbe.* (2017) 21:494–506.e4. doi: 10.1016/j.chom.2017.03.008

Sharaf R, Lee GQ, Sun X, Etemad B, Aboukhater LM, Hu Z, et al. HIV-1 proviral landscapes distinguish posttreatment controllers from noncontrollers. *J Clin Invest.* (2018) 128:4074–85. doi: 10.1172/JCI120549

Das AT, Pasternak AO, Berkhout B. On the generation of the MSD- \II class of defective HIV proviruses. *Retrovirology.* (2019) 16:19. doi: 10.1186/s12977-019-0481-2

Avettand-Fenoel V, Hocqueloux L, Ghosn J, Cheret A, Frange P, Melard A, et al. Total HIV-1 DNA, a marker of viral reservoir dynamics with clinical implications. *Clin Microbiol Rev.* (2016) 29:859–80. doi: 10.1128/CMR.00015-16

Douek DC. Disrupting T-cell homeostasis: how HIV-1 infection causes disease. *AIDS Rev.* (2003) 5:172–7.

Baxter AE, O'Doherty U, Kaufmann DE. Beyond the replication-competent HIV reservoir: transcription and translation-competent reservoirs. *Retrovirology.* (2018) 15:18. doi: 10.1186/s12977-018-0392-7

Karn J, Stoltzfus CM. Transcriptional and posttranscriptional regulation of HIV-1 gene expression. *Cold Spring Harb Perspect Med.* (2012) 2:a006916. doi: 10.1101/cshperspect.a006916

Khoury G, Darcis G, Lee MY, Bouchat S, Van Driessche B, Purcell DFJ, et al. The molecular biology of HIV latency. *Adv Exp Med Biol.* (2018) 1075:187–212. doi: 10.1007/978-981-13-0484-2_8

Kula A, Guerra J, Knezevich A, Kleva D, Myers MP, Marcello A. Characterization of the HIV-1 RNA associated proteome identifies Matrin 3 as a nuclear cofactor of Rev function. *Retrovirology.* (2011) 8:60. doi: 10.1186/1742-4690-8-60

Sarracino A, Gharu L, Kula A, Pasternak AO, Avettand-Fenoel V, Rouzioux C, et al. Posttranscriptional regulation of HIV-1 gene expression during replication and reactivation from latency by nuclear matrix protein MATR3. *MBio.* (2018) 9:e02158-18. doi: 10.1128/mBio.02158-18

DeMaster LK, Liu XH, VanBelzen DJ, Trinite B, Zheng LJ, Agosto LM, et al. A subset of CD4/CD8 double-negative T cells expresses HIV proteins in patients on antiretroviral therapy. *J Virol.* (2016) 90:2165–79. doi: 10.1128/JVI.01913-15

Baxter AE, Niessl J, Fromentin R, Richard J, Porichis F, Charlebois R, et al. Single-cell characterization of viral translation-competent reservoirs in HIV-infected individuals. *Cell Host Microbe.* (2016) 20:368–80. doi: 10.1016/j.chom.2016.07.015

Grau-Expósito J, Serra-Peinado C, Miguel L, Navarro J, Curran A, Burgos J, et al. A novel single-cell FISH-flow assay identifies effector memory CD4(+) T cells as a major niche for HIV-1 transcription in HIV-infected patients. *MBio.* (2017) 8:e00876-17. doi: 10.1128/mBio.00876-17

Pasternak AO, de Bruin M, Jurriaans S, Bakker M, Berkhout B, Prins JM, et al. Modest nonadherence to antiretroviral therapy promotes residual HIV-1 replication in the absence of virological rebound in plasma. *J Infect Dis.* (2012) 206:1443–52. doi: 10.1093/infdis/jis502

Van Gulck E, Bracke L, Heyndrickx L, Coppens S, Atkinson D, Merlin C, et al. Immune and viral correlates of "secondary viral control" after treatment interruption in chronically HIV-1 infected patients. *PLoS ONE.* (2012) 7:e37792. doi: 10.1371/journal.pone.0037792

Pasternak AO, Lukashov VV, Berkhout B. Cell-associated HIV RNA: a dynamic biomarker of viral persistence. *Retrovirology.* (2013) 10:41. doi: 10.1186/1742-4690-10-41

Pace MJ, Agosto L, Graf EH, O'Doherty U. HIV reservoirs and latency models. *Virology.* (2011) 411:344–54. doi: 10.1016/j.virol.2010.12.041

Pasternak AO, Berkhout B. What do we measure when we measure cell-associated HIV RNA. *Retrovirology.* (2018) 15:13. doi: 10.1186/s12977-018-0397-2

Trejbalova K, Kovarova D, Blazkova J, Machala L, Jilich D, Weber J, et al. Development of 5' LTR DNA methylation of latent HIV-1 provirus in cell line models and in long-term-infected individuals. *Clin Epigenetics.* (2016) 8:19. doi: 10.1186/s13148-016-0185-6

Pinzone MR, VanBelzen DJ, Weissman S, Bertuccio MP, Cannon L, Venanzi- Rullo E, et al. Longitudinal HIV sequencing reveals reservoir expression leading to decay which is obscured by clonal expansion. *Nat Commun.* (2019) 10:728. doi: 10.1038/s41467-019-08431-7

Einkauf KB, Lee GQ, Gao C, Sharaf R, Sun X, Hua S, et al. Intact HIV-1 proviruses accumulate at distinct chromosomal positions during prolonged antiretroviral therapy. *J Clin Invest.* (2019) 129:988–98. doi: 10.1172/JCI124291

Telwatte S, Lee S, Somsouk M, Hatano H, Baker C, Kaiser P, et al. Gut and blood differ in constitutive blocks to HIV transcription, suggesting tissue-specific differences in the mechanisms that govern HIV latency. *PLoS Pathog.* (2018) 14:e1007357. doi: 10.1371/journal.ppat.10 07357

Bruel T, Schwartz O. Markers of the HIV-1 reservoir: facts and controversies. *Curr Opin HIV AIDS.* (2018) 13:383–8. doi:10.1097/COH.0000000000000482

Sharaf RR, Li JZ. The alphabet soup of HIV reservoir markers. *Curr HIV/AIDS Rep.* (2017) 14:72–81. doi: 10.1007/s11904-017-0355-y

Jameson SC, Masopust D. Understanding subset diversity in T cell memory. *Immunity.* (2018) 48:214–26. doi: 10.1016/j.immuni.2018.02.010

Lee GQ, Lichterfeld M. Diversity of HIV-1 reservoirs in CD4+ T-cell subpopulations. *Curr Opin HIV AIDS.* (2016) 11:383–7. doi:10.1097/COH.0000000000000281

Wightman F, Solomon A, Khoury G, Green JA, Gray L, Gorry PR, et al. Both CD31(+) and CD31$^-$ naive CD4(+) T cells are persistent HIV type 1-infected reservoirs in individuals receiving antiretroviral therapy. *J Infect Dis.* (2010) 202:1738–48. doi: 10.1086/656721

Chomont N, El-Far M, Ancuta P, Trautmann L, Procopio FA, Yassine- Diab B, et al. HIV reservoir size and persistence are driven by T cell survival and homeostatic proliferation. *Nat Med.* (2009) 15:893–900. doi:10.1038/nm.1972

Khoury G, Anderson JL, Fromentin R, Hartogenesis W, Smith MZ, Bacchetti P, et al. Persistence of integrated HIV DNA in CXCR3 + CCR6 + memory CD4+ T cells in HIV-infected individuals on antiretroviral therapy. *AIDS.* (2016) 30:1511–20. doi: 10.1097/QAD.0000000000 001029

Buzon MJ, Sun H, Li C, Shaw A, Seiss K, Ouyang Z, et al. HIV-1 persistence in CD4+ T cells with stem cell-like properties. *Nat Med.* (2014) 20:139–42. doi: 10.1038/nm.3445

Gattinoni L, Lugli E, Ji Y, Pos Z, Paulos CM, Quigley MF, et al. A human memory T cell subset with stem cell-like properties. *Nat Med.* (2011) 17:1290–7. doi: 10.1038/nm.2446

Zerbato JM, McMahon DK, Sobolewski MD, Mellors JW, Sluis-Cremer N. Naive CD4+ T cells harbor a large inducible reservoir of latent, replication-competent HIV-1. *Clin Infect Dis.* (2019). doi: 10.1093/cid/ciz108. [Epub ahead of print].

Venanzi Rullo E, Cannon L, Pinzone MR, Ceccarelli M, Nunnari G, O'Doherty U. Genetic evidence that Naïve T cells can contribute significantly to the HIV intact reservoir: time to re-evaluate their role. *Clin Infect Dis.* (2019) ciz378. doi: 10.1093/cid/ciz378. [Epub ahead of print].

Hiener B, Horsburgh BA, Eden JS, Barton K, Schlub TE, Lee E, et al. Identification of genetically intact HIV-1 proviruses in specific CD4(+) T cells from effectively treated participants. *Cell Rep.* (2017) 21:813–22. doi: 10.1016/j.celrep.2017.09.081

Takeshita M, Suzuki K, Kassai Y, Takiguchi M, Nakayama Y, Otomo Y, et al. Polarization diversity of human CD4+ stem cell memory T cells. *Clin Immunol.* (2015) 159:107–17. doi: 10.1016/j.clim.2015.04.010

Lee GQ, Orlova-Fink N, Einkauf K, Chowdhury FZ, Sun X, Harrington S, et al. Clonal expansion of genome-intact HIV-1 in functionally polarized Th1 CD4+ T cells. *J Clin Invest.* (2017) 127:2689–96. doi: 10.1172/JCI93289

Gosselin A, Wiche Salinas TR, Planas D, Wacleche VS, Zhang Y, Fromentin R, et al. HIV persists in CCR6+CD4+ T cells from colon and blood during antiretroviral therapy. *AIDS.* (2017) 31:35–48. doi:10.1097/QAD.0000000000001309

Muranski P, Restifo NP. Essentials of Th17 cell commitment and plasticity. *Blood.*

(2013) 121:2402–14. doi: 10.1182/blood-2012-09-378653

Sun H, Kim D, Li X, Kiselinova M, Ouyang Z, Vandekerckhove L, et al. Th1/17 polarization of CD4 T cells supports HIV-1 persistence during antiretroviral therapy. *J Virol.* (2015) 89:11284–93. doi: 10.1128/JVI.01595-15

Couturier J, Lewis DE. HIV persistence in adipose tissue reservoirs. *Curr HIV/AIDS Rep.* (2018) 15:60–71. doi: 10.1007/s11904-018-0378-z

Abreu CM, Veenhuis RT, Avalos CR, Graham S, Queen SE, Shirk EN, et al. Infectious virus persists in CD4+ T cells and macrophages in ART-suppressed SIV-infected Macaques. *J Virol.* (2019) 93:e00065-19. doi: 10.1128/JVI.00065-19

Kumar A, Darcis G, Van Lint C, Herbein G. Epigenetic control of HIV-1 post integration latency: implications for therapy. *Clin Epigenetics.* (2015) 7:103. doi: 10.1186/s13148-015-0137-6

Avalos CR, Price SL, Forsyth ER, Pin JN, Shirk EN, Bullock BT, et al. Quantitation of productively infected monocytes and macrophages of simian immunodeficiency virus-infected macaques. *J Virol.* (2016) 90:5643–56. doi: 10.1128/JVI.00290-16

Ganor Y, Real F, Sennepin A, Dutertre CA, Prevedel L, Xu L, et al. HIV-1 reservoirs in urethral macrophages of patients under suppressive antiretroviral therapy. *Nat Microbiol.* (2019) 4:633–44. doi:10.1038/s41564-018-0335-z

Darcis G, Coombs RW, Van Lint C. Exploring the anatomical HIV reservoirs: role of the testicular tissue. *AIDS.* (2016) 30:2891–3. doi: 10.1097/QAD.0000000000001281

Jenabian MA, Costiniuk CT, Mehraj V, Ghazawi FM, Fromentin R, Brousseau J, et al. Immune tolerance properties of the testicular tissue as a viral sanctuary site in ART-treated HIV-infected adults. *AIDS.* (2016) 30:2777–86. doi: 10.1097/QAD.0000000000001282

Wong JK, Yukl SA. Tissue reservoirs of HIV. *Curr Opin HIV AIDS.* (2016) 11:362–70. doi: 10.1097/COH.0000000000000293

Wong ME, Jaworowski A, Hearps AC. The HIV reservoir in monocytes and macrophages. *Front Immunol.* (2019) 10:1435. doi: 10.3389/fimmu.2019.01435

Frank I, Acharya A, Routhu NK, Aravantinou M, Harper JL, Maldonado S, et al. A Tat/Rev induced limiting dilution assay to measure viral reservoirs in non-human primate models of HIV infection. *Sci Rep.* (2019) 9:12078. doi: 10.1038/s41598-019-48354-3

Nixon CC, Mavigner M, Silvestri G, Garcia JV. *In vivo* models of human immunodeficiency virus persistence and cure strategies. *J Infect Dis.* (2017) 215(Suppl. 3):S142–51. doi: 10.1093/infdis/jiw637

Pillai SK, Deeks SG. Signature of the sleeper cell: a biomarker of HIV latency revealed. *Trends Immunol.* (2017) 38:457–8. doi: 10.1016/j.it.2017.04.007

Dahabieh MS, Battivelli E, Verdin E. Understanding HIV latency: the road to an HIV cure. *Annu Rev Med.* (2015) 66:407–21. doi: 10.1146/annurev-med-092112-152941

Wherry EJ. T cell exhaustion. *Nat Immunol.* (2011) 12:492–9. doi: 10.1038/ni.2035

Chew GM, Fujita T, Webb GM, Burwitz BJ, Wu HL, Reed JS, et al. TIGIT marks exhausted T cells, correlates with disease progression, and serves as a target for immune restoration in HIV and SIV infection. *PLoS Pathog.* (2016) 12:e1005349. doi: 10.1371/journal.ppat.1005349

Fromentin R, Bakeman W, Lawani MB, Khoury G, Hartogensis W, DaFonseca S, et al. CD4+ T cells expressing PD-1, TIGIT and LAG-3 contribute to HIV persistence during ART. *PLoS Pathog.* (2016) 12:e1005761. doi: 10.1371/journal.ppat.1005761

Pardons M, Baxter AE, Massanella M, Pagliuzza A, Fromentin R, Dufour C, et al. Single-cell characterization and quantification of translation-competent viral reservoirs in treated and untreated HIV infection. *PLoS Pathog.* (2019) 15:e1007619. doi: 10.1371/journal.ppat.1007619

Fromentin R, DaFonseca S, Costiniuk CT, El-Far M, Procopio FA, Hecht FM, et al. PD-1 blockade potentiates HIV latency reversal *ex vivo* in CD4(+) T cells from ART-suppressed individuals. *Nat Commun.* (2019) 10:814. doi: 10.1038/s41467-019-08798-7

Bui JK, Cyktor JC, Fyne E, Campellone S, Mason SW, Mellors JW. Blockade of the PD-1 axis alone is not sufficient to activate HIV-1 virion production from CD4+ T cells of individuals on suppressive ART. *PLoS ONE.* (2019) 14:e0211112. doi: 10.1371/journal.pone.0211112

Hurst J, Hoffmann M, Pace M, Williams JP, Thornhill J, Hamlyn E, et al. Immunological biomarkers predict HIV-1 viral rebound after treatment interruption. *Nat Commun.* (2015) 6:8495. doi: 10.1038/ncomm s9495

Banga R, Procopio FA, Ruggiero A, Noto A, Ohmiti K, Cavassini M, et al. Blood CXCR3+ CD4 T cells are enriched in inducible replication competent HIV in aviremic antiretroviral therapy-treated individuals. *Front Immunol.* (2018) 9:144. doi: 10.3389/fimmu.2018.00144

Banga R, Procopio FA, Noto A, Pollakis G, Cavassini M, Ohmiti K, et al. PD-1(+) and follicular helper T cells are responsible for persistent HIV-1 transcription in treated aviremic individuals. *Nat Med.* (2016) 22:754–61. doi: 10.1038/nm.4113

Perreau M, Savoye AL, De Crignis E, Corpataux JM, Cubas R, Haddad EK, et al. Follicular helper T cells serve as the major CD4 T cell compartment for HIV-1 infection, replication, and production. *J Exp Med.* (2013) 210:143–56. doi: 10.1084/jem.20121932

Fukazawa Y, Lum R, Okoye AA, Park H, Matsuda K, Bae JY, et al. B cell follicle sanctuary permits persistent productive simian immunodeficiency virus infection in elite controllers. *Nat Med.* (2015) 21:132–9. doi: 10.1038/nm.3781

Rothenberger M, Nganou-Makamdop K, Kityo C, Ssali F, Chipman JG, Beilman GJ, et al. Impact of Integrase Inhibition compared to non- nucleoside inhibition on HIV reservoirs in Lymphoid Tissues. *J Acquir Immune Defic Syndr.* (2019) 81:355–60. doi: 10.1097/QAI.00000000000 02026

Estes JD, Kityo C, Ssali F, Swainson L, Makamdop KN, Del Prete GQ, et al. Defining total-body AIDS-virus burden with implications for curative strategies. *Nat Med.* (2017) 23:1271–6. doi: 10.1038/nm.4411

Fletcher CV, Staskus K, Wietgrefe SW, Rothenberger M, Reilly C, Chipman JG, et al. Persistent HIV-1 replication is associated with lower antiretroviral drug concentrations in lymphatic tissues. *Proc Natl Acad Sci USA.* (2014) 111:2307–12. doi: 10.1073/pnas.1318249111

McGary CS, Deleage C, Harper J, Micci L, Ribeiro SP, Paganini S, et al. CTLA-4+PD-1- Memory CD4+ T cells critically contribute to viral persistence in antiretroviral therapy-suppressed, SIV-infected rhesus macaques. *Immunity.* (2017) 47:776–88.e5. doi: 10.1016/j.immuni.2017.09.018

Yi JS, Cox MA, Zajac AJ. T-cell exhaustion: characteristics, causes and conversion. *Immunology.* (2010) 129:474–81. doi:10.1111/j.1365-2567.2010.03255.x

Boyer Z, Palmer S. Targeting immune checkpoint molecules to eliminate latent HIV. *Front Immunol.* (2018) 9:2339. doi: 10.3389/fimmu.2018.02339

Zerbato JM, Purves HV, Lewin SR, Rasmussen TA. Between a shock and a hard place: challenges and developments in HIV latency reversal. *Curr Opin Virol.* (2019) 38:1–9. doi: 10.1016/j.coviro.2019.03.004

Guihot A, Marcelin AG, Massiani MA, Samri A, Soulié C, Autran B, et al. Drastic decrease of the HIV reservoir in a patient treated with nivolumab for lung cancer. *Ann Oncol.* (2018) 29:517–8. doi: 10.1093/annonc/mdx696

Scully EP, Rutishauser RL, Simoneau CR, Delagrèverie H, Euler Z, Thanh C, et al. Inconsistent HIV reservoir dynamics and immune responses following anti-PD-1 therapy in cancer patients with HIV infection. *Ann Oncol.* (2018) 29:2141–2. doi: 10.1093/annonc/mdy259

Day D, Hansen AR. Immune-related adverse events associated with immune checkpoint inhibitors. *BioDrugs.* (2016) 30:571–84. doi: 10.1007/s40259-016-0204-3

Marini A, Harper JM, Romerio F. An *in vitro* system to model the establishment and reactivation of HIV-1 latency. *J Immunol.* (2008) 181:7713–20. doi: 10.4049/jimmunol.181.11.7713

Iglesias-Ussel M, Vandergeeten C, Marchionni L, Chomont N, Romerio F. High levels of CD2 expression identify HIV-1 latently infected resting memory CD4+ T cells in virally suppressed subjects. *J Virol.* (2013) 87:9148–58. doi: 10.1128/JVI.01297-13

Biswas P, Mantelli B, Delfanti F, Ferrarini M, Poli G, Lazzarin A. CD30 ligation differentially affects CXCR4-dependent HIV-1 replication and soluble CD30 secretion in non-Hodgkin cell lines and in gamma delta T lymphocytes. *Eur J Immunol.* (2003) 33:3136–45. doi: 10.1002/eji.200324344

Romagnani S, Annunziato F, Manetti R, Almerigogna F, Biagiotti R, Giudizi MG, et al. Role for CD30 in HIV expression. *Immunol Lett.* (1996) 51:83–8. doi: 10.1016/0165-2478(96)02559-X

Hogan LE, Vasquez J, Hobbs KS, Hanhauser E, Aguilar-Rodriguez B, Hussien R, et al. Increased HIV-1 transcriptional activity and infectious burden in peripheral blood and gut-associated CD4+ T cells expressing CD30. *PLoS Pathog.* (2018) 14:e1006856. doi: 10.1371/journal.ppat.1006856

Wang CC, Thanh C, Gibson EA, Ball-Burack M, Hogan LE, Descours B, et al. Transient loss of detectable HIV-1 RNA following brentuximab vedotin anti-CD30 therapy for Hodgkin lymphoma. *Blood Adv.* (2018) 2:3479–82. doi: 10.1182/bloodadvances.2018024364

Serra-Peinado C, Grau-Expósito J, Luque-Ballesteros L, Astorga-Gamaza A, Navarro J, Gallego-Rodriguez J, et al. Expression of CD20 after viral reactivation renders HIV-reservoir cells susceptible to Rituximab. *Nat Commun.* (2019) 10:3705. doi: 10.1038/s41467-019-11556-4

Hogarth PM, Pietersz GA. Fc receptor-targeted therapies for the treatment of inflammation, cancer and beyond. *Nat Rev Drug Discov.* (2012) 11:311–31. doi: 10.1038/nrd2909

Holgado MP, Sananez I, Raiden S, Geffner JR, Arruvito L. CD32 ligation promotes the activation of CD4+ T cells. *Front Immunol.* (2018) 9:2814. doi: 10.3389/fimmu.2018.02814

Descours B, Petitjean G, López-Zaragoza JL, Bruel T, Raffel R, Psomas C, et al. CD32a is a marker of a CD4 T-cell HIV reservoir harbouring replication- competent proviruses. *Nature.* (2017) 543:564–7. doi: 10.1038/nature21710

Abdel-Mohsen M, Kuri-Cervantes L, Grau-Exposito J, Spivak AM, Nell RA, Tomescu C, et al. CD32 is expressed on cells with transcriptionally active HIV but does not enrich for HIV DNA in resting T cells. *Sci Transl Med.* (2018) 10:eaar6759. doi: 10.1126/scitranslmed.aar6759

Martin GE, Pace M, Thornhill JP, Phetsouphanh C, Meyerowitz J, Gossez M, et al. CD32-expressing CD4 T cells are phenotypically diverse and can contain proviral HIV DNA. *Front Immunol.* (2018) 9:928. doi: 10.3389/fimmu.2018.00928

Badia R, Ballana E, Castellví M, García-Vidal E, Pujantell M, Clotet B, et al. CD32 expression is associated to T-cell activation and is not a marker of the HIV-1 reservoir. *Nat Commun.* (2018) 9:2739. doi:10.1038/s41467-018-05157-w

Pérez L, Anderson J, Chipman J, Thorkelson A, Chun TW, Moir S, et al. Conflicting evidence for HIV enrichment in CD32. *Nature.* (2018) 561:E9–16. doi: 10.1038/s41586-018-0493-4

Bertagnolli LN, White JA, Simonetti FR, Beg SA, Lai J, Tomescu C, et al. The role of CD32 during HIV-1 infection. *Nature.* (2018) 561:E17–9. doi: 10.1038/s41586-018-0494-3

Osuna CE, Lim SY, Kublin JL, Apps R, Chen E, Mota TM, et al. Evidence that CD32a does not mark the HIV-1 latent reservoir. *Nature.* (2018) 561:E20–8. doi: 10.1038/s41586-018-0495-2

Darcis G, Kootstra N, Hooibrink B, van Montfort T, Groen K, Jurriaans S, et al. CD32+CD4+ T cells are enriched in HIV DNA. In: *Conference on Retroviruses and Opportunistic Infections.* Seattle, WA (2019).

Thornhill JP, Pace M, Martin GE, Hoare J, Peake S, Herrera C, et al. CD32 expressing doublets in HIV-infected gut-associated lymphoid tissue are associated with a T follicular helper cell phenotype. *Mucosal Immunol.* (2019) 12:1212–9. doi: 10.1038/s41385-019-0180-2

Noto A, Procopio FA, Banga R, Suffiotti M, Corpataux JM, Cavassini M, et al. CD32(+) and PD-1(+) lymph node CD4 T cells support persistent HIV-1 transcription in treated aviremic individuals. *J Virol.* (2018) 92:e00901–18. doi: 10.1128/JVI.00901-18

Wittner M, Dunay GA, Kummer S, Bockhorn M, Hüfner A, Schmiedel S, et al. CD32 Expression of different memory T cell subpopulations in the blood and lymph nodal tissue of HIV patients and healthy controls correlates with immune activation. *J Acquir Immune Defic Syndr.* (2018) 77:345–9. doi: 10.1097/QAI.0000000000001622

Chavez L, Calvanese V, Verdin E. HIV latency is established directly and early in both resting and activated primary CD4 T cells. *PLoS Pathog.* (2015) 11:e1004955. doi: 10.1371/journal.ppat.1004955

van der Sluis RM, van Montfort T, Pollakis G, Sanders RW, Speijer D, Berkhout B, et al. Dendritic cell-induced activation of latent HIV-1 provirus in actively proliferating primary T lymphocytes. *PLoS Pathog.* (2013) 9:e1003259. doi: 10.1371/journal.ppat.10 03259

Kaiser P, Joos B, Niederost B, Weber R, Gunthard HF, Fischer M. Productive human immunodeficiency virus type 1 infection in peripheral blood predominantly takes place in CD4/CD8 double-negative T lymphocytes. *J Virol.* (2007) 81:9693–706. doi: 10.1128/JVI.00492-07

Chun TW, Nickle DC, Justement JS, Large D, Semerjian A, Curlin ME, et al. HIV-infected individuals receiving effective antiviral therapy for extended periods of time continually replenish their viral reservoir. *J Clin Invest.* (2005) 115:3250–5. doi: 10.1172/JCI26197

Vásquez JJ, Aguilar-Rodriguez BL, Rodriguez L, Hogan LE, Somsouk M, McCune JM, et al. CD32-RNA co-localizes with HIV-RNA in CD3+ cells found within gut tissues from viremic and ART-suppressed individuals. *Pathog Immun.* (2019) 4:147–60. doi: 10.20411/pai.v4i1.271

Lorenzo-Redondo R, Fryer HR, Bedford T, Kim EY, Archer J, Pond SLK, et al. Persistent HIV-1 replication maintains the tissue reservoir during therapy. *Nature.* (2016) 530:51–6. doi: 10.1038/nature16933

Thompson CG, Rosen EP, Prince HMA, White N, Sykes C, de la Cruz G, et al. Heterogeneous antiretroviral drug distribution and HIV/SHIV detection in the gut of three species. *Sci Transl Med.* (2019) 11:eaap8758. doi:10.1126/scitranslmed.aap8758

Moir S, Malaspina A, Li Y, Chun TW, Lowe T, Adelsberger J, et al. B cells of HIV-1-infected patients bind virions through CD21-complement interactions and transmit infectious virus to activated T cells. *J Exp Med.* (2000) 192:637–46. doi: 10.1084/jem.192.5.637

Rappocciolo G, Piazza P, Fuller CL, Reinhart TA, Watkins SC, Rowe DT, et al. DC-SIGN on B lymphocytes is required for transmission of HIV-1 to T lymphocytes. *PLoS Pathog.* (2006) 2:e70. doi: 10.1371/journal.ppat.00 20070

13

Specific Biological Features of Adipose Tissue and their Impact on HIV Persistence

Christine Bourgeois[1], Jennifer Gorwood[2], Aurélie Barrail-Tran[1,3], Claire Lagathu[2], Jacqueline Capeau[2], Delphine Desjardins[1], Roger Le Grand[1], Abderaouf Damouche[1], Véronique Béréziat[2] and Olivier Lambotte[1,3]*

[1] Center for Immunology of Viral Infections and Autoimmune Diseases, IDMIT Department, IBFJ, CEA, Université Paris Sud, INSERM U1184, Fontenay-aux-Roses, France, [2] INSERM UMR_S 938, Centre de Recherche Saint-Antoine, Institut Hospitalo-Universitaire de Cardio-Métabolisme et Nutrition (ICAN), Sorbonne Université, Paris, France, [3] AP-HP, Service de Médecine Interne et Immunologie Clinique, Hôpital Bicêtre, Groupe Hospitalier Universitaire Paris Sud, Le Kremlin-Bicêtre, France

***Correspondence:**
Christine Bourgeois
christine.bourgeois@u-psud.fr

Although white AT can contribute to anti-infectious immune responses, it can also be targeted and perturbed by pathogens. The AT's immune involvement is primarily due to strong pro-inflammatory responses (with both local and paracrine effects), and the large number of fat-resident macrophages. Adipocytes also exert direct antimicrobial responses. In recent years, it has been found that memory T cells accumulate in AT, where they provide efficient secondary responses against viral pathogens. These observations have prompted researchers to re-evaluate the links between obesity and susceptibility to infections. In contrast, AT serves as a reservoir for several persistence pathogens, such as human adenovirus Ad-36, *Trypanosoma gondii*, *Mycobacterium tuberculosis*, influenza A virus, and cytomegalovirus (CMV). The presence and persistence of bacterial DNA in AT has led to the concept of a tissue-specific microbiota. The unexpected coexistence of immune cells and pathogens within the specific AT environment is intriguing, and its impact on anti-infectious immune responses requires further evaluation. AT has been recently identified as a site of HIV persistence. In the context of HIV infection, AT is targeted by both the virus and the antiretroviral drugs. AT's intrinsic metabolic features, large overall mass, and wide distribution make it a major tissue reservoir, and one that may contribute to the pathophysiology of chronic HIV infections. Here, we review the immune, metabolic, viral, and pharmacological aspects that contribute to HIV persistence in AT. We also evaluate the respective impacts of both intrinsic and HIV-induced factors on AT's involvement as a viral reservoir. Lastly, we examine the potential consequences of HIV persistence on the metabolic and immune activities of AT.

Keywords: adipose tissue, fat, HIV, infectious disease, resident memory T cells, T lymphocyte, reservoir, immune response

INTRODUCTION

The three types of adipose tissue (AT: brown, white, and beige) each have specific functional properties (Cinti, 2012, 2018). Unless otherwise stated, the term "AT" will henceforth refer to white AT. The biology of AT is complex; this tissue exerts a range of metabolic, regenerative, immune, and other specific functions (Britton and Fox, 2011; Guerrero-Juarez and Plikus, 2018). The immune potential of AT is currently under renewed scrutiny. Historically, the strong pro-inflammatory responses within AT (exerting both local and paracrine effects), and the high number of fat-resident macrophages suggested that AT contributed to anti-infectious innate immune responses. The presence and persistence of bacterial DNA further suggests that a broad range of pathogens persists in AT (Burcelin et al., 2013). AT is a site of HIV persistence and appears as a crucial cofactor in both viral persistence and chronic immune activation/inflammation during HIV infection (Damouche et al., 2015; Gorwood et al., 2019). Concomitantly, studies on the AT's immune compartment have highlighted the non-negligible contribution of resident immune cells [and particularly AT memory (Trm) CD8 T cells] to anti-infectious responses (Han et al., 2017). Here, we first review AT's specific properties (independently of HIV infection) and, notably, its contribution to anti-infectious immune responses. We then discuss the changes in AT induced by HIV infection and/or antiretroviral therapy (ART). Lastly, we consider the potential consequences of HIV infection on the metabolic and immune functions of AT.

SPECIFIC FEATURES OF ADIPOSE TISSUE

The Anatomic and Functional Heterogeneity of Adipose Tissue

In healthy males and females, AT accounts for, respectively, 15 and 25% of the body weight, and is distributed across a large number of discrete anatomic sites (Shen et al., 2003; Lee et al., 2013; **Table 1**). Subcutaneous AT (SAT, accounting for over 80% of total body fat) and visceral AT (VAT) are the best-studied depots (**Figure 1**). The classification of the various types of AT reflects differences in the tissues' ontogeny (Chau et al., 2014) and metabolic profiles. SAT and VAT differ with regard to their metabolic activity and immune cell content (Wajchenberg, 2000; Fain et al., 2004; Ibrahim, 2009; Madani et al., 2009; Altintas et al., 2011). Furthermore, SAT can be divided into superficial SAT and deep SAT, which again differ with regard to their metabolic properties (Smith et al., 2001). Likewise, VAT depots can be subclassified as omental fat (protective layer surrounding the intestine), retroperitoneal fat (near the kidney), and mesenteric fat (close to the intestine), which again have different activities (Wronska and Kmiec, 2012). In addition to SAT and VAT, AT is present in multiple locations, and may exhibit even more specialized functions related to the associated tissue. Dermal AT (dAT) is a specialized adipose depot that is distinct from SAT. Lastly, perivascular AT (pAT) has a role in the homeostasis of the cardiovascular system (Cheng et al., 2018).

Adipose tissue can also surround lymphoid structures [notably lymph nodes (LNs)] or even infiltrate them [e.g., the bone marrow (BM) and thymus]. The physiologic impact of AT also differs from one lymphoid site to another. For example, the infiltration of fat into the thymus is always associated with age-associated thymic involution and the loss of thymic function (Hale, 2004; Coín Aragüez et al., 2013), whereas fat infiltration into the BM (the third largest fat depot after SAT and VAT) is a physiologic feature initially required for hematopoiesis. However, an age-related increase in fat infiltration into the BM is associated with defective hematopoiesis – suggesting that too much fat is harmful. The AT that surrounds the LNs (perinodal fat) does not appear to infiltrate them (Knight, 2008). Perinodal AT is thought to deliver nutrients (such as fatty acids) to immune cells; this prevents activated lymphocytes from competing for blood nutrients, and improves immune responses (Pond, 2002). Conversely, chronic stimulation of LNs also influences the cellular composition of the perinodal AT (Mattacks et al., 2003). Inducible lymphoid structures have been identified at mucosal sites (i.e., mucosal-associated lymphoid tissue) and also in AT: in addition to the milky spots (MSs) previously described in the omentum, fat-associated lymphoid clusters (FALCs) are found in mesenteric and pericardial AT (Beelen, 1991; Cruz-Migoni and Caamaño, 2016). In contrast to fat-embedded LNs, FALCs and MSs are found at points of direct contact between immune cells and metabolic cells (Moro et al., 2010). It is not yet clear whether MSs and FALCs are different immune clusters (they can differ in their composition and size) (Moro et al., 2010; Lolmède et al., 2011; Meza-Perez and Randall, 2017; Bénézech and Jackson-Jones, 2019), although both have immune functions (Rangel-Moreno et al., 2009; Bénézech and Jackson-Jones, 2019). Group 2 innate lymphoid cells (ILC2s) and B cells are crucial components of FALCs, since they coordinate local immune responses in fat depots and contribute to AT homeostasis (Bénézech and Jackson-Jones, 2019) and anti-infectious responses (Jones et al., 2015). These immune clusters provided the first evidence of a direct role of fat immune cells in anti-infectious responses, and also highlight the "regionalization" of AT. In fact, AT is a vascularized tissue that is organized into several lobular unit (Tang et al., 2008; Walker et al., 2008; Chi et al., 2018; Dichamp et al., 2019). These partitioned areas exhibit specific metabolic (and probably immune) activities. As a general rule, it is important to take account of AT's heterogeneity on two levels (i.e., the lymphoid structure considered, and the region within each AT depot). This heterogeneity may be associated with differences in the interactions between metabolic and immune cells (Mahlakõiv et al., 2019).

From an immunologic point of view, AT is close to most of the physical barriers in the organism [i.e., the digestive tract, respiratory tract (Chen et al., 2019), and skin] and lymphoid tissues. The proximity between AT and the immune sites raises the question of whether AT contributes significantly to local immune responses after the first physical barrier or mucosa has been breached. In fact, AT may act both passively and actively as a second line of defense against microbial invasion. Given that the

TABLE 1 | The anatomical and functional heterogeneity of adipose tissues.

Anatomical location/Sublocation	Functions	References
Major metabolic sites		
Subcutaneous AT (SAT)	Metabolic activity	Lee et al., 2013; Chau et al., 2014
Superficial SAT		Smith et al., 2001
Deep SAT		
Visceral AT (VAT)	More active metabolically More strongly associated with metabolic diseases	Wronska and Kmiec, 2012
Omental		
Retroperitoneal		
Mesenteric		
Adipose tissue associated with primary and secondary immune sites		
Bone marrow AT (MAT)	Contributing to hematopoiesis Deleterious in excess	Hardouin et al., 2014; Scheller et al., 2016
AT embedding LN	Delivering nutrients to immune cells Favoring immune responses	Knight, 2008
Thymic AT	Associated to age-associated thymic involution and the loss of thymic function	Coín Aragüez et al., 2013
Additional specialized adipose tissue		
Dermal AT (dAT)	– Wound healing, hair follicle cycling, thermoregulation – Immune responses	Chase et al., 1953; Moffat, 1968; Alexander et al., 2015; Guerrero-Juarez and Plikus, 2018
Perivascular AT (pAT)	– Vascular homeostasis	Rajsheker et al., 2010; Britton and Fox, 2011; Szasz and Webb, 2012; Gu et al., 2019

various AT depots also differ in their immune cell composition, they may also differ in their role in immune responses.

Metabolic Functions, Plasticity, and Expandability of Adipose Tissue

Physiological Metabolic Plasticity

Adipose tissue was initially defined as a metabolic site; it constitutes the body's major energy storage site and is also an endocrine tissue that directly modulates systemic lipid and glucose metabolism and insulin sensitivity. AT is composed of two cell fractions: the adipocytes that represent approximately 80% of the volume of AT and 60% of the total cell population, and the stromal vascular fraction (SVF), both surrounded by extracellular matrix (ECM) (**Figure 1**). All these three compartments are responsible for the pleiotropic roles of AT. In physiological conditions, AT must be viewed primary as a protective tissue that stores and prevents excessive exposure of other organs to fatty acids. One key feature of AT is its ability to adapt and expand in response to energy needs or surpluses thanks to its cellular heterogeneity. The response to metabolic cues is based on adipocyte hypertrophy (increase in adipocyte volume) and/or hyperplasia (increase in adipocyte number by recruitment and proliferation of precursor cells and adipogenesis). Adipocyte volume reflects the specific function of adipocyte to store energy in the form of lipids, and thus, the cell capacity to dramatically modulate its size in response to changes in energy balance. Lipid accumulation is determined by the balance between lipogenesis and lipolysis. This plasticity also includes vascular remodeling and ECM remodeling to allow adequate tissue expansion, oxygenation, and mobilization of nutrients (Pellegrinelli et al., 2016).

The adipocyte's metabolic activity is primarily modulated by insulin. When the energy balance is positive, insulin favors adipogenesis, lipogenesis from non-lipid precursor such as glucose, and the uptake of circulating free fatty acids (FFAs) to synthesize triacylglycerols (TGs) that will accumulate within the lipid droplets. In response to insulin, adipocytes secrete the lipoprotein lipase (that process TG into FFA and glycerol phosphate), but also favor glucose and glycerol influx by translocation of glucose transporter type 4 (GLUT4) to the plasma membrane and upregulation of glycerol channels. At the opposite, in time of energy shortage, adipocytes release FFA back in the circulation during lipolysis through the action of different lipases. It results in the efflux of glycerol-phosphate and FFA that serve as a source of energy for most tissues. Hence, under physiological conditions, adipocytes adapt rapidly to metabolic changes. Regional variations in the metabolic activity of adipocytes have been observed in healthy subjects, especially in regards to regulation of lipolysis and lipogenesis.

Even in non-expanding AT, adipocytes are renewed frequently to compensate for adipocyte death, with a turnover of approximately 10% annually (Spalding et al., 2008), indicating that committed adipocyte progenitors/precursors exist within AT. Adipose-derived mesenchymal stem cells (ASCs), defined as mesenchymal stem cells (MSCs) with similar clinical potential as MSCs from BM, were discovered. ASCs were identified as multipotent cells capable of *in vitro* differentiation into adipocytes, osteoblasts, chondrocytes, and myoblasts (Rodriguez et al., 2005; Cawthorn et al., 2012). Adipocyte differentiation starts with a first phase called determination, during which a multipotent precursor (ASCs) commits itself to adipocyte lineage and becomes a preadipocyte, unable to differentiate into any other cell type. Adipogenic cascade and molecular regulation of adipogenesis requires the coordination of multiple regulatory and signaling pathways. During the second phase, called adipogenesis, the preadipocyte differentiates into a mature adipocyte that acquires all the machinery required

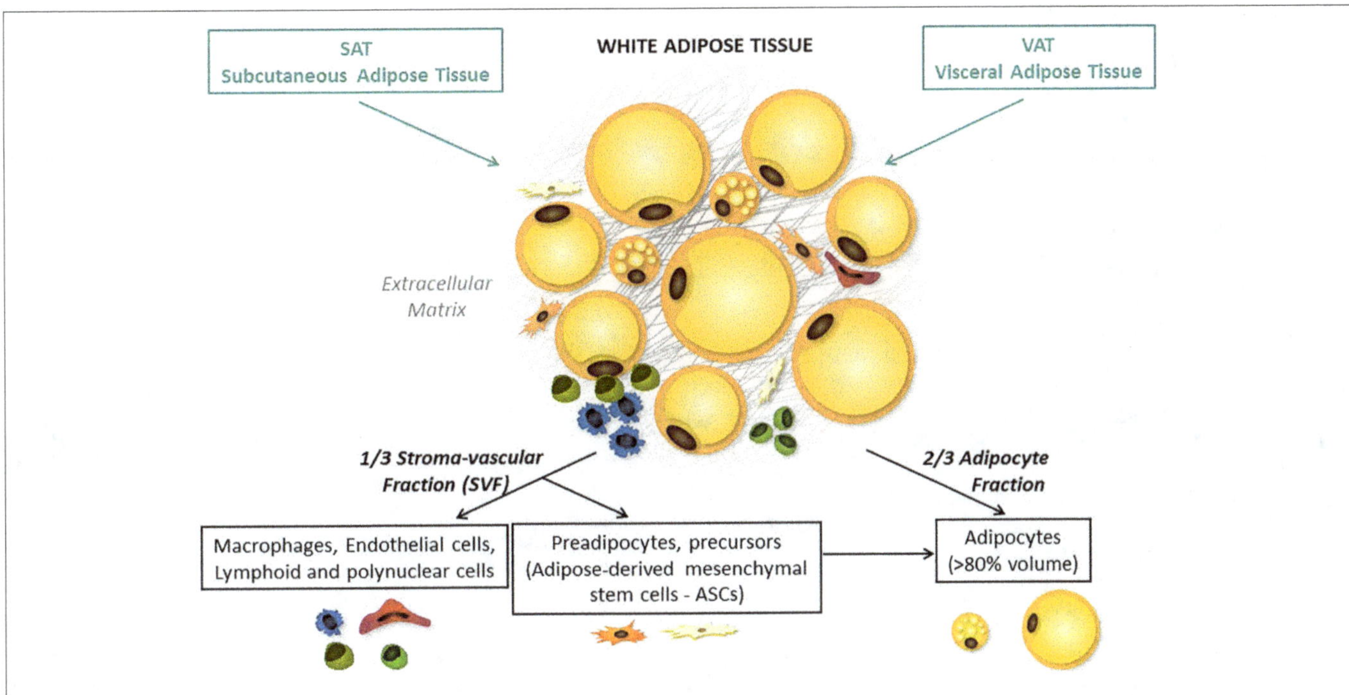

FIGURE 1 | Adipose tissue distribution and composition. Adipose tissue is composed of two cell fractions that can be easily separated through collagenase digestion: the adipocytes and the stromal vascular fraction (SVF), both surrounded by extracellular matrix (ECM). All these three compartments are responsible for the pleiotropic roles of AT. Adipocytes are the main cellular component crucial for both energy storage and endocrine activity. The other cell type that are present are precursors (such as adipose-derived mesenchymal stem cells – ASCs), fibroblasts, vascular cells, and immune cells. AT is distributed across a large number of discrete anatomic sites (Shen et al., 2003; Lee et al., 2013). Subcutaneous AT (SAT, accounting for over 80% of total body fat) and visceral AT (VAT) are the best-studied depots.

for lipid transport and synthesis, insulin sensitivity, and adipokine secretion. Adipogenesis is characterized by cell cycle arrest and the induction of a transcriptional cascade: Peroxisome proliferator-activated receptor gamma (PPAR-γ), the master regulator of adipogenesis (Shao et al., 2016), several members of the CCAAT-enhancer binding protein (C/EBP) following a strict temporal regulation, C/EBPβ and C/EBPδ inducing C/EBPα (Rosen and MacDougald, 2006), and sterol regulatory element binding protein 1c (SREBP1c) (Peirce et al., 2014; **Figure 2**).

Studies of obesity have uncovered the presence of metabolically active immune cells within AT (Mathis et al., 2011). Under physiological conditions, immune cells in the AT [notably anti-inflammatory M2 macrophages (Morris et al., 2011) and CD4 regulatory T cells (Tregs) (Feuerer et al., 2009; Cipolletta, 2014; Kolodin et al., 2015)] ensure homeostasis by remodeling the ECM (Odegaard and Chawla, 2013), eliminating dying adipocytes, and limiting inflammation. Natural killer T (NKT) cells (Lynch et al., 2012, 2015), ILCs (Flach and Diefenbach, 2015; Lee et al., 2016; O'Sullivan et al., 2016; Boulenouar et al., 2017), and eosinophils (Wu et al., 2011; Lee E.-H. et al., 2018) have also been reported, although their net activity to metabolic homeostasis is subject to debate. In essence, all types of immune cell have now been found in AT, although the AT's specific immune content appears to vary from one anatomic site to another. Furthermore, it is not clear whether the immune compartment of AT changes transiently in response to metabolic cues during the physiological cycle between fasting and satiety.

Defects in Adipose Tissue Expandability

When the AT's buffering capacity is exceeded (as a consequence of sustained lipid/nutrient overload, for example), a wide range of disorders can result (de Ferranti and Mozaffarian, 2008): ectopic accumulation of lipids within the body, insulin resistance, and the associated metabolic complications (Lionetti et al., 2009) (such as obesity and type II diabetes). These disorders are associated with major changes in the metabolic and immune compartments of AT. Adipose hypertrophy and hyperplasia are both associated with intracellular dysfunction in adipocytes (molecular changes in the lipolytic and lipogenic pathways, endoplasmic reticulum, and mitochondrial stresses). In turn, these changes lead to the release of pro-inflammatory adipokines, free fatty acids, and inflammatory mediators that exacerbate the dysfunction in AT. Changes in macrophage polarization (Lumeng et al., 2007), a reduction in the proportion of Treg cells (Feuerer et al., 2009), and an accumulation of CD8 T cells (Nishimura et al., 2009b) have been reported in mice, and these immune alterations participate in the development of metabolic alterations within AT. In the context of obesity, the interaction between adipocytes and macrophages is crucial. Firstly, obesity is associated with the recruitment of macrophages to the AT – although the exact mechanism has yet to be characterized (Weisberg et al., 2003; Nishimura et al., 2009b).

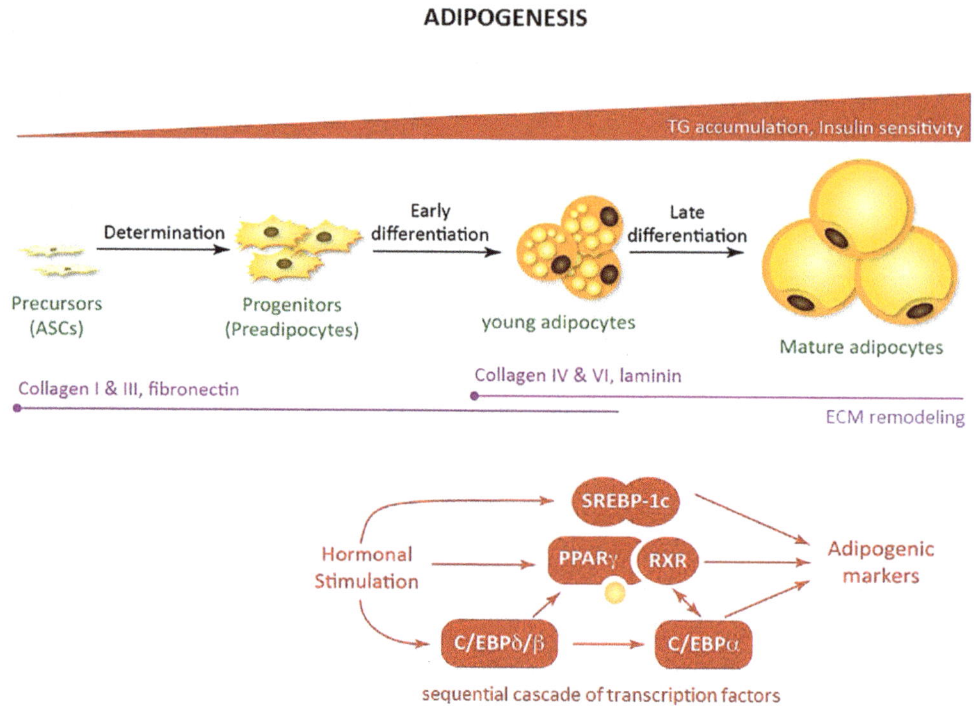

FIGURE 2 | Adipogenesis. Schematic figure of the regulation of adipogenesis from mesenchymal precursors. Adipogenesis is a sequential cascade of transcription factors leading to lipid accumulation and the acquisition of insulin sensitivity. Adipogenesis also involves extracellular matrix remodeling.

These macrophages produce pro-inflammatory cytokines, which in turn diminish the adipocytes' insulin sensitivity [described for TNF-α in rodents (Xu et al., 2003)]. Lastly, insulin resistance impairs the hormone's ability to suppress lipolysis (Bastard et al., 2006). The accumulation of large body of data on the critical interactions between metabolic cells and immune cells has prompted the emergence of a new field of research: immunometabolism.

Adipose Tissue Senses and Sends Multiple Signals

Adipose tissue sense a number of hormonal, metabolic, and/or inflammatory signals (Kim et al., 2014; Cousin et al., 2015), as well as neuronal signals (Chi et al., 2018) and infectious episodes (Casteilla et al., 2011). The main modulator of AT is the nutritional status. Studies of obesity have demonstrated that AT is extremely flexible; it can exert anti- or pro-inflammatory actions, depending on the metabolic context. AT also differs when comparing males and females (Poglio et al., 2010; Luche et al., 2015) due to hormonal influences. AT is also innervated by both sympathetic and parasympathetic systems, regulating AT growth (Engela et al., 2013). In turn, AT-derived signals regulate food intake and peripheral metabolism. The endocrine activity of AT is a pivotal pathway of interactions between AT and other organs. In that way, the brain–gut–AT axis is a significant communication pathway (Franquesa et al., 2015). Interestingly, germ-free animals have 40% less fat mass than mice raised under conventional microbial conditions (Puissant et al., 2005), suggesting a gut microbiota's direct contribution to AT biology. Pioneering studies have demonstrated that lean and obese animals differ with regard to their gut microbiota. Microbial dysbiosis in obese animals may subsequently affect the efficiency of calorie harvesting from the diet, and calorie storage in AT (Puissant et al., 2005; Le Blanc and Mougiakakos, 2012; Luz-Crawford et al., 2013). Accordingly, certain strains of microbes appear to induce obesity (Prockop and Oh, 2012; Wang et al., 2014) and impair immune functions, which may increase the organism's susceptibility to infections (Bornstein et al., 2000; Poglio et al., 2012; Lee Y.S. et al., 2018; **Figure 3**). Lastly, AT is also a site of accumulation of persistent organic pollutants and various lipophilic drugs (Kintscher et al., 2008) that makes AT a potential sensor of environmental toxicity.

The Accumulation of Hematopoietic Stem and Precursor Cells and Mesenchymal Stem Cells in Adipose Tissue

In addition to AT's involvement in metabolic homeostasis, this tissue also contains large numbers of both hematopoietic stem and precursor cells (HSPCs) and ASCs (Baglioni et al., 2009; Kim et al., 2014; Cousin et al., 2015). These cells confer AT with a high regenerative potential, which is currently being investigated for therapeutic purposes (Poglio et al., 2010; Casteilla et al., 2011; Luche et al., 2015). Importantly, ASCs enable tissue repair but also regulate inflammation, and their immunomodulatory properties have been extensively studied

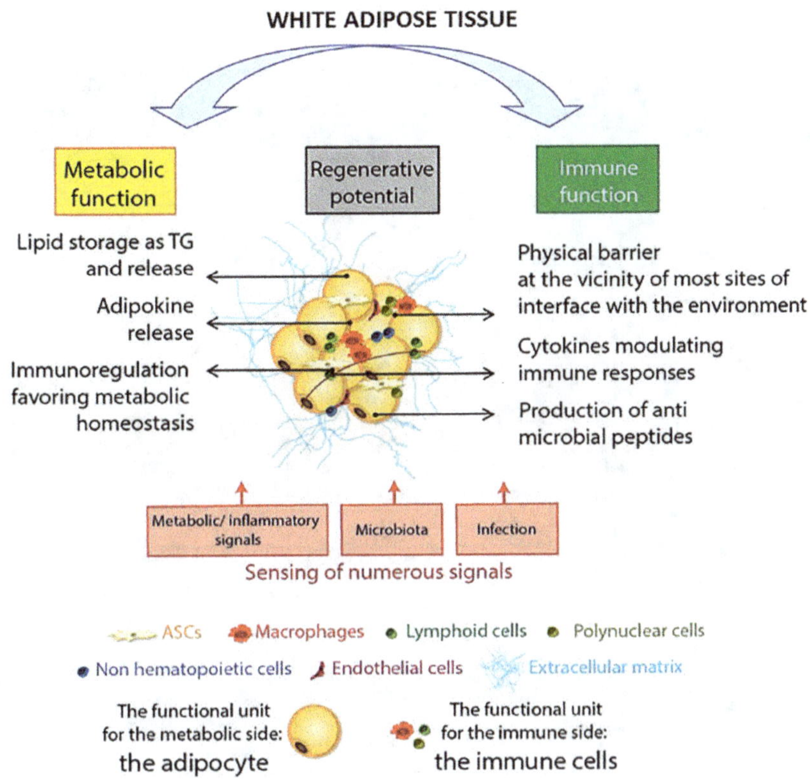

FIGURE 3 | The adipose tissue as a sensor: the AT immune and metabolic sides. Adipose tissue has many functional activities, including metabolic functions, immune responses, and regeneration. The large, ubiquitous depots of AT provide local storage for stem cell progenitors, and innate and adaptive immune cells. The adipocyte is the functional unit in the AT's metabolic activity. Immune cells ensure adipose tissue homeostasis by providing a controlled environment that favors adipogenesis and metabolic homeostasis. Interestingly, AT components are also involved in anti-infectious immune responses: adipocytes exert an anti-infectious response by producing antimicrobial peptides such as the cathelicidins while both innate and adaptive immune cells contribute to anti-infectious responses. Another important feature of AT is its high sensitivity to environmental cues, such as metabolic and inflammatory signals, the microbiota, and infectious episodes.

(Puissant et al., 2005; Le Blanc and Mougiakakos, 2012; Prockop and Oh, 2012; Engela et al., 2013; Luz-Crawford et al., 2013; Franquesa et al., 2015). ASCs appear to affect both innate and adaptive immunity. However, recent data suggest that this immunosuppressive profile may not be constitutive, and may depend on the pathophysiologic context (Wang et al., 2014). In contrast, data on HSPCs and the latter's regenerative potential are scarce (Cousin et al., 2015). However, Poglio et al. (2010) demonstrated that AT is a reservoir of functional mast cell progenitors and these progenitors may renew innate immunity in AT but also support innate immunity in other organs (Poglio et al., 2012). AT may thus constitute an alternate source of immune precursors, which might be involved in the development of long-term, sustained immune responses.

The Intrinsic Coexistence of Metabolic Cells and Immune Cells in Adipose Tissue: The Concept of Immunometabolism

Immunometabolism refers to the interplay between immune processes and metabolic pathways (Mathis et al., 2011; Lee Y.S. et al., 2018). AT is the prototypic immunometabolic tissue in which immune and metabolic cells interact (**Figure 3**). The SVF contains a broad range of immune cells, such as macrophages [detected in the early 2000s (Bornstein et al., 2000; Weisberg et al., 2003)] and T lymphocytes (Wu et al., 2007; Kintscher et al., 2008). Characterization of the immune compartment in AT has confirmed or revealed the presence of DCs (Bertola et al., 2012), neutrophils (Elgazar-Carmon et al., 2008), eosinophils (Wu et al., 2011), mast cells (Liu et al., 2009), and (for the lymphoid compartment) NK cells (Boulenouar et al., 2017), invariant NKT cells (Lynch et al., 2012), B cells (Nishimura et al., 2013), γδT cells (Zúñiga et al., 2010), and ILCs (Ferrante, 2013; **Figure 4**). In healthy individuals, AT is mainly described as an anti-inflammatory site, due to the high proportion of cells with an immunosuppressive phenotype. Given that immune cells in AT and their role as metabbolic modulators have been exhaustively reviewed elsewhere (Nishimura et al., 2009a; Schaffler and Scholmerich, 2010; Lolmède et al., 2011; de Jong et al., 2014; Guzik et al., 2017), we shall focus on the AT-derived parameters that may be linked to anti-infectious properties.

Metabolic and immune cells obviously have different functional activities, and are also at opposite ends of the spectrum with regard to their metabolic strategies and energy needs. Whereas metabolic cells have large intracellular energy

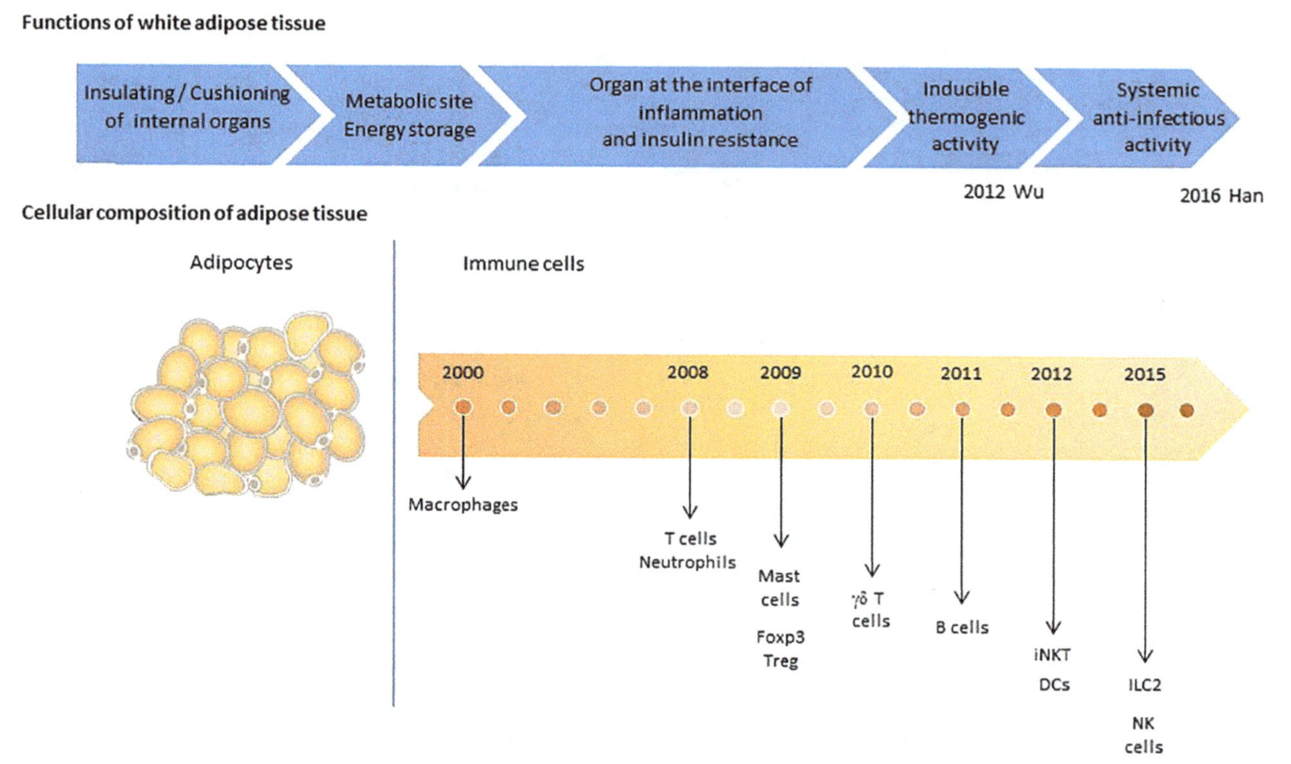

FIGURE 4 | The detection of immune cells in adipose tissue: a time line. Adipose tissue was initially defined as a cushioning site, and subsequently as a metabolic site mainly composed of adipocytes. The AT's immune function has emerged progressively. The first cell subset to be identified was the macrophage population (Bornstein et al., 2000; Weisberg et al., 2003; Xu et al., 2003), which contributes to the homeostasis of AT *via* the clearance of cellular debris, lipid buffering, and immune surveillance. T cell populations were then also described (Wu et al., 2007; Kintscher et al., 2008; Rausch et al., 2008), followed by neutrophils (Elgazar-Carmon et al., 2008), mast cells (Liu et al., 2009), regulatory T cells (Tregs) (Feuerer et al., 2009), B cells (Winer et al., 2011), eosinophils (Wu et al., 2011), dendritic cells (DCs) (Bertola et al., 2012), iNKT cells (Lynch et al., 2012), natural killer (NK) cells (Wensveen et al., 2015; Lee et al., 2016), and innate lymphoid cells (ILCs) (Brestoff et al., 2015; Lee et al., 2015; O'Sullivan et al., 2016). The cell types' respective roles in local metabolic homeostasis have been documented, although data on their potential anti-infectious activities are scarce. The recent publication of Han et al. (2017) provide a significant evidence of the contribution of AT immune cells to anti-infective immune responses.

storage vesicles, immune cells mainly rely on external energy supplies. Indeed, immune cells and immune responses depend closely on external energy supplies. However, one can consider that this strategy is well suited to the rapid changes in metabolic status that accompany immune activation and proliferation.

Summary of the Biological Features of Adipose Tissue

In brief, AT comprises many different depots, some of which make specific contributes to the homeostasis of various tissues (BM, skin, blood vessels, etc.). The main AT depots (SAT and VAT) are capable of integrating signals from various sources and modulating their biology accordingly (**Figure 1**). A depot's functional properties depend on its location (SAT vs. VAT) and may be partitioned within a given location. The AT's sensitivity to metabolic and inflammatory signals also influences the tissue's immune cell composition and properties. In rodent models of obesity, massive changes in the composition of the SVF has been described. One might think that adipocytes' metabolic plasticity is related to changes in the AT's immune functions. In fact, these two phenomena are relatively disconnected. Immune plasticity appears to be rather associated with the loss of adipocyte plasticity and the lipid spillover that initiates local inflammation. The AT's high sensitivity to environmental cues complicates studies of human samples. The highly heterogeneous metabolic context and history of infections in clinical trial participants constitute a major limitation.

ADIPOSE TISSUE AND INFECTIONS

As always in research on AT, the initial datasets emerged from studies of obesity. Interestingly, obesity and susceptibility to infections appears to have a two-way link, and AT has a key role in the dialog between metabolism and the immune system. On the one hand, it has been shown that infection impacts AT biology both indirectly (*via* the bystander effect of inflammation) and/or directly (*via* the impact of local pathogen persistence). These findings strengthen the "infectobesity" hypothesis, in which obesity has an infectious etiology. On the other hand, a growing body of evidence indicates that the obesity-induced disruption of AT direct influences the patients' susceptibility to infection.

AT therefore appears to contribute to anti-infectious immune responses and, at the same time, constitute a target for pathogens and a site at which infections induce perturbations. Both of these aspects will be reviewed below – firstly in contexts unrelated to HIV, and secondly in the specific context of HIV infection.

Our understanding of AT's contribution to anti-infectious immune responses has changed over time (**Figure 4**). AT was initially considered to be an inert mechanical barrier – a buffer site that protects against mechanical trauma and thus protects organs from breach and subsequent infections. In the early 2000s, innate immune cells were found in AT (Zeyda and Stulnig, 2007; Schaffler and Scholmerich, 2010). In particular, the AT-resident macrophage fraction was found to contribute to strong pro-inflammatory responses with both local and paracrine effects (Hotamisligil, 2006; Ouchi et al., 2011; Jackson et al., 2017). Other immune cells (CD8 T cells and NK cells) have been identified more recently, although the cells' local effects have mainly been studied with regard to metabolic homeostasis. Our knowledge of AT's anti-infectious potential has also benefited from research showing that adipocytes *per se* exert antimicrobial responses (Nippe et al., 2011; Alcorn and Kolls, 2015). Lastly, the discovery of memory T cell accumulation in AT as a means of providing efficient secondary responses against pathogens constituted a major breakthrough; it became clear that AT is an immune partner in both local and systemic immune responses (Han et al., 2017; **Figure 5**). However, AT is a reservoir for pathogens in various infectious contexts (Nishimura et al., 2000; Neyrolles et al., 2006; Desruisseaux et al., 2007; Dhurandhar, 2011; Nagajyothi et al., 2012; Couturier et al., 2015, 2016; Damouche et al., 2015; Trindade et al., 2016; Beigier-Bompadre et al., 2017; Tanowitz et al., 2017; Couturier and Lewis, 2018; Contreras et al., 2019; **Table 2**). The detection of various bacterial DNAs in AT also constitutes an argument in favor of the tissue-specific microbiota hypothesis (Burcelin et al., 2013). The

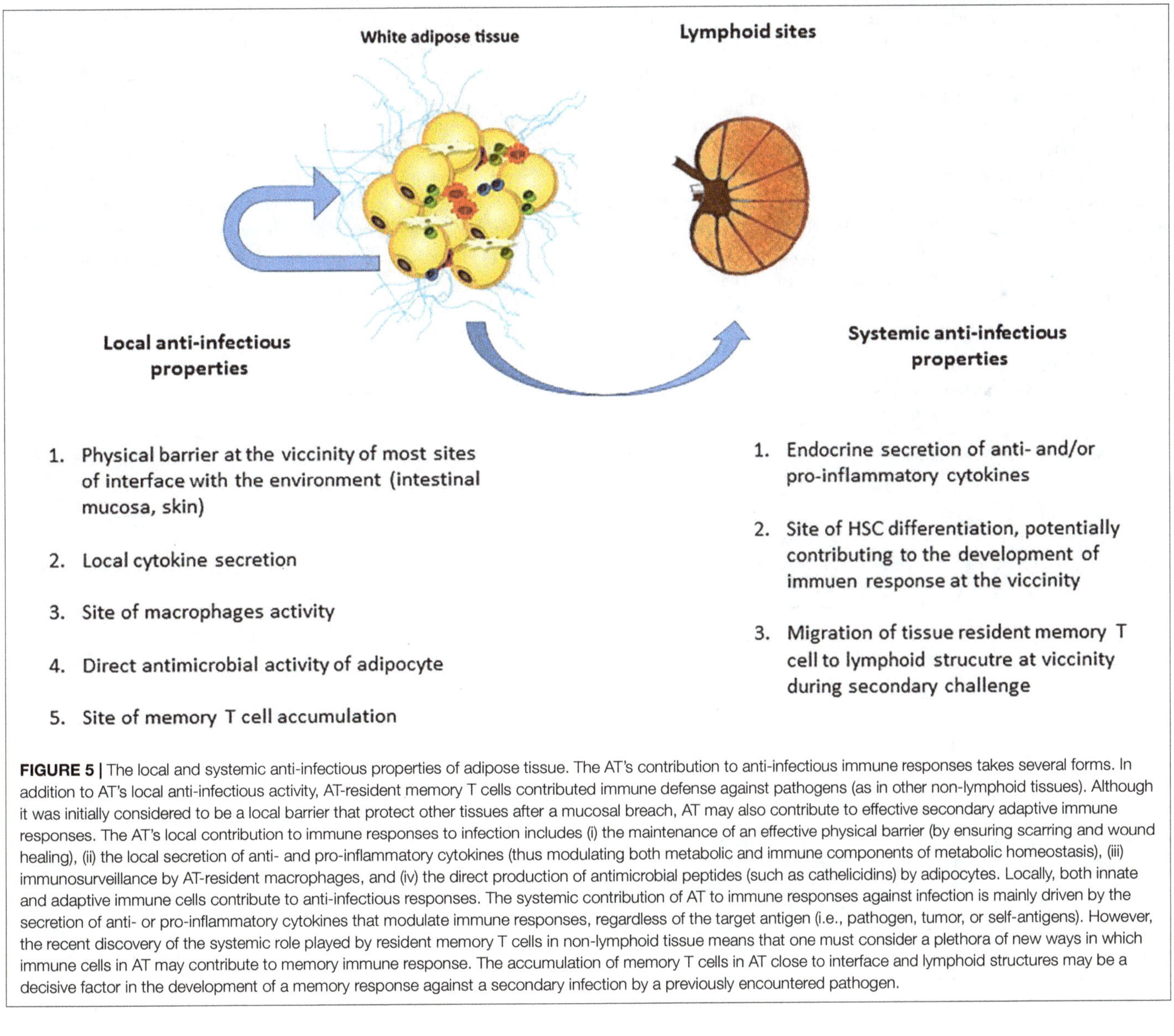

FIGURE 5 | The local and systemic anti-infectious properties of adipose tissue. The AT's contribution to anti-infectious immune responses takes several forms. In addition to AT's local anti-infectious activity, AT-resident memory T cells contributed immune defense against pathogens (as in other non-lymphoid tissues). Although it was initially considered to be a local barrier that protect other tissues after a mucosal breach, AT may also contribute to effective secondary adaptive immune responses. The AT's local contribution to immune responses to infection includes (i) the maintenance of an effective physical barrier (by ensuring scarring and wound healing), (ii) the local secretion of anti- and pro-inflammatory cytokines (thus modulating both metabolic and immune components of metabolic homeostasis), (iii) immunosurveillance by AT-resident macrophages, and (iv) the direct production of antimicrobial peptides (such as cathelicidins) by adipocytes. Locally, both innate and adaptive immune cells contribute to anti-infectious responses. The systemic contribution of AT to immune responses against infection is mainly driven by the secretion of anti- or pro-inflammatory cytokines that modulate immune responses, regardless of the target antigen (i.e., pathogen, tumor, or self-antigens). However, the recent discovery of the systemic role played by resident memory T cells in non-lymphoid tissue means that one must consider a plethora of new ways in which immune cells in AT may contribute to memory immune response. The accumulation of memory T cells in AT close to interface and lymphoid structures may be a decisive factor in the development of a memory response against a secondary infection by a previously encountered pathogen.

unexpected coexistence of immune cells and pathogens within AT is intriguing, and warrants further evaluation with regard to anti-infectious immune responses. Here are some points to discuss for considering a role in immunity of AT besides its close proximity to sites of entry for infective agents.

Anti-infectious Immunity in Adipose Tissue

We will distinguish the local and systemic immune responses developed by AT. Indeed, the systemic activity of AT was initially related to the endocrine cytokine production but need to be reconsidered with the contribution of AT CD8 T cells to anti-infectious secondary responses.

Local Immunity

Soluble factors and adipokines

Adipose tissue produces a broad range of molecules referred to as adipokines. Although some adipokines (such as adiponectin) are produced solely by adipocytes, most (including cytokines and chemokines) are produced by AT-resident immune cells (Fain et al., 2004) [notably macrophages (Ouchi et al., 2011)]. Although the endocrine activity of AT is pivotal, the local effect of the adipokines is non-negligible. Some adipokine such as TNF-α are not secreted into the circulation and exert local activity (Mohamed-Ali et al., 1997; Braune et al., 2017). Low-grade local inflammation is essential for remodeling healthy AT and healing wounds efficiently (Wernstedt Asterholm et al., 2014), whereas higher-grade inflammation helps to modulate immune responses against pathogens. Leptin (whose primary role is to regulate metabolism) is probably a prototypic example of the close link between the metabolism and the immune system (Matarese and La Cava, 2004). Leptin promotes T-cell proliferation, T-cell activation, and T-helper cell polarization *in vitro*. As a whole, AT inflammation is described in various models of infection (Nagajyothi et al., 2012; Contreras et al., 2019), underscoring that anti-infectious responses develop in AT.

The stromal vascular fraction

Little information is available on the anti-infective properties of TA, as studies have mainly evaluated their contribution to metabolic functions (**Table 3**). Healthy AT is associated to an anti-inflammatory environment, that may theoretically limit the anti-infectious potential of AT. Among type 2 immune subsets present in AT, Tregs and ILC2 are central partners of AT regulation, providing anti-inflammatory signals by different pathways. One specific feature of non-obese VAT is the high proportion of CD4 Tregs, which account for up to 50–70% of CD4 T cells in VAT in 25-week-old male mice (Feuerer et al., 2009). Interestingly, the Tregs in AT express the transcription factor PPAR-γ that regulates fatty acid storage and glucose metabolism (Cipolletta et al., 2012). Adipocytes express PPAR-γ, the most notable function of which is the regulation of adipogenesis. The presence of a PPAR-γ signature in AT Tregs has been considered as a marker of these cells' functional plasticity; the Tregs express the very same transcription factor produced by the cells on which they exert a modulatory effect (Cipolletta et al., 2011; Cipolletta, 2014). In contrast to peripheral Tregs, rodent adipose Tregs also express transcripts coding for

TABLE 2 | Metabolic and anti-infectious activity of immune cells in adipose tissue.

Cell subsets	Modulation associated with obesity	Metabolic activity	Anti-infectious activity	References
Macrophages	↗ Shift from M2 to M1	Subset-dependent M2: Phagocytosis of dying adipocytes Lipid buffering Limiting inflammation M1: TNF-α production inducing insulin resistance in adipocytes Favoring angiogenesis	M1: TNF-α, MIP-1α producer	Weisberg et al., 2003; Lumeng et al., 2007; Catrysse and van Loo, 2018; Ivanov et al., 2018; Lumeng et al., 2007; Morris et al., 2013; Suganami et al., 2007; Pang et al., 2008
CD4 T cells	Shift from Th2 to Th1	Subset dependent Th2: maintaining glucose homeostasis Th1: promoting inflammation		
CD8 T cells	↗	Rare at steady state, may contribute to the elimination of compromised adipocyte Early promoter of obesity-induced inflammation	Increased proportion in various contexts of AT infection Contributing to anti-infectious memory responses	Rausch et al., 2008; Nishimura et al., 2009b; Han et al., 2017
NKT cells	↘	Regulator of adipose tissue function Th2 cell type cytokine production		
Treg	↘	Regulator of adipose tissue function	Control of adipocyte function Lipid uptake and metabolism	Feuerer et al., 2009; Cipolletta et al., 2012, 2015; Kolodin et al., 2015; Laparra et al., 2019
NK cells	↗ Stimulated phenotype	Subset dependent Early sensor of adipose stress – At steady state, eliminating macrophage – When activated, triggering M1 macrophage accumulation and adipose fibrosis		
ILC2	↘	Regulator of adipose tissue function Favoring beiging (Met-Enk, IL4) Favoring Type 2 innate immunity	Promoting B cell response, IgM production	Moro et al., 2010; Brestoff et al., 2015; Lee et al., 2015

TABLE 3 | Microbes detected in adipose tissue.

Pathogens	Species	Infected cell subset	Impact on AT biology	References
Human adenovirus	m			Dhurandhar, 2011
Trypanosoma gondii	m			Machado et al., 2012; Nagajyothi et al., 2012; Trindade et al., 2016; Tanowitz et al., 2017
Plasmodium berghei	m			Franke-Fayard et al., 2010
Plasmodium falciparum	Hu			Seydel et al., 2006
Leishmania parasites	m	ASCs		Allahverdiyev et al., 2011
Nippostrongylus brasiliensis			↗ Eosinophils	Wu et al., 2011; Hussaarts et al., 2015
Mycobacterium tuberculosis	m, Hu	Adipocytes SVF cells	↗ CD8 T cells and NK cells, ↗ IFN-g production	Neyrolles et al., 2006; Beigier-Bompadre et al., 2017
Microbiota/bacterial DNA				Burcelin et al., 2013
Chlamydia pneumoniae	*In vitro*			Bouwman et al., 2008
Rickettsia prowazekii				Bechah et al., 2010
Staphylococcus aureus	*In vitro*	Adipocytes		Hanses et al., 2011
Influenza virus	Hu			Nishimura et al., 2000
Respiratory syncytial virus	*In vitro*			Bouwman et al., 2008
HIV	NHP, Hu		↗ CD8 T cells	Couturier et al., 2015; Damouche et al., 2015
Cytomegalovirus	m	Adipocytes Endothelial cells	Metabolic changes ↗ CD8 T cells	Price et al., 1990; Sacher et al., 2011; Contreras et al., 2019

Species in which the microbes have been identified are indicated (m, mouse; Hu, human; NHP, non-human primate). When available, the cell subset targeted by the microbes and the impact on the immune compartment is indicated.

several proteins involved in lipid metabolism (Pcyt1a and Dgat1), and are capable of lipid uptake (Cipolletta et al., 2012, 2015; Kolodin et al., 2015). Unfortunately, the high proportion of Tregs in VAT has not been confirmed in humans or non-human primates (NHPs) (Damouche et al., 2017). Given that the immune cell populations in AT are strongly modulated by inflammatory and/or metabolic signals and microbiota, the lower proportion of Tregs in human VAT (relative to murine VAT) might reflect differences in the metabolic and microbial challenges faced by humans vs. rodents. However, subsequent analyses of Treg counts in various mouse strains revealed that the high observed values were restricted to the VAT of male C57Bl/6 mice of a certain age (Laparra et al., 2019). Whereas the proportion of AT Tregs is much lower in obese rodents than in lean rodents [which presumably influences ongoing, obesity-associated inflammation (Cipolletta et al., 2012)], there is less agreement about whether this is true in humans. Although this disparity may reflect the fact that Foxp3 staining is less specific for human Tregs than for mouse Tregs (which could explain the preserved expression of Foxp3+ cells in obesity due to the accumulation of effector cells) and/or different metabolic and infectious histories in humans and mice, it may also reflect a model-specific difference in the contribution of the Treg subset in AT. Therefore, the potential immunosuppressive role of Tregs (i.e., limiting the development of an efficient anti-infectious immune responses) may not be as relevant in humans as first thought. The role of AT Tregs in the maintenance of human metabolic homeostasis is also subject to debate.

Group 2 innate lymphoid cells are also a crucial subset involved in the regulation of AT function (Molofsky et al., 2013). First described in FALCs in the mesentery, their identification has been extended to the whole AT. ILC2s contribute to the conversion of white to beige AT by directly impacting adipocyte progenitors (Brestoff et al., 2015) and thus preventing excessive energy storage. They also act indirectly by favoring eosinophils and M2 macrophages maintenance (Lee et al., 2015). Interestingly, ILC2 also provide help to B cells and contribute to IgA production, thus potentially contributing to immune responses.

Importantly, these cells are subjected and strongly regulated by the metabolic context. A detailed analysis of anti-infective immune responses would require the study of immune responses in both healthy and obese AT. Increases in macrophages, Th1 CD4 T cells, and CD8 T cells are described in most metabolic (McLaughlin et al., 2014; Liu and Nikolajczyk, 2019) and infectious episode affecting AT (Nagajyothi et al., 2012; Beigier-Bompadre et al., 2017), as well as inductive lymphoid structures (Rangel-Moreno et al., 2009; Bénézech et al., 2015, Bénézech and Jackson-Jones, 2019). These similarities question the potential synergy between obesity and anti-infectious immune responses. As in any non-lymphoid sites, the recruitment of innate and adaptive immune cell defines AT anti-infectious local responses but the AT local properties may impact their anti-infectious potential.

Adipocytes: The Immune Side of the Metabolic Cells

A number of studies have found that adipocyte lineage cells possess innate immune activity. Early-stage adipocyte precursors (such as preadipocytes) are known to have certain macrophage-like properties (Cousin et al., 1999; Charrière et al., 2003; Saillan-Barreau et al., 2003). The adipocytes' direct contribution to the immune response during infection is also suggested by the cell surface expression of Toll-like receptors (which sense conserved microbial motifs) on adipocytes. Stimulation of these receptors induces the production of pro-inflammatory cytokines (Lin et al., 2000). The expression of MHC class II molecules (crucial for CD4 T cell survival and activation) at the surface of adipocytes has also been described (Meijer et al., 2011; Deng et al., 2013). Deng et al. (2013) demonstrated that MHC class II expression on adipocytes was essential for the development of obesity-induced adipose inflammation. Adipocytes may act as antigen-presenting cells for T lymphocytes, although they do not enable full activation (Deng et al., 2013; Hruskova and Biswas, 2013). Zhang et al. (2015) recent report is even more striking; the researchers demonstrated that dermal adipocytes exerted direct antimicrobial activity against *Staphylococcus aureus* by producing cathelicidins – thus unequivocally confirming AT as a crucial component of innate responses to infection (Alcorn and Kolls, 2015; Kugelberg, 2015; Zhang et al., 2015).

Systemic Immunity

The endocrine activity of adipose tissue

Once the AT's endocrine activity had been demonstrated, the impact of various adipokines (including hormones, cytokines, and chemokines produced in AT) on the immune system was widely documented. Leptin, IL-1, IL-6, IL-8, interferon gamma (IFN-γ), transforming growth factor beta (TGF-β), and chemokines (such as monocyte chemotactic protein-1 and macrophage inflammatory protein-1) produced by AT interfere with the remote immune system. T cells and antigen-presenting cells are influenced by leptin, IL-6, and insulin. Conversely, in a context of calorie restriction and starvation, levels of pro-inflammatory adipokines fall and those of anti-inflammatory adipokines rise, which contributes to immunosuppression. Although not specific to the immune responses directed against pathogens, AT, by the secretion of various adipokines modulate immune responses.

Various murine models indicated that obesity (i.e., excessive adiposity) increases susceptibility to infection. Obese mice are more susceptible to bacterial infections due to greater microbial load and/or impaired clearance (*Klebsiella*, *Mycobacterium tuberculosis*, *Staphylococcus*) (Mancuso et al., 2002; Ikejima et al., 2005; Wieland et al., 2005), impaired resistance to listeria monocytogenes infection (Ikejima et al., 2005). However, most of these results were obtained using leptin-deficient *ob/ob* mice which are resistant to a variety of experimental models of inflammation/autoimmunity (La Cava et al., 2004; Matarese and La Cava, 2004), and therefore cannot be considered as a model which fully recapitulates the pathophysiology of obesity. Overall, obesity appears to be associated with higher susceptibility to infection (Karlsson and Beck, 2010; Huttunen and Syrjänen, 2013) even if the mechanisms involved remain unclear.

Adipose-tissue-resident memory T cells

It has been consistently observed that CD8 T cells accumulated in AT when the latter is exposed to metabolic or infectious insults. Whereas the clonal specificity of these cells is not clear in a metabolic context, pathogen-specific CD8 T cells have been found in AT. Although AT exhibits some very specific features, it is tempting to speculate that AT-Trm cells behave in much the same way as other memory T cells resident in non-lymphoid tissues. The literature on the biology of Trm cells is extensive (Gebhardt et al., 2009; Mueller et al., 2013; Sathaliyawala et al., 2013). Beura et al. (2018) recently described how CD8 Trm cells (but not CD4 Trm cells) (Beura et al., 2019) migrate from non-lymphoid tissue to nearby lymphoid sites. Resident memory T cells may thus support a secondary immune response produced at lymphoid sites during rechallenge. If this phenomenon occurs in AT, it would highlight the tissue as a major partner in memory T cell responses. Interestingly, Han et al.'s (2017) important study demonstrated that CD8 T cells from AT can indeed produce secondary immune responses. By grafting AT collected from animals infected with *Toxoplasma gondii*, the researchers demonstrate that CD8 T cells in the graft protected the naïve recipients from what would normally be a lethal challenge with the same pathogens (Han et al., 2017).

The phenotypic characterization of Trm cells is ongoing (Walsh et al., 2019), and it is not yet clear whether or not the memory CD8 T cells found in AT are indeed resident. In non-lymphoid sites, the expression of surface markers like CD103 and CD69 is usually considered to be a marker of residency. CD69 is strongly expressed by CD4 and CD8 T cells in AT (Couturier et al., 2015; Damouche et al., 2017). However, given that CD69 is also an activation marker, the expression of CD69 on memory T cells in AT has been linked to activation as well as residency. Importantly, the two notions are not necessarily exclusive; the tissue-specific expression of CD69 may reflect the low-grade stimulation and activation of T cells, which would favor their persistence. The results of parabiosis experiments tend to support the existence of Trm cells in AT (Han et al., 2017).

In conclusion, AT's potential role in innate and adaptive immune responses to infection is based on the tissue's immune cell content, pro-inflammatory potential, and proximity to sites with immune activity. Lastly, the recent realization that Trm T cells contribute to memory responses at lymphoid sites drastically broadens the anti-infectious potential of AT; this tissue might support local and systemic cell-based anti-infectious responses (**Figure 4**).

Adipose Tissue as a Pathogen Reservoir, and Pathogen-Induced Perturbations

Our group and others have demonstrated that AT is a reservoir for HIV (Couturier et al., 2015, 2016, 2018; Damouche et al., 2015; Hsu et al., 2017). Interestingly, a number of pathogens persist in AT – prompting the question of whether HIV's persistence in AT relies on a specific targeting mechanism or reflects the AT's broader, intrinsic ability to store pathogens. Although the marked accumulation of pathogens in AT is striking, the cell subsets that define the cellular reservoir differ (**Table 2**) – suggesting the presence of pathogen-specific mechanisms.

Pathogens frequently reported in HIV co-infections [such as *M. tuberculosis* (Beigier-Bompadre et al., 2017) and *Leishmania* parasites (Allahverdiyev et al., 2011)] have been detected in

AT. Interestingly, the cytomegalovirus (CMV, a herpes virus that infects most people worldwide) has been also detected in AT (Contreras et al., 2019). The impact of CMV infection on aging has been widely documented (Solana et al., 2012; Wertheimer et al., 2014), and HIV infection has also been linked to accelerated aging (Appay et al., 2007, 2011). In a context of HIV, interaction with other pathogens present in AT might accentuate the specific effects of the viral infection. Conversely, HIV may accentuate a preexisting chronic tuberculosis (TB) or *Leishmania* infection locally.

Mycobacterium tuberculosis in Adipose Tissue

Tuberculosis is one of the most common co-infections in people living with HIV. In non-treated patients with latent TB, the immunosuppression associated with HIV infection is particularly harmful because it may trigger the development of an active TB infection. Treating a TB and HIV co-infection is clinically challenging; drug interference and toxicity prevents the respective treatments from being combined, leading clinicians to favor one treatment over the other (Djimeu and Heard, 2019). It has been shown that TB-associated immune reconstitution inflammatory syndrome can develop when ART is initiated (Worodria et al., 2011; Abay et al., 2015; Haridas et al., 2015; Boulougoura and Sereti, 2016). Importantly, ART-controlled HIV infection appears to interfere with TB infection (Worodria et al., 2018; Holmberg et al., 2019).

Mycobacterium tuberculosis can be detected in both SVF cells (macrophages) and adipocytes. Furthermore, the transfer of AT lysates from infected mice to naïve recipients can induce a TB infection. The local persistence of *M. tuberculosis* is associated with changes in the AT's immune compartment, with infiltration of CD8 T cells and NK cells and the production of IFN-γ (Neyrolles et al., 2006; Beigier-Bompadre et al., 2017).

Cytomegalovirus in Adipose Tissue

As mentioned above, CMV is a herpesvirus that infects most of the world's population. The long-term impact of chronic CMV persistence has been extensively studied. Infection by CMV is associated with immune senescence, and is a prognostic component of the immune risk profile in elderly adults. CMV and HIV infections are interlinked; accentuated CMV-specific memory T-cell responses associated with an immune risk phenotype constitute a prominent immunologic feature of accelerated aging in HIV infection (Barrett et al., 2012). Conversely, the efficacy of ART treatment (restoration of the CD4 T cell count) depends on the patient's CMV status (Appay et al., 2011; Sauce et al., 2011). The reason for the connection between HIV and CMV is subject to debate but may be related to the viruses' apparent colocalization in AT.

Cytomegalovirus infection of AT is also associated with the infiltration and/or local expansion of CD8 T cells, the development of pro-inflammatory responses, and metabolic alterations (Contreras et al., 2019). Interestingly, signs of aging have also been associated with HIV infection; it remains to be established whether a synergistic effect of the various local infections may aggravate alterations in AT's metabolic functions.

Human Immunodeficiency Virus in Adipose Tissue

The link between AT and HIV infection has long been known. People infected with HIV suffer from metabolic alterations (including dyslipidemia, insulin resistance, and lipodystrophy) that were initially considered to be adverse reactions to the first classes of antiretroviral drugs (ARVs) to be developed [i.e., nucleoside reverse transcriptase inhibitors (NRTIs) and protease inhibitors (PIs)] (Samaras et al., 2007; Falutz, 2011). However, the presence of metabolic alterations in treatment-naïve HIV-infected people suggests that the virus has a direct impact. Accordingly, researchers sought to determine whether HIV infects adipocytes, since infection might explain the broad disruption of fat biology (either alone or by accentuating the toxicity of ARV drugs). These studies were performed in the early 2000s. Although adipocytes (i) express the co-receptors required for HIV entry (Hazan et al., 2002), and (ii) can be infected *in vitro* (Maurin et al., 2005), HIV has never been directly detected in these cells (Dupin et al., 2002; Munier et al., 2003). The spread of viral proteins has also been studied, and viral proteins such as Vpr have indeed been found in AT from HIV-infected patients. The viral proteins' contribution to adipose dysfunction has been studied (Muthumani et al., 2005; Shrivastav et al., 2008; Agarwal et al., 2013). In the meantime, however, studies of AT alterations in obesity revealed the high proportion of immune cells (and notably CD4 T cells and macrophages, HIV's two main targets) in AT. When considering the SVF in particular, a different picture emerged: HIV (or SIV, in macaque models) was detected (Couturier et al., 2015, 2016; Damouche et al., 2015) in both viremic and controlled ART-treated patients. The virus was also found in the macrophage fraction in the viremic macaque model but not in samples from ART-treated HIV-infected patients. The low macrophage count in these patients precluded any conclusions as to the respective levels of macrophage infection during the viremic and aviremic phases.

Several research groups have confirmed that HIV infects CD4 T cells in AT (Damouche et al., 2015; Couturier et al., 2016) and that this virus is replication-competent (Damouche et al., 2015; Couturier et al., 2018; **Table 4**). However, these and other findings raise a number of questions. Firstly, there are few data on the time course of AT infection and the mechanism that underlies HIV infection and persistence in AT cells. It appears that AT cells are infected quite rapidly (within 4 weeks: personal data). Secondly, the CD4 T cell fractions in SAT and VAT exhibit similar level of HIV DNA during the chronic phase of the infection – suggesting that the common features of SAT and VAT (rather than the specific properties of each type of AT) favor viral infection and/or persistence. However, the specific factors that allow viral persistence in AT have yet to be defined. Thirdly, viral persistence of HIV in many other AT depots (e.g., perivascular, dermal, and BM depots) has not been evaluated. Fourthly, there are few data on the impact of obesity on HIV infections and the establishment of the HIV reservoir in AT. From a technical

TABLE 4 | Studies of the presence of HIV (or the simian form, SIV/SHIV) in adipose tissue in humans and simians, indicating the detection strategies and pathogens.

Year	Species	Detection of viral nucleic acids in adipose tissue	References
2002	Hu	No HIV DNA in adipose tissue lysate	Dupin et al., 2002
2015	Hu	SHIV DNA in SVF cells	Couturier et al., 2015
	Cyno Ms, Hu	SIV DNA and RNA in SVF cells, SVF CD4 T cells and SVF macrophages HIV DNA and RNA in SVF cells, SVF CD4 T cells *in vitro* reactivation assay	Damouche et al., 2015
2016	Rh Ms	SHIV DNA in SVF cells	Couturier et al., 2016
2017	Rh Ms	SHIV RNA in SVF and SVF CD4 T cells at week 2	Hsu et al., 2017
2018	Hu	HIV DNA in SVF CD4 T cells	Koethe et al., 2017
2018	Hu	*In vitro* reactivation assay	Couturier et al., 2018

Cyno Ms, cynomolgus macaque; Rh Ms, rhesus macaques.

standpoint, studies of most of these questions are limited by the small number of cells recovered from AT samples.

MECHANISMS THAT MAY FAVOR THE PERSISTENCE OF HIV IN ADIPOSE TISSUE

Very little information is available on the mechanisms that may favor HIV persistence but various hypotheses may be formulated (**Table 5**).

Immunologic Parameters

Both of HIV's main targets (CD4 T cells and macrophages) are present in AT. Both cell types are predominantly in a resting phase, which may favor the latency of HIV. The proximity to a major site of viral replication (such as the gut mucosae) may also contribute to the direct infection of AT. However, SAT or VAT do not differ significantly with regard to the level of HIV DNA in CD4 T cells (Damouche et al., 2015) – suggesting that environmental factors (e.g., low-grade inflammation, local microbial inflammation, and the viral load) do not drastically affect the level of infection of the CD4 T cell compartment.

Adipose Tissue as an Immunosuppressive Environment

One possible mechanism for HIV persistence in AT would involve local immunosuppression and thus failure to eliminate HIV-infected cells. An obvious candidate for this immunosuppression is the Foxp3+ CD4 Treg subset. We compared the distribution of the various cell subtypes associated with immunosuppression in the AT of mice, NHPs, and macaques (Laparra et al., 2019). In AT from adult male humans and NHPs, we found a low proportion of Tregs, MSCs, and other subsets with immunosuppressive functions – thus ruling out a major role of Treg inhibition in the persistence of HIV in AT. Importantly, we observed a small but statistically significant increase in the proportion of Foxp3+ Treg cells in SAT from ART-treated HIV-infected patients, relative to SAT from non-infected control subjects (Damouche et al., 2017) – suggesting that the changes induced by HIV infection in AT may also contribute to viral persistence. Adipocytes may represent the main Ag-presenting cells subset in AT (representing >50% of AT cell), but may lack costimulatory signals that are required for efficient presentation and immune cell activation (Meijer et al., 2011; Deng et al., 2013). However, data demonstrating that adipocytes ensure efficient T cell stimulation (Xiao et al., 2016) and the presence of DCs in AT emphasize the need to decipher the capacity for Ag presentation by AT.

T Cell Exhaustion and Senescence

Another intrinsic property of AT is the high surface expression of PD-1 (an exhaustion marker) on both CD4 and CD8 T cells. Although it is not known whether or not cells in AT cells express PD-L1 or PD-L2, the presence of PD-1 indicates high susceptibility to exhaustion. The difference in PD-1 expression between AT-resident T cells and circulating T cells is observed on both CD4 and CD8 T cell subsets, but reflect two distinct processes. Indeed, the high PD-1 expression on CD4 T cells in AT is due to the higher proportion of memory CD4 T cells which intrinsically express PD-1, and not to a higher expression level in CD4 T cells in AT compared with blood. At the opposite, memory CD8 T cells collected from AT or blood differ with regard to PD-1 expression – suggesting that a phenotypic change within CD8 T cell subsets is associated with the cells' persistence in the AT environment. Regardless of the mechanisms, AT resident T cells exhibit high proportion of PD-1 expressing cells.

Similarly, AT resident CD4 and CD8 T cells also expressed high proportion of CD57 expressing cells (Koethe et al., 2017; Wanjalla et al., 2019). CD57 expression is associated with both terminal differentiation and replicative senescence, providing mixed signals regarding their functional potential.

CD4 and CD8 T Cells Are Not Colocalized in AT

We have studied the distribution of CD4 and CD8 T cells in AT from ART patients (Damouche et al., 2015). In both HIV-infected and non-infected donors, we observed that CD4 and CD8 T cells were generally not colocalized. This provides a strong rationale for the persistence of HIV-infected CD4 T cells, which could not be reached by CD8 T cells. This observation obviously parallels the situation described in LNs, whereas follicular helper CD4 T cells are also out of reach of CD8 T cells and thus persist in the germinal center. It remains to be determined whether or not metabolic alterations that disturb the AT architecture can modify this non-colocalization and thus induce clusters with direct contact between CD4 and CD8 T cells. The absence of CD4–CD8 T cell contact may have a direct

TABLE 5 | Mechanisms that may favor the persistence of HIV in adipose tissue.

Parameters potentially favoring viral persistence in adipose tissue		References
Immunological parameters	**Mechanisms/observations**	
AT as an Immunosuppressive environment		Wan et al., 2008; Khairoun and Korevaar, 2013; Yousefi et al., 2016
ASC	Limiting T cell proliferation	Khairoun and Korevaar, 2013
	Favoring Treg (generation and accumulation)	Yousefi et al., 2016
Th2-like cells and cytokines		
Limited efficiency of Ag presenting cells		
Distinct local distribution of CD4 and CD8 T cells		Damouche et al., 2015
Defective T cell responses		Wronska and Kmiec, 2012
Exhaustion	High percentage of PD-1 expressing cells	Shirakawa et al., 2016; Damouche et al., 2017
Senescence	High percentage of CD57 expressing cells	Koethe et al., 2017
Metabolic reprogramming		
Resident memory T cell		Pan et al., 2017
CD36 expression on AT T cell		Couturier et al., 2019
Metabolic parameters		
Interaction between adipocyte and immune cells		Mazzon and Mercer, 2014
The consequences of a lipid-rich environment		
Oxidative stress		Malmberg et al., 2001; Ivanov et al., 2016
Hypoxia in adipose tissue		Tao et al., 2015
Insulin sensitivity		Tsai et al., 2018
Viral and pharmacological parameters		
HIV viral proteins		Boya et al., 2004; Debaisieux et al., 2012; Clark et al., 2017; Jacob et al., 2017
Adipose tissue remodeling and fibrosis		Sun et al., 2013; Vila et al., 2014; Marcelin et al., 2017
Antiretroviral diffusion (ARV)		Dupin et al., 2002; Couturier et al., 2018

impact on the persistence of HIV-infected CD4 T cells, and might also interfere with the effective differentiation of memory cells. Indeed, CD4 T cell help is a crucial factor in the differentiation and maintenance of CD8 T cells.

HIV Viral Proteins Affecting Immune Cells

The immune compartment can be modulated not only by AT's intrinsic properties but also by HIV infection. It has been shown that the HIV proteins Tat, Nef, gp120, and Vpr can modulate immune cells, notably by inducing the apoptosis of non-infected CD4 T cells as a bystander effect (Boya et al., 2004). Nef binds to CXCR4 and modulates T cell activation (Jacob et al., 2017), and so may also be involved in HIV persistence. Tat induces apoptosis in non-infected CD8 and CD4 T cells, and alters the metabolic, morphologic, and biochemical properties of CD4 T cells (Debaisieux et al., 2012; Faller et al., 2014; Clark et al., 2017). Vpr lengthens the lifespan of HIV-infected macrophages by modulating glutamate metabolism in the mitochondria (Datta et al., 2016).

Metabolic Reprogramming of Immune Cells in AT

Recent research has characterized the metabolic requirements of functionally effective immune cells. Metabolic reprogramming of immune cells is a crucial aspect related to their differentiation status. Resting, memory, and regulatory T cells have different metabolic requirements: activation of T cells is accompanied by a switch from oxidative metabolism to intensified glucose metabolism *via* aerobic glycolysis. Tregs have reduced ability to activate the PI3K/Akt pathway (Palmer et al., 2016a,b). Metabolic reprograming of immune cells is also described in non-lymphoid tissues: Trm cell survival depends on exogenous lipid uptake (Pan et al., 2017). T lymphocytes in AT express high levels of CD36, a scavenger receptor for lipid uptake (Couturier et al., 2019).

Viruses are obligate parasites that are completely reliant on host cell metabolism. They manipulate cellular metabolism including glycolysis, fatty acid synthesis, and glutaminolysis to create an intracellular metabolic niche, which supports virion production and promotes survival of infected cells. Increased Glut1 expression on CD4 T cells in culture increases cellular permissivity to HIV-1 infection, while suppression of glucose metabolism by PI3K inhibitors inhibits infection (Loisel-Meyer et al., 2012). Lastly, Saez-Cirion et al.'s recent study (Valle-Casuso et al., 2019) showed that HIV specifically targets highly metabolically active CD4 T cells (i.e., enabling the virus to multiply more rapidly). HIV-1 selectively infects CD4 T cells with high levels of oxidative phosphorylation and glycolysis, independently of their activation phenotype. In a similar way to carcinogenesis, it is also now admitted the existence of a metabolic reprogramming upon HIV infection, related to modifications in glucose metabolism (Ahmed et al., 2018).

In this respect, AT provides very specific metabolic cues whose effects on the local immune responses (and the virus cycle) requires further investigation. Whether AT immune cells in AT may be sensible to these HIV-induced reprogramming or favor viral latency remain to be evaluated.

Metabolic Parameters

Initially, the term "immunometabolism" referred to the two-way interaction between the metabolism and the immune system. This entity has now been subdivided into "tissue immunometabolism" (the impact of immune cells on both local and systemic metabolic homeostasis, and vice versa) (Matarese and La Cava, 2004; Ferrante, 2013) and "cellular immunometabolism" (the intracellular metabolic changes associated with immune cell responses and survival) (Wang and Wu, 2018). Importantly, viruses need to subvert the cell's metabolism to develop, and so virus–metabolism interactions are now also considered. With regard to the specific metabolic properties of AT, various factors (including the ECM in AT) may directly or indirectly favor viral infection and/or persistence.

The Consequences of a Lipid-Rich Environment

Lipids fulfill three general functions: (i) energy storage, principally as TG and steryl esters in lipid droplets, (ii) structural components of the cell (plasma and organelle membranes, and membrane component of budding and intracellular trafficking), and (iii) first and second messengers in signal transduction (van Meer et al., 2008). With regard to the latter point, several studies have found that the type and quantity of fatty acids and lipid mediators can influence the immune system in a potent manner (Pal et al., 2012). Saturated fatty acids are able to activate Toll-like receptors on adipocytes *via* endogenous ligand fetuin-A (Pal et al., 2012), and are involved in inflammation. Unsaturated fatty acids can be oxidized to generate potent pro-inflammatory or pro-resolving lipid mediators. High concentrations of fatty acids are toxic for T cells, whereas non-toxic concentrations can induce proliferation and cytokine production. This aspect of the interaction between immune cells and metabolic signals is probably the best documented (Ferrante, 2013), although the direct influence of the AT environment on immune responses during infection requires further investigation. Furthermore, studies of the interactions between viruses and host cells have also revealed the role played by structural lipids during each step in the viral lifecycle (binding, internalization, fusion, genome uncoating, replication, particle assembly, and budding) (Mazzon and Mercer, 2014). In the early stages of infection, viruses subvert cellular lipids and use lipid-based signaling mechanisms for entry and trafficking. Once an infection has developed and viral genes have been expressed, lipid synthesis is extensively reprogrammed and the lipid distribution is remodeled to promote viral replication, assembly, and egress. It is known that HIV actively modulates lipid rafts by increasing the synthesis and trafficking of cholesterol to these sites. Furthermore, soluble HIV-1 proteins can enter cells through lipid rafts (Mañes et al., 2003). These observations suggest that the lipid-rich environment in AT may have a direct impact on plasma membrane composition and plasticity (notably the lipid rafts). In the context of tumors, an increase in circulating cholesterol levels is associated with an increase in the cholesterol content of lipid rafts; in turn, this alters raft-mediated downstream signaling and promotes tumor growth (Mollinedo and Gajate, 2015). It is not clear whether the structural composition and plasticity of plasma and organelle membranes of the main cellular targets of HIV differ in AT (relative to other tissues), although these factors might contribute to preferential infection by HIV and facilitated viral latency. Unfortunately, very little is known about the putative specific influence of the AT's lipid-rich environment on the lifecycle of HIV.

Oxidative Stress

Adipose tissue produces reactive oxygen species (ROS) under various circumstances, and especially in a context of obesity. Both chronic and acute exposure to oxidative stress affects adipocyte and T cells (Malmberg et al., 2001), and also appears to impact HIV's lifecycle (Ivanov et al., 2016). In fact, HIV infection triggers pronounced oxidative stress, which subsequently enhances viral transcription and creates a positive feedback loop. The Vpr protein induces hypoxia inducible factor 1 (HIF-1) and then the ROS-dependent activation of HIV's long terminal repeat. Pro-inflammatory cytokines (such as TNF-α) also enhance viral transcription. Importantly, glutathione treatment of chronically infected cells during the later stages of the HIV life cycle leads to the abrogation of virion budding and release (Beura et al., 2018), which potentially favors viral latency. The direct impact of oxidative stress in the AT on the HIV and HIV-infected cells has yet to be evaluated in detail. Given the known functional impact of oxidative stress on the immune cells and adipocytes in AT, ROS production may also affect HIV's infectivity and persistence.

Hypoxia in Adipose Tissue

As adipocytes expand, the interstitial oxygen tension falls. The subsequent activation of HIF-1 inhibits pre-adipocyte differentiation and initiates AT fibrosis. HIF-1 is also expressed by T cells and other immune cells, and is a potent regulator of T cell survival, activation, and differentiation (McNamee et al., 2013; Tao et al., 2015). It is known that HIF-1 drives pro-inflammatory Th17 cell function and longevity. Lastly, low oxygen levels inhibit the replication of HIV-1 and its reactivation from latent reservoirs (Charles et al., 2009; Loisel-Meyer et al., 2012; Nekhai et al., 2013). As previously described for the lipid-rich environment and oxidative stress, the intrinsic impact of the AT environment must be taken into account.

Insulin Sensitivity

Insulin has a critical role in maintaining the homeostasis of energy metabolism, and coordinates the storage and utilization of fuel molecules in AT and in other insulin-sensitive peripheral tissues. Recent research has highlighted the two-way link between insulin and immune cells (Dalmas et al., 2017; Tsai et al., 2018), and has confirmed that metabolic parameters can indirectly influence immune responses. However, this two-way link has not been observed in AT, and a direct relationship between insulin sensitivity and the HIV life cycle has not been demonstrated at the cellular level.

Adipose Tissue Remodeling and Fibrosis

In addition to intrinsic metabolic–immune interactions in healthy AT, metabolic and immune remodeling can also be induced by HIV infection and ART treatment. Remodeling of the ECM is a key event in HIV infection, and HIV infection has a specific role in AT fibrosis. Macrophages and

ASCs are major players in the onset of AT fibrosis (Vila et al., 2014; Marcelin et al., 2017), notably by the production of TGF-β. It has been reported that SIV-infected macaques upregulated TGF-β expression in the SAT and VAT (Gorwood et al., 2019). The HIV-1 proteins Tat and Nef are secreted by infected cells and then induce a profibrotic phenotype in ASCs. The increase in collagen production and TGF-β secretion associated with HIV infection may be involved in AT fibrosis. The TGF-β produced by profibrotic adipose-derived MSCs might also have an impact on the Tregs in AT, although this topic requires further investigation. The persistence of an inflammatory stimulus and/or hypoxia in AT may be responsible for the excessive synthesis of ECM components and the subsequent interstitial deposition of fibrotic material (Sun et al., 2013). This collagen deposition is accompanied by the infiltration of macrophages and other immune cells (Spencer et al., 2010). Although fibrosis directly impacts adipocyte biology and immune cell migration, a direct link between the HIV lifecycle and the severity of the induced fibrosis has not been described.

Pharmacologic Parameters

The adipose toxicity of the first generation of ARVs (notably in *in vitro* assays) has been extensively described (Koethe, 2017). Nevertheless, the pharmacokinetics and intracellular metabolism of ARVs in adipocytes have not been extensively characterized. It is known that NRTIs and PIs accumulate in murine and human adipocytes *in vitro* (Janneh et al., 2003, 2010; Vernochet et al., 2005; Couturier et al., 2018) but only two *in vivo* studies (Dupin et al., 2002; Couturier et al., 2018) have reported on ARV concentrations in the AT of HIV-infected patients. Further studies of ARV penetration in AT are needed, and it remains to be established whether or not the tissue concentrations of the various ARVs in AT are therapeutic.

Indeed, the penetration of ARVs into AT is influenced by several physiochemical and pharmacokinetics factors, including the blood perfusion rate, molecular size, ionization state, plasma protein binding, lipophilicity, and efflux/influx transporter affinity.

The perfusion rate varies considerably from one tissue to another. AT is a poorly vascularized compartment with a low perfusion rate [approximately 200 mL/min or 0.025 mL/g tissue) (Derendorf et al., 2019)],which might limit the diffusion of ARVs. However, all of the ARVs except enfuvirtide are small molecules, and so can penetrate AT more easily. Given that only unbound, non-ionized drugs can cross cell membranes, the degree of binding to plasma proteins and the pKa are likely to influence AT penetration. It should be borne in mind that an ARV's ionization state can differ from one tissue to another as a result of the local pH. In contrast to other tissues, penetration into AT did not appears to be related to the protein binding of ARVs (Dupin et al., 2002; Couturier et al., 2018). For example, most NRTIs penetrate genital and colorectal tissue extensively, notably as a result of their low plasma protein binding (<0.7–49%). In contrast, PIs, non-NRTIs, and integrase strand transfer inhibitors bind readily to plasma proteins (except for indinavir, nevirapine, and raltegravir in each of the three classes, respectively); >90% of the drug molecules are bound to albumin or alpha-1 acid glycoprotein, which thus may partly limit their access to genital and colorectal tissues (Trezza et al., 2015). Lipid solubility appears to be the most important factor in AT penetration. Hence, the relatively hydrophilic NRTIs (such as abacavir, lamivudine, emtricitabine, and tenofovir) are rarely or not detected in AT cells (Dupin et al., 2002; Couturier et al., 2018). In contrast, the more hydrophobic dolutegravir penetrates into AT in HIV-infected patients (Couturier et al., 2018). Lastly, the ARVs' affinity for efflux or influx transporters [such as the ATP-binding cassette (ABC) and solute carrier transporter families] and the presence of transporters in AT may influence drug penetration. Although these transporters have been well characterized in various tissues (Kis et al., 2010), only one study of AT has been published; it found that P-glycoprotein (ABCB1) was expressed on pre-adipocytes and limits the accumulation of zidovudine (Janneh et al., 2010).

Other important factors include the complex structure of adipocyte tissue and the relationships between adipocytes and other cells. In SIV-infected macaques, Damouche et al. (2015) showed that CD4 T cells are distal to blood vessels in AT – implying that ARVs have to cross additional barriers if they are to reach infected immune cells in AT. Couturier et al. (2018) reported that the *in vitro* accumulation of tenofovir-diphosphate (the intracellular, active form of tenofovir) was low in CD4 T cells and was associated with increased HIV production.

The low levels of ARVs in AT and the corresponding impact on HIV replication suggest that AT is a pharmacological sanctuary in which high tissue concentrations of ARVs are required to suppress local HIV replication.

CONSEQUENCES OF AT INFECTION

Special focuses have been obviously given to the metabolic consequences of fat tissue infection that will be only briefly discussed in this review [see the excellent review on the subject (Desruisseaux et al., 2007; Koethe, 2017; Couturier and Lewis, 2018; Godfrey et al., 2019)]. Works are still ongoing notably to decipher the respective impact of the local viral infection and antiretroviral treatment. The question is even more relevant with the recent description of weight gain in patients (and notably women) treated with integrase inhibitors (Norwood et al., 2017; Bourgi et al., 2019; Kerchberger et al., 2019). However, more recent data suggest an even broader impact of fat tissue infection, potentially affecting systemic secondary immune responses and contributing to the accelerated aging, two defects commonly associated with chronic HIV infection.

Metabolic Alterations Associated With Viral Persistence in AT

In treatment-naïve patients infected with HIV, we observed a number of metabolic alterations: a decrease in the amount of AT (Visnegarwala et al., 2005), AT redistribution (Madge et al., 1999), changes in adipogenic markers (Giralt et al., 2006; Vidal et al., 2012), and mitochondrial damage (Garrabou et al., 2011). Experiments in SIV-infected macaques have shown that chronic viral infection is associated with the presence of small adipocytes and elevated fibrosis – suggesting a specific impact of HIV infection on AT (Gorwood et al., 2019). Secreted viral proteins (such as Tat, Nef, Vpr, and gp120) have also been shown to influence the AT, although their secretion within the AT has never been observed. In a mouse model, Vpr induced metabolic changes in AT (Agarwal et al., 2013). Tat and Nef induced a profibrotic phenotype in adipose-derived MSCs, and Nef altered adipogenesis (Gorwood et al., 2019). The effect of Tat on adipogenesis is subject to debate (Cotter et al., 2011; Díaz-Delfín et al., 2012; Gorwood et al., 2019). The impact of Tat and Nef on MSCs has been studied extensively. Tat and Nef induce premature senescence in MSCs; Nef inhibits autophagy by binding to Beclin1, whereas Tat activates nuclear factor kappa B and this increases inflammation (Beaupere et al., 2015). Tat has been implicated in inflammation and elevated expression of pro-inflammatory cytokines in the AT (Díaz-Delfín et al., 2012), and activates nuclear factor kappa B in MSCs and CD4 T cells (Fiume et al., 2012). Taken as a whole, these studies suggest that HIV has a role in metabolic impairments in AT. Furthermore, various classes of ARVs (NRTIs, PIs, and now integrase strand transfer inhibitors) have long been implicated in the modification and redistribution of AT – suggesting that ART and HIV have an additional and/or synergistic impact.

Immune Effects of Viral Persistence in AT

In the cynomolgus macaque model of intravenous infection with SIVmac 251, major changes in the CD4 T cell compartment in SAT and VAT were not observed; the CD4 T cell counts were unchanged, suggesting that limited depletion occurs in AT (Damouche et al., 2015). The main change was a significantly elevated CD8 T cell count. The specificity of CD8 T cell accumulation in AT remains to be evaluated, notably with regard to the recruitment of HIV-specific CD8 T cells. Changes in CD4 and CD8 T cell counts have been reported in ART-treated HIV-infected patients (Wanjalla et al., 2019). Given the putative role of AT as a site of memory T cell accumulation for lymphoid secondary immune responses, the nature of the change in the T cell compartment needs to be determined. One can reasonably hypothesize that HIV's targeting of AT has both metabolic and immunologic consequences, with impaired memory responses against other pathogens (and not just HIV).

In contrast to the changes observed in a context of obesity, viral persistence does not appear to greatly modify the macrophage count. Phenotypically, the macrophages shift toward an M1 profile but less so than in a context of obesity. This intermediate profile suggests that the local inflammation associated with HIV infection differs from the "metabolic inflammation" associated with obesity. Similarly, viral persistence does not lead to great changes in the level of pro-inflammatory cytokine secretion. Overall, HIV-associated inflammation in AT may differ qualitatively and/or quantitatively from that one observed in the extreme context of obesity. The characteristics of AT in HIV infection vs. obesity have recently been nicely reviewed (Wanjalla et al., 2018).

Accelerated Aging

Infection by HIV is thought to lead to the premature aging of AT, although further investigation is required. For example, the prevalence of comorbidities usually associated with aging (such as cardiometabolic disease) and the trunk fat accumulation phenotype are more prevalent in ART-treated HIV-infected patients (Caron-Debarle et al., 2010). Risk factors include HIV infection itself, and the duration and type of ART. The pathophysiologic mechanisms are poorly understood, although several factors are likely to be involved. ECM remodeling, inflammation, and redistribution have been observed in the AT of HIV-infected patients treated with first-generation ARVs (Bastard et al., 2002; Lagathu et al., 2005, 2007, 2017; Caron et al., 2007; Caron-Debarle et al., 2010; Béréziat et al., 2011). Interestingly, normal aging is also associated with fibrosis, inflammation, and AT redistribution (Tchkonia et al., 2010). Thus, one can hypothesize that HIV led to the premature aging of AT in these patients, and had cardiovascular and metabolic consequences. Immunosenescence has also been observed during chronic HIV-infection; this promotes immune activation and inflammation, which in turn might enhance HIV persistence and accelerate aging in a positive feedback loop (Appay and Sauce, 2008).

PERSPECTIVES

The Immune Properties of Adipose Tissue

Due to the physical size of AT and its critical location close to immune sites (i.e., interface sites or lymphoid sites), a better understanding of the tissue's local and systemic properties is essential. Both metabolic and infectious signals may change the homeostasis of AT and then directly impair the effectiveness of secondary immune responses. A growing body of evidence points to an anti-infectious role for AT. Research in this field may highlight novel mechanistic links between obesity and susceptibility to infections.

Another feature of AT is its potential modulation by pharmacologic modulators of metabolism. Indeed, AT is doubtless a valuable model in which strategies aimed at correcting viral-induced defects and/or reducing the size of the viral reservoir can be evaluated.

Therapeutic Strategies Based on Metabolic Pathways

At present, ART usually controls HIV replication in infected people. Nevertheless, cellular and tissue reservoirs of HIV are always present; it is still impossible to cure HIV and eradicate the virus from the body completely. The size of the HIV reservoir depends on several factors, including the time interval between the infection and the initiation of ART, the CD4/CD8 ratio, and the level of inflammation (even in patients on ART). To reduce systemic and local inflammation, pravastatin is already being used to treat HIV-infected patients (Toribio et al., 2017). Another possible treatment option is metformin, an antidiabetic, senolytic drug that might promote metabolic function in the AT, decrease inflammation, and modulate T cell activation (Moyo et al., 2014). Metformin's effects have been studied in HIV-infected people with diabetes, and the drug is currently being tested clinically in non-diabetic HIV-infected patients (Routy et al., 2019). Another therapeutic strategy for controlling the HIV reservoir involves targeting immunometabolic checkpoints; metformin targets the 5′-adenosine monophosphate-activated protein kinase and the mammalian target of rapamycin (mTOR) (Routy et al., 2015), and the monoclonal antibody pembrolizumab targets PD-1 on infected CD4 T cells. This PD-1 blockade was initially used in cancer treatment but has been shown to reduce CD4 T cell HIV reservoirs *ex vivo* (Evans et al., 2018). Other immune checkpoint inhibitors (such as anti-CTLA4, mTORC1/2 inhibitors) used primarily to treat cancer might also be of value in reducing HIV reservoirs and persistence (Adashek et al., 2019). Two main strategies for reducing reservoirs and persistence are currently being investigated. Firstly, HIV "shock and kill" strategies are based on treatment with latency reversal agents (LRAs) and then immune clearance through cytopathic effects or immune-mediated responses. The HIV proteins Tat and Nef can be used as LRAs for latent CD4 T cells (Kuang and Brockman, 2018; Tang et al., 2018), whereas Nef inhibitors could be used as HIV-specific immune adjuvants for curative vaccines (Dekaban and Dikeakos, 2017). Anti-Bcl-2 drugs can also target and kill HIV-latent T cells, and thus direct reduce the HIV reservoir (Cummins et al., 2017). Secondly, the "deep latency" strategy adopt the opposite approach; proviral HIV is silenced so that it cannot rebound (Elsheikh et al., 2019). Lastly, recent studies have isolated several neutralizing monoclonal antibodies from HIV-infected patients – opening up the use of broadly neutralizing antibodies (bnAbs) as a potentially curative treatment for HIV (Possas et al., 2018). It has been suggested that bnAbs can control HIV replication and reactivate latent cells, although the use of these antibodies to specifically target HIV-1 in humans constitutes a major challenge (Shen et al., 2019). These cutting-age therapeutic strategies are currently under development. However, it remains to be seen whether these therapies can reach all the cellular and tissue reservoirs and, in particular, all the infected cells within the AT and other HIV sanctuaries (i.e., the central nervous system, spleen, and LNs).

CONCLUSION

It is now well established that HIV infects AT, although the respective effects of the virus and ARVs on AT remain to be evaluated. This infection probably has more consequences than initially supposed. AT's metabolic, immune, and regenerative properties mean that HIV infection triggers multiple defects in regenerative and/or immune functions. Regarding the mechanisms involved in HIV's infection of (and then persistence in) AT, it is important to note that many pathogens are now known to persist in AT – suggesting the existence of an intrinsic mechanism that strongly favors their persistence. HIV persistence in AT may depend on various mechanisms; some may be intrinsic to the biology of AT, whereas others may be more closely related to virus-induced perturbations. Importantly, the AT's metabolic activity may provide a means of therapeutically reducing or even eradicating the viral load in AT. A growing number of studies have demonstrated the effectiveness of metabolic approaches to immune modulation; this may be particularly relevant for decreasing the HIV reservoir in AT.

AUTHOR CONTRIBUTIONS

All authors, by their respective field of expertise (immunology, pharmacology, metabolism, and infectiology) contributed to the writing of the article.

REFERENCES

Abay, S. M., Deribe, K., Reda, A. A., Biadgilign, S., Datiko, D., Assefa, T., et al. (2015). The effect of early initiation of antiretroviral therapy in TB/HIV-coinfected patients. *J. Int. Assoc. Provid. AIDS Care* 14, 560–570. doi: 10.1177/2325957415599210

Adashek, J. J., Junior, P. N. A., Galanina, N., and Kurzrock, R. (2019). Remembering the forgotten child: the role of immune checkpoint inhibition in patients with human immunod eficiency virus and cancer. *J. Immunother. Cancer* 7:130. doi: 10.1186/s40425-019-0618-9

Agarwal, N., Iyer, D., Patel, S. G., Sekhar, R. V., Phillips, T. M., Schubert, U., et al. (2013). HIV-1 Vpr induces adipose dysfunction *in vivo* through reciprocal effects on PPAR/GR co-regulation. Sci. *Transl. Med.* 5:213ra164. doi: 10.1126/scitranslmed.3007148

Ahmed, D., Roy, D., and Cassol, E. (2018). Examining relationships between metabolism and persistent inflammation in HIV patients on antiretroviral therapy. *Mediators Inflamm.* 2018, 1–14. doi: 10.1155/2018/6238978

Alcorn, J. F., and Kolls, J. K. (2015). Killer fat. *Science* 347, 26–27. doi: 10.1126/science.aaa4567

Alexander, C. M., Kasza, I., Yen, C.-L., Reeder, S. B., Hernando, D., Gallo, R. L., et al. (2015). Dermal white adipose tissue: a new component of the thermogenic response. *J. Lipid Res.* 56, 2061–2069. doi: 10.1194/jlr.R062893

Allahverdiyev, A. M., Bagirova, M., Elcicek, S., Koc, R. C., Baydar, S. Y., Findikli, N., et al. (2011). Adipose tissue-derived mesenchymal stem cells as a new host cell in latent leishmaniasis. *Am. J. Trop. Med. Hyg.* 85, 535–539. doi: 10.4269/ajtmh.2011.11-0037

Altintas, M. M., Azad, A., Nayer, B., Contreras, G., Zaias, J., Faul, C., et al. (2011). Mast cells, macrophages, and crown-like structures distinguish subcutaneous from visceral fat in mice. *J. Lipid Res.* 52, 480–488. doi: 10.1194/jlr.M011338

Appay, V., Almeida, J. R., Sauce, D., Autran, B., and Papagno, L. (2007). Accelerated immune senescence and HIV-1 infection. *Exp. Gerontol.* 42, 432–437. doi: 10.1016/j.exger.2006.12.003

Appay, V., Fastenackels, S., Katlama, C., Ait-Mohand, H., Schneider, L., Guihot, A., et al. (2011). Old age and anti-cytomegalovirus immunity are associated with altered T-cell reconstitution in HIV-1-infected patients. *AIDS* 25, 1813–1822. doi: 10.1097/QAD.0b013e32834640e6

Appay, V., and Sauce, D. (2008). Immune activation and inflammation in HIV-1 infection?: causes and consequences. *J. Pathol.* 214, 231–241. doi: 10.1002/path.2276

Baglioni, S., Francalanci, M., Squecco, R., Lombardi, A., Cantini, G., Angeli, R., et al. (2009). Characterization of human adult stem-cell populations isolated from. (visceral)and subcutaneous adipose tissue. *FASEB J.* 23, 3494–3505. doi: 10.1096/fj.08-126946

Barrett, L., Fowke, K. R., and Grant, M. D. (2012). Cytomegalovirus, aging,. (and)HIV: a perfect storm. *AIDS Rev.* 14, 159–167.

Bastard, J.-P., Caron, M., Vidal, H., Jan, V., Auclair, M., Vigouroux, C., et al. (2002). Association between altered expression of adipogenic factor SREBP1 in lipoatrophic adipose tissue from HIV-1-infected patients and abnormal adipocyte differentiation and insulin resistance. *Lancet* 359, 1026–1031. doi: 10.1016/s0140-6736(02)08094-7

Bastard, J.-P., Maachi, M., Lagathu, C., Kim, M. J., Caron, M., Vidal, H., et al. (2006). Recent advances in the relationship between obesity, inflammation, and insulin resistance. *Eur. Cytokine Netw.* 17, 4–12.

Beaupere, C., Garcia, M., Larghero, J., Fève, B., Capeau, J., and Lagathu, C. (2015). The HIV proteins Tat and Nef promote human bone marrow mesenchymal stem cell senescence and alter osteoblastic differentiation. *Aging Cell* 14, 534–546. doi: 10.1111/acel.12308

Bechah, Y., Paddock, C. D., Capo, C., Mege, J.-L., and Raoult, D. (2010). Adipose tissue serves as a reservoir for recrudescent rickettsia prowazekii infection in a mouse model. *PLoS One* 5:e8547. doi: 10.1371/journal.pone.0008547

Beelen, R. H. (1991). The greater omentum: physiology and immunological concepts. *Neth. J. Surg.* 43, 145–149.

Beigier-Bompadre, M., Montagna, G. N., Kühl, A. A., Lozza, L., Weiner, J., Kupz, A., et al. (2017). Mycobacterium tuberculosis infection modulates adipose tissue biology. *PLoS Pathog.* 13:e1006676. doi: 10.1371/journal.ppat.1006676

Bénézech, C., and Jackson-Jones, L. H. (2019). ILC2 Orchestration of local immune function in adipose tissue. *Front. Immunol.* 10:171. doi: 10.3389/fimmu.2019.00171

Bénézech, C., Luu, N.-T., Walker, J. A., Kruglov, A. A., Loo, Y., Nakamura, K., et al. (2015). Inflammation-induced formation of fat-associated lymphoid clusters. *Nat. Immunol.* 16, 819–828. doi: 10.1038/ni.3215

Béréziat, V., Cervera, P., Le Dour, C., Verpont, M.-C., Dumont, S., Vantyghem, M.-C., et al. (2011). LMNA mutations induce a non-inflammatory fibrosis and a brown fat-like dystrophy of enlarged cervical adipose tissue. *Am. J. Pathol.* 179, 2443–2453. doi: 10.1016/j.ajpath.2011.07.049

Bertola, A., Ciucci, T., Rousseau, D., Bourlier, V., Duffaut, C., Bonnafous, S., et al. (2012). Identification of adipose tissue dendritic cells correlated with obesity-associated insulin-resistance and inducing Th17 responses in mice and patients. *Diabetes Metab. Res. Rev* 61, 2238–2247. doi: 10.2337/db11-1274

Beura, L. K., Fares-Frederickson, N. J., Steinert, E. M., Scott, M. C., Thompson, E. A., Fraser, K. A., et al. (2019). CD4 + resident memory T cells dominate immunosurveillance and orchestrate local recall responses. *J. Exp. Med.* 216, 1214–1229. doi: 10.1084/jem.20181365

Beura, L. K., Wijeyesinghe, S., Thompson, E. A., Macchietto, M. G., Rosato, P. C., Pierson, M. J., et al. (2018). T Cells in nonlymphoid tissues give rise to lymph-node-resident memory T Cells. *Immunity* 48:327-338.e5. doi: 10.1016/j.immuni.2018.01.015

Bornstein, S. R., Abu-Asab, M., Glasow, A., Päth, G., Hauner, H., Tsokos, M., et al. (2000). Immunohistochemical and ultrastructural localization of leptin and leptin receptor in human white adipose tissue and differentiating human adipose cells in primary culture. *Diabetes Metab. Res. Rev.* 49, 532–538. doi: 10.2337/diabetes.49.4.532

Boulenouar, S., Michelet, X., Duquette, D., Alvarez, D., Hogan, A. E., Dold, C., et al. (2017). Adipose type one innate lymphoid cells regulate macrophage homeostasis through targeted cytotoxicity. *Immunity* 46, 273–286. doi: 10.1016/j.immuni.2017.01.008

Boulougoura, A., and Sereti, I. (2016). HIV infection and immune activation. *Curr. Opin. HIV AIDS* 11, 191–200. doi: 10.1097/COH.0000000000000241

Bourgi, K., Rebeiro, P. F., Turner, M., Castilho, J. L., Hulgan, T., Raffanti, S. P., et al. (2019). Greater weight gain in treatment naïve persons starting dolutegravir-based antiretroviral therapy. *Clin. Infect. Dis.* doi: 10.1093/cid/ciz407 [Epub ahead of print].

Bouwman, J. J., Visseren, F. L., Bouter, K. P., and Diepersloot, R. J. (2008). Infection-induced inflammatory response of adipocytes in vitro. *Int. J. Obes.* 32, 892–901. doi: 10.1038/ijo.2008.36

Boya, P., Pauleau, A.-L., Poncet, D., Gonzalez-Polo, R.-A., Zamzami, N., and Kroemer, G. (2004). Viral proteins targeting mitochondria: controlling cell death. *Biochim. Biophys. Acta Bioenerg.* 1659, 178–189. doi: 10.1016/j.bbabio.2004.08.007

Braune, J., Weyer, U., Hobusch, C., Mauer, J., Brüning, J. C., Bechmann, I., et al. (2017). IL-6 regulates M2 polarization and local proliferation of adipose tissue macrophages in obesity. *J. Immunol.* 198, 2927–2934. doi: 10.4049/jimmunol.1600476

Brestoff, J. R., Kim, B. S., Saenz, S. A., Stine, R. R., Monticelli, L. A., Sonnenberg, G. F., et al. (2015). Group 2 innate lymphoid cells promote beiging of white adipose tissue and limit obesity. *Nature* 519, 242–246. doi: 10.1038/nature14115

Britton, K. A., and Fox, C. S. (2011). Perivascular adipose tissue and vascular disease. *Clin. Lipidol.* 6, 79–91. doi: 10.2217/clp.10.89

Burcelin, R., Serino, M., Chabo, C., Garidou, L., Pomié, C., Courtney, M., et al. (2013). Metagenome and metabolism: the tissue microbiota hypothesis. *Diabetes. Obes. Metab.* 15(Suppl. 3), 61–70. doi: 10.1111/dom.12157

Caron, M., Auclair, M., Donadille, B., Béréziat, V., Guerci, B., Laville, M., et al. (2007). Human lipodystrophies linked to mutations in A-type lamins and to HIV protease inhibitor therapy are both associated with prelamin A accumulation, oxidative stress and premature cellular senescence. *Cell Death Differ.* 14, 1759–1767. doi: 10.1038/sj.cdd.4402197

Caron-Debarle, M., Lagathu, C., Boccara, F., Vigouroux, C., and Capeau, J. (2010). HIV-associated lipodystrophy: from fat injury to premature aging. *Trends Mol. Med.* 16, 218–229. doi: 10.1016/j.molmed.2010.03.002

Casteilla, L., Planat-Benard, V., Laharrague, P., and Cousin, B. (2011). Adipose-derived stromal cells: their identity and uses in clinical trials, an update. *World J. Stem Cells* 3, 25–33. doi: 10.4252/wjsc.v3.i4.25

Catrysse, L., and van Loo, G. (2018). Adipose tissue macrophages and their polarization in health and obesity. *Cell. Immunol.* 330, 114–119. doi: 10.1016/j.cellimm.2018.03.001

Cawthorn, W. P., Scheller, E. L., and MacDougald, O. A. (2012). Adipose tissue stem cells: the great WAT hope. *Trends Endocrinol. Metab.* 23, 270–277. doi: 10.1016/j.tem.2012.01.003

Charles, S., Ammosova, T., Cardenas, J., Foster, A., Rotimi, J., Jerebtsova, M., et al. (2009). Regulation of HIV-1 transcription at 3% versus 21% oxygen concentration. *J. Cell. Physiol.* 221, 469–479. doi: 10.1002/jcp.21882

Charrière, G., Cousin, B., Arnaud, E., André, L., Bacou, F., Penicaud, L., et al. (2003). Preadipocyte conversion to macrophage. evidence of plasticity. *J. Biol. Chem.* 278, 9850–9855. doi: 10.1074/jbc.m210811200

Chase, H. B., Montagna, W., and Malone, J. D. (1953). Changes in the skin in relation to the hair growth cycle. *Anat. Rec.* 116, 75–81. doi: 10.1002/ar.1091160107

Chau, Y.-Y., Bandiera, R., Serrels, A., Martínez-Estrada, O. M., Qing, W., Lee, M., et al. (2014). Visceral and subcutaneous fat have different origins and evidence supports a mesothelial source. *Nat. Cell Biol.* 16, 367–375. doi: 10.1038/ncb2922

Chen, Y.-Y., Kao, T.-W., Fang, W.-H., Wang, C.-C., Chang, Y.-W., Yang, H.-F., et al. (2019). Body fat percentage in relation to lung function in individuals with normal weight obesity. *Sci. Rep.* 9:3066. doi: 10.1038/s41598-019-38804-3

Cheng, C. K., Bakar, H. A., Gollasch, M., and Huang, Y. (2018). Perivascular adipose tissue: the sixth man of the cardiovascular system. *Cardiovasc. Drugs Ther.* 32, 481–502. doi: 10.1007/s10557-018-6820-z

Chi, J., Wu, Z., Choi, C. H. J., Nguyen, L., Tegegne, S., Ackerman, S. E., et al. (2018). Three-dimensional adipose tissue imaging reveals regional variation in beige fat biogenesis and PRDM16-dependent sympathetic neurite density. *Cell Metab.* 27:226-236.e3. doi: 10.1016/j.cmet.2017.12.011

Cinti, S. (2012). The adipose organ at a glance. *Dis. Model. Mech.* 5, 588–594. doi: 10.1242/dmm.009662

Cinti, S. (2018). *Adipose Organ Development and Remodeling. In Comprehensive Physiology.* Hoboken, NJ: John Wiley & Sons, Inc.

Cipolletta, D. (2014). Adipose tissue-resident regulatory T cells: phenotypic specialization, functions and therapeutic potential. *Immunology* 142, 517–525. doi: 10.1111/imm.12262

Cipolletta, D., Cohen, P., Spiegelman, B. M., Benoist, C., and Mathis, D. (2015). Appearance and disappearance of the mRNA signature characteristic of Treg cells in visceral adipose tissue: age, diet, and PPARγ effects. *Proc. Natl. Acad. Sci. U.S.A.* 112, 482–487. doi: 10.1073/pnas.1423486112

Cipolletta, D., Feuerer, M., Li, A., Kamei, N., Lee, J., Shoelson, S. E., et al. (2012). PPAR-γ is a major driver of the accumulation and phenotype of adipose tissue Treg cells. *Nature* 486, 549–553. doi: 10.1038/nature11132

Cipolletta, D., Kolodin, D., Benoist, C., and Mathis, D. (2011). Seminars in Immunology Tissular T regs?: a unique population of adipose-tissue-resident Foxp3 + CD4 + T cells that impacts organismal metabolism. *Semin. Immunol.* 23, 431–437. doi: 10.1016/j.smim.2011.06.002

Clark, E., Nava, B., and Caputi, M. (2017). Tat is a multifunctional viral protein that modulates cellular gene expression and functions. *Oncotarget* 8, 27569–27581. doi: 10.18632/oncotarget.15174

Coín Aragüez, L., Murri, M., Oliva Olivera, W., Salas, J., Mayas, M. D., Delgado-Lista, J., et al. (2013). Thymus fat as an attractive source of angiogenic factors in elderly subjects with myocardial ischemia. *Age* 35, 1263–1275. doi: 10.1007/s11357-012-9418-6

Contreras, N. A., Sitnik, K. M., Jeftic, I., Coplen, C. P., Èièin-Šain, L., and Nikolich-Žugich, J. (2019). Life-long control of cytomegalovirus (CMV) by T resident memory cells in the adipose tissue results in inflammation and hyperglycemia. *PLoS Pathog.* 15:e1007890. doi: 10.1371/journal.ppat.1007890

Cotter, E. J., Chew, N., Powderly, W. G., and Doran, P. P. (2011). HIV type 1 alters mesenchymal stem cell differentiation potential and cell phenotype ex *Vivo*. *AIDS Res. Hum. Retroviruses* 27, 187–199. doi: 10.1089/aid.2010.0114

Cousin, B., Casteilla, L., Laharrague, P., Luche, E., Lorsignol, A., Cuminetti, V., et al. (2015). Immuno-metabolism and adipose tissue: the key role of hematopoietic stem cells. *Biochimie* 124, 21–26. doi: 10.1016/j.biochi.2015.06.012

Cousin, B., Munoz, O., Andre, M., Fontanilles, A. M., Dani, C., Cousin, J. L., et al. (1999). A role for preadipocytes as macrophage-like cells. *FASEB J.* 13, 305–312. doi: 10.1096/fasebj.13.2.305

Couturier, J., Agarwal, N., Nehete, P. N., Baze, W. B., Barry, M. A., Jagannadha Sastry, K., et al. (2016). Infectious SIV resides in adipose tissue and induces metabolic defects in chronically infected rhesus macaques. *Retrovirology* 13:30. doi: 10.1186/s12977-016-0260-2

Couturier, J., and Lewis, D. E. (2018). HIV persistence in adipose tissue reservoirs. *Curr. HIV/AIDS Rep.* 15, 60–71. doi: 10.1007/s11904-018-0378-z

Couturier, J., Nuotio-Antar, A. M., Agarwal, N., Wilkerson, G. K., Saha, P., Kulkarni, V., et al. (2019). Lymphocytes upregulate CD36 in adipose tissue and liver. *Adipocyte* 8, 154–163. doi: 10.1080/21623945.2019.1609202

Couturier, J., Suliburk, J. W., Brown, J. M., Luke, D. J., Agarwal, N., Yu, X., et al. (2015). Human adipose tissue as a reservoir for memory CD4+ T cells and HIV. *AIDS* 29, 667–674. doi: 10.1097/QAD.0000000000000599

Couturier, J., Winchester, L. C., Suliburk, J. W., Wilkerson, G. K., Podany, A. T., Agarwal, N., et al. (2018). Adipocytes impair efficacy of antiretroviral therapy. *Antiviral Res.* 154, 140–148. doi: 10.1016/j.antiviral.2018.04.002

Cruz-Migoni, S., and Caamaño, J. (2016). Fat-associated lymphoid clusters in inflammation and immunity. *Front. Immunol.* 7:612. doi: 10.3389/fimmu.2016.00612

Cummins, N. W., Sainski-Nguyen, A. M., Natesampillai, S., Aboulnasr, F., Kaufmann, S., and Badley, A. D. (2017). Maintenance of the HIV reservoir is antagonized by selective BCL2 inhibition. *J. Virol.* 91:e00012-17. doi: 10.1128/JVI.00012-17

Dalmas, E., Lehmann, F. M., Dror, E., Wueest, S., Thienel, C., Borsigova, M., et al. (2017). Interleukin-33-activated islet-resident innate lymphoid cells promote insulin secretion through myeloid cell retinoic acid production. *Immunity* 47:928-942.e7. doi: 10.1016/j.immuni.2017.10.015

Damouche, A., Lazure, T., Avettand-Fènoël, V., Huot, N., Dejucq-Rainsford, N., Satie, A.-P., et al. (2015). Adipose tissue is a neglected viral reservoir and an inflammatory site during chronic HIV and SIV infection. *PLoS Pathog.* 11:e1005153. doi: 10.1371/journal.ppat.1005153

Damouche, A., Pourcher, G., Pourcher, V., Benoist, S., Busson, E., Lataillade, J.-J., et al. (2017). High proportion of PD-1-expressing CD4 + T cells in adipose tissue constitutes an immunomodulatory microenvironment that may support HIV persistence. *Eur. J. Immunol.* 47, 2113–2123. doi: 10.1002/eji.201747060

Datta, P. K., Deshmane, S., Khalili, K., Merali, S., Gordon, J. C., Fecchio, C., et al. (2016). Glutamate metabolism in HIV-1 infected macrophages: role of HIV-1 Vpr. *Cell Cycle* 15, 2288–2298. doi: 10.1080/15384101.2016.1190054

de Ferranti, S., and Mozaffarian, D. (2008). The perfect storm: obesity, adipocyte dysfunction, and metabolic consequences. *Clin. Chem.* 54, 945–955. doi: 10.1373/clinchem.2007.100156

de Jong, A. J., Kloppenburg, M., Toes, E. M. R., and Ioan-Facsinay, A. (2014). Fatty acids, lipid mediators, and T-cell function. *Front. Immunol.* 5:483. doi: 10.3389/fimmu.2014.00483

Debaisieux, S., Rayne, F., Yezid, H., and Beaumelle, B. (2012). The ins and outs of HIV-1 Tat. *Traffic* 13, 355–363. doi: 10.1111/j.1600-0854.2011.01286.x

Dekaban, G. A., and Dikeakos, J. D. (2017). HIV-I Nef inhibitors: a novel class of HIV-specific immune adjuvants in support of a cure. *AIDS Res. Ther.* 14:53. doi: 10.1186/s12981-017-0175-6

Deng, T., Lyon, C. J., Minze, L. J., Lin, J., Zou, J., Liu, J. Z., et al. (2013). Article class II major histocompatibility complex plays an essential role in obesity-induced adipose inflammation. *Cell Metab.* 17, 411–422. doi: 10.1016/j.cmet.2013.02.009

Derendorf, H., Schmidt, S., and Preceded, M. (2019). *Rowland. Rowland, and Tozer's Clinical Pharmacokinetics, and. (Pharmacodynamics)?: Concepts and Applications*. Philadelphia, PE: LWW.

Desruisseaux, M. S., Trujillo, M. E., Tanowitz, H. B., and Scherer, P. E. (2007). Adipocyte, Adipose Tissue, and Infectious Disease. *Infect Immun.* 75, 1066-1078.

Dhurandhar, N. V. (2011). A framework for identification of infections that contribute to human obesity. *Lancet. Infect. Dis.* 11, 963–969. doi: 10.1016/S1473-3099(11)70274-2

Díaz-Delfín, J., Domingo, P., Wabitsch, M., Giralt, M., and Villarroya, F. (2012). HIV-1 Tat protein impairs adipogenesis and induces the expression and secretion of proinflammatory cytokines in human SGBS adipocytes. *Antivir. Ther.* 17, 529–540. doi: 10.3851/IMP2021

Dichamp, J., Barreau, C., Guissard, C., Carrière, A., Martinez, Y., Descombes, X., et al. (2019). 3D analysis of the whole subcutaneous adipose tissue reveals a complex spatial network of interconnected lobules with heterogeneous browning ability. *Sci. Rep.* 9:6684. doi: 10.1038/s41598-019-43130-9

Djimeu, E. W., and Heard, A. C. (2019). Treatment of HIV among tuberculosis patients: a replication study of timing of antiretroviral therapy for HIV-1-associated tuberculosis. *PLoS One* 14:e0210327. doi: 10.1371/journal.pone.0210327

Dupin, N., Buffet, M., Marcelin, A.-G., Lamotte, C., Gorin, I., Ait-Arkoub, Z., et al. (2002). HIV and antiretroviral drug distribution in plasma and fat tissue of HIV-infected patients with lipodystrophy. *AIDS* 16, 2419–2424. doi: 10.1097/00002030-200212060-00006

Elgazar-Carmon, V., Rudich, A., Hadad, N., and Levy, R. (2008). Neutrophils transiently infiltrate intra-abdominal fat early in the course of high-fat feeding. *J. Lipid Res.* 49, 1894–1903. doi: 10.1194/jlr.M800132-JLR200

Elsheikh, M. M., Tang, Y., Li, D., and Jiang, G. (2019). Deep latency: a new insight into a functional HIV cure. *EBio. Med.* 45, 624–629. doi: 10.1016/j.ebiom.2019.06.020

Engela, A. U., Hoogduijn, M. J., Boer, K., Litjens, N. H., Betjes, M. G., Weimar, W., et al. (2013). Human adipose-tissue derived mesenchymal stem cells induce functional de-novo regulatory T cells with methylated FOXP3 gene DNA. *Clin. Exp. Immunol.* 173, 343–354. doi: 10.1111/cei.12120

Evans, V. A., van der Sluis, R. M., Solomon, A., Dantanarayana, A., McNeil, C., Garsia, R., et al. (2018). Programmed cell death-1 contributes to the establishment and maintenance of HIV-1 latency. *AIDS* 32, 1491–1497. doi: 10.1097/QAD.0000000000001849

Fain, J. N., Madan, A. K., Hiler, M. L., Cheema, P., and Bahouth, S. W. (2004). Comparison of the release of adipokines by adipose tissue, adipose tissue matrix, and adipocytes from visceral and subcutaneous abdominal adipose tissues of obese humans. *Endocrinology* 145, 2273–2282. doi: 10.1210/en.2003-1336

Faller, E. M., McVey, M. J., and MacPherson, P. A. (2014). IL-7 receptor recovery on CD8 T-cells isolated from HIV+ patients is inhibited by the HIV Tat protein. *PLoS One* 9:e102677. doi: 10.1371/journal.pone.0102677

Falutz, J. (2011). HIV infection, body composition changes and related metabolic complications: contributing factors and evolving management strategies. *Curr. Opin. Clin. Nutr. Metab. Care* 14, 255–260. doi: 10.1097/MCO.0b013e3283457a8f

Ferrante, A. W. Jr. (2013). The immune cells in adipose tissue. *Diabetes. Obes. Metab.* 15(Suppl. 3), 34–38. doi: 10.1111/dom.12154

Feuerer, M., Herrero, L., Cipolletta, D., Naaz, A., Wong, J., Nayer, A., et al. (2009). Lean, but not obese, fat is enriched for a unique population of regulatory T cells that affect metabolic parameters. *Nat. Med.* 15, 1–11.

Fiume, G., Vecchio, E., De Laurentiis, A., Trimboli, F., Palmieri, C., Pisano, A., et al. (2012). Human immunodeficiency virus-1 Tat activates NF-κB *via* physical interaction with IκB-α and p65. *Nucleic Acids Res.* 40, 3548–3562. doi: 10.1093/nar/gkr1224

Flach, M., and Diefenbach, A. (2015). Adipose tissue: ILC2 Crank Up the Heat. *Cell Metab.* 21, 152–153. doi: 10.1016/j.cmet.2015.01.015

Franke-Fayard, B., Fonager, J., Braks, A., Khan, S. M., and Janse, C. J. (2010). Sequestration and tissue accumulation of human malaria parasites: can we learn anything from rodent models of malaria? *PLoS Pathog.* 6:e1001032. doi: 10.1371/journal.ppat.1001032

Franquesa, M., Mensah, F. K., Huizinga, R., Strini, T., Boon, L., Lombardo, E., et al. (2015). Human adipose tissue-derived mesenchymal stem cells abrogate plasmablast formation and induce regulatory B cells independently of T helper cells. *Stem Cells* 33, 880–891. doi: 10.1002/stem.1881

Garrabou, G., López, S., Morén, C., Martínez, E., Fontdevila, J., Cardellach, F., et al. (2011). Mitochondrial damage in adipose tissue of untreated HIV-infected patients. *AIDS* 25, 165–170. doi: 10.1097/QAD.0b013e3283423219

Gebhardt, T., Wakim, L. M., Eidsmo, L., Reading, P. C., and Heath, W. R. (2009). Memory T cells in nonlymphoid tissue that provide enhanced local immunity during infection with herpes simplex virus. *Nat. Immunol.* 10, 524–530. doi: 10.1038/ni.1718

Giralt, M., Domingo, P., Guallar, J. P., Rodriguez de la Concepción, M. L., Alegre, M., and Domingo, J. C. (2006). HIV-1 infection alters gene expression in adipose tissue, which contributes to HIV- 1/HAART-associated lipodystrophy. *Antivir. Ther.* 11, 729–740.

Godfrey, C., Bremer, A., Alba, D., Apovian, C., Koethe, J. R., Koliwad, S., et al. (2019). Obesity and fat metabolism in HIV-infected individuals: immunopathogenic mechanisms and clinical implications. *J.Infect.Dis.* 220, 420–431. doi: 10.1093/infdis/jiz118

Gorwood, J., Bourgeois, C., Mantecon, M., Atlan, M., Pourcher, V., Pourcher, G., et al. (2019). Impact of HIV/SIV infection and viral proteins on adipose tissue fibrosis and adipogenesis. *AIDS* 33, 953–964. doi: 10.1097/qad.0000000000002168

Gu, W., Nowak, W. N., Xie, Y., Le Bras, A., Hu, Y., Deng, J., et al. (2019). Single-cell RNA-sequencing and metabolomics analyses reveal the contribution of perivascular adipose tissue stem cells to vascular remodeling. *Arterioscler. Thromb. Vasc. Biol.* 39, 2049–2066. doi: 10.1161/ATVBAHA.119.312732

Guerrero-Juarez, C. F., and Plikus, M. V. (2018). Emerging nonmetabolic functions of skin fat. *Nat. Rev. Endocrinol.* 14, 163–173. doi: 10.1038/nrendo.2017.162

Guzik, T. J., Skiba, D. S., Touyz, R. M., and Harrison, D. G. (2017). The role of infiltrating immune cells in dysfunctional adipose tissue. *Cardiovasc. Res.* 113, 1009–1023. doi: 10.1093/cvr/cvx108

Hale, L. P. (2004). Histologic and molecular assessment of human thymus. *Ann. Diagn. Pathol.* 8, 50–60. doi: 10.1016/j.anndiagpath.2003.11.006

Han, S.-J., Glatman Zaretsky, A., Andrade-Oliveira, V., Collins, N., Dzutsev, A., Shaik, J., et al. (2017). White adipose tissue is a reservoir for memory T Cells and promotes protective memory responses to infection. *Immunity* 47:1154-1168.e. doi: 10.1016/j.immuni.2017.11.009

Hanses, F., Kopp, A., Bala, M., Buechler, C., Falk, W., Salzberger, B., et al. (2011). Intracellular survival of *Staphylococcus aureus* in adipocyte-like differentiated 3T3-L1 cells is glucose dependent and alters cytokine, chemokine, and adipokine secretion. *Endocrinology* 152, 4148–4157. doi: 10.1210/en.2011-0103

Hardouin, P., Pansini, V., and Cortet, B. (2014). Bone marrow fat. *Joint. Bone Spine* 81, 313–319. doi: 10.1016/j.jbspin.2014.02.013

Haridas, V., Pean, P., Jasenosky, L. D., Madec, Y., Laureillard, D., Sok, T., et al. (2015). TB-IRIS, T-cell activation, and remodeling of the T-cell compartment in highly immunosuppressed HIV-infected patients with TB. *AIDS* 29, 263–273. doi: 10.1097/QAD.0000000000000546

Hazan, U., Romero, I. A., Cancello, R., Valente, S., Perrin, V., Mariot, V., et al. (2002). Human adipose cells express CD4, CXCR4, and CCR5 [corrected] receptors: a new target cell type for the immunodeficiency virus-1? *FASEB J.* 16, 1254–1256. doi: 10.1096/fj.01-0947fje

Holmberg, V., Soini, H., Kivelä, P., Ollgren, J., and Ristola, M. (2019). Epidemiology and outcome of HIV patients in finland co-infected with tuberculosis 1998–2015. *BMC Infect. Dis.* 19:264. doi: 10.1186/s12879-019-3890-x

Hotamisligil, G. S. (2006). Inflammation and metabolic disorders. *Nature* 44, 860–867.

Hruskova, Z., and Biswas, S. K. (2013). Previews a new "‘ Immunological ’" role for adipocytes in obesity. *Cell. Metab.* 17, 315–317. doi: 10.1016/j.cmet.2013.02.015

Hsu, D. C., Wegner, M. D., Sunyakumthorn, P., Silsorn, D., Tayamun, S., and Inthawong, D. (2017). CD4+ Cell infiltration into subcutaneous adipose tissue is not indicative of productively infected cells during acute SHIV infection. *J. Med. Primatol.* 46, 154–157. doi: 10.1111/jmp.12298

Hussaarts, L., García-Tardón, N., van Beek, L., Heemskerk, M. M., Haeberlein, S., van, G. C., et al. (2015). Chronic helminth infection and helminth-derived egg antigens promote adipose tissue M2 macrophages and improve insulin sensitivity in obese mice. *FASEB J.* 29, 3027–3039. doi: 10.1096/fj.14-266239

Huttunen, R., and Syrjänen, J. (2013). Obesity and the risk and outcome of infection. *Int. J. Obes.* 37, 333–340. doi: 10.1038/ijo.2012.62

Ibrahim, M. M. (2009). Subcutaneous and visceral adipose tissue: structural and functional differences. *Obes. Rev.* 11, 11–18. doi: 10.1111/j.1467-789X.2009.00623.x

Ikejima, S., Sasaki, S., Sashinami, H., Mori, F., Ogawa, Y., Nakamura, T., et al. (2005). Impairment of host resistance to Listeria monocytogenes infection in liver of db/db and ob/ob mice. *Diabetes Metab. Res. Rev.* 54, 182–189. doi: 10.2337/diabetes.54.1.182

Ivanov, A. V., Valuev-Elliston, V. T., Ivanova, O. N., Kochetkov, S. N., Starodubova, E. S., Bartosch, B., et al. (2016). Oxidative stress during HIV Infection: mechanisms and consequences. *Oxid. Med. Cell. Longev.* 2016:8910396.

Ivanov, S., Merlin, J., Lee, M. K. S., Murphy, A. J., and Guinamard, R. R. (2018). Biology and function of adipose tissue macrophages, dendritic cells and B cells. *Atherosclerosis* 271, 102–110. doi: 10.1016/j.atherosclerosis.2018.01.018

Jackson, E., Shoemaker, R., Larian, N., and Cassis, L. (2017). *Adipose Tissue as a Site of Toxin Accumulation. In Comprehensive Physiology.* Hoboken, NJ: John Wiley & Sons, Inc.

Jacob, R. A., Johnson, A. L., Pawlak, E. N., Dirk, B. S., Van Nynatten, L. R., Haeryfar, S., et al. (2017). The interaction between HIV-1 Nef and adaptor protein-2 reduces Nef-mediated CD4+ T cell apoptosis. *Virology* 509, 1–10. doi: 10.1016/j.virol.2017.05.018

Janneh, O., Hoggard, P. G., Tjia, J. F., Jones, S. P., Khoo, S. H., Maher, B., et al. (2003). Intracellular disposition and metabolic effects of zidovudine, stavudine and four protease inhibitors in cultured adipocytes. *Antivir. Ther.* 8, 417–426.

Janneh, O., Owen, A., Bray, P. G., Back, D. J., and Pirmohamed, M. (2010). The accumulation and metabolism of zidovudine in 3T3-F442A pre-adipocytes. *Br. J. Pharmacol.* 159, 484–493. doi: 10.1111/j.1476-5381.2009.00552.x

Jones, D. D., Racine, R., Wittmer, S. T., Harston, L., Papillion, A. M., Dishaw, L. M., et al. (2015). The omentum is a site of protective IgM production during intracellular bacterial infection. *Infect. Immun.* 83, 2139–2147. doi: 10.1128/IAI.00295-15

Karlsson, E. A., and Beck, M. A. (2010). The burden of obesity on infectious disease. *Exp. Biol. Med.* 235, 1412–1424. doi: 10.1258/ebm.2010.010227

Kerchberger, A. M., Sheth, A. N., Angert, C. D., Mehta, C. C., Summers, N. A., Ofotokun, I., et al. (2019). Weight gain associated with integrase stand transfer inhibitor use in women. *Clin. Infect. Dis.* doi: 10.1093/cid/ciz853 [Epub ahead of print].

Khairoun, M., and Korevaar, S. S. (2013). Human bone marrow- and adipose tissue-derived mesenchymal stromal cells are immunosuppressive *In vitro* and in a humanized allograft rejection model. *J. Stem Cell Res. Ther.* 6:20780.

Kim, H., Darwish, I., Monroy, M.-F., Prockop, D. J., Liles, W. C., and Kain, K. C. (2014). Mesenchymal stromal (stem) cells suppress pro-inflammatory cytokine production but fail to improve survival in experimental staphylococcal toxic shock syndrome. *BMC Immunol.* 15:1. doi: 10.1186/1471-2172-15-1

Kintscher, U., Hartge, M., Hess, K., Foryst-Ludwig, A., Clemenz, M., Wabitsch, M., et al. (2008). T-lymphocyte infiltration in visceral adipose tissue: a primary event in adipose tissue inflammation and the development of obesity-mediated insulin resistance. *Arterioscler. Thromb. Vasc. Biol.* 28, 1304–1310. doi: 10.1161/ATVBAHA.108.165100

Kis, O., Robillard, K., Chan, G. N. Y., and Bendayan, R. (2010). The complexities of antiretroviral drug-drug interactions: role of ABC and SLC transporters. *Trends Pharmacol. Sci.* 31, 22–35. doi: 10.1016/j.tips.2009.10.001

Knight, S. C. (2008). Specialized perinodal fat fuels and fashions immunity. *Immunity* 28, 135–138. doi: 10.1016/j.immuni.2008.01.003

Koethe, J. R. (2017). *Adipose Tissue in HIV Infection. In Comprehensive Physiology.* Hoboken, NJ: John Wiley & Sons, Inc.

Koethe, J. R., McDonnell, W., Kennedy, A., Abana, C. O., Pilkinton, M., Setliff, I., et al. (2017). Adipose tissue is enriched for activated and late-differentiated CD8+ T cells, and shows distinct CD8+ receptor usage, compared to blood in HIV-infected persons. *JAIDS J. Acquir. Immune Defic. Syndr.* 77:1. doi: 10.1097/QAI.0000000000001573

Kolodin, D., van Panhuys, N., Li, C., Magnuson, A. M., Cipolletta, D., Miller, C. M., et al. (2015). Antigen- and cytokine-driven accumulation of regulatory T cells in visceral adipose tissue of lean mice. *Cell Metab.* 21, 543–557. doi: 10.1016/j.cmet.2015.03.005

Kuang, X., and Brockman, M. (2018). Implications of HIV-1 Nef for "Shock and Kill" strategies to eliminate latent viral reservoirs. *Viruses* 10:677. doi: 10.3390/v10120677

Kugelberg, E. (2015). Infection: double skin protection. *Nat. Rev. Immunol.* 15, 68–69. doi: 10.1038/nri3811

La Cava, A., Alviggi, C., and Matarese, G. (2004). Unraveling the multiple roles of leptin in inflammation and autoimmunity. *J. Mol. Med.* 82, 4–11. doi: 10.1007/s00109-003-0492-1

Lagathu, C., Cossarizza, A., Béréziat, V., Nasi, M., Capeau, J., and Pinti, M. (2017). Basic science and pathogenesis of ageing with HIV. *AIDS* 31, S105–S119. doi: 10.1097/QAD.0000000000001441

Lagathu, C., Eustace, B., Prot, M., Frantz, D., Gu, Y., Bastard, J.-P., et al. (2007). Some HIV antiretrovirals increase oxidative stress and alter chemokine, cytokine or adiponectin production in human adipocytes and macrophages. *Antivir. Ther.* 12, 489–500.

Lagathu, C., Kim, M., Maachi, M., Vigouroux, C., Cervera, P., Capeau, J., et al. (2005). HIV antiretroviral treatment alters adipokine expression and insulin sensitivity of adipose tissue in vitro and *in vivo*. *Biochimie* 87, 65–71. doi: 10.1016/j.biochi.2004.12.007

Laparra, A., Tricot, S., Le Van, M., Damouche, A., Gorwood, J., Vaslin, B., et al. (2019). The frequencies of immunosuppressive cells in adipose tissue differ in human, non-human primate, and mouse models. *Front. Immunol.* 10:117. doi: 10.3389/fimmu.2019.00117

Le Blanc, K., and Mougiakakos, D. (2012). Multipotent mesenchymal stromal cells and the innate immune system. *Nat. Rev. Immunol.* 12, 383–396. doi: 10.1038/nri3209

Lee, B.-C., Kim, M.-S., Pae, M., Yamamoto, Y., Eberlé, D., Shimada, T., et al. (2016). Adipose natural killer cells regulate adipose tissue macrophages to promote insulin resistance in obesity. *Cell Metab.* 23, 685–698. doi: 10.1016/j.cmet.2016.03.002

Lee, E.-H., Itan, M., Jang, J., Gu, H.-J., Rozenberg, P., Mingler, M. K., et al. (2018). Eosinophils support adipocyte maturation and promote glucose tolerance in obesity. *Sci. Rep.* 8:9894. doi: 10.1038/s41598-018-28371-4

Lee, M.-J., Wu, Y., and Fried, S. K. (2013). Adipose tissue heterogeneity: implication of depot differences in adipose tissue for obesity complications. *Mol. Aspects Med.* 34, 1–11. doi: 10.1016/j.mam.2012.10.001

Lee, M.-W., Odegaard, J. I., Mukundan, L., Qiu, Y., Molofsky, A. B., Nussbaum, J. C., et al. (2015). Activated type 2 innate lymphoid cells regulate beige fat biogenesis. *Cell* 160, 74–87. doi: 10.1016/j.cell.2014.12.011

Lee, Y. S., Wollam, J., and Olefsky, J. M. (2018). An integrated view of immunometabolism. *Cell* 172, 22–40. doi: 10.1016/j.cell.2017.12.025

Lin, Y., Lee, H., Berg, A. H., Lisanti, M. P., Shapiro, L., and Scherer, P. E. (2000). The lipopolysaccharide-activated toll-like receptor (TLR)-4 induces synthesis of the closely related receptor TLR-2 in adipocytes. *J. Biol. Chem.* 275, 24255–24263. doi: 10.1074/jbc.m002137200

Lionetti, L., Mollica, M. P., Lombardi, A., Cavaliere, G., Gifuni, G., and Barletta, A. (2009). From chronic overnutrition to insulin resistance: the role of fat-storing capacity and inflammation. *Nutr. Metab. Cardiovasc. Dis.* 19, 146–152. doi: 10.1016/j.numecd.2008.10.010

Liu, J., Divoux, A., Sun, J., Zhang, J., Clément, K., Glickman, J. N., et al. (2009). Genetic deficiency and pharmacological stabilization of mast cells reduce diet-induced obesity and diabetes in mice. *Nat. Med.* 15, 940–945. doi: 10.1038/nm.1994

Liu, R., and Nikolajczyk, B. S. (2019). Tissue immune cells fuel obesity-associated inflammation in adipose tissue and beyond. *Front. Immunol.* 10:1587. doi: 10.3389/fimmu.2019.01587

Loisel-Meyer, S., Swainson, L., Craveiro, M., Oburoglu, L., Mongellaz, C., Costa, C., et al. (2012). Glut1-mediated glucose transport regulates HIV infection. *Proc. Natl. Acad. Sci. U.S.A.* 109, 2549–2554. doi: 10.1073/pnas.1121427109

Lolmède, K., Duffaut, C., and Bouloumié, A. (2011). Immune cells in adipose tissue?: key players in metabolic disorders. *Diabetes Metab.* 37, 283–290. doi: 10.1016/j.diabet.2011.03.002

Luche, E., Sengenès, C., Arnaud, E., Laharrague, P., Casteilla, L., and Cousin, B. (2015). Differential hematopoietic activity in white adipose tissue depending on its localization. *J. Cell. Physiol.* 230, 3076–3083. doi: 10.1002/jcp.25045

Lumeng, C. N., Bodzin, J. L., and Saltiel, A. R. (2007). Obesity induces a phenotypic switch in adipose tissue macrophage polarization. *J. Clin. Invest.* 117, 175–184. doi: 10.1172/jci29881

Luz-Crawford, P., Kurte, M., Bravo-Alegría, J., Contreras, R., Nova-Lamperti, E., Tejedor, G., et al. (2013). Mesenchymal stem cells generate a CD4+CD25+Foxp3+ regulatory T cell population during the differentiation process of Th1 and Th17 cells. *Stem Cell Res. Ther.* 4:65. doi: 10.1186/scrt216

Lynch, L., Michelet, X., Zhang, S., Brennan, P. J., Moseman, A., Lester, C., et al. (2015). Regulatory iNKT cells lack expression of the transcription factor PLZF and control the homeostasis of T(reg) cells and macrophages in adipose tissue. *Nat. Immunol.* 16, 85–95. doi: 10.1038/ni.3047

Lynch, L., Nowak, M., Varghese, B., Clark, J., Hogan, A. E., Toxavidis, V., et al. (2012). Adipose tissue invariant NKT cells protect against diet-induced obesity and metabolic disorder through regulatory cytokine production. *Immunity* 37, 574–587. doi: 10.1016/j.immuni.2012.06.016

Machado, F. S., Dutra, W. O., Esper, L., Gollob, K. J., Teixeira, M. M., Factor, S. M., et al. (2012). Current understanding of immunity to *Trypanosoma cruzi* infection and pathogenesis of Chagas disease. *Semin. Immunopathol.* 34, 753–770. doi: 10.1007/s00281-012-0351-7

Madani, R., Karastergiou, K., Ogston, N. C., Miheisi, N., Bhome, R., Haloob, N., et al. (2009). RANTES release by human adipose tissue in vivo and evidence for depot-specific differences. *Am. J. Physiol. Endocrinol. Metab.* 296, E1262–E1268. doi: 10.1152/ajpendo.90511.2008

Madge, S., Kinloch-de-Loes, S., Mercey, D., Johnson, M. A., and Weller, I. V. (1999). Lipodystrophy in patients naive to HIV protease inhibitors. *AIDS* 13, 735–737.

Mahlakõiv, T., Flamar, A. L., Johnston, L. K., Moriyama, S., Putzel, G. G., Bryce, P. J., et al. (2019). Stromal cells maintain immune cell homeostasis in adipose tissue *via* production of interleukin-33. *Sci. Immunol.* 4:eaax0416. doi: 10.1126/sciimmunol.aax0416

Malmberg, K. J., Arulampalam, V., Ichihara, F., Petersson, M., Seki, K., Andersson, T., et al. (2001). Inhibition of activated/memory (CD45RO(+)) T cells by oxidative stress associated with block of NF-kappaB activation. *J. Immunol.* 167, 2595–2601. doi: 10.4049/jimmunol.167.5.2595

Mancuso, P., Gottschalk, A., Phare, S. M., Peters-Golden, M., Lukacs, N. W., and Huffnagle, G. B. (2002). Leptin-deficient mice exhibit impaired host defense in Gram-negative pneumonia. *J. Immunol.* 168, 4018–4024. doi: 10.4049/jimmunol.168.8.4018

Mañes, S., del Real, G., and Martínez, C.-A. (2003). Pathogens: raft hijackers. *Nat. Rev. Immunol.* 3, 557–568. doi: 10.1038/nri1129

Marcelin, G., Ferreira, A., Liu, Y., Atlan, M., Aron-Wisnewsky, J., Pelloux, V., et al. (2017). A PDGFRα-mediated switch toward CD9 high adipocyte progenitors controls obesity-induced adipose tissue fibrosis. *Cell Metab.* 25, 673–685. doi: 10.1016/j.cmet.2017.01.010

Matarese, G., and La Cava, A. (2004). The intricate interface between immune system and metabolism. *Trends Immunol.* 25, 193–200. doi: 10.1016/j.it.2004.02.009

Mathis, D., Shoelson, S. E., Lugus, J. J., Walsh, K., Shoelson, S. E., and Cantrell, D. A. (2011). Immunometabolism: an emerging frontier. *Nat. Rev. Immunol.* 11:81. doi: 10.1038/nri2922

Mattacks, C. A., Sadler, D., and Pond, C. M. (2003). The cellular structure and lipid/protein composition of adipose tissue surrounding chronically stimulated lymph nodes in rats. *J. Anat.* 202, 551–561. doi: 10.1046/j.1469-7580.2003.00188.x

Maurin, T., Saillan-Barreau, C., Cousin, B., Casteilla, L., Doglio, A., and Pénicaud, L. (2005). Tumor necrosis factor-alpha stimulates HIV-1 production in primary culture of human adipocytes. *Exp. Cell Res.* 304, 544–551. doi: 10.1016/j.yexcr.2004.12.003

Mazzon, M., and Mercer, J. (2014). Lipid interactions during virus entry and infection. *Cell. Microbiol.* 16, 1493–1502. doi: 10.1111/cmi.12340

McLaughlin, T., Liu, L.-F., Lamendola, C., Shen, L., Morton, J., Rivas, H., et al. (2014). T-cell profile in adipose tissue is associated with insulin resistance and systemic inflammation in humans. *Arterioscler. Thromb. Vasc. Biol.* 34, 2637–2643. doi: 10.1161/ATVBAHA.114.304636

McNamee, E. N., Korns Johnson, D., Homann, D., and Clambey, E. T. (2013). Hypoxia and hypoxia-inducible factors as regulators of T cell development, differentiation, and function. *Immunol. Res.* 55, 58–70. doi: 10.1007/s12026-012-8349-8

Meijer, K., de Vries, M., Al-Lahham, S., Bruinenberg, M., Weening, D., Dijkstra, M., et al. (2011). Human primary adipocytes exhibit immune cell function: adipocytes prime inflammation independent of macrophages. *PLoS One* 6:e17154. doi: 10.1371/journal.pone.0017154

Meza-Perez, S., and Randall, T. D. (2017). Immunological Functions of the Omentum. *Trends Immunol.* 38, 526–536. doi: 10.1016/j.it.2017.03.002

Moffat, G. H. (1968). The growth of hair follicles and its relation to the adjacent dermal structures. *J. Anat.* 102, 527–540.

Mohamed-Ali, V., Goodrick, S., Rawesh, A., Katz, D. R., Miles, J. M., Yudkin, J. S., et al. (1997). Subcutaneous adipose tissue releases interleukin-6, but not tumor necrosis factor-alpha, in vivo. *J. Clin. Endocrinol. Metab.* 82, 4196–4200. doi: 10.1210/jc.82.12.4196

Mollinedo, F., and Gajate, C. (2015). Lipid rafts as major platforms for signaling regulation in cancer. *Adv. Biol. Regul.* 57, 130–146. doi: 10.1016/j.jbior.2014.10.003

Molofsky, A. B., Nussbaum, J. C., Liang, H.-E., Van Dyken, S. J., Cheng, L. E., Mohapatra, A., et al. (2013). Innate lymphoid type 2 cells sustain visceral adipose tissue eosinophils and alternatively activated macrophages. *J. Exp. Med.* 210, 535–549. doi: 10.1084/jem.20121964

Moro, K., Yamada, T., Tanabe, M., Takeuchi, T., Ikawa, T., Kawamoto, H., et al. (2010). Innate production of T(H)2 cytokines by adipose tissue-associated c-Kit(+)Sca-1(+) lymphoid cells. *Nature* 463, 540–544. doi: 10.1038/nature08636

Morris, D. L., Cho, K. W., DelProposto, J. L., Oatmen, K. E., Geletka, L. M., Martinez-Santibanez, G., et al. (2013). Adipose tissue macrophages function as antigen-presenting cells and regulate adipose tissue CD4 + T cells in mice. *Diabetes Metab. Res. Rev.* 62, 2762–2772. doi: 10.2337/db12-1404

Morris, D. L., Singer, K., and Lumeng, C. N. (2011). Adipose tissue macrophages: phenotypic plasticity and diversity in lean and obese states. *Curr. Opin. Clin. Nutr. Metab. Care* 14, 341–346. doi: 10.1097/MCO.0b013e328347970b

Moyo, D., Tanthuma, G., Cary, M. S., Mushisha, O., Kwadiba, G., Chikuse, F., et al. (2014). Cohort study of diabetes in HIV-infected adult patients: evaluating the effect of diabetes mellitus on immune reconstitution. *Diabetes Res. Clin. Pract.* 103, e34–e36. doi: 10.1016/j.diabres.2013.12.042

Mueller, S. N., Gebhardt, T., Carbone, F. R., and Heath, W. R. (2013). Memory T cell subsets, migration patterns, and tissue residence. *Annu. Rev. Immunol.* 31, 137–161. doi: 10.1146/annurev-immunol-032712-095954

Munier, S., Borjabad, A., Lemaire, M., Mariot, V., and Hazan, U. (2003). In vitro infection of human primary adipose cells with HIV-1: a reassessment. *AIDS* 17, 2537–2539. doi: 10.1097/00002030-200311210-00019

Muthumani, K., Choo, A. Y., Premkumar, A., Hwang, D. S., Thieu, K. P., Desai, B. M., et al. (2005). Human immunodeficiency virus type 1 (HIV-1) Vpr-regulated cell death: insights into mechanism. *Cell Death. Differ.* 12(Suppl. 1), 962–970. doi: 10.1038/sj.cdd.4401583

Nagajyothi, F., Desruisseaux, M. S., Machado, F. S., Upadhya, R., Zhao, D., Schwartz, G. J., et al. (2012). Response of adipose tissue to early infection with *Trypanosoma cruzi* (Brazil strain). *J. Infect. Dis.* 205, 830–840. doi: 10.1093/infdis/jir840

Nekhai, S., Kumari, N., and Dhawan, S. (2013). Role of cellular iron and oxygen in the regulation of HIV-1 infection. *Future Virol.* 8, 301–311. doi: 10.2217/fvl.13.6

Neyrolles, O., Herná Ndez-Pando, R., Pietri-Rouxel, F., Fornè, P., Tailleux, L., and Barrios, J. A. (2006). Is adipose tissue a place for mycobacterium tuberculosis persistence? *PLoS One* 1:e43. doi: 10.1371/journal.pone.0000043

Nippe, N., Varga, G., Holzinger, D., Löffler, B., Medina, E., Becker, K., et al. (2011). Subcutaneous infection with S. aureus in mice reveals association of resistance with influx of neutrophils and *Th2* response. *J. Invest. Dermatol.* 131, 125–132. doi: 10.1038/jid.2010.282

Nishimura, H., Itamura, S., Iwasaki, T., Kurata, T., and Tashiro, M. (2000). Characterization of human influenza A (H5N1) virus infection in mice: neuro-, pneumo- and adipotropic infection. *J. Gen. Virol.* 81, 2503–2510. doi: 10.1099/0022-1317-81-10-2503

Nishimura, S., Manabe, I., and Nagai, R. (2009a). Adipose tissue inflammation in obesity and metabolic syndrome. *Discov. Med.* 8, 55–60.

Nishimura, S., Manabe, I., Nagasaki, M., Eto, K., Yamashita, H., Ohsugi, M., et al. (2009b). CD8+ effector T cells contribute to macrophage recruitment and adipose tissue inflammation in obesity. *Nat. Med.* 15, 914–920. doi: 10.1038/nm.1964

Nishimura, S., Manabe, I., Takaki, S., Nagasaki, M., Otsu, M., Yamashita, H., et al. (2013). Adipose Natural Regulatory B cells negatively control adipose tissue inflammation. *Cell Metab.* 18, 759–766. doi: 10.1016/j.cmet.2013.09.017

Norwood, J., Turner, M., Bofill, C., Rebeiro, P., Shepherd, B., Bebawy, S., et al. (2017). Brief report: weight gain in persons with HIV switched from efavirenz-based to integrase strand transfer inhibitor-based regimens. *J. Acquir. Immune Defic. Syndr.* 76, 527–531. doi: 10.1097/QAI.0000000000001525

Odegaard, J. I., and Chawla, A. (2013). Pleiotropic actions of insulin resistance and inflammation in metabolic homeostasis. *Science* 339, 172–177. doi: 10.1126/science.1230721

O'Sullivan, T. E., Rapp, M., Fan, X., Weizman, O.-E., Bhardwaj, P., Adams, N. M., et al. (2016). Adipose-resident group 1 innate lymphoid cells promote obesity-associated insulin resistance. *Immunity* 45, 428–441. doi: 10.1016/j.immuni.2016.06.016

Ouchi, N., Parker, J. L., Lugus, J. J., and Walsh, K. (2011). Adipokines in inflammation and metabolic disease. *Nat. Publ. Gr.* 11, 85–97. doi: 10.1038/nri2921

Pal, D., Dasgupta, S., Kundu, R., Maitra, S., Das, G., Mukhopadhyay, S., et al. (2012). Fetuin-A acts as an endogenous ligand of TLR4 to promote lipid-induced insulin resistance. *Nat. Med.* 18, 1279–1285. doi: 10.1038/nm.2851

Palmer, C. S., Cherry, C. L., Sada-Ovalle, I., Singh, A., and Crowe, S. M. (2016a). Glucose metabolism in T cells and monocytes: new perspectives in HIV pathogenesis. *EBio. Med.* 6, 31–41. doi: 10.1016/j.ebiom.2016.02.012

Palmer, C. S., Hussain, T., Duette, G., Weller, T. J., Ostrowski, M., Sada-Ovalle, I., et al. (2016b). Regulators of glucose metabolism in CD4 + and CD8 + T cells. *Int. Rev. Immunol.* 35, 477–488. doi: 10.3109/08830185.2015.1082178

Pan, Y., Tian, T., Park, C. O., Lofftus, S. Y., Mei, S., Liu, X., et al. (2017). Survival of tissue-resident memory T cells requires exogenous lipid uptake and metabolism. *Nature* 543, 252–256. doi: 10.1038/nature21379

Pang, C., Gao, Z., Yin, J., Zhang, J., Jia, W., and Ye, J. (2008). Macrophage infiltration into adipose tissue may promote angiogenesis for adipose tissue remodeling in obesity. *Am. J. Physiol. Endocrinol. Metab.* 295, E313–E322. doi: 10.1152/ajpendo.90296.2008

Peirce, V., Carobbio, S., and Vidal-Puig, A. (2014). The different shades of fat. *Nature* 510, 76–83. doi: 10.1038/nature13477

Pellegrinelli, V., Carobbio, S., and Vidal-Puig, A. (2016). Adipose tissue plasticity: how fat depots respond differently to pathophysiological cues. *Diabetologia* 59, 1075–1088. doi: 10.1007/s00125-016-3933-4

Poglio, S., De Toni, F., Lewandowski, D., Minot, A., Arnaud, E., Barroca, V., et al. (2012). In situ production of innate immune cells in murine white adipose tissue. *Blood* 120, 4952–4962. doi: 10.1182/blood-2012-01-406959

Poglio, S., De Toni-Costes, F., Arnaud, E., Laharrague, P., Espinosa, E., Casteilla, L., et al. (2010). Adipose tissue as a dedicated reservoir of functional mast cell progenitors. *Stem Cells* 28, 2065–2072. doi: 10.1002/stem.523

Pond, C. M. (2002). Paracrine interactions of mammalian adipose tissue. *J. Exp. Zool. Part A Comp. Exp. Biol.* 295A, 99–110. doi: 10.1002/jez.a.10215

Possas, C., Antunes, A. M. S., Lins Mendes, F. M., Veloso, V., Martins, R. M., and Homma, A. (2018). HIV cure: global overview of bNAbs' patents and related scientific publications. *Expert Opin. Ther. Pat.* 28, 551–560. doi: 10.1080/13543776.2018.1495708

Price, P., Eddy, K. S., Papadimitriou, J. M., Robertson, T. A., and Shellam, G. R. (1990). Cytomegalovirus infection of adipose tissues induces steatitis in adult mice. *Int. J. Exp. Pathol.* 71, 557–571.

Prockop, D. J., and Oh, J. Y. (2012). Mesenchymal stem/stromal cells (MSCs): role as guardians of inflammation. *Mol. Ther.* 20, 14–20. doi: 10.1038/mt.2011.211

Puissant, B., Barreau, C., Bourin, P., Clavel, C., Corre, J., Bousquet, C., et al. (2005). Immunomodulatory effect of human adipose tissue-derived adult stem cells: comparison with bone marrow mesenchymal stem cells. *Br. J. Haematol.* 129, 118–129. doi: 10.1111/j.1365-2141.2005.05409.x

Rajsheker, S., Manka, D., Blomkalns, A. L., Chatterjee, T. K., Stoll, L. L., and Weintraub, N. L. (2010). Crosstalk between perivascular adipose tissue and blood vessels. *Curr. Opin. Pharmacol.* 10, 191–196. doi: 10.1016/j.coph.2009.11.005

Rangel-Moreno, J., Moyron-Quiroz, J. E., Carragher, D. M., Kusser, K., Hartson, L., Moquin, A., et al. (2009). Omental milky spots develop in the absence of lymphoid tissue-inducer cells and support B and T cell responses to peritoneal antigens. *Immunity* 30, 731–743. doi: 10.1016/j.immuni.2009.03.014

Rausch, M. E., Weisberg, S., Vardhana, P., and Tortoriello, D. V. (2008). Obesity in C57BL/6J mice is characterized by adipose tissue hypoxia and cytotoxic T-cell infiltration. *Int. J. Obes.* 32, 451–463. doi: 10.1038/sj.ijo.0803744

Rodriguez, A.-M., Elabd, C., Amri, E. Z., Ailhaud, G., and Dani, C. (2005). The human adipose tissue is a source of multipotent stem cells. *Biochimie* 87, 125–128. doi: 10.1016/j.biochi.2004.11.007

Rosen, E. D., and MacDougald, O. A. (2006). Adipocyte differentiation from the inside out. *Nat. Rev. Mol. Cell Biol.* 7, 885–896. doi: 10.1038/nrm2066

Routy, J.-P., Isnard, S., Mehraj, V., Ostrowski, M., Chomont, N., Ancuta, P., et al. (2019). Effect of metformin on the size of the HIV reservoir in non-diabetic ART-treated individuals: single-arm non-randomised Lilac pilot study protocol. *BMJ Open* 9:e028444. doi: 10.1136/bmjopen-2018-028444

Routy, J. P., Mehraj, V., Vyboh, K., Cao, W., Kema, I., and Jenabian, M. A. (2015). Clinical relevance of kynurenine pathway in HIV/AIDS: an immune checkpoint at the crossroads of metabolism and inflammation. *AIDS Rev.* 17, 96–106.

Sacher, T., Andrassy, J., Kalnins, A., Dölken, L., Jordan, S., Podlech, J., et al. (2011). Shedding light on the elusive role of endothelial cells in cytomegalovirus dissemination. *PLoS Pathog.* 7:e1002366. doi: 10.1371/journal.ppat.1002366

Saillan-Barreau, C., Cousin, B., André, M., Villena, P., Casteilla, L., and Pénicaud, L. (2003). Human adipose cells as candidates in defense and tissue remodeling phenomena. *Biochem. Biophys. Res. Commun.* 309, 502–505. doi: 10.1016/j.bbrc.2003.08.034

Samaras, K., Wand, H., Law, M., Emery, S., Cooper, D., and Carr, A. (2007). Prevalence of metabolic syndrome in HIV-infected patients receiving highly active antiretroviral therapy using International diabetes foundation and adult treatment panel III criteria: associations with insulin resistance, disturbed body fat compartmental. *Diabetes Care* 30, 113–119. doi: 10.2337/dc06-1075

Sathaliyawala, T., Kubota, M., Yudanin, N., Turner, D., Camp, P., Thome, J., et al. (2013). Distribution and compartmentalization of human circulating and tissue-resident memory T cell subsets. *Immunity* 38, 187–197. doi: 10.1016/j.immuni.2012.09.020

Sauce, D., Larsen, M., Fastenackels, S., Pauchard, M., Ait-Mohand, H., Schneider, L., et al. (2011). HIV disease progression despite suppression of viral replication is associated with exhaustion of lymphopoiesis. *Blood* 117, 5142–5151. doi: 10.1182/blood-2011-01-331306

Schaffler, A., and Scholmerich, J. (2010). Innate immunity and adipose tissue biology. *Trends Immunol.* 31, 228–235. doi: 10.1016/j.it.2010.03.001

Scheller, E. L., Cawthorn, W. P., Burr, A. A., Horowitz, M. C., and Macdougald, O. A. (2016). Marrow adipose tissue: trimming the fat. *Trends Endocrinol Metab.* 27, 392–403. doi: 10.1016/j.tem.2016.03.016

Seydel, K. B., Milner, D. A. Jr., Kamiza, S. B., Molyneux, M. E., and Taylor, T. E. (2006). The distribution and intensity of parasite sequestration in comatose malawian children. *J. Infect. Dis.* 194, 208–215.

Shao, X., Wang, M., Wei, X., Deng, S., Fu, N., Peng, Q., et al. (2016). Peroxisome proliferator-activated receptor-γ: master regulator of adipogenesis and obesity. *Curr. Stem Cell Res. Ther.* 11, 282–289. doi: 10.2174/1574888x10666150528144905

Shen, S., Tian, W., Ji, Y., Gao, Y., Zhang, M., Han, X., et al. (2019). Higher genetic diversity and viral evolution on key regions of envelope gene are associated with broader neutralizing antibody responses: report of two chronic HIV infected cases. *JPN. J. Infect. Dis.* 72, 312–317. doi: 10.7883/yoken.JJID.2018.336

Shen, W., Wang, Z., Punyanita, M., Lei, J., Sinav, A., Kral, J. G., et al. (2003). Adipose tissue quantification by imaging methods: a proposed classification. *Obes. Res.* 11, 5–16. doi: 10.1038/oby.2003.3

Shirakawa, K., Yan, X., Shinmura, K., Endo, J., Kataoka, M., Katsumata, Y., et al. (2016). Obesity accelerates T cell senescence in murine visceral adipose tissue. *J. Clin. Invest.* 126, 4626–4639. doi: 10.1172/JCI88606

Shrivastav, S., Kino, T., Cunningham, T., Ichijo, T., Schubert, U., Heinklein, P., et al. (2008). Human immunodeficiency virus (HIV)-1 viral protein R suppresses transcriptional activity of peroxisome proliferator-activated receptor {gamma} and inhibits adipocyte differentiation: implications for HIV-associated lipodystrophy. *Mol. Endocrinol.* 22, 234–247. doi: 10.1210/me.2007-0124

Smith, S. R., Lovejoy, J. C., Greenway, F., Ryan, D., deJonge, L., de la Bretonne, J., et al. (2001). Contributions of total body fat, abdominal subcutaneous adipose tissue compartments, and visceral adipose tissue to the metabolic complications of obesity. *Metabolism* 50, 425–435. doi: 10.1053/meta.2001.21693

Solana, R., Tarazona, R., Aiello, A. E., Akbar, A. N., Appay, V., Beswick, M., et al. (2012). CMV and Immunosenescence: from basics to clinics. *Immun. Ageing* 9:23. doi: 10.1186/1742-4933-9-23

Spalding, K. L., Arner, E., Westermark, P. O., Bernard, S., Buchholz, B. A., Bergmann, O., et al. (2008). Dynamics of fat cell turnover in humans. *Nature* 453, 783–787. doi: 10.1038/nature06902

Spencer, M., Yao-Borengasser, A., Unal, R., Rasouli, N., Gurley, C. M., Zhu, B., et al. (2010). Adipose tissue macrophages in insulin-resistant subjects are associated with collagen VI and fibrosis and demonstrate alternative activation. *Am. J. Physiol. Endocrinol. Metab.* 299, E1016–E1027. doi: 10.1152/ajpendo.00329.2010

Suganami, T., Tanimoto-Koyama, K., Nishida, J., Itoh, M., Yuan, X., Mizuarai, S., et al. (2007). Role of the Toll-like receptor 4/NF-kappaB pathway in saturated fatty acid-induced inflammatory changes in the interaction between adipocytes and macrophages. *Arterioscler. Thromb. Vasc. Biol.* 27, 84–91. doi: 10.1161/01.atv.0000251608.09329.9a

Sun, K., Tordjman, J., Clément, K., and Scherer, P. E. (2013). Fibrosis and adipose tissue dysfunction. *Cell Metab.* 18, 470–477. doi: 10.1016/j.cmet.2013.06.016

Szasz, T., and Webb, R. C. (2012). Perivascular adipose tissue: more than just structural support. *Clin. Sci.* 122, 1–12. doi: 10.1042/CS20110151

Tang, W., Zeve, D., Suh, J. M., Bosnakovski, D., Kyba, M., Hammer, R. E., et al. (2008). White fat progenitor cells reside in the adipose vasculature. *Science* 322, 583–586. doi: 10.1126/science.1156232

Tang, X., Lu, H., Dooner, M., Chapman, S., Quesenberry, P. J., and Ramratnam, B. (2018). Exosomal Tat protein activates latent HIV-1 in primary, resting CD4+ T lymphocytes. *JCI Insight* 3:95676. doi: 10.1172/jci.insight.95676

Tanowitz, H. B., Scherer, P. E., Mota, M. M., and Figueiredo, L. M. (2017). Adipose tissue: a safe haven for parasites? *Trends Parasitol.* 33, 276–284. doi: 10.1016/j.pt.2016.11.008

Tao, J.-H., Barbi, J., and Pan, F. (2015). Hypoxia-inducible factors in T lymphocyte differentiation and function. a review in the theme: cellular responses to hypoxia. *Am. J. Physiol. Cell Physiol.* 309, C580–C589. doi: 10.1152/ajpcell.00204.2015

Tchkonia, T., Morbeck, D. E., Von Zglinicki, T., Van Deursen, J., Lustgarten, J., Scrable, H., et al. (2010). Fat tissue, aging, and cellular senescence. *Aging Cell* 9, 667–684. doi: 10.1111/j.1474-9726.2010.00608.x

Toribio, M., Fitch, K. V., Sanchez, L., Burdo, T. H., Williams, K. C., Sponseller, C. A., et al. (2017). Effects of pitavastatin and pravastatin on markers of immune activation and arterial inflammation in HIV. *AIDS* 31, 797–806. doi: 10.1097/QAD.0000000000001427

Trezza, C., Ford, S. L., Spreen, W., Pan, R., and Piscitelli, S. (2015). Formulation and pharmacology of long-acting cabotegravir. *Curr. Opin. HIV AIDS* 10, 239–245. doi: 10.1097/COH.0000000000000168

Trindade, S., Rijo-Ferreira, F., Carvalho, T., Pinto-Neves, D., Guegan, F., Aresta-Branco, F., et al. (2016). *Trypanosoma brucei* parasites occupy and functionally adapt to the adipose tissue in mice. *Cell Host Microbe* 19, 837–848. doi: 10.1016/j.chom.2016.05.002

Tsai, S., Clemente-Casares, X., Zhou, A. C., Lei, H., Ahn, J. J., Chan, Y. T., et al. (2018). Insulin receptor-mediated stimulation boosts T cell immunity during inflammation and infection. *Cell Metab.* 28, 1–13. doi: 10.1016/j.cmet.2018.08.003

Valle-Casuso, J. C., Angin, M., Volant, S., Passaes, C., Monceaux, V., Mikhailova, A., et al. (2019). Cellular metabolism is a major determinant of HIV-1 reservoir seeding in CD4+ T cells and offers an opportunity to tackle infection. *Cell Metab.* 29:611-626.e5. doi: 10.1016/j.cmet.2018.11.015

van Meer, G., Voelker, D. R., and Feigenson, G. W. (2008). Membrane lipids: where they are and how they behave. *Nat. Rev. Mol. Cell Biol.* 9, 112–124. doi: 10.1038/nrm2330

Vernochet, C., Azoulay, S., Duval, D., Guedj, R., Cottrez, F., Vidal, H., et al. (2005). Human immunodeficiency virus protease inhibitors accumulate into cultured human adipocytes and alter expression of adipocytokines. *J. Biol. Chem.* 280, 2238–2243. doi: 10.1074/jbc.m408687200

Vidal, F., Domingo, P., Villarroya, F., Giralt, M., López-Dupla, M., Gutiérrez, M., et al. (2012). Adipogenic/lipid, inflammatory, and mitochondrial parameters in subcutaneous adipose tissue of untreated HIV-1-infected long-term nonprogressors: significant alterations despite low viral burden. *J. Acquir. Immune Defic. Syndr.* 61, 131–137. doi: 10.1097/qai.0b013e31825c3a68

Vila, I. K., Badin, P.-M., Marques, M.-A., Monbrun, L., Lefort, C., Mir, L., et al. (2014). Immune cell Toll-like receptor 4 mediates the development of obesity- and endotoxemia-associated adipose tissue fibrosis. *Cell Rep.* 7, 1116–1129. doi: 10.1016/j.celrep.2014.03.062

Visnegarwala, F., Raghavan, S. S., Mullin, C. M., Bartsch, G., Wang, J., Kotler, D., et al. (2005). Sex differences in the associations of HIV disease characteristics and body composition in antiretroviral-naive persons. *Am. J. Clin. Nutr.* 82, 850–856. doi: 10.1093/ajcn/82.4.850

Wajchenberg, B. (2000). Subcutaneous and visceral adipose tissue?: their relation to the metabolic syndrome. *Endocr. Rev.* 21, 697–738. doi: 10.1210/edrv.21.6.0415

Walker, G. E., Marzullo, P., Verti, B., Guzzaloni, G., Maestrini, S., Zurleni, F., et al. (2008). Subcutaneous abdominal adipose tissue subcompartments: potential role in rosiglitazone effects. *Obesity* 16, 1983–1991. doi: 10.1038/oby.2008.326

Walsh, D. A., Borges da Silva, H., Beura, L. K., Peng, C., Hamilton, S. E., Masopust, D., et al. (2019). The functional requirement for CD69 in establishment of resident memory CD8 + T cells varies with tissue location. *J. Immunol.* 203, 946–955. doi: 10.4049/jimmunol.1900052

Wan, C.-D., Cheng, R., Wang, H.-B., and Liu, T. (2008). Immunomodulatory effects of mesenchymal stem cells derived from adipose tissues in a rat orthotopic liver transplantation model. *Hepatobil. Pancreat. Dis. Int.* 7, 29–33.

Wang, Q., and Wu, H. (2018). T Cells in adipose tissue: critical players in immunometabolism. *Front. Immunol.* 9:2509. doi: 10.3389/fimmu.2018.02509

Wang, Y., Chen, X., Cao, W., and Shi, Y. (2014). Plasticity of mesenchymal stem cells in immunomodulation: pathological and therapeutic implications. *Nat. Immunol.* 15, 1009–1016. doi: 10.1038/ni.3002

Wanjalla, C. N., McDonnell, W. J., Barnett, L., Simmons, J. D., Furch, B. D., Lima, M. C., et al. (2019). Adipose tissue in persons With HIV Is enriched for CD4+ T effector memory and T effector memory RA+ cells, which show higher CD69 expression and CD57, CX3CR1, GPR56 Co-expression with increasing glucose intolerance. *Front. Immunol.* 10:408. doi: 10.3389/fimmu.2019.00408

Wanjalla, C. N., McDonnell, W. J., and Koethe, J. R. (2018). Adipose tissue T cells in HIV/SIV infection. *Front. Immunol.* 9:2730. doi: 10.3389/fimmu.2018.02730

Weisberg, S. P., Mccann, D., Desai, M., Rosenbaum, M., Leibel, R. L., and Ferrante, A. W. (2003). Obesity is associated with macrophage accumulation in adipose tissue. *J. Clin. Invest.* 112, 1796–1808. doi: 10.1172/jci19246

Wensveen, F. M., Jelenèiæ, V., Valentiæ, S., Šestan, M., Wensveen, T. T., Theurich, S., et al. (2015). NK cells link obesity-induced adipose stress to inflammation and insulin resistance. *Nat. Immunol.* 16, 376–385. doi: 10.1038/ni.3120

Wernstedt Asterholm, I., Tao, C., Morley, T. S., Wang, Q. A., Delgado-Lopez, F., Wang, Z. V., et al. (2014). Adipocyte inflammation is essential for healthy adipose tissue expansion and remodeling. *Cell Metab.* 20, 103–118. doi: 10.1016/j.cmet.2014.05.005

Wertheimer, A. M., Bennett, M. S., Park, B., Uhrlaub, J. L., Martinez, C., Pulko, V., et al. (2014). Aging and cytomegalovirus infection differentially and jointly affect distinct circulating T cell subsets in humans. *J. Immunol.* 192, 2143–2155. doi: 10.4049/jimmunol.1301721

Wieland, C. W., Florquin, S., Chan, E. D., Leemans, J. C., Weijer, S., Verbon, A., et al. (2005). Pulmonary Mycobacterium tuberculosis infection in leptin-deficient ob/ob mice. *Int. Immunol.* 17, 1399–1408. doi: 10.1093/intimm/dxh317

Winer, D. A., Winer, S., Shen, L., Wadia, P. P., Yantha, J., Paltser, G., et al. (2011). B cells promote insulin resistance through modulation of T cells and production of pathogenic IgG antibodies. *Nat. Med.* 17, 610–617. doi: 10.1038/nm.2353

Worodria, W., Massinga-Loembe, M., Mazakpwe, D., Luzinda, K., Menten, J., Van Leth, F., et al. (2011). Incidence and predictors of mortality and the effect of tuberculosis immune reconstitution inflammatory syndrome in a cohort of TB/HIV patients commencing antiretroviral therapy. *J. Acquir. Immune Defic. Syndr.* 58, 32–37. doi: 10.1097/QAI.0b013e3182255dc2

Worodria, W., Ssempijja, V., Hanrahan, C., Ssegonja, R., Muhofwa, A., Mazapkwe, D., et al. (2018). Opportunistic diseases diminish the clinical benefit of immediate antiretroviral therapy in HIV–tuberculosis co-infected adults with low CD4+ cell counts. *AIDS* 32, 2141–2149. doi: 10.1097/QAD.0000000000001941

Wronska, A., and Kmiec, Z. (2012). Structural and biochemical characteristics of various white adipose tissue depots. *Acta Physiol.* 205, 194–208. doi: 10.1111/j.1748-1716.2012.02409.x

Wu, D., Molofsky, A. B., Liang, H. E., Ricardo-Gonzalez, R. R., Jouihan, H. A., Bando, J. K., et al. (2011). Eosinophils sustain adipose alternatively activated macrophages associated with glucose homeostasis. *Science* 332, 243–247. doi: 10.1126/science.1201475

Wu, H., Ghosh, S., Perrard, X. D., Feng, L., Garcia, G. E., Perrard, J. L., et al. (2007). T-cell accumulation and regulated on activation, normal T cell expressed and secreted upregulation in adipose tissue in obesity. *Circulation* 115, 1029–1038. doi: 10.1161/circulationaha.106.638379

Xiao, L., Yang, X., Lin, Y., Li, S., Jiang, J., Qian, S., et al. (2016). Large adipocytes function as antigen-presenting cells to activate CD4 + T cells *via* upregulating MHCII in obesity. *Int. J. Obes.* 40, 112–120. doi: 10.1038/ijo.2015.145

Xu, H., Barnes, G. T., Yang, Q., Tan, G., Yang, D., Chou, C. J., et al. (2003). Chronic inflammation in fat plays a crucial role in the development of obesity-related insulin resistance. *J. Clin. Invest.* 112, 1821–1830. doi: 10.1172/jci200319451

Yousefi, F., Ebtekar, M., Soudi, S., Soleimani, M., and Hashemi, S. M. (2016). In vivo immunomodulatory effects of adipose-derived mesenchymal stem cells conditioned medium in experimental autoimmune encephalomyelitis. *Immunol. Lett.* 172, 94–105. doi: 10.1016/j.imlet.2016.02.016

Zeyda, M., and Stulnig, T. M. (2007). Adipose tissue macrophages. *Immunol Lett.* 112, 61–67. doi: 10.1016/j.imlet.2007.07.003

Zhang, L.-J. L., Guerrero-Juarez, C. F., Hata, T., Bapat, S. P., Ramos, R., Plikus, M. V., et al. (2015). Innate immunity. dermal adipocytes protect against invasive *Staphylococcus aureus* skin infection. *Science* 347, 67–71. doi: 10.1126/science.1260972

Zúñiga, L. A., Shen, W.-J., Joyce-Shaikh, B., Pyatnova, E. A., Richards, A. G., Thom, C., et al. (2010). IL-17 regulates adipogenesis, glucose homeostasis, and obesity. *J. Immunol.* 185, 6947–6959. doi: 10.4049/jimmunol.1001269

14

Killing of Latently HIV-Infected CD4 T Cells by Autologous CD8 T Cells is Modulated by Nef

Ziv Sevilya[1,2], *Ehud Chorin*[2,3], *Orit Gal-Garber*[4], *Einat Zelinger*[4], *Dan Turner*[2,3], *Boaz Avidor*[2,3], *Gideon Berke*[5] *and David Hassin*[1,2,3,6*]

[1] Internal Medicine Department A, Assuta Ashdod Medical Center, Ashdod, Israel, [2] Crusaid Kobler AIDS center, Tel-Aviv Sourasky Medical Center, Tel-Aviv, Israel, [3] Sackler Faculty of Medicine, Tel-Aviv University, Tel-Aviv, Israel, [4] Interdepartmental Equipment Facility, Robert H. Smith Faculty of Agriculture, Food and Environment, the Hebrew University, Rehovot, Israel, [5] Department of Immunology, Weizmann Institute of Science, Rehovot, Israel, [6] Faculty of Health Sciences, Ben Gurion University of the Negev, Beer-Sheva, Israel

***Correspondence:**
David Hassin
hassindavid@gmail.com

The role of HIV-specific CD8 T cell activity in the course of HIV infection and the way it affects the virus that resides in the latent reservoir resting memory cells is debated. The PBMC of HIV-infected patients contain HIV-specific CD8 T cells and their potential targets, CD4 T cells latently infected by HIV. CD4 T cells and CD8 T cells procured from PBMC of HIV-infected patients were co-incubated and analyzed: Formation of CD8 T cells and HIV-infected CD4 T cell conjugates and apoptosis of these CD4 T cells were observed by fluorescence microscopy with *in situ* PCR of HIV LTR DNA. Furthermore, conjugation of CD8 T cells with CD4 T cells and apoptosis of CD4 T cells was observed and quantified by imaging flow cytometry using anti-human activated caspase 3 antibody and TUNEL assay. The conjugation activity and apoptosis were found to be much higher in patients with acute HIV infection or AIDS compared to patients in chronic infection on antiretroviral therapy (ART) or not. Patients on ART had low grade conjugation and apoptosis of isolated CD69, CD25, and HLA-DR-negative CD4 T cells (latent reservoir cells) by CD8 T cells. Using *in situ* PCR The latent reservoir CD4 T cells were shown to contain most of the HIV DNA. We demonstrate in HIV-infected patients, that CD8 T cells conjugate with and kill HIV-infected CD4 T cells, including HIV-infected resting memory CD4 T cells, throughout the course of HIV infection. We propose that in HIV-infected patients CD4 T cell annihilation is caused in part by ongoing activity of HIV-specific CD8 T cells. HIV Nef protein interacts with ASK 1 and inhibits its pro-apoptotic death signaling by Fas/FasL, thus protecting HIV-infected cells from CD8 T cells killing. A peptide that interrupts Nef-ASK1 interaction that had been delivered into CD4 T cells procured from patients on ART resulted in the increase of their apoptosis inflicted by autologous CD8 T cells. We suggest that elimination of the HIV-infected latent reservoir CD4 T cells can be achieved by Nef inhibition.

Keywords: CD8 T cells, cellular immunology, HIV, virology, latent reservoir HIV infected CD4 T cells, apoptosis of HIV infected CD4 T cells

INTRODUCTION

HIV-infected patients are currently treated by antiretroviral therapy (ART), which achieves viral suppression but not a cure. Latent reservoirs of resting memory HIV-infected CD4 T cells are established very early after infection and result in a viral rebound upon treatment interruption. The biology of latent reservoirs cells is poorly understood (1, 2). The CD8 T cell receptor (TCR) recognize a viral epitope presented in the HLA class 1 receptor, resulting in the formation of an immunological synapse between the CD8 T cells and the target cells, which can be observed as a CD8 T cell-target cell conjugate. This conjugate formation was found to be antigen and TCR specific; CD8 T cells conjugate with and kill only peptide-MHC restricted target cells that the immune system was previously exposed to (3–6). Immunological synapse formation results in the apoptosis of the target cell by the interaction of cell surface receptors, Fas-FasL, and by perforin and granzymes secreted from the CD8 T cells. Perforin expression in the CD8 T cells decays very rapidly upon the disappearance of the target cells, it can therefore serve as a marker of ongoing activation and killing capacity of CD8 T cells (3, 7). The role of CD8 T cells in the course of HIV infection and their possible effects on the latent reservoir of CD4 T cells is unknown.

The appearance of HIV-specific CD8 T cells in acute HIV infection correlates with the decline in both viral load and number of CD4 T cells (8–11). Depletion of CD8 T cells in simian immunodeficiency virus (SIV)-infected macaques resulted in a rapid rise in the plasma viral load (8, 11). The frequency of CD8 T cells that target multiple HIV proteins in the peripheral blood mononuclear cells (PBMC) of untreated HIV-infected patients is 8.7 ± 1.38% (12). Functional HIV-specific CD8 T cells can be identified in the PBMC of patients on prolonged ART with undetectable viral load (12–15). A broad HIV-specific CD8 T cell response against Gag and Nef proteins in ART-treated patients was observed recently; suggesting preservation of active CD8 T cells immune function (15, 16). These data imply that viral proteins are expressed and presented by resting memory CD4 T cells recognized by CD8 T cells.

PBMC of HIV-infected patients contain HIV-specific CD8 T cells and their potential targets, HIV-infected CD4 T cells. The frequency of cells harboring HIV pro-viral DNA in lymph nodes and gut biopsies is comparable to the frequency of chronic HIV-infected memory CD4 T cells in the PBMC of HIV infected patients (17). We previously studied the interaction between CD8 and CD4 T cells in untreated HIV-infected patients. CD4 and CD8 T cells were directly procured from the PBMC of acute and chronic untreated HIV-infected patients and co-incubated (the cells were neither manipulated nor stimulated *in vitro*). Formation of CD8-CD4 T cell conjugates and CD4 T cells apoptosis were observed by fluorescence microscopy and by continuous recording in tissue culture. It emerged that 6% of the CD4 T cells from acute HIV-infected patients were conjugated by autologous CD8 T cells, while 3% of the CD4 T cells were conjugated by autologous CD8 T cells in chronic untreated HIV-infected patients. Annexin binding and cell morphology typical of apoptosis were observed in the conjugated CD4 T cells. The majority of CD8 T cells that had conjugated to CD4 T cells expressed perforin. Apoptosis was significantly elevated in acute HIV infection and more modest during the chronic phase of untreated HIV infection. The CD4 T cells conjugated by autologous CD8 T cells procured from chronic untreated HIV-infected patients were positive for HIV DNA, as observed by *in situ* PCR (5).

It has been suggested that the HIV Nef protein may play an important role in the ability of HIV to evade the immune system (18). The HIV Nef protein down regulates HLA expression and protects HIV-infected cells from being killed by cytotoxic T lymphocytes (CTL) (19). Nef was associated with Apoptosis Signal regulating Kinase 1 (ASK1) which protected the Nef transfected CD4 T cells from apoptosis by FasL and TNF-α (20, 21).

We studied the interaction between CD8 and CD4 T cells procured from the PBMC of AIDS, acute, and chronic untreated and treated HIV-infected patients. The cells were studied by fluorescent microscopy, *in situ* PCR of HIV DNA and imaging flow cytometry. We found that CD8 T cells form conjugates and kill HIV-infected CD4 T cells in all stages of the infection, including in HIV-infected patients on ART. The conjugation activity and apoptosis rates were much higher in patients with acute infection or AIDS than in chronic untreated and treated patients. Most of the CD4 T cells from chronic and treated HIV-infected patients that were positive for HIV DNA by *in situ* PCR were resting memory cells. The autologous CD8 T cells were shown to conjugate with and kill latent reservoir CD4 T cells. A peptide that interrupts Nef-ASK1 interaction that had been delivered into CD4 T cells procured from patients on ART resulted in the increase of their apoptosis inflicted by autologous CD8 T cells.

MATERIALS AND METHODS

Study Subjects

Twenty-eight HIV-infected patients in acute, chronic untreated, treated by ART and AIDS patients as well as 14 matched healthy controls were enrolled into this study at the Crusaid Kobler AIDS Center, Tel Aviv Sourasky Medical Center, Israel (**Table 1**). Acute HIV-infected patients were defined 3–12 weeks after clinical presentation. Chronic untreated HIV-infected subjects were defined as patients at least 1 year after HIV infection. AIDS patients were late presenters with CD4 T cell counts below 200 cell/μl. All the patients on ART had an undetectable viral load <20 copies/ml and a CD4 T cell count above 360 cell/μl. Plasma viral load and CD4 and CD8 T lymphocyte counts were determined as previously described (5). All subjects provided written informed consent for participation in the study, which was approved by the institutional ethics committee in accordance with the ethical standards laid down in the 1964 Declaration of Helsinki and its later amendments.

Abbreviations: PBMC, Peripheral blood mononuclear cells; HIV, Human immunodeficiency virus; LTR, Long terminal repeat; ART, Antiretroviral therapy; TCR, T cell receptor; CTL, Cytotoxic T lymphocyte; HLA, Human leukocyte antigen; MHC, Major histocompatibility complex; TUNEL, Terminal deoxynucleotidyl transferase dUTP nick end labeling.

TABLE 1 | Characteristics of the patients enrolled in this study.

Case	Age	CD4 (cells/μl)	CD8 (cells/μl)	Viral load (copies/ml)		
ACUTE HIV INFECTED PATIENTS						
1	26	609	2523	60148		
2	53	419	550	88088		
3	55	504	1584	876323		
Case	**Age**	**CD4 (cells/μl)**	**CD8 (cells/μl)**	**Viral load**		
AIDS PATIENTS						
1	32	84	1032	65540		
2	36	72	204	490565		
3	28	42	504	273074		
Case	**Age**	**CD4 (cells/μl)**	**CD8 (cells/μl)**	**Viral load (copies/ml)**	**Time from infection (years)**	
CHRONIC HIV INFECTED PATIENTS						
1	32	624	656	2801	3	
2	34	713	897	989	2	
3	26	546	957	19611	1	
Case	**Age**	**CD4 (cells/μl)**	**CD8 (cells/μl)**	**Viral load**	**Time from infection (years)**	**Time on ART (years)**
PATIENTS ON ANTIRETROVIRAL THERAPY						
1	50	666	630	TND	8	8
2	63	506	546	TND	9	8
3	40	736	1664	TND	10	7
4	48	612	680	TND	7	4
5	45	624	1182	TND	13	9
6	48	738	360	TND	1	0.5
7	43	903	736	TND	6	4
8	51	408	799	TND	8	6
9	51	544	621	TND	20	17
10	49	945	588	TND	5	4
11	46	1131	1218	TND	8	6
12	42	1128	962	TND	7	6
13	26	850	1462	TND	1	0.5
14	42	750	1000	TND	2.5	2
15	44	507	390	TND	10	9
16	37	1131	986	TND	4	3
17	36	680	510	TND	5	4
18	43	1196	667	TND	16	15
19	25	1000	625	TND	3	2

Isolation of CD8 T Cells and CD4 T Cells From PBMC

Thirty milliliters of whole blood were collected in EDTA and the PBMC were separated over a Ficoll-Hypaque density gradient. CD8 T cells were positively selected using CD8 MicroBeads kit (Miltenyi Biotech), according to the manufacturer's protocol. CD4 T cells were separated from the CD8 T cell-depleted PBMC by negative selection of CD4 T cells (CD4 T cell isolation kit, Miltenyi Biotech). Purity of the CD4 and CD8 T cells was tested by Imaging flow cytometer (ImageStream) and determined to be above 95%.

Separating Resting From Activated CD4 T Cells

Resting CD4 T cells were separated from activated CD4 T cells using a two-step negative selection method based on the activated cells surface markers CD25, CD69, and HLA-DR, (22–24) using CD69 MicroBead kit II, Anti-HLA-DR MicroBeads, and anti-human CD25 conjugated to microbeads (MicroBeads II, Miltenyi Biotech) according to the manufacturer's protocol (Miltenyi Biotech). The purity of the separated cells was demonstrated by staining with anti-CD69 (Enzo), anti-HLA-DR (Enzo), and anti-CD25 (Enzo) antibodies conjugated to APC and analyzed by the ImageStream. Typical purities of resting CD4 T cells were 95–98.5% with <1.5% contamination by activated CD4 T cells (**Figure 4**).

Conjugate Formation of CD8-CD4 T Cells

CD4 T cells were labeled with 2 μM calcein AM (Molecular probes C1430). Freshly isolated 1×10^6 CD4 and 1×10^6 CD8 T cells were mixed in 1 ml PBS containing 0.9 mM $CaCl_2$ and 0.5 mM $MgCl_2$, incubated for 15 min at 37°C, and then co-centrifuged at 185 g for 20 min at room temperature. They were re suspended in cold PBS containing 0.9 mM $CaCl_2$ and 0.5 mM $MgCl_2$ and placed on ice. Conjugates of the CD8 T cells with CD4 T cells were immediately quantified in the hemocytometer by fluorescence microscopy (5). Conjugated CD4 and CD8 T cells were fixed in 4% PFA (15 min, 22°C). The fixed cells were incubated with 2% fetal bovine serum (FBS) in PBS (1 h, 4°C) followed by staining with anti-human CD8 antibody conjugated to APC (clone HIT8a, Biolegend). The slides were visualized by a confocal microscope. At least 1,000 cells were scored for each patient. The percent conjugation is the number of conjugated CD4 T cells divided by the total number of CD4 T cells X100. Counting CTL target cell conjugates under a microscope has been shown to be both accurate and specific (3–5).

In situ PCR of HIV DNA

The method was adopted from the protocols published (5, 25–28). Following conjugation of CD4 T cells with CD8 T cells, 1×10^5 cells were fixed with 4% PFA on slides and an *in-situ* PCR amplification reaction in a thermal cycler was performed for 30 cycles. The primers are from the HIV LTR: Forward primer (NEC 152) 5′-GCCTCAATAAAGCTTGCCTTGA-3′. Reverse primer (NEC 131) - 5′-GGCGCCACTGCTAGAGATTTT-3′ (27–29). After amplification, fluorescein-tagged 56nt probe was used to identify the amplified HIV DNA: 5′-CACAACAGACGGGCACACACCTACTTTAAGCACTCAAGG CAAGCTTTATTGAGGCA-3′ (5). When indicated, after the *in-situ* PCR the slides were labeled with anti-human perforin antibody (clone dG9 Biolegend 308109) conjugated to AlexaFlour 647. The slides were observed on a confocal microscope, and 1,000 cells were screened for cells harboring HIV DNA and CD4-CD8 T cell conjugates in each slide.

Immunological Synapse Proteins in CD8-CD4 T Cells Conjugates

Conjugated CD8-CD4 T cells procured from patients on ART were fixed with 4% PFA, permeabilized and stained with anti-human CD8 antibody conjugated to PerCP/Cy5.5 (clone HIT8a, Biolegend), anti-human perforin antibody clone dG9 conjugated with B.V.510 (Biolegend), anti-human γ-tubulin (clone D-10, Santa Cruz) conjugated with PE, anti-human LCK antibody (Y123 RabMab, abcam) and observed by a confocal microscope.

CD4-CD8 T Cells Conjugation Analyzed by Multispectral Imaging Flow Cytometry (Imagestream)

After conjugation, the cells were fixed with 4% PFA, they were incubated with anti-human CD8 antibody conjugated with APC (clone HIT8a, Biolegend), anti-human CD4 antibody PE/Cy7 conjugated (clone OKT, Biolegend) and 1.4 μM DAPI. The cells were imaged by a multispectral imaging flow cytometer (ImageStreamX flow-cytometer; Amnis Corp., Seattle, WA). A total of $2–5 \times 10^4$ cells were collected from each sample and the data were analyzed using image analysis software (IDEA 6.0; Amnis Corp.). The images were compensated for fluorescent dye overlap by using single-stained controls. Gating strategy for CD8-CD4 T cell conjugates analysis is based on the manufacturer's protocol and it was performed as follows: the aspect ratio vs. the area of the bright field image was plotted to identify conjugates. Only conjugates that contained two cells; one cell positive for both CD8 and DAPI and one cell DAPI-positive were considered as true conjugates. Further confirmation of the gated conjugates was done for each CD8-CD4 conjugated T cell by direct observation and photography using the ImageStream. Gating based on CD4 staining was not consistent and it was therefore not used in our gating strategy.

CD4 T Cells Apoptosis Analyzed by the Imagestream

For the apoptosis assay, the conjugates were incubated for 120 min at 37°C and then fixed and permeabilized. Apoptosis was evaluated using both a DNA fragmentation TUNEL assay (BioVision, Apo-BrdU-Red™ K404) and labeling with anti-human active capase-3 antibody (rabbit polyclonal, Enzo ALX-210-807). The cells were also stained with anti-human CD8 antibody conjugated to PerCP/Cy5.5 (clone HIT8a, Biolegend), anti-human CD4 antibody conjugated to PE/Cy7 (clone OKT, Biolegend) and 1.4 μM DAPI (Enzo, BML-AP402-0010). A total of 50,000 cells were analyzed in the ImagStream: those that were CD8-negative, DAPI-positive and positive for either caspase-3 active or TUNEL assay were defined as CD4 T cells in apoptosis.

Internalization of the ASK1 Peptide Into CD4 T Cells

ASK1 amino acid sequence 152-DEVGEANN-159 that was shown to interact with the Nef protein (21) was synthesized and HPLC purified to 95.07%.(Genemed Synthesis Inc.). 4×10^6 CD4 T cells procured from patients on ART and matching healthy controls were incubated in RPMI supplemented with 1% penicillin/streptomycin and 10% FBS in 10 cm plates. Cells from healthy controls or from patients on ART were incubated with or without 10 μM ASK1 peptide for 16 h at 37°C in 5% CO2 (21). Following incubation, the CD4 T cells were harvested and mixed with equal numbers of autologous CD8 T cells for the apoptosis assay.

Sample Size

The sample size was calculated from the percent conjugated CD4 T cells means and standard deviations reported in our previous study for acute and chronic untreated patients (5), which were found to be similar to the results obtained in the present study. The type 1 error probability was $\alpha = 0.05$ and the power ($1-\beta$) was 0.90. This result was obtained in a minimum sample size of 3 patients at each different disease stage. In patients on ART, which are in the focus of the present study the sample size was 12.

Statistical Analysis

Differences between HIV patients and controls and between HIV patient subgroups were compared using a Student *t*-test (for comparison of two groups) or a one-way ANOVA (for comparison of more than two groups). Differences were considered significant when $p \leq 0.01$(*) and very significant when $p \leq 0.001$ (**). All calculations were done using SPSS v15.0 by IBM and MedCalc V14.8 by MedCalc software. Values are presented as mean ± standard error of the mean.

RESULTS

HIV DNA Observed in CD4 T Cells Interacting With Autologous CD8 T Cells Throughout the Course of HIV Infection

We studied CD4 T cells conjugated with autologous CD8 T cells procured from the PBMC of AIDS, acute, and chronic untreated and treated HIV-infected patients as well as healthy controls (**Tables 1, 2; Figure 1**). The CD4 and CD8 T cells were procured directly from the PBMC of HIV-infected patients by means of magnetic beads, followed by co-incubation and fixation on slides. The cells were neither manipulated nor stimulated *in vitro*. *In situ* PCR was performed on the fixed cells by means of primers from the HIV long terminal repeat (LTR). The same primers were used for the identification of HIV provirus in CD4 T cells in various studies (27–29). The probe was a conserved sequence of 56nt labeled by FITC (5). Anti-perforin APC-labeled antibodies were used after the *in-situ* PCR to look for the perforin content in the CD8 T cells.

TABLE 2 | Quantification of HIV DNA-positive CD4 T cells and CD4-CD8 T cell conjugates throughout the course of HIV infection observed by *in-situ* PCR.

HIV Infection	Acute	Chronic untreated	Chronic on ART	AIDS
Number of patients	3	3	12	3
HIV-DNA-positive CD4 T cells, %	11 ± 3.0	10 ± 2.0	12 ± 1.5	9.5 ± 2.0
Conjugated CD4 T cells, %	6.5 ± 1.0	3 ± 0.6	3 ± 0.3	7.0 ± 0.9
Conjugated HIV-DNA-positive CD4 T cells, %	70 ± 3.0	30 ± 5	25 ± 3.0	75 ± 8.0

HIV DNA was detected in ~10% of CD4 T cells procured from all stages of HIV infection. From 25 to 30% of the HIV-infected CD4 T cells were conjugated by CD8 T cells in chronic untreated patients and patients on ART, which are 3 ± 0.6 and 3 ± 0.3% of the CD4 T cells, respectively (**Table 2; Figures 1B,C**). In contrast, from 70 to 75% of the HIV-infected CD4 T cells were conjugated by autologous CD8 T cells in acute HIV infection and AIDS patients, which are 6.5 ± 1.0 and 7.0 ± 0.9% of the CD4 T cells, respectively (**Table 2; Figures 1A,D**). The CD4 T cells procured from healthy controls were negative for HIV DNA (**Figure 1G**). The conjugation results for acute and chronic untreated HIV-infected patients as observed by *in situ* PCR were similar to those observed previously by directly interacting CD8 T cells with calcein-labeled CD4 T cells (5). Calcein-labeled CD4 T cells and autologous CD8 T cells procured from the PBMC of AIDS patients were co-incubated and observed directly by fluorescent microscopy: similar to the *in-situ* PCR results (**Table 2**), 7.0 ± 0.65 % of the CD4 T cells were conjugated by CD8 T cells compared to 0.9 ± 0.07% of the cells of the matched healthy controls.

CD4 T cells and autologous CD8 T cells procured from AIDS patients and co-incubated revealed robust apoptotic morphology of the HIV-infected CD4 T cells with numerous apoptotic bodies (**Figures 1D,E**). In contrast, the CD4 T cells that were incubated without the autologous CD8 T cells demonstrated no apoptotic morphology (**Figure 1F**). Very rare apoptotic events were observed in HIV-infected CD4 T cells incubated with autologous CD8 T cells of chronic untreated HIV-infected patients and patients on ART. It is worth noting that in an earlier study (5) with 11 chronic untreated HIV patients the conjugation and apoptosis rates were observed with wide range of viral loads (189-96,389 copies/ml). Hence the copy by itself had no influence on the outcome of conjugation and lysis.

Interaction of CD8 and Autologous CD4 T Cells in HIV-Infected Patients on ART

CD4 T cells procured from seven HIV-infected patients on ART with undetectable viral load were labeled with calcein, incubated with an equal number of autologous CD8 T cells, and screened by fluorescence microscopy: 2.3 ± 0.3% of the CD4 T cells were conjugated by autologous CD8 T cells compared to 0.8 ± 0.1% in the healthy controls. The four-fold increase of the CD8 T cells interacting with the CD4 T cells resulted in an increase of the conjugation: 5.7 ± 1.3% compared to 1.2 ± 0.3% in the healthy controls (**Table 3; Figure 2A**). The CD4-CD8 T cells interaction was further quantified after labeling the CD8 T cells with anti-CD8 antibody (APC labeled), and the results showed that 3% of the CD4 T cells were conjugated by the CD8 T cells (**Figure 2B**). Calcein-labeled CD4 T cells interacting with non-autologous CD8 T cells procured from patients on ART resulted in only 1 ± 0.2 % conjugation, similar to the healthy controls.

Multi-spectral imaging flow cytometer (ImagStream, Amnis) was used to study the conjunction of CD8 T cells with autologous CD4 T cells procured from an additional five patients on ART and compared to matched healthy controls. The ImageStream combines flow cytometry with single-cell microscopy for the

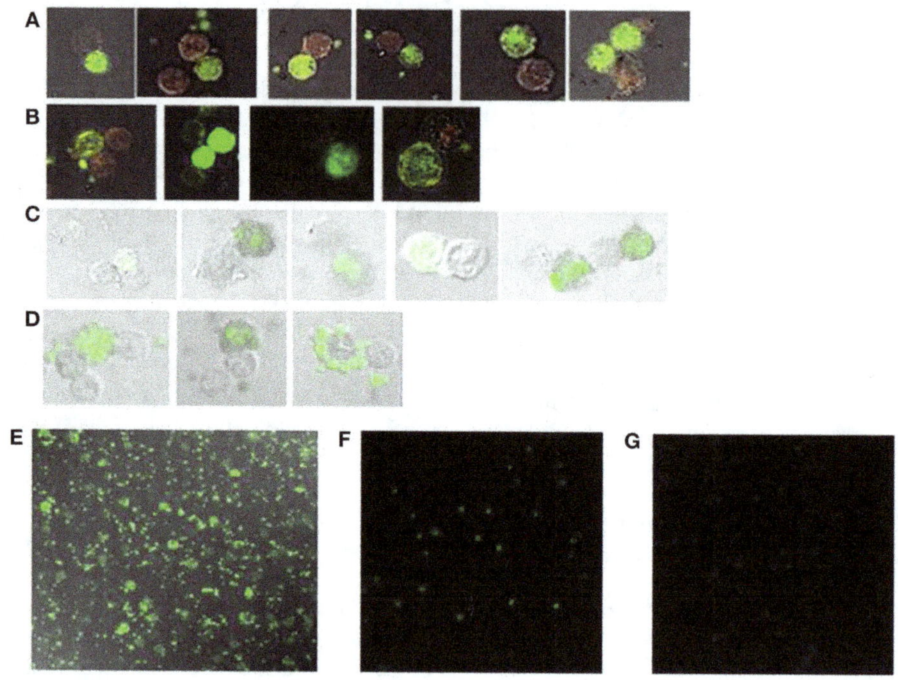

FIGURE 1 | HIV DNA observed in CD4 T cells interacting with autologous CD8 T cells throughout the course of HIV infection. Following incubation of CD4 T cells with autologous CD8 T cells *in situ* PCR of HIV LTR DNA was performed, followed by hybridization with a 56nt long FITC-labeled DNA probe (green). Anti-perforin antibody labeled by Alexa Fluor 647 (red) was used for immunohistochemistry **(A, B)**. The slides were then observed by confocal microscopy (x63). CD4 T cells were conjugated by autologous CD8 T cells, as observed in: **(A)** acute HIV infection, **(B)** chronic HIV infection, **(C)** a chronic HIV-infected patient on ART, **(D,E)** an AIDS patient, **(F)** CD4 T cells from an AIDS patient incubated without CD8 T cells, **(G)** a healthy control.

TABLE 3 | Conjugation of CD8 T cells with autologous CD4 T cells procured from chronic HIV-infected patients on ART.

Method	CD4:CD8 T cell ratio	Sample type	Number	%Conjugation
Calcein-labeled CD4 T cells interacting with CD8 T cells	1:01	Patients on ART	7	2.3 ± 0.3
		Controls	7	0.8 ± 0.1
	1:04	Patients on ART	3	5.7 ± 1.3
		Controls	3	1.2 ± 0.3
CD4/CD8 T cells observed by ImageStream	1:01	Patients on ART	5	2.5 ± 0.5
		Controls	5	0.9 ± 0.2
	1:04	Patients on ART	2	4.8 ± 0.4
		Controls	2	1.4 ± 0.3

analysis and quantification of fluorescent signals for thousands of cells per sample. Following conjugation, the cells were fixed by 4% PFA and labeled with anti-CD4 antibody (PE/Cy7-labeled), anti-CD8 antibody (PerCP/Cy5.5 labeled) and DAPI. A total of 50,000 cells from each sample were analyzed. The gating strategy to identify and quantify the conjugates is based on the aspect ratio plotted against the area and it was confirmed by directly observing the selected cell populations. Each selected conjugate was observed and photographed by the ImageStream (**Figure 2C**). By the ImageStream analysis 2.5 ± 0.5% of the CD4 T cells procured from patients on ART were conjugated with autologous CD8 T cells compared to 0.9 ± 0.2% in the healthy controls. Four-fold increases of the CD8 T cells interacting with CD4 T cells resulted in an increase in the conjugation of the CD4 T cells to 4.8 ± 0.4% compared to 1.4 ± 0.3% in the healthy controls (**Table 3**).

The CD4-CD8 T cell conjugates from patients on ART were studied to identify known specific immunological synapse proteins (30). After the conjugation of CD4 T cells with autologous CD8 T cells, the cells were fixed (4% PFA), permeabilized and labeled with anti-CD8, anti γ-tubulin, and anti-perforin antibodies (**Figure 2D**). Additionally, the synapse was studied by anti-CD4, anti-CD8, and anti-LCK antibodies (**Figure 2E**). Both γ-tubulin and perforin localized in the

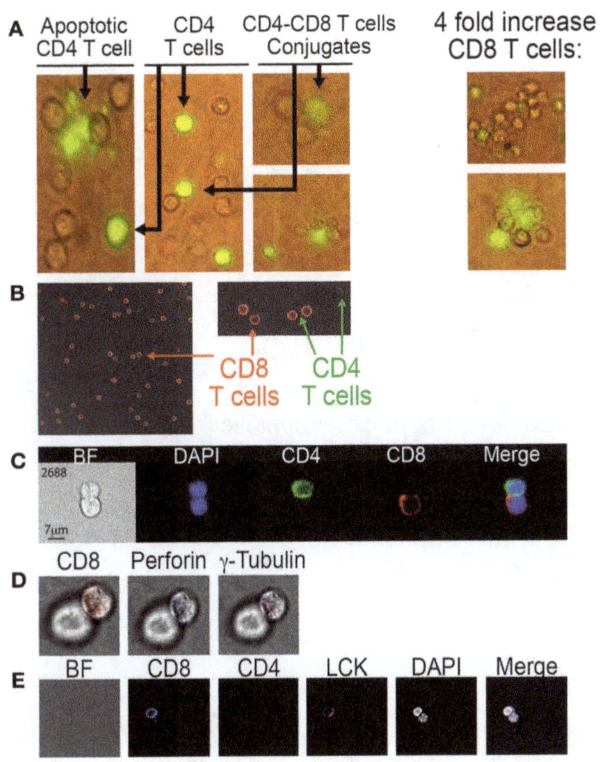

FIGURE 2 | Conjugation and immunological synapse formation between CD8 T cells and autologous CD4 T cells procured from patients on ART. **(A)** Calcein-labeled CD4 T cells co-incubated with autologous CD8 T cells as observed by fluorescent microscopy (x40). **(B)** CD8-CD4 T cell conjugates labeled with anti-CD8 antibody (APC, red) and observed by confocal microscopy (x63). **(C)** CD8-CD4 T cell conjugates labeled with anti-CD8 antibody (APC, red) and anti-CD4 antibody (PE-Cy7, green) and observed by the ImageStream. **(D)** Immunological synapse formation between CD8 and CD4 T cells. The conjugates were labeled with: anti-CD8 antibody,anti-perforin antibody and anti-γ tubulin antibody. **(E)** anti-CD8 antibody, anti-CD4 antibody and anti-LCK antibody.

interface between the CD8 T cell and the conjugated CD4 T cell. It has been reported that γ-tubulin, the centrosome, polarizes toward the synapse and docks at the plasma membrane once the TCR is engaged (30). Perforin expression indicates activation and killing capacity of CD8 T cells, and perforin co-localizes with granzyme B in cytotoxic granules that are polarizing to the immunological synapse (3, 31). LCK, which is a key protein tryosine kinase that initiates intracellular signaling by the TCR (32), was also observed at the synapse between CD8 and CD4 T cells procured from HIV-infected patients on ART (**Figure 2E**).

Apoptosis of CD4 T Cells Caused by Autologous CD8 T Cells Procured From HIV-Infected Patients on ART

CD4 T cells procured from HIV-infected patients on ART or healthy controls were mixed with equal number of autologous CD8 T cells and incubated at 37°C for 120 min (5). The cells were then fixed with 4% PFA, permeablized, and labeled with anti-CD8 antibody (APC-labeled) and the apoptotic markers: anti-active caspase-3 antibody (AF568-labeled) and terminal deoxynucleotidyl transferase dUTP nick end labeling (TUNEL) assay (Ex/Em = 488/576). Apoptosis was defined as being positive by the gating of one or both of the apoptotic markers. Conjugation was quantified in the ImageStream by gating the aspect ratio vs. area of the bright field image and identifying both CD4 and CD8 signals in the conjugates. A total of 50,000 cells from each sample were analyzed both by FACS and by single-cell microscopy. **Figure 3A** demonstrates an apoptotic assay of autologous CD8 and CD4 T cells procured from a 43-year-old female patient who had been on ART for over 10 years and who had an undetectable viral load and CD4 T cells of 507 cells/mm^3 (39%). Both apoptotic markers, caspase-3 activation (orange) and DNA fragmentation by TUNEL assay yellow), can be seen in the CD4 T cells conjugated with autologous CD8 T cells.

Quantitative analysis by the ImageStream of conjugation and apoptosis of CD4 T cells in five patients on ART was performed and compared to matched healthy controls. Apoptotic CD4 T cells comprised 2.1 ± 0.4% of the CD4 T cells, compared to 0.6 ± 0.3% of the cells in the healthy controls. Additionally, 2.5 ± 0.4% of the CD4 T cells were conjugated by the CD8 T cells. Only 6.6% of the conjugated CD4 T cells were positive for the apoptotic markers compared to 2.5 ± 0.6% of the conjugated cells in the healthy controls (**Figure 3B**), suggesting a possible inhibition of apoptosis in the HIV-infected CD4 T cells.

Latent Reservoir CD4 T Cells Can Be Conjugated By Autologous CD8 T Cells Which May Lead to Their Apoptosis

HIV persists in both treated and untreated infected patients in a stable pool of resting CD4 T cells as a latent but replication competent provirus (2). These proviruses can express some but not all gene products in the absence of virion production (33–35). To study the resting memory CD4 T cells population, we separated resting from activated CD4 T cells procured from HIV-infected patients both untreated and treated by ART by a published two-step bead depletion procedure (22, 24). After separating the CD8 T cells using magnetic beads, the CD4 T cells were negatively selected using magnetic beads coated with a cocktail of monoclonal antibodies (Miltenyi CD4 T cell isolation kit). The purified CD4 T cells were further separated into resting and activated cells by beads coated with CD69, CD25, and HLA-DR antibodies as the activated CD4 T cell population. The CD69, CD25, and HLA-DR negative cells are the resting memory cells. The purity of the resting memory CD4 T cells was routinely assessed by staining them with antibodies against CD69, CD25, and HLA-DR and analyzing 50,000 cells using the ImageStream. Typical purities of resting CD4 T cells were 95–98.5% with <1.5% contamination by activated CD4 T cells (**Figure 4A**). The fraction of resting and activated CD4 T cells before cell separation was evaluated by staining CD4 T cell samples with APC-labeled antibodies against CD69, CD25, and HLA-DR followed by ImageStream analysis of 50,000 cells. Activated cells (CD25, CD69, and HLA-DR positive) were 51% of the CD4 T cells and

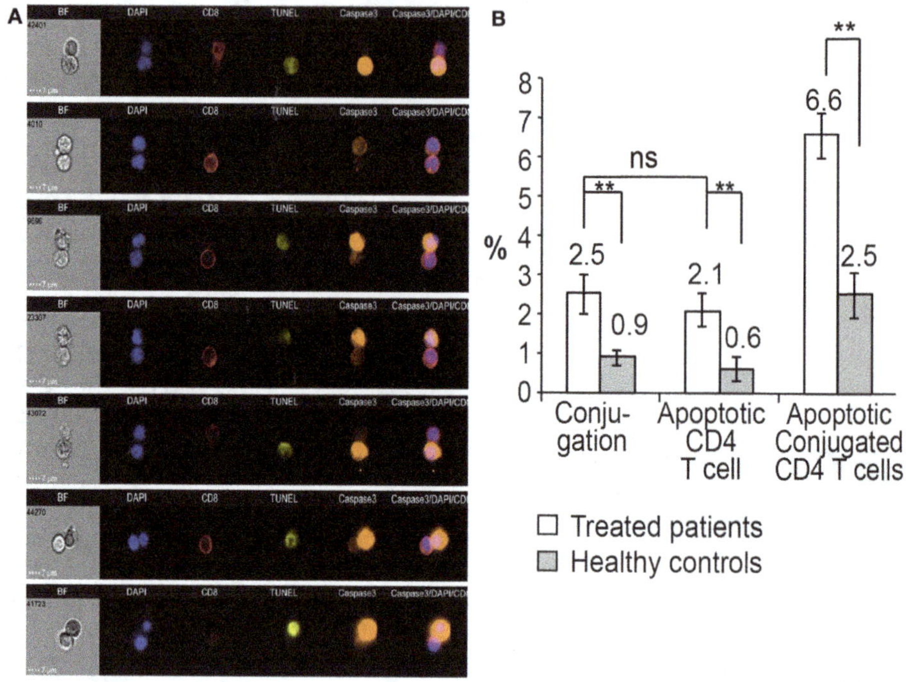

FIGURE 3 | Conjugation and apoptosis of CD4 T cells by autologous CD8 T cells procured from patients on ART and analyzed by the ImageStream. **(A)** Apoptosis assay of CD4 T cells with CD8 T cells procured from a 43-year-old female patient on ART with undetectable viral load and a CD4 T cell count of 507 cells/mm^3 (39%). The CD4 T cells in apoptosis are positive for activated caspase 3 (orange) and DNA fragmentation, TUNEL assay (yellow), CD8 T cells (red), DAPI (purple). **(B)** Quantitative analysis of conjugation and apoptosis of CD4 and CD8 T cells in five patients on ART compared to five healthy controls. ** indicate *P*-values < 0.01, two-tailed paired *t*-test.

49% were resting cells (CD25, CD69, and HLA-DR negative; **Figure 4B**).

In-situ PCR of HIV DNA was performed on resting and activated CD4 T cells procured from a 52-year-old male patient on ART and a 55-year-old male untreated patient. A total of 1000 cells were screened in the *in situ* PCR slides by confocal microscopy. Four percent of the activated CD4 T cells of the patient on ART contained HIV DNA and 5% of the activated CD4 T cells in the untreated patient contained HIV DNA. In contrast, most of the HIV DNA was found in the resting memory CD4 T cells: 30% in the patient on ART and 22% in the untreated patient. Our results indicate that 88 and 81% of the CD4 T cells containing HIV DNA are resting memory cells as opposed to 12 and 19% of the activated CD4 T cells in the patient on ART and in the untreated patient, respectively (**Figure 5A**). In those patients, the ImageStream analysis revealed that about 50% of the CD4 T cells were activated and that 50% of them were resting, findings that are comparable to published data in their age group (36).

Conjugation and apoptosis of resting and activated CD4 T cells by autologous CD8 T cells procured from three patients treated by ART and three healthy controls were analyzed by the ImagStream (**Figures 5B–D**). Following the separation of the activated and resting CD4T cells, they were incubated with autologous CD8 T cells for 2 h (5) and then fixed by 4% PFA and stained with anti-CD4 antibody, anti-CD8 antibody, anti-active caspase-3 antibody, and DNA fragmentation assay (TUNEL assay). ImageStream analysis was performed on 50,000 cells from each sample. Conjugation of resting CD4 T cells with autologous CD8 T cells was comparable to un-separated CD4 T cells (1.9 ± 0.3 and 2.3 ± 0.3%, respectively). The conjugation of the activated CD4 T cells was not significantly different from that of the control (1.2 ± 0.2 and 0.9 ± 0.2%, respectively), probably due to the very low content of HIV DNA in the activated CD4 T cells as demonstrated by *in situ* PCR (**Figure 5A**).

The apoptosis of the total CD4 T cells was comparable with that of the resting CD4 T cells after incubation with autologous CD8 T cells (2.2 ± 0.4 and 2.1 ± 0.5%, respectively), at levels significantly higher than those in healthy controls (0.6 ± 0.2 and 0.8 ± 0.3%, respectively). The activated CD4 T cells after incubation with autologous CD8 T cells demonstrated significantly higher apoptosis (4.3% ± 0.3) than that of the resting cells, indicating that activated CD4 T cells are more susceptible to CD8 T cell-induced apoptosis. The ImageStream clearly demonstrated that the resting memory cells can be conjugated by autologous CD8 T cells and undergo apoptosis (**Figures 5D,E**).

Inhibition of HIV Nef Interaction With ASK1 in the CD4 T Cells Procured From Patients on Art Results in Increased Susceptibility to Killing by Autologous CD8 T Cells

HIV Nef protein interacts with ASK 1 and inhibits its pro-apoptotic death signaling by Fas/FasL and TNFα, thus protecting

A

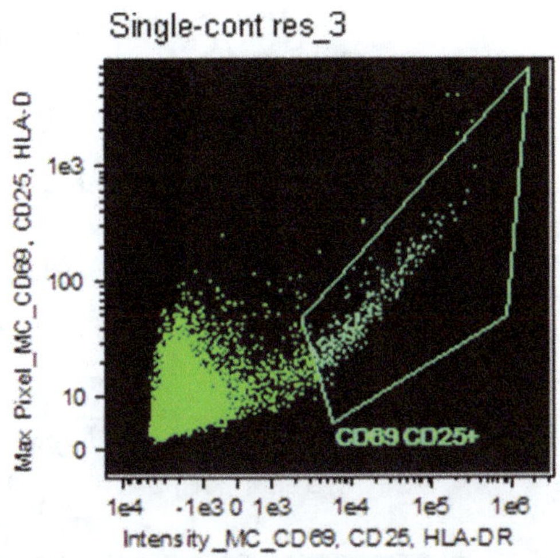

Intensity_MC_CD69, CD25, HLA-DR, Max Pixel_MC_CD69, CD25, HLA-D

Population	Count	%Gated
Single	39327	100
CD69 CD25+ & Single	590	1.5

B

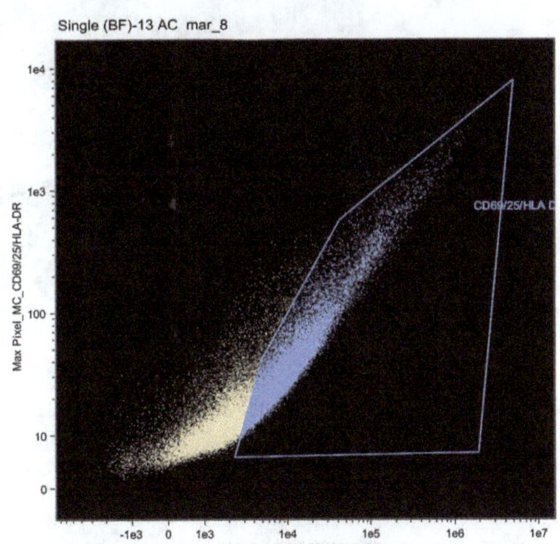

Intensity_MC_CD69/25/HLA-DR, Max Pixel_MC_CD69/25/HLA-DR

Population	Count	%Gated	Mean	Median	Std. Dev.	Geo. Mean
Single (BF)	43304	100	11005.31, 42.57	3578.99, 17.76	41697.19, 124.96	4026.46, 21.66
CD69/25/HLA DR+ & Single (BF)	22066	51	19538.83, 66.05	8186.56, 28.95	54977.31, 152.3	9876.29, 36.19

FIGURE 4 | Resting CD4 T cells procured from HIV infected patients on ART. **(A)** Representative analysis indicating the purity of resting CD4 T cells. Resting CD4 T cells procured from the PBMC of HIV infected patients on ART were purified using a two-step negative selection, stained with anti-human CD25, anti-human CD69 and anti-human HLA-DR antibodies and analyzed by the ImageStream. **(B)** The fraction of resting and activated CD4 T cells. CD4 T cells procured from the PBMC of HIV infected patients on ART were labeled with antibodies against CD25, CD69 and HLA-DR followed by ImageStream analysis. 51% of the CD4 T cells were CD25, CD69, and HLA-DR positive (activated cells) and 49% were CD25, CD69, and HLA-DR negative (resting cells).

HIV-infected cells from being killed by CD8 T cells (19). A peptide derived from ASK1 protein sequence, amino acids 152 to 159 (DEVGEANN) inhibited the interaction between Nef and ASK1 and circumvented the anti-apoptotic effect of Nef, restoring ASK1 pro-apoptotic function induced by TNFα (21). The possible role of HIV Nef protein in protecting the latent reservoir cells from being killed by CD8 T cells was investigated by using the peptide (DEVGEANN). CD4 T cells and autologous CD8 T cells were procured from the PBMC of four HIV-infected patients on ART and matched healthy controls. The CD4 T cells were incubated with 10 μM peptide (DEVGEANN) for 16 h at 37°C in 5% CO2 (20). CD4 T cells procured from the same patients on ART and healthy controls were incubated without the peptide as a control. Following the incubation, the CD4 T

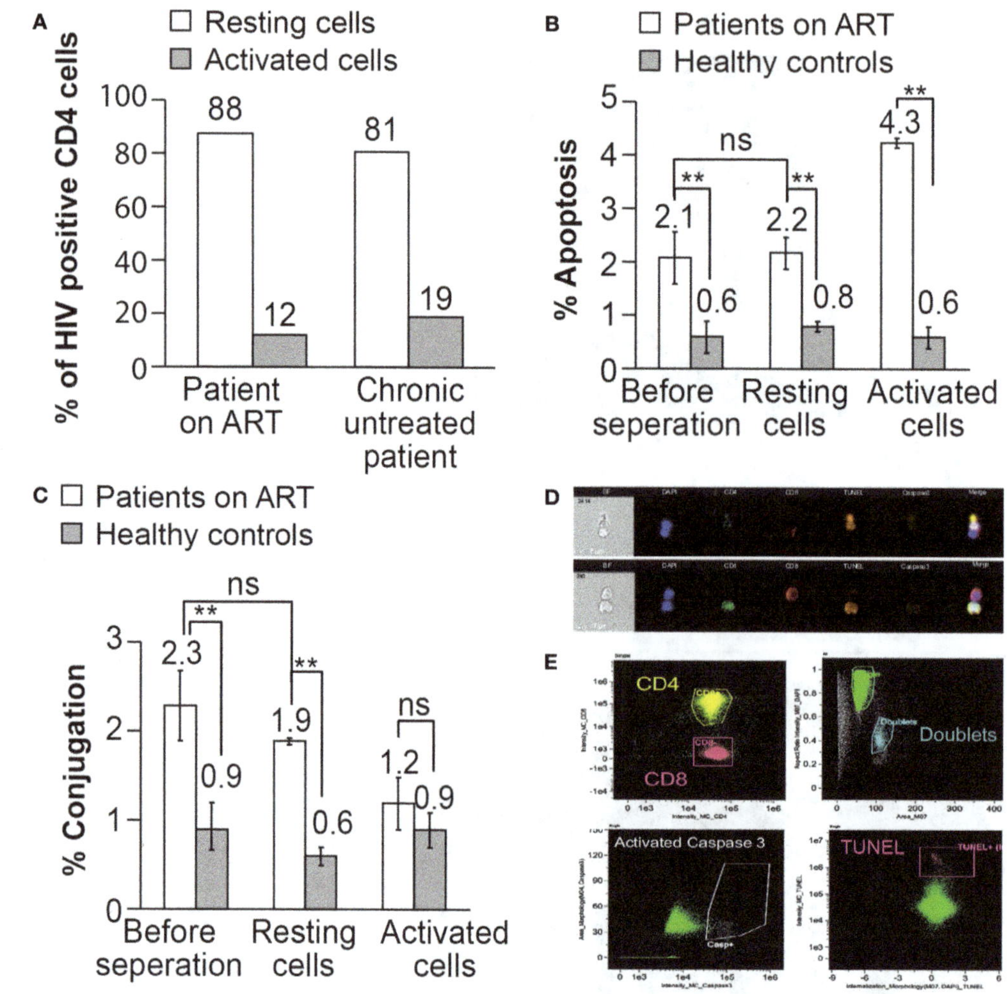

FIGURE 5 | The resting memory CD4 T cells can be recognized and undergo apoptosis by autologous CD8 T cells in patients on ART. **(A)** *In situ* PCR was performed on resting and activated CD4 T cells procured from an untreated HIV-infected patient and from a patient on ART. The percent of HIV-infected CD4 T cells was calculated out of 1000 resting or activated CD4 T cells. **(B)** The apoptosis of un-separated, resting, and activated CD4 T cells by autologous CD8 T cells was analyzed in 3 patients on ART by ImageStream analysis. The apoptotic cells were gated and observed by anti-activated caspase 3 antibody and TUNEL assay. **(C)** The conjugation of CD8 T cells with autologous CD4 T cells before or after separation to resting or activated cells was analyzed in 3 patients on ART by ImageStream analysis. The conjugates were gated by plotting the aspect ratio against the area and the results were confirmed by directly observing the selected cell populations. **(D)** Representative images obtained by the ImagStream analysis of resting memory CD4 T cells conjugated by autologous CD8 T cells undergoing apoptosis. CD4 in green, CD8 in red, TUNEL in orange, and activated caspase 3 in yellow. **(E)** Representative imaging flow cytometry plots of resting memory CD4 T cells conjugated by autologous CD8 T cells undergoing apoptosis. $^{**}P < 0.01$, as obtained in two-tailed paired t-test.

cells were mixed with autologous CD8 T cells and incubated for 120 min at 37°C for the cytotoxic assay. The cells were then fixed by 4% PFA and labeled with anti-CD4 antibody, anti-CD8 antibody, anti-active caspase-3 antibody, and DNA fragmentation assay (TUNEL assay). Between 10,000 and 50,000 cells from each sample were analyzed by the ImageStream.

The incubation with the peptide did not affect the conjugation between the CD4 and CD8 T cells both in HIV-infected patients on ART (2.6 ± 0.3 % without the peptide and 3.2 ± 0.8% with the peptide) and healthy controls (0.7 ± 0.1 without the peptide and 0.6 ± 0.3 with the peptide; **Figure 6A**). The apoptosis of the CD4 T cells incubated with the peptide was significantly higher than the apoptosis of CD4 T cells without the peptide (4.0 ± 0.4 and 2.1 ± 0.5%, respectively). The peptide did not have any effect on the apoptosis of CD4 T cells procured from healthy controls 0.9 ± 0.2% without the peptide and 1.2 ± 0.3% with the peptide.

DISCUSSION

HIV infection is currently treatable but not curable because anti-retroviral therapy (ART) suppresses HIV viral load without affecting the viral "latent reservoir." The role of CTL in the course of HIV infection and the way they affect the virus that resides in the latent reservoir is unknown. There are ~10% of HIV-specific CD8 T cells in the peripheral blood mononuclear cells (PBMC) of HIV-infected patients (12) and their potential

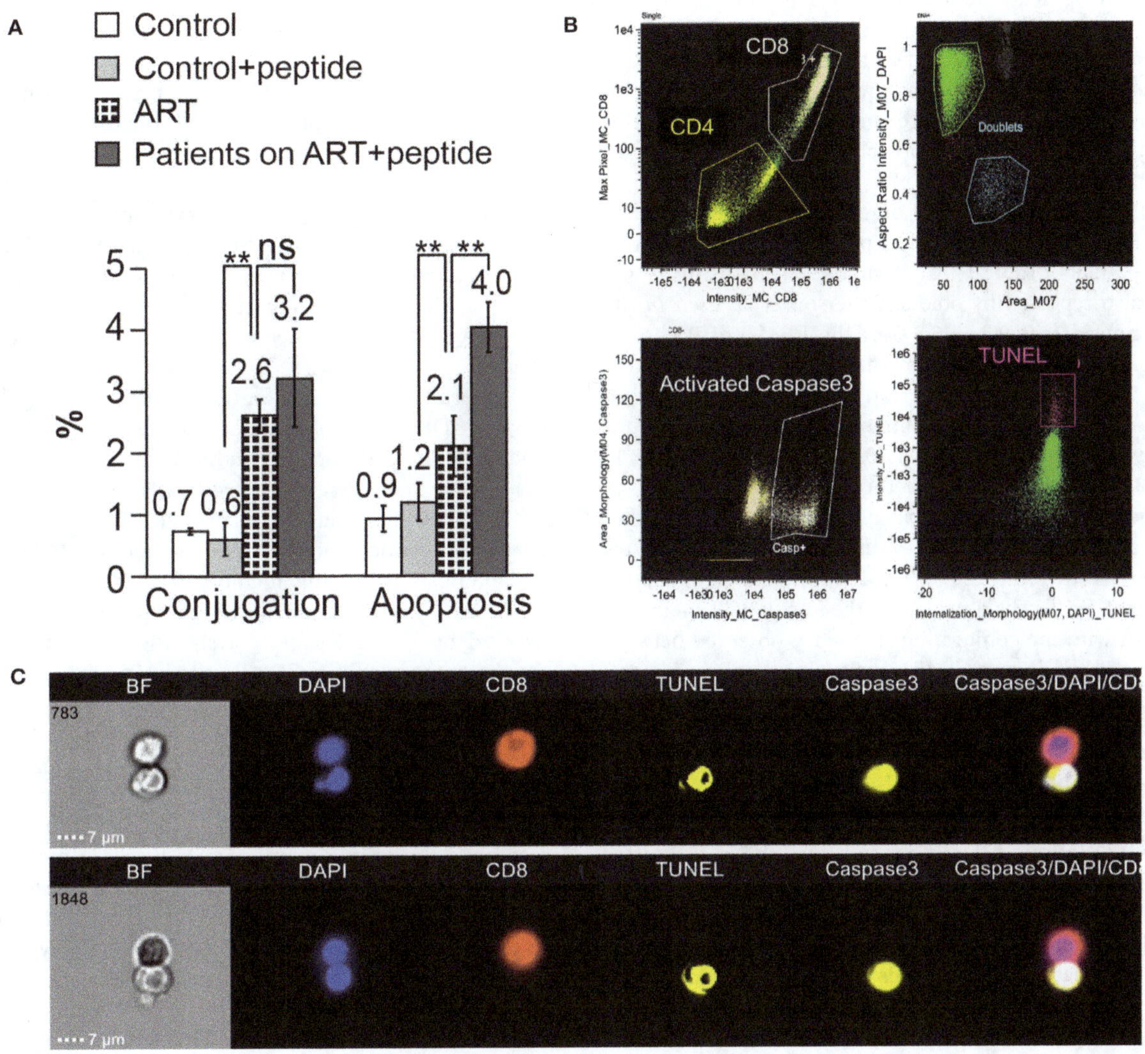

FIGURE 6 | Inhibition of HIV Nef interaction with ASK1 in the CD4 T cells procured from patients on ART results in increased susceptibility to killing by autologous CD8 T cells. CD4 T cells and autologous CD8 T cells were procured from the PBMC of four HIV-infected patients on ART and matched healthy controls. The CD4 T cells were incubated with ASK1 peptide that interferes with Nef-ASK1 interaction. Following the incubation with or without the peptide, the CD4 T cells were mixed with autologous CD8 T cells for the cytotoxic assay. The cells were then fixed and labeled with anti-CD4 antibody, anti-CD8 antibody, anti-active caspase-3 antibody and DNA fragmentation assay (TUNEL assay) and analyzed by the ImageStream. **(A)** Four independent conjugation and apoptosis assays are presented. ** indicate *P*-values < 0.01, as obtained by two-tailed paired *t*-test. **(B)** Representative imaging flow cytometry plots of CD4 T cells incubated with the peptide and interacted with CD8 T cells. **(C)** ImageStream images of TUNEL and activated caspase-3 positive CD4 T cells treated with ASK1 peptide conjugated with autologous CD8 T cells.

targets HIV-infected CD4 T cells (17, 25, 37). We investigated the interaction between CD8 T cells and autologous CD4 T cells procured from the blood of HIV-infected patients. The cells were neither manipulated nor stimulated *in vitro*. We had previously shown that PBMC of acute and chronic HIV-infected patients who were not treated by ART contain HIV-specific CD8 T cells that conjugate with and kill HIV-infected autologous CD4 T cells (5). The results of the present study demonstrate that CD8 T cells conjugate with and kill autologous HIV-infected CD4 T cells throughout the course of HIV infection, including those of patients on ART. The conjugation activity and apoptosis during acute HIV infection and AIDS were much higher compared to chronic HIV-infected patients untreated or treated by ART. We demonstrated that the latent reservoir cells can also be targeted by autologous CD8 T cells. This interaction is of low magnitude and considered as being "controlled" during the chronic stage of HIV infection in patients who are untreated or treated by ART. Our results suggest that the HIV Nef protein plays a role in protecting the latent reservoir cells from the killing of CD8 T cells.

CD8 T cells interacting with autologous CD4 T cells were fixed on slides and studied by *in situ* PCR of HIV DNA. The *in situ* PCR primers (NEC152 and NEC131) are conserved in the HIV LTR sequence and were described before (27, 28, 38). The primers are currently in use by the central virology laboratory of the

Israeli Ministry of Health to identify HIV DNA in lymphocytes of newborns from HIV-infected mothers. We used a 56nt probe, which was conserved in the amplified DNA. The LTR is expected to be present in most of the integrated viral DNA, and the method that we used to recognize it should not be affected by the abundance of internal deletions and hypermutations of the described integrated virus (39). HIV DNA was demonstrated in about 10% of the CD4 T cells obtained from acute infected patients, chronic untreated infected patients, patients on ART, and AIDS patients (**Table 1**). Comparable results using *in situ* PCR were also reported by others: Patterson et al. used *in situ* PCR and showed that 9.3 ± 3.3% of the PBMC of 9 chronic untreated HIV infected patients have amplified HIV DNA within them (37). Bagasra et al. reported on HIV DNA in the PBMC procured from chronic infected patients and AIDS patients: the HIV-positive cells ranged between 0.1 and 13.5% of all cells (average 4.3 ± 3.0%) (25, 40). A method that quantify the *in-situ* PCR product by flow cytometry was developed by Re et al. They reported that the frequency of HIV infected CD4 T cells in the PBMC range from 0.6 to 20% (29, 41, 42). The frequency of HIV-infected CD4 T cells obtained by the *in situ* PCR method is in agreement with the conjugation frequency observed between CD8 T cells and autologous CD4 T cells during the various stages of HIV infection reported here and by Chorin et al. (5).

We separated active CD4 T cells (CD69-, CD25-, and HLA-DR-positive) from resting memory CD4 T cells (CD69-, CD25-, and HLA-DR-negative) procured from chronic untreated and treated HIV-infected patients and assayed them by *in situ* PCR of HIV DNA. We found that the majority of the HIV-infected CD4 T cells in those patients reside in the resting memory (latent reservoir) cell compartment. There was no decline of HIV-infected CD4 T cells in patients on ART, indicating a high level of stability of the latent reservoir cells even in the absence of viral replication (1).

Formation of CD8-CD4 T-cell conjugates and apoptosis of the CD4 T cells were observed by fluorescence microscopy, imaging flow cytometry (ImageStream) and *in situ* PCR of HIV DNA of the conjugated CD4 T cells (**Tables 2, 3; Figure 2**). In addition to a high conjugation rate, there was robust apoptosis of the HIV-positive CD4 T cells after incubation with autologous CD8 T cells in AIDS patients (**Figure 1**). In contrast, the conjugation and apoptosis rates were much lower in the chronic untreated and ART-treated HIV-infected patients. Similar results were observed in studies of acute compared to chronic untreated HIV infection where conjugation and apoptosis were significantly higher in acute HIV-infected patients (5). These results suggest a possible inhibition of conjugation and apoptosis of the CD4 T cells interacting with autologous CD8 T cells in chronic HIV-infected patients and patients on ART. The apoptotic activity is apparently unleashed in AIDS as well as in acute HIV infection.

At present, all the patients infected by HIV are treated by ART, and most of them have an undetectable viral load. Markers of inflammation have been documented in those patients, suggesting continuous response of the immune system against the latent reservoir cells (43). The latent reservoir cells are not affected by treatment with ART, and the virus rebounds rapidly once treatment is stopped. We found continuous interaction of CD8 T cells with autologous CD4 T cells in patients on ART. Conjugation of CD8 with CD4 T cells was measured and found to be similar by three different assays: *in situ* PCR of HIV DNA in the CD4 T cells (**Table 1; Figure 1**), calcein-labeled CD4 T cells conjugation assay and ImageStream analysis of conjugated cells marked by antibodies (**Table 2; Figure 2**). The presence of an active immunological synapse between the CD8 and the autologous CD4 T cells was confirmed using specific markers of an immunological synapse that were observed with confocal microscopy (**Figure 2**). A significant level of apoptosis of the CD4 T cells following incubation with autologous CD8 T cells procured from patients on ART was observed by the ImageStream (**Figure 3**).

Our results demonstrate for the first-time ongoing interaction between CD8 and autologous CD4 T cells even in HIV-infected patients on ART. Assuming that the interaction is between CD8 T cells and the latent reservoir CD4 T cells, highly purified resting CD4 T cells were isolated from the PBMC of patients on ART using a negative depletion isolation method (22, 24). Conjugation and apoptosis of resting memory CD4 T cells by autologous CD8 T cells were comparable to unseparated CD4 T cells, as observed by ImageStream analysis (**Figures 5B,C**), suggesting that the activity of the CD8 T cells is against latent reservoir CD4 T cells.

The biology of latent reservoir CD4 T cells is still a mystery. We observed interactions between CD8 T cells and autologous CD4 T cells that contain HIV DNA within them. We assume that CD8 T cells recognize HIV epitopes presented by the HLA receptor of the resting memory CD4 T cells. Ho et al. analyzed the structure of integrated HIV DNA in latent reservoir cells and found that 11.7% of them consist of the whole viral genome, with the majority consisting of large deletions and hypermutations (39). Fromentin et al. reported expression of unspliced HIV RNA in CD4 T cells in patients on ART (44). Imamichi et al. found defective HIV proviruses that produce novel coding RNA species involving elements of gag, pol, env, rev, and nef maintaining translationally competent open reading frames in HIV-infected patients on ART (45). Pace et al. documented that resting cells that had been spinoculated by w/ NL4-3 *in vitro* were capable of producing HIV Gag protein without supporting productive infection (35). Using a primary cell model of latency Thomas et al. found that a Nef-specific CD8 T-cell clone exhibited low-level recognition of this latently HIV infected cells prior to their reactivation. Moreover, they observed Nef specific CD8 T cell response in the PBMC of ART treated patients, which indicate an ongoing expression of Nef during prolong ART treatment (15). This data can suggest that low-grade viral proteins are expressed and presented by resting memory CD4 T cells that are recognized by CD8 T cells.

We found significant apoptosis in acute HIV infection and AIDS, while patients in chronic stages of HIV infection and patients on ART had low-grade apoptotic activity of the CD4 T cells, including resting memory cells. Such low-grade apoptotic activity was observed even in the conjugated CD4 T cells (**Figure 3B**). The HIV Nef protein interferes with CTL activity by down-regulating HLA expression, expressing FasL molecules on the surface of the HIV-infected CD4 T cells and protecting the HIV-infected CD4 T cells from the killing of CTL by the interaction of Nef with ASK1 protein (19, 20). Infection of rhesus macaques with Nef-defective SIV resulted in low viral load and caused a substantial delay in the onset of disease (46). Rare individuals infected by HIV containing Nef deletion are observed to have low viral loads and stable CD4 T cell counts for many years even in the absence of treatment by ART (47). Inhibition of Nef interaction with ASK1 was designed to study the possibility that HIV Nef protein is involved in the inhibition of apoptosis in the CD4 T cells. Kumar et al. identified the domain in the ASK1 that interacts with HIV Nef protein. This 8-amino acid peptide inhibited ASK1-Nef interaction and abolished the Nef protection of cells from apoptosis induced by tumor necrosis factor α (TNFα) (21). We found that the delivery of the peptide to the CD4 T cells before the interaction with autologous CD8 T cells resulted in a 2-fold increase of the apoptosis of the CD4 T cells in the apoptotic assay (**Figure 6**). These data suggest that the virus keeps the latent reservoir CD4 T cells protected from the immune system by expressing HIV Nef protein. Viral proteins that interfere with CTL activity resulting in the maintenance of latency were described in herpes viruses, adenoviruses, cowpox virus, vaccinia virus, and HTLV-1. Similar to Nef activity, these proteins act by down-regulating HLA expression, interfering with the virally infected cellular apoptotic machinery and manipulating Fas/FasL interaction (18, 48). Immune checkpoint molecules, PD-1, TIGIT and LAG-3, are positively associated with the frequency of CD4 T cells harboring integrated HIV DNA in patients on ART. This serves as evidence for continuous interaction with and evasion from the CTL in patients on ART (43, 48). Further studies are needed to understand the viral and cellular mechanisms that up-regulate those immune checkpoints in latently infected HIV CD4 T cells.

Mathematical modeling of CTL activity during HIV infection is consistent with lytic control by CTL, and predicts that most productively infected cells are killed by CTL (10, 49). Apart from their positive effects of controlling viral spread, CTL have been shown to cause tissue damage in viral infections, such as in viral myocarditis (50) and viral hepatitis. We propose that CD4 T cell annihilation in HIV-infected patients results from the ongoing interaction of CD8 T cells with HIV-infected CD4 T cells. We assume that a dynamic balance is established between HIV-infected CD4 T cells and HIV-specific CD8 T cells during the chronic stage of HIV infection, resulting in restrained apoptosis of the CD4 T cells and leading to their gradual decline. The virus manipulates the immune system to maintain a low-grade infection, thus achieving prolonged survival combined with efficient viral spread. We suggest that Nef have a role in maintaining this balance based on our findings that inhibition of Nef resulted in significant increase in the killing of CD4 T cells by autologous CD8 T cells. We propose that CTL activity following Nef inhibition may help eliminate the latently HIV- infected CD4 T cells reservoir. An additional definitive study that includes a larger population of HIV infected patients should be done. In addition, the study of the role of Nef in HIV infected patients could be expended to elucidate the molecular effect of Nef in response to CD8 T cells conjugation.

ETHICS STATEMENT

This study was carried out in accordance with the recommendations of the institutional Tel-Aviv Medical center ethics committee in accordance with the ethical standards laid down in the 1964 Declaration of Helsinki and its later amendments. The protocol was approved by the Tel-Aviv Medical center ethics committee. All subjects gave written informed consent in accordance with the Declaration of Helsinki.

AUTHOR CONTRIBUTIONS

ZS design the research, acquired the data performed the experiments, analyzed the data, performed the statistical analysis and drafted the manuscript. EC design the research, contributed to the interpretation of the results and edited the manuscript. OG-G design the research, contributed to the interpretation of the results. EZ contributed to the interpretation of the results. DT and BA provided samples and contributed to the interpretation of the results. GB design the research and contributed to the interpretation of the results. DH design and oversaw the research, analyzed, and interpreted the data, wrote the manuscript and revised the final version of the manuscript.

REFERENCES

Ruelas DS, Greene WC. An integrated overview of HIV-1 latency. *Cell (*2013) 155:519–29. doi: 10.1016/j.cell.2013.09.044

Donahue DA, Wainberg MA. Cellular and molecular mechanisms involved in the establishment of HIV-1 latency. *Retrovirology* (2013) 10:11. doi: 10.1186/1742-4690-10-11

Hassin D, Garber OG, Meiraz A, Schiffenbauer YS, Berke G. Cytotoxic T lymphocyte perforin and Fas ligand working in concert even when Fas ligand lytic action is still not detectable. *Immunology* (2011) 133:190–6. doi: 10.1111/j.1365-2567.2011.03426.x

Berke G and Clark W. Killer lymphocytes. Berlin: Springer (2005).

Chorin E, Garber OG, Yagel Y, Turner D, Avidor B, Berke G, et al. Peripheral blood mononuclear cells of HIV-infected patients contain CD8 T cells that form conjugates with and kill HIV-infected autologous CD4 T cells. *Immunology* (2015) 144:412–21. doi: 10.1111/imm.12385

Hassin D, Fixler R, Bank H, Klein AS, Hasin Y. Cytotoxic T lymphocytes and natural killer cell activity in the course of mengo virus infection of mice. *Immunology* (1985) 56:701–5.

Meiraz A, Garber OG, Harari S, Hassin D, Berke G. Switch from perforin-expressing to perforin-deficient CD8+ T cells accounts for two distinct types of effector cytotoxic T lymphocytes *in vivo*. *Immunology* (2009) 128:69–82. doi: 10.1111/j.1365-2567.2009. 03072.x

Jin X, Baur DE, Tuttleton SE, Lewin S, Gettie A, Blanchard J, et al. Dramatic rise in plasma viremia after CD8+ T cell depletion in simian immunodeficiency virus-infected macaques. *J Exp Med.* (1999). 189:991–8. doi: 10.1084/jem.189.6.991

Borrow P, Lewicki H, Hahn BH, Shaw GM, Oldstone MB. Virus-specific CD8+ cytotoxic T-lymphocyte activity associated with control of viremia in primary human immunodeficiency virus type 1 infection. *J Virol.* (1994) 68: 6103–10.

Gadhamsetty JB, de Boer RJ. What do mathematical models tell us about killing rates during HIV-1 infection? *Immunol Lett.* (2015) 168:1–6. doi: 10.1016/j.imlet.2015.07.009

Schmitz JE, Kuroda MJ, Santra S, Sasseville VG, Simon MA, Lifton MA, et al. Control of viremia in simian immunodeficiency virus infection by CD8+ lymphocytes. *Science* (1999) 283:857–60. doi: 10.1126/science.283. 5403.857

Migueles SA, Laborico AC, Shupert WL, Sabbaghian MS, Rabin R, Hallahan CW, et al. HIV-specific CD8+ T cell proliferation is coupled to perforin expression and is maintained in nonprogressors. *Nat Immunol.* (2002) 3:1061–8. doi: 10.1038/ni845

Migueles SA, Osborne CM, Royce C, Compton AA, Joshi RP, Weeks KA, et al. Lytic granule loading of CD8+ T cells is required for HIV-infected cell elimination associated with immune control. *Immunity* (2008) 29:1009–1. doi: 10.1016/j.immuni.2008.10.010

Oxenius A, Price DA, Dawson SJ, Gunthard HF, Fisher M, Perrin L, et al. Residual HIV-specific CD4 abd CD8 T cell frequencies after prolonged antiretroviral therapy reflect pretreatment plasma virus load. *AIDS* (2002) 16:2317–22. doi: 10.1097/00002030-200211220- 00012

Thomas AS, Jones KL, Gandhi RT, McMahonDK, Cyktor JC, Chan D, et al. T cell responses targeting HIV Nef uniquely correlate with infected cell frequencies after long-term antiretroviral therapy. *PLoSPathog* (2017) 13:e1006629. doi: 10.1371/journal.ppat.1006629

Grützner EM, Hoffmann T, Wolf E, Gersbacher E, Neizert A, Stirner R, et al. Treatment intensification in HIV-infected patients is associated with reduced frequencies of regulatory T cells. *Front Immunol.* (2018) 9:811. doi: 10.3389/fimmu.2018.00811

Chomont N, El-Far M, Ancuta P, Trautmann L, Procopio FA, Yassine-Diab B et al. HIV reservoir size and persistence are driven by T cell survival and homeostatic proliferation. *Nat Med.* (2009) 15:893–900. doi: 10.1038/nm.1972

Xu XN, Screaton GR, McMichael AJ. Virus infection: escape, resistance and counterattack. *Immunity* (2001) 15:867–70. doi: 10.1016/S1074-7613(01)00255-2

Collins KL, Chen BK, Kalams SA, Wallker BD, Baltimore D. HIV-Nef protein protects infected primary cells against killing by cytotoxic T lymphocytes. *Nature* (1998) 391:397–401. doi: 10.1038/34929

Geleziunas R, Xu W, Takeda K, Ichhijo H, Greene WC. HIV-1 Nef inhibits ASK1-dependent death signaling providing a potential mechanism for protecting the infected host cell. *Nature* (2001) 410:242–6. doi: 10.1038/35071111

Kumar B, Tripathi C, Kanchan RK, Tripathi JK, Ghosh JK, Ramachandran R, et al. Dynamics of Physical Interaction between HIV-1 Nef and ASK1: Identifying the Interacting Motif(S). *PLoS ONE* (2013) 8:e67586. doi: 10.1371/journal.pone.0067586

Laird GM, Eisele EE, Rabi SA, Lai J, Chioma S, Blankson JN, et al. Rapid quantification of the latent reservoir for HIV-1 using a viral outgrowth assay. *PLoS Pathog* (2013). 9:e1003398. doi: 10.1371/journal.ppat. 1003398

Fehse B, Frerk O, Goldmann M, Bulduk M, Zander AR. Efficient depletion of alloreactive donor T lymphocytes based on expression of two activation-induced antigens (CD25 and CD69). *Br J Haematol.* (2000) 109:644–51. doi: 10.1046/j.1365-2141.2000.02074.x

Laird G M, Bullen CK, Rosenbloom DIS, Martin AR, Hill AL, Durand CM, et al. *Ex vivo* analysis identifies effective HIV-1 latency–reversing drug combinations. *J Clin Invest.* (2015) 125:1901–12. doi: 10.1172/ JCI80142

Bagasra O, Hauptman SP, Lischner HW, Sachs M, Pomerantz RJ. Detection of human immunodeficiency virus type 1 provirus in mononuclear cells by in situpolymerase chain reaction. *N Engl J Med.* (1992) 326:1385–91. doi: 10.1056/NEJM199205213262103

Bagasra O. Protocols for the *in situ* PCR-amplification and detection of mRNA and DNA sequences. *Nat Protoc.* (2007) 2:2782–95. doi: 10.1038/nprot.2007.395

Legoff J, Bouhlal H, Grésenguet G, Weiss H, Khonde N, Hocini H, et al. Real time PCR quantification of genital shedding of herpes simplex virus (HSV) and humanimmunodeficiency virus (HIV) in women coinfected with HSV and HIV. *J Clin Microbiol.* (2006) 44:423–32. doi: 10.1128/JCM.44.2.423-432.2006

N-Ngo-Giang-Huong N, Khamduang W, Leurent B, Collins I, Nantasen I, Leechanachai P, et al. Early HIV-1 diagnosis using in-house real time PCR amplification on dried blood spots for infants in remote and resource limited settings. *J Acquir Imm Def Syndromes* (2008) 49:465–71. doi: 10.1097/QAI.0b013e31818e2531

Gibellini D, Zauli G, Re MC, Furlini G, La Placa M. Flow cytometry *in situ* polymerase chain reaction as an innovative approach to HIV-1 proviral DNA detection. *Eur J Histochem.* (1998). 42:137–41.

Dustin ML, Long EO. Cytotoxic immunological synapses. *Immunol Rev.* (2010) 235:24–34. doi: 10.1111/j.0105-2896.2010.00904.x

Voskoboinik I, Whisstock JC, Joseph A. Perforin and granzymes: function, dysfunction and human pathology. *Nat Rev Immunol.* (2015) 15:388–400. doi: 10.1038/nri3839

Tsun A, Qureshi I, Stinchcombe JC, Jenkins MR, de la Roche M, Kleczkowska Zamoyska R. et al. Centrosome docking at the immunological synapse is controlled by Lck signaling. *J Cell Biol.* (2011) 192:663–74. doi: 10.1083/jcb.201008140

Lassen KG, Ramyar KX, Bailey JR, Zhou Y, Siliciano RF. Nuclear retention of multiply spliced HIV-1 RNA in resting CD4+ T cells. *PLoS Pathog* (2006) 2:e68. doi: 10.1371/journal.ppat.0020068

Saleh S, Wightman F, Ramanayake S, Alexander M, Kumar N, Khoury G, et al. Expression and reactivation of HIV in a chemokine induced model of HIV latency in primary resting CD4+ T cells. *Retrovirology* (2011) 8:80. doi: 10.1186/1742-4690-8-80

Pace MJ, Graf EH, Agosto LM, Mexas AM, Male F, Brady T, et al. Directly Infected resting CD4+T cells can produce HIV gag without spreading infection in a model of HIV latency. *PLoS Pathog* (2012) 8:e1002818. doi: 10.1371/journal.ppat.1002818

Farber D L, Yudanin NA, Restifo NP. Human memory T cells: generation, compartmentalization and homeostasis. *Nat Rev Immunol.* (2014) 14:24–35. doi: 10.1038/nri3567

Patterson BK, Till M, Otto P, Goolsby C, Furtado MR, McBride LJ, Wolinsky SM. Detection of HIV-1 DNA and messenger RNA in individual cells by PCR- driven *in situ* hybridization and flow cytometry. *Science* (1993) 260:976–9. doi: 10.1126/science.8493534

Rozera G, Fabbri G, Lorenzini P, Mastrorosa I, Timelli L, Zaccarelli M, et al. Peripheral blood HIV-1 DNA dynamics in antiretroviral-treated HIV/HCV co-infected patients receiving directly-acting antivirals. *PLoS ONE* (2017)12:e0187095. doi: 10.1371/journal.pone.0187095

Ho YC, Shan L, Hosmane NN, Wang J, Laskey SB, Rosenbloom DIS, et al. Replication-competent non-induced proviruses in the latent reservoir increase barrier to HIV-1 cure. *Cell* (2013) 155:540–51. doi: 10.1016/j.cell.2013.09.020

Bagasra O, Seshamma T, Oakes JW, Pomerantz RJ. High percentages of CD4-positive lymphocytes harbor the HIV-1 provirus in the blood of certain infected individuals. *AIDS* (1993) 11:1419–25. doi: 10.1097/00002030-199311000-00003

Re MC, Furlini G, Gibellini D, Vignoli M, Ramazzotti E, Lolli E, et al. Quantification of human immunodeficiency virus type 1-infected mononuclear cells in peripheral blood of seropositive subjects by newly developed flow cytometry analysis of the product of an *in situ* PCR assay. *J Clin Microbiol.* (1994) 32:2152–7.

Gibellini DE, Re MC, Furlini G, La Placa M. Flow cytometry analysis of an *in situ* PCR for the detection of human immunodeficiency virus type-1 (HIV- proviral DNA. In: Gosden JR, editor. *PRINS and In Situ PCR Protocols. Methods in Molecular Biology*^{TM}*, Vol 71.* Humana Press (1997).

Funderburq NT. Markers of coagulation and inflammation often remain elevated in ART-treated HIV-infected patients. *Curr Opin HIV AIDS.* (2014) 9:80–6. doi: 10.1097/COH.0000000000000019

Fromentin R, Bakeman W, Lawani MB, Khoury G, Hartogensis W, DaFonseca S, et al. CD4+ T cells expressing PD-1, TIGIT and LAG-3 contribute to HIV persistence during ART. *PLoS Pathog* (2016) 12:e1005761. doi: 10.1371/journal.ppat.1005761

Imamichi H, Dewar RL, Adelsberger JW, Rehm CA, O'Doherty U, Paxinos EE, et al. Defective HIV-1 proviruses produce novel protein-coding RNA species in HIV-infected patients on combination antiretroviral therapy. *Proc Natl Acad Sci USA.* (2016) 113:8783–8. doi: 10.1073/pnas.1609057113

Kestler HW III, Ringler DJ, Mori K, Panicali DL, Sehgal PK, Daniel MD, et al. Importance of the nef gene for maintenance of high virus loads and for development of AIDS. *Cell* (1991) 65:651–62. doi: 10.1016/0092-8674(91)90097-I

Kirchhoff F, Greenough TC, Brettler DB, Sullivan JL, Desrosiers RC. Absence of intact nef sequences in a long-term survivor with nonprogressive HIV-1 infection. *N Engl J Med.* (1995) 332:228–32. doi:10.1056/NEJM199501263320405

Pawlak EN, Dikeakos JD. HIV-1 Nef: a master manipulator of the membrane trafficking machinery mediating immune evasion. *Biochim Biophys Acta.* (2015) 1850:733–41. doi: 10.1016/j.bbagen.2015.01.003

Gadhamsetty S, Coorens T, de Boer RJ. Notwithstanding circumstantial alibis, cytotoxic T cells can be major killers of HIV-1-infected cells. *J Virol.* (2016) 90:7066–83. doi: 10.1128/JVI.00306-16

Hassin D, Fixler R, Shimoni Y, Rubinstein E, Raz S, Gotsman MS et al. Physiological changes induced in cardiac myocytes by cytotoxic T lymphocytes. *Am J Physiol.* (1987) 252:C10–6. doi:10.1152/ajpcell.1987.252.1.C10

15

HIV-1 Productively Infects and Integrates in Bronchial Epithelial Cell

Dinesh Devadoss[1†], Shashi P. Singh[2†], Arpan Acharya[3], Kieu Chinh Do[4], Palsamy Periyasamy[3], Marko Manevski[1], Neerad Mishra[2], Carmen S. Tellez[4], Sundaram Ramakrishnan[5], Steven A. Belinsky[4], Siddappa N. Byrareddy[3], Shilpa Buch[3], Hitendra S. Chand[1] and Mohan Sopori[2*]*

[1] Department of Immunology and Nano-Medicine, Herbert Wertheim College of Medicine, Florida International University, Miami, FL, United States, [2] Respiratory Immunology Division, Lovelace Respiratory Research Institute, Albuquerque, NM, United States, [3] Department of Pharmacology & Experimental Neuroscience, University of Nebraska Medical Center, Omaha, NE, United States, [4] Lung Cancer Program, Lovelace Respiratory Research Institute, Albuquerque, NM, United States, [5] Department of Surgery, University of Miami Miller School of Medicine, Miami, FL, United States

Correspondence:
Mohan Sopori
msopori@lrri.org
Hitendra S. Chand
hchand@fiu.edu

[†]These authors have contributed equally to this work

Background: The role of lung epithelial cells in HIV-1-related lung comorbidities remains unclear, and the major hurdle in curing HIV is the persistence of latent HIV reservoirs in people living with HIV (PLWH). The advent of combined antiretroviral therapy has considerably increased the life span; however, the incidence of chronic lung diseases is significantly higher among PLWH. Lung epithelial cells orchestrate the respiratory immune responses and whether these cells are productively infected by HIV-1 is debatable.

Methods: Normal human bronchial epithelial cells (NHBEs) grown on air–liquid interface were infected with X4-tropic HIV-1_{LAV} and examined for latency using latency-reversing agents (LRAs). The role of CD4 and CXCR4 HIV coreceptors in NHBEs were tested, and DNA sequencing analysis was used to analyze the genomic integration of HIV proviral genes, Alu-HIVgag-pol, HIV-nef, and HIV-LTR. Lung epithelial sections from HIV-infected humans and SHIV-infected macaques were analyzed by FISH for HIV-gag-pol RNA and epithelial cell-specific immunostaining.

Results and Discussion: NHBEs express CD4 and CXCR4 at higher levels than A549 cells. NHBEs are infected with HIV-1 basolaterally, but not apically, by X4-tropic HIV-1_{LAV} in a CXCR4/CD4-dependent manner leading to HIV-p24 antigen production; however, NHBEs are induced to express CCR5 by IL-13 treatment. In the presence of cART, HIV-1 induces latency and integration of HIV provirus in the cellular DNA, which is rescued by the LRAs (endotoxin/vorinostat). Furthermore, lung epithelial cells from HIV-infected humans and SHIV-infected macaques contain HIV-specific RNA transcripts. Thus, lung epithelial cells are targeted by HIV-1 and could serve as potential HIV reservoirs that may contribute to the respiratory comorbidities in PLWH.

Keywords: lung epithelial cells, HIV receptors, genomic integration, HIV *gag-pol*, Nested-PCR, Fluorescent *in-situ* hybridization

INTRODUCTION

In the era of combined antiretroviral therapy (cART), the life span of PLWH has increased considerably; however, the incidence of obstructive lung diseases (OLDs) is significantly higher in PLWH (Maitre et al., 2018; Singhvi et al., 2019). A major hurdle in curing HIV is the persistence of latent HIV reservoirs in PLWH (Richman et al., 2009; Vanhamel et al., 2019). While CD4+ memory T cells are the recognized HIV reservoirs (Chun et al., 1997), recent evidence has demonstrated the presence of a minor macrophage subpopulation, which harbors HIV-1 in cART-treated HIV-infected subjects (Andrade et al., 2020). Lungs are established reservoirs of HIV-1 (Almodovar, 2014); however they may also be one of the preferred HIV sanctuaries in cART-treated subjects. Thus, bronchoalveolar lavage (BAL) is enriched in memory T cells and BAL cells contain 13-fold higher HIV-DNA than peripheral blood mononuclear cells (Costiniuk et al., 2018). The role of epithelial cells as HIV-1 targets is ambiguous. For example, the foreskin epithelial cells are known to express HIV coreceptors (Liu et al., 2014), and upon coculturing, transfers the HIV to lymphocytes (Yasen et al., 2017). NHBEs express CXCR4 and respond to X4-tropic gp120 treatment (Gundavarapu et al., 2013), and herein, we show that they also express CCR5 after IL-13 treatment; however, whether these cells are productively infected by HIV-1 remains debatable (Brune et al., 2016; Chinnapaiyan et al., 2017). Previously, we reported that lung tissues of cynomolgus macaques (CMs) infected with simian-adapted HIV (SHIV) had significantly higher HIV-gp120-positive epithelial cells (Chand et al., 2018); however, the source of gp120 was not established. In this study, we demonstrate that HIV-infected NHBEs, grown on the air–liquid interphase (ALI) produce HIV-p24, and the surviving HIV-1-infected cells harbor the HIV-provirus integrated within the host cell genome, which is activated by latency-reversing agents (LRAs). Moreover, *ex-vivo* analysis of lung epithelial cells from HIV-infected human subjects and SHIV-infected macaque lungs harbor HIV-specific RNA, suggesting a productive infection of lung epithelial cells by HIV-1 in both *in-vitro* and *in-vivo*.

MATERIALS AND METHODS

Normal Human Bronchial Epithelial Cells and ALI culture

Normal Human Bronchial Epithelial cells (NHBEs) were obtained from MatTek Incorp (EpiAirway^{TM}, Ashland, MA) and cultured as described previously (Hussain et al., 2018). The apical surface of the cells was exposed to air, and the cells were incubated in the media (provided by MatTek) for 48 h at 37°C before infection with HIV-1.

HIV-Infected Lung Tissue Sections

The archived lung tissue sections were kindly provided by the National NeuroAIDS Tissue Consortium (NNTC) and Lung Tissue Research Consortium (LTRC) of NIH. The formalin-fixed and paraffin-embedded human patient samples were from HIV-1-negative (HIV−) donors and HIV-1-positive (HIV+) subjects, and from HIV+ subjects on HAART (HIV+HAART). The lung tissue sections from SHIV-infected (SHIV+) and cigarette smoke (CS)-exposed SHIV+ macaques (CS+SHIV) were obtained from the study reported previously (Chand et al., 2018).

HIV Infection and p24 Analysis

The X4-tropic viral strain HIV-1_{LAV} was employed in these studies. NHBEs grown in air–liquid-interface (ALI) in transwells were infected either basolaterally (BL) or apically (AP) with X4-tropic HIV-1_{LAV} (5 ng/ml p24 equivalent). Control cultures received only the medium. Control and infected transwells were incubated for 2 h at 37°C in 5% CO_2 atmosphere. At 2 h post-infection, BL-infected cells were washed 4× with 2 ml PBS and the apically AP-infected cells with 0.5 ml PBS. The fourth wash from all cultures was analyzed for HIV-1-p24 level to ensure removal of the residual virus; this time point was designated as 0-time. Fresh medium was added to the cultures, and the plates were incubated at 37°C in 5% CO_2; the cultures were harvested at the indicated times.

The p24 concentration in the transwell culture media was measured using a p24 capture ELISA kit as per manufacturer's instructions (ZeptoMetrix Corp. Cat # 0801200 or Advance Bioscience Laboratories, Rockville, MD, USA). To promote latently in HIV-infected AECs, following infection of NHBEs with HIV-1, where indicated, the cells were transferred to the medium containing cART (a cocktail of ritonavir, tenofovir, and emtricitabine) for 6 days. The cells were washed, transferred to the culture medium without cART and, where indicated, treated with the latency-reversing agents (LRAs) vorinostat and LPS, as described before (Archin et al., 2012; Alvarez-Carbonell et al., 2017). At 24 h after the transfer, culture media were harvested and assayed for p24 levels.

Immunostaining and Fluorescent Imaging Analysis

For immunohistochemical staining, deparaffinized and hydrated lung tissue sections were washed with PBS containing 0.05% Brij-35 (pH 7.4) and immunostained for antigen expression as described previously (Chand et al., 2018). Briefly, the antigens were unmasked by steaming the sections in 10 mM citrate buffer (pH 6.0) followed by incubation in a blocking solution containing 3% BSA, 1% Gelatin, and 1% normal donkey serum with 0.1% Triton X-100 and 0.1% Saponin; the sections were stained with antibodies to CD4 (Abcam, #ab133616), CXCR4 (Abcam, #ab181020), HIV-Tat (Abcam, #ab63957) and pan-CK

Abbreviations: ALI, Air-liquid interface; AP, Apical side; BECs, Bronchial epithelial cells; BL, Basolateral side; cART, Combined antiretroviral therapy; CD4, Cluster of differentiation 4; CMs, Cynomolgus macaques; COPD, Chronic obstructive pulmonary disease; CS, Cigarette smoke; CXCR4, C-X-C chemokine receptor type 4; FISH, Fluorescent *In-Situ* Hybridization; Gag, Group specific antigen; HAART, Highly active antiretroviral therapy; HDACi, Histone deacetylase inhibitor; HIV-1, Human immunodeficiency virus type-1; LDH, Lactate dehydrogenase; LPS, Lipopolysaccharide; LRAs, Latency-reversing agents; LTRs, Long-terminal repeats; Nef, Negative regulatory factor; NHBEs, Normal human bronchial epithelial cells; OLD, Obstructive lung diseases; pCK, Pan cytokeratin; PLWH, People living with HIV; SHIV, Simian-adapted HIV.

(#4545, Cell Signaling Technologies, Danvers, MA). Similarly, to stain NHBEs, the cells were grown on coated coverslips or the coated Labtek-II slides (Thermo Fisher Inc.) and fixed in 4% paraformaldehyde. The slides were washed with PBS containing 0.05% Brij-35 (pH 7.4) and immunostained as described previously (Chand et al., 2017). Briefly, non-specific binding sites on the cells were blocked by a solution containing 3% BSA, 1% Gelatin, and 1% normal donkey serum with 0.1% Triton X-100 and 0.1% Saponin. The cells were then treated with antibodies to CD4, CXCR4, and pan-CK, as described above. The labeled cells/tissue sections were stained with appropriate second antibodies conjugated with fluorescent dyes (Jackson ImmunoResearch Lab Inc., West Grove, PA). The slides were treated with 4′,6-diamidino-2-phenylindole (DAPI) containing Fluormount-GTM (SouthernBiotech, Birmingham, AL) to visualize cell nuclei. Immunofluorescent images were captured using BZX700 Microscopy system (Keyence Corp., Japan) and analyzed using NIH Image J software.

DNA Isolation

To isolate DNA from the transwell-grown NHBEs, cells were dislodged from the filters and digested in 2.0 ml Eppendorf tubes containing 1.5 ml of digestion buffer (pH 8.0) comprising SDS, EDTA, and proteinase K as per manufacturer's instructions (MatTek Corp, MA, USA). Total DNA from the control and HIV-1 treated NHBEs was isolated using Qiagen DNA extraction kit (Germantown, MD, USA) and quantified using Nanodrop (Applied Biosystems, ThermoFisher).

HIV-1 Gag DNA Quantification

The HIV-1 infected NHBEs were collected from the transwells at different time points (0, 2, 4, 24, 48, and 96 h) after infection. DNA was isolated from the cells using Qiagen DNA extraction kit per manufacturer's instructions (QIAGEN Germantown, MD, USA), and cell associated HIV-1 gag DNA was quantified as described by Pasternak et al. (2008). using Applied Biosystems QuantStudio 3 Real-Time PCR System (Applied Biosystems, Waltham, MA, USA), and the data was used to calculate HIV-1 gag copies/ng of DNA.

Alu-Gag PCR and Nucleotide Sequencing

We utilized the methods as described previously (Liszewski et al., 2009) in which a two-step Alu-gag PCR assay was used to determine the presence of integrated HIV-1 proviral DNA. This method utilizes a nested PCR approach. Briefly, during the 1st round PCR, the region between HIV-1 gag gene and nearest Alu repeat element of host genome was amplified. The primer sequences used in the 1st step PCR were: Alu Forward: 5′-GCCTCCCAAAGTGCTGGGATTACAG-3′ and HIV gag reverse: 5′-GTTCCTGCTATGTCACTTCC-3′ which corresponds to nucleotide (nt) 1,505–1,486 of HIV-1 HXB2 genome. The reactions were carried out in 50 μl and contained 1.5 mM $MgCl_2$, 0.2 mM dNTPs mix, 100 nM Alu Forward primer, 600 nM HIV gag reverse primer and 5 U of Platinum Taq DNA polymerase (Life Technologies; USA). In the 2nd round PCR, the 5′ LTR region of HIV-1 was amplified using 1 μl of the 1st round PCR amplicon as the template. The primers for the second round were: 5′ LTR Forward: 5′-TTAAGCCTCA ATAAAGCTTGCC-3′ and 5′ LTR Reverse: 5′-GTTCCTGCTA TGTCACTTCC-3′. The PCR amplification was carried out in Applied Biosystem 9700 thermal cycler under the following conditions, 1st round of PCR: 95°C for 2 m, followed by 40 cycles at 95°C for 15 s, 50°C (T_m) for 15 s, and 72°C for 3.5 min; 2nd round of PCR: 95°C for 2 m, followed by 40 cycles at 95°C for 15 s, 60°C (T_m) for 15 s and 72°C for 30 s. PCR amplicons were resolved on a 2% agarose gel (Promega Corporation, Madison, USA) pre-stained with Ethidium bromide (0.5 μg/ml). The gel images were documented using a Bio Rad gel documentation system (BIORAD, USA).

The PCR amplicons were purified using QIAGEN PCR purification kit (QIAGEN, Germany) as per the manufacturer's instructions and subjected to Sanger sequencing using BigDye Terminator v3.1 Cycle Sequencing Kit (Applied Biosystems, California; USA). Automated capillary electrophoresis was performed on an ABI PRISM® 3500 Genetic Analyzer (Applied Biosystems, California; USA) using data collection software v.3.1 at the University of Nebraska Medical Center DNA Sequencing Core facility. The raw sequence data were manually edited, spliced, and assembled by Sequencher v4.9 to generate the final contig. Multiple sequence alignment of edited sequence was performed with HIV-1_{LAV} reference sequence of HIV-1 using Clustal W (Aiyar, 2000).

HIV-1 Gag DNA Amplification and Sequencing

HIV-1 gag DNA from infected NHBEs was amplified essentially using the primers, probes, and PCR protocol described previously (Khoja et al., 2008). Briefly, primers used in first round of PCR on cellular DNA were forward primer (5′-CTCTCGACGCAGGACTCGGCTTGC-3′, nt 683–706, HXB2) and reverse primer (5′-CCAATTCCCCCTATCATTTTTGG-3′, nt 2,382–2,404) with a T_m of 58°C. For the second round of amplification, forward primer (5′-GAGGCTAGAAGGA GAGAGATGGG-3′, nt 772–794, HXB2) and GIPR (5′-TTATT GTGACGAGGGGTCGTTGCC-3′, nt 2,269–2,292) with a T_m of 60°C were used. The amplicon (1,520 bp) was analyzed on 1.2% agarose gels following ethidium bromide staining. For sequencing, the amplified DNA product was extracted from the agarose gel, and purified, using QIAquick Gel Extraction kit (Cat#28704, Qiagen Inc.) based on the manufacturer's instructions. The product was sent for sequencing to Sequetech Corp (Mountain View, CA).

HIV-1 Nef DNA Amplification and Sequencing

Nef DNA was also amplified by a two-step nested PCR strategy as described previously (Shugars et al., 1993). Briefly, the two sets of amplification primers were designed to anneal to highly conserved segments flanking the HIV-1 nef gene. The primers used for the first round of amplification were, forward primer (5′-AATAGAGTTAGGCAGGGATA-3′, nt 8,338-8,358, HXB2) and reverse primer (5′-CTGGTCTAACCAGAGAGACCC AGTAC-3′, nt 9,533-9,558) with a T_m of 55°C. For the second round of amplification, forward primer (5′-CTCGCAGT

CTAGAAGAATAAGACAGGGCTTGGAAAGG-3′, nt 8,754-8,782, HXB2) and reverse primer (5′-CGTCCAGAATTCGGA AAGTCCCCAGCGGAAAGTC-3′, nt 9,436–9,457) were used that included the restriction sites for XbaI and EcoR1, respectively and amplified at the T_m of 55°C. The PCR product from the first round of amplification (1,200 bp) was diluted 1:100 for the second round of amplification using 30 PCR cycles. The PCR product (703 bp) was visualized by ethidium bromide staining and agarose gel electrophoresis. The amplified Nef DNA was extracted from the agarose gel, purified using QIAquick Gel Extraction Kit, and sent for sequencing to Sequetech Corp (Mountain View, CA).

Quantitative Real-Time RT-PCR

Total RNA was isolated from the experimental cells using RNAeasy kit (Qiagen, Germantown, MD) as per manufacturer's instruction. RNA concentration was determined using the Synergy HTX Multi-Mode reader (BioTek, Winooski, VT), and cDNA was synthesized using iScript advanced cDNA kit (BioRad, Hercules, CA). The primer/probe sets for CD4, HIV-LTR RNA, and MUC5AC were obtained from Applied Biosystems (Thermo Fisher Inc.). The amplified cDNA was quantified by qPCR using the TaqMan Gene expression kit (Thermo Fisher Inc.) in the Stratagene Mx3000P Real-Time PCR System (Agilent, Santa Clara, CA). Relative quantities were calculated by normalizing the averaged C_T values to CDKN1B or GAPDH to obtain ΔC_T, and the fold-change ($\Delta\Delta C_T$) over the controls was determined as described previously (Chand et al., 2017).

Lactate Dehydrogenase Release Assay

The loss of plasma membrane integrity is considered as a maker of cell death and is measured as the release of cytosolic LDH in culture media after the rupture of plasma membrane. The concentration of LDH in the culture supernatants collected from HIV-1 infected NHBE transwells was measured by using CytoTox96 assay (Promega, Madison, WI) as per manufacturer's instructions.

RNA Fluorescent *In-Situ* Hybridization

RNA FISH was essentially performed using the RNAscope® Fluorescent Multiplexed reagent kit (Advanced Cell Diagnostics, Newark, CA) as per the manufacturer's protocol and as reported recently (Devadoss et al., 2020). Briefly, the probe set for HIVgag-pol consisted of 20 dual probes targeting different segments within the whole transcript (Advanced Cell Diagnostics). Deparaffinized and permeabilized lung sections were hybridized with probes for 2 h at 40°C using a HyBEZ® oven (Advanced Cell Diagnostics), and the signal was amplified by serial incubation in amplification buffers and HRP-tagged probe (Thermo Fisher Inc), at 40°C using a HyBEZ® oven. Probes were detected using Tyramide signal amplification (TSA) reaction using an Alexa-flour-labeled TSA kit (PerkinElmer Bioscience) according to the manufacturer's instructions. The sections were processed for immunostaining of panCK as described above, followed by mounting with 4′,6-diamidino-2-phenylindole (DAPI) containing Fluormount-G (SouthernBiotech, Birmingham, AL) to visualize the nuclei. Immunofluorescence images were captured with BZX700 Microscopy system (Keyence Corp, Japan) and analyzed by NIH ImageJ software. RNA FISH expression was quantified by the analysis and as reported recently (Devadoss et al., 2020). Briefly, signals (dots/cell) for each transcript probe were counted and allocated to separate bins with Bin 0 (0 Dots/Cell); Bin 1 (1–3 Dots/Cell); Bin 2 (4–9 Dots/Cell); Bin 3 (10–15 Dots/Cell); Bin 4 (>15 Dots/Cell). The histology score (H-Score) was calculated as Sum of each (bin number × percentage of cells per bin) that ranged from 0 to 400 based on the transcript's expression.

Western Blot Analysis

Cell extracts were prepared using RIPA buffer (20 mM Tris, pH 7.4, 137 mM NaCl, 1% NP-40, 0.25% Deoxycholate, 0.1% SDS, 1 mM EDTA and 1% protease inhibitor). Protein concentration was determined by BCA kit (Pierce; Rockford, IL), and 50 µg of protein was analyzed by western blotting as described previously (Hussain et al., 2018). Proteins were detected by ECL and visualized by chemiluminescence (Perkin Elmer, Waltham, MA) using the BioRad Chemidoc Imaging system (Hercules, CA).

Statistical Analysis

Grouped results were expressed as means ± SEM. Data were analyzed using GraphPad Prism Software (GraphPad Software, Inc., San Diego, CA). Grouped results were analyzed using two-way analysis of variance. When the effects were significant ($p \le 0.05$), the Fisher's least significant difference test was used to determine differences between groups.

RESULTS AND DISCUSSION

Human Bronchial Epithelial Cells Intrinsically Express CD4 and CXCR4, and Express CCR5 Upon IL-13 Treatment

CD4, CXCR4, and CCR5 are HIV-1 receptors/coreceptors (Brelot and Chakrabarti, 2018). NHBEs express CXCR4 (Eddleston et al., 2002; Gundavarapu et al., 2013), and it is X4- but not the R5-tropic HIV-gp120 that induces airway inflammatory mucus in these cells (Gundavarapu et al., 2013). Based on the qPCR and immunoblot analysis, compared to A549 (a human alveolar epithelial cell line), NHBEs showed >50-fold higher expression of *CD4* mRNA (**Figure 1A**) and >5-fold higher CD4 protein levels (**Figures 1B, C**). Immunocytometry staining indicated that, in addition to CXCR4 (**Figure 1D**), NHBEs exhibited high levels of CD4 expression (**Figure 1E**), and the CD4 levels were approximately 3.5-fold higher than CXCR4 (**Figure 1F**). Thus, NHBEs express HIV-1 receptor CD4 and coreceptor CXCR4, rendering them as potential HIV-1 targets.

The expression CCR5 on NHBEs is not unequivocal (Brune et al., 2016; Chinnapaiyan et al., 2017). During carcinogenesis, epithelial cells have been shown to express CCR5 that enhances their resistance to cytotoxicity (Jiao et al., 2019). Th2 responses in the lung are common and are induced by infections and exposure to allergens (Hansbro et al., 2014). IL-13 is a key Th2 cytokine, which is strongly upregulated in the lungs of SHIV-infected macaques (Chand et al., 2018). Moreover, CCR5 plays a critical role in the IL-13-induced lung pathogenesis (Ma et al., 2006). Therefore, we determined whether IL-13 affects the

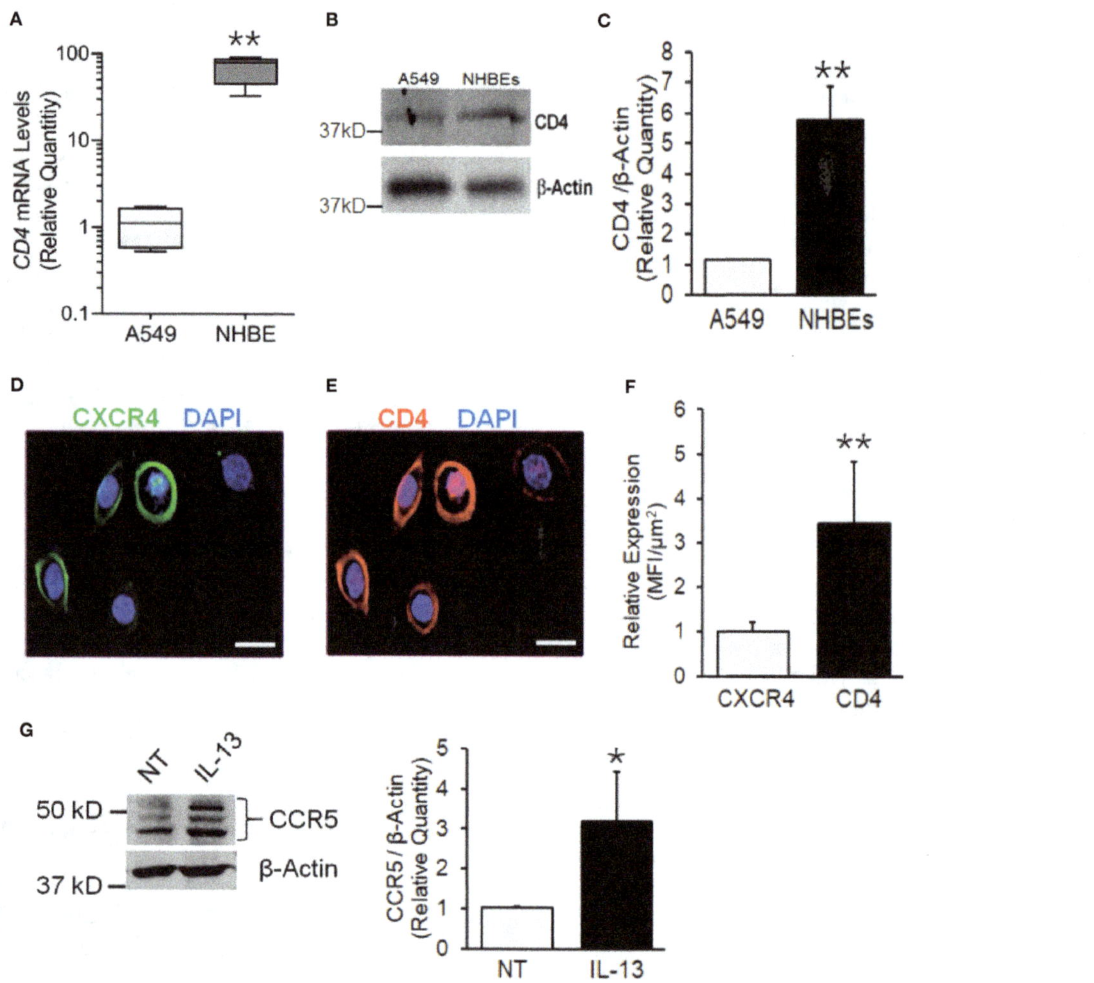

FIGURE 1 | Human airway epithelial cells express HIV receptor and co-receptors. **(A)** qPCR analysis of CD4 mRNA levels in NHBEs compared to A549 cells. **(B)** Western blot analysis of CD4 protein levels in NHBE and A549 cells with β-actin as the loading control. **(C)** Densitometric analysis of CD4 protein levels compared to A549 cells. Representative micrographs of NHBE cells showing **(D)** CXCR4 (green) and **(E)** CD4 (red) immunopositivity along with DAPI-stained nuclei (blue); scale—5μ. **(F)** Relative expression of CXCR4 and CD4 in NHBEs as assessed by measuring the Mean Fluorescence Intensity (MFI) per unit area. **(G)** Western blot analysis of CCR5 protein levels in NHBE cells treated with IL-13 (1 ng/ml) for 48 h compared to non-treated (NT) control cells and densitometric analysis of CCR5 levels normalized to β-actin levels compared to controls. Data shown as mean ± SEM; n = 3/group and are representative of three different experiments; $^*p < 0.05$; $^{**}p < 0.01$.

expression of CCR5 on NHBE cells. As shown in **Figure 1G**, IL-13 (1 ng/ml) treatment induced the significant levels of CCR5 in NHBEs. Therefore, it is likely that *in-vivo* lung epithelial cells are primed to express CCR5.

X4-Tropic HIV-1$_{LAV}$ Infects NHBEs

Among the HIV-1 patients, the R5 (CCR5-tropic) HIV-1 variants predominate over the course of infection, and the X4 (CXCR4-tropic) variants arise later (Poon et al., 2012); however, nearly 22% of patients on cART principally harbor the X4 variants (Ferrer et al., 2014). Moreover, a recent study indicated that X4 variants are mainly associated with pulmonary arterial hypertension—a lung condition quite prevalent among PLWH (Almodovar et al., 2020). Most importantly, NHBEs explicitly express CXCR4 (Eddleston et al., 2002; Gundavarapu et al., 2013), and the X4-but not the R5-tropic HIV-gp120 induces inflammatory mucus response in NHBEs (Gundavarapu et al., 2013). Therefore, to ascertain whether NHBEs are productively infected by HIV-1, ALI-differentiated NHBEs were infected with X4-tropic HIV-1$_{LAV}$. Cellular DNA was isolated and assayed for HIV-gag by qPCR at denoted time points (**Figure 2A**), and the culture supernatants were analyzed for HIV-p24 levels (**Figure 2B**). Both HIV-1 titer (HIV-1 cell-associated DNA) and p24 levels reached maximum at 24 h and declined thereafter to very low levels at 96 h post-infection. HIV-1 infection induces cell death (Cooper et al., 2013), and HIV-1 infection of NHBEs showed increased levels of the cell-death marker lactate dehydrogenase (LDH) (**Figure S1**).

Transmission of HIV-1 *via* oral or oropharyngeal route is highly unlikely (CDC Report August 6, 2019: www.cdc.gov/hiv/basics),

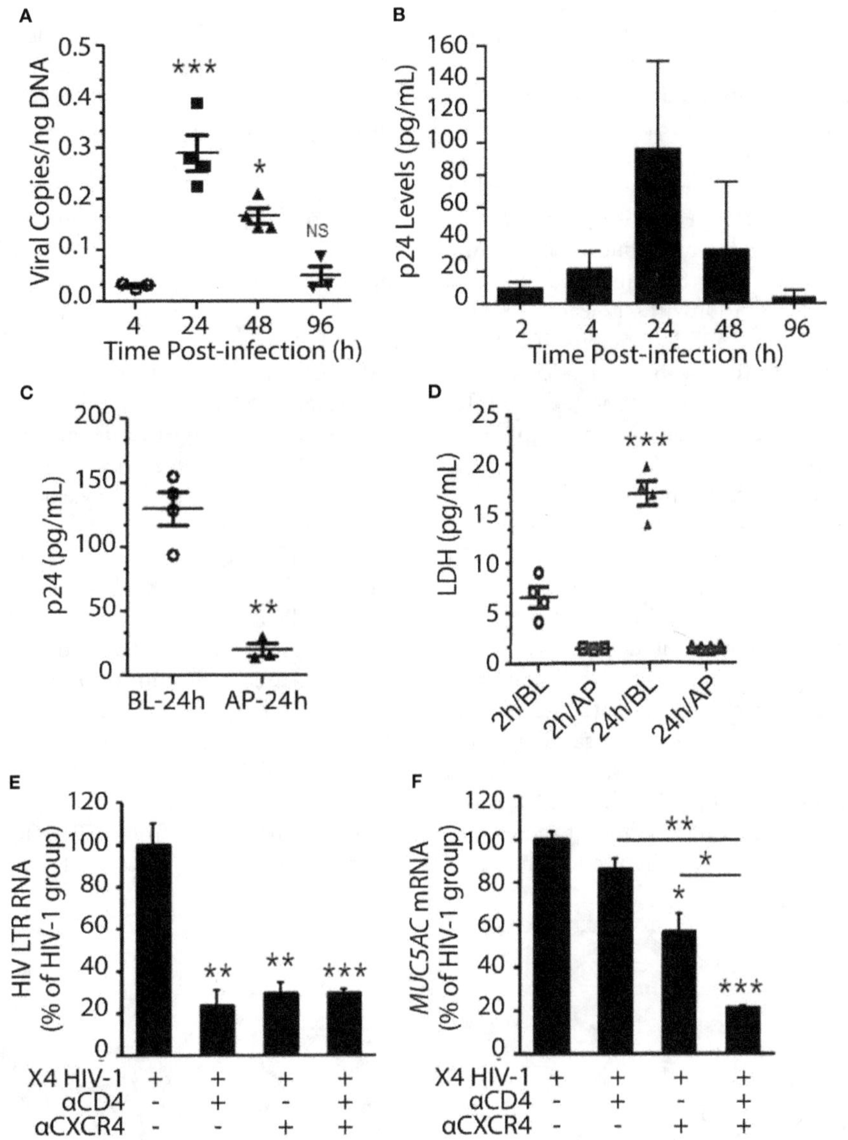

FIGURE 2 | Differentiated NHBE cells were infected by X4-tropic HIV-1 and blocking HIV-coreceptors inhibits HIV infectivity. **(A)** Expression kinetics of HIV-1 gag DNA levels (viral copies per ng of cellular DNA) in NHBE cell lysates analyzed at 2, 4, 24, 48, and 96 h post X4-tropic HIV-1_{LAV} infection. **(B)** Expression kinetics of p24 (pg/ml) measured in cell culture media collected from the bottom of transwells at the denoted time post infection. **(C)** HIV-1 p24 levels at 24 h post-infection in NHBEs that were infected *via* basolateral (BL) or apical (AP) surfaces; and **(D)** LDH release quantification at 2 and 24 h post-infection in BL- or AP-infected cells. Relative quantities of **(E)** HIV-1 LTR RNA levels and **(F)** *MUC5AC* mRNA levels in NHBE cells pre-treated with either anti-CD4 or anti-CXCR4 antibodies followed by infection with X4-tropic HIV-1_{LAV} and 48 h post- infection cells were harvested and analyzed. Data shown as mean ± SEM; n = 3/group; *$p < 0.05$; **$p < 0.01$; ***$p < 0.001$.

and the saliva may inactivate HIV-1 (Baron et al., 1999). We analyzed the susceptibility of NHBEs to HIV-1 infection *via* basolateral (BL) *versus* AP apical (AP) side. NHBEs grown on ALI were infected with HIV-1 from either AP or BL surfaces, and p24 levels were measured at 24 h. LDH levels assessed at 2 and 24 h post-infection indicated that NHBEs are mainly sensitive to HIV-1 from BL side and relatively resistant to HIV infection from AP side (**Figure 2C**); and BL infection with HIV-1 showed increased LDH release (**Figure 2D**). Thus, the apical side of differentiated lung epithelial cells is essentially refractory to HIV-1 infection.

Next, to verify that basolateral HIV-1 infection is mediated *via* HIV receptors/coreceptors, NHBEs were pre-incubated with anti-CXCR4 and/or anti-CD4 antibodies. The HIV-LTR RNA levels were potently inhibited in cells pre-incubated with antibodies to CD4 and/or CXCR4 compared to control HIV-1 infected cells (**Figure 2E**). Similarly, HIV-1-induced MUC5AC mucin expression was significantly reduced in cells pretreated with CD4- and/or CXCR4-antibodies (**Figure 2F**). These data suggest that HIV-1 infection of bronchial epithelial cells is dependent on classical HIV-1 receptors/coreceptors.

HIV-1 Establishes Latency With Proviral DNA Integration Into NHBE Genome

Although HIV-1-induced cell death is associated with genomic integration of HIV-1 DNA (Cooper et al., 2013); the proviral integration in BECs remains uncertain. Treatment with antiretroviral drugs suppresses HIV-1 below detection limits but also promotes infected-cell survival and establishes HIV-1 latency (Dahabieh et al., 2015). The latent cells harbor replication-competent integrated HIV-1 provirus; however, the cells remain transcriptionally silent establishing them as viral reservoirs (Margolis and Archin, 2017; Sengupta and Siliciano, 2018). LRAs activate latent HIV-1 proviruses, leading to the production of the virus (Takahama and Yamamoto, 2020). We observed that the treatment of NHBEs with cART (a cocktail of ritonavir, tenofovir, and emtricitabine) at 0-time (*i.e.*, 2h after HIV-1 infection), inhibited but failed to eliminate p24 expression at 8 h post-infection (**Figure S1B**).

To demonstrate that HIV-1 infects and establishes latency, NHBEs were infected with HIV-1_{LAV} at 24 h after HIV-1 infection and the culture media were replaced with cART-containing media. Infected NHBEs were culture d for 6 more days, washed, and replenished with the culture media without cART and treated with the LRAs comprised of LPS, a gram-negative bacterial wall component and Vorinostat, a histone deacetylase inhibitor (HDACi) (Archin et al., 2012), After 24 h, the culture supernatants were harvested and assayed for p24 levels. As shown in **Figure 3A**, before the removal of cART, cells had very low levels of p24 (day 6 with cART); however, at 24 h after cART removal, there is a small but significant increase in p24 levels (7 day media control). Media harvested from cells treated with LRAs (7 day-HDACi/LPS) had significantly higher p24 levels suggesting that, in the presence of cART, NHBEs are latently infected by HIV-1, and the latency is reversed by LPS and vorinostat. Together, these results suggest that in the presence of cART, HIV-1 infection of NHBEs yields latently infected cells and the latent HIV-1 provirus is activated by LRAs, leading to the reemergence of proviral factors.

For productive infection and proviral latency, HIV-1 DNA needs to be integrated into the host genome (Craigie and Bushman, 2012). To demonstrate that HIV-1 DNA is integrated into NHBEs, we analyzed genes in 5′- and 3′-LTR of HIV (*i.e.* gag and Nef genes, respectively). DNA isolated from control and HIV-infected NHBEs was used to amplify HIV-gag in a nested PCR, and there was a single 1.52 kb amplicon present in the infected cells (**Figure S2A**). The amplicon was isolated and sequenced (**Figure S2B**); the sequence alignment confirmed >99% identity to the HIV-1 gag sequence. Similarly, Nef gene was amplified using the nested-PCR approach that yielded a single amplicon of 703 bp (**Figure S3A**). The sequencing analysis confirmed >99% identity to HIV-1 Nef sequence (**Figure S3B**). In the second approach, a two-step Alu-gag PCR assay was employed (**Figure 3B**). The two rounds of PCRs resulted in a 130 bp amplicon of 5′-LTR of HIV-1 genome (**Figure 3C**), and the amplicon was sequenced (**Figure 3D**). The sequence alignment of the raw sequencing data exactly matched with the reference sequence of LTR-gag region of HIV-1 strain used for the infection (**Figure 3E**), confirming the chromosomal integration of HIV provirus in NHBEs. Taken together, these data support the presence of several HIV-1 genes in the cellular DNA from HIV-infected NHBE cells and the association of Alu sequences with the LTR DNA. Alu sequences

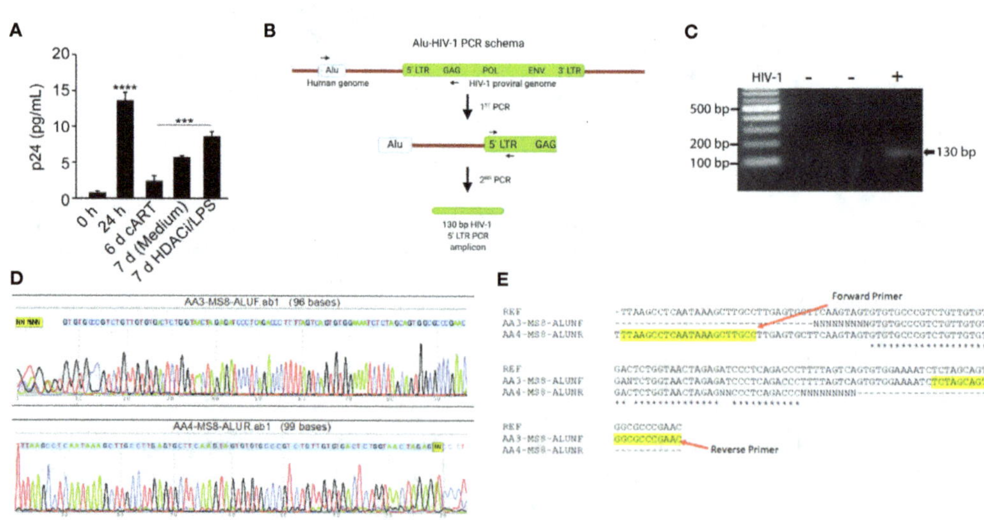

FIGURE 3 | Differentiated NHBE cells act as HIV-1 reservoir and Alu-PCR analysis confirming the integration of HIV-1 proviral genome in NHBEs. **(A)** HIV-1 p24 levels after latency-reversing agents, vorinostat and LPS, treatment of HIV-1 infected cells. **(B)** Schematics of the nested-PCR approach used to confirm the HIV DNA integration in infected NHBEs. **(C)** Agarose gel analysis of the nested PCR amplicon showing amplification of 130 bp band from 5′ LTR region of HIV-1. **(D)** Electropherogram of the 130 bp PCR amplicon generated using Forward and Reverse primers confirms the presence of the HIV proviral genome (The 5′-LTR sequence of HIV is indicated with blue shade). **(E)** Multiple sequence alignment of edited HIV-1 5′-LTR sequence obtained from the sequencing of the 130 bp PCR amplicon along with the sequence of HIV-1_{LAV} used to infect the NHBEs. The primer sequences used are highlighted in yellow. Data shown as mean ± SEM; n = 3/group; ***p < 0.001; ****p < 0.0001.

are present only in primate DNA (Quentin and Fichant, 1994) and represent at least 20% of human genome (Schmid, 1996). Thus, the association of Alu sequences with HIV-specific LTR DNA clearly indicates that HIV is integrated within the NHBE cellular DNA.

HIV RNA Present in Lung Epithelial Cells From SHIV-Infected Macaques and HIV-Infected Human Subjects

To ascertain whether HIV replicates *in-vivo* in airway epithelial cells, we evaluated lung sections for HIV-specific RNA by FISH using RNAScope® and HIV-gag-pol probes (ACD Biotechne Inc.). HIV-specific gag-pol RNA showed 20-fold higher expression in SHIV-infected pan-cytokeratin (pCK)-positive BECs than uninfected control lungs (**Figures 4A, B**). Moreover, SHIV infection of cigarette smoke (CS)-exposed macaques (CS+SHIV) showed about three-fold higher levels of HIV-specific RNA than HIV-infected controls, thus, supporting the evidence that combined exposure of CMs to CS and SHIV is more injurious to the lung than independent exposures to either SHIV or CS (Chand et al., 2018). Similarly, the lung sections from HIV-infected subjects showed >25-fold higher levels of HIV-specific RNA in pCK-positive epithelial cells, and the high levels of the RNAs persisted (14-fold higher than controls) in HIV subjects undergoing HAART (HIV+HAART) compared to uninfected human airway control sections (**Figures 4C, D**). These results underscore the inference that both in humans and in macaques, the lung epithelial cells are targets of HIV-1 infection and might be responsible for the higher respiratory comorbidities among PLWH.

Lung is an important reservoir for HIV-1 (Almodovar, 2014; Costiniuk et al., 2018), and herein, we demonstrate that the airway epithelial cells are targets of HIV-1 infection in both *in-vitro* and *in-vivo* settings and that in the presence of cART the cells harbor latent HIV-1 provirus. Lung bronchial epithelial cells are crucial innate immune cells and the first line of defense against airborne pathogens (Wu et al., 2011). In the respiratory tract, airway epithelial cells are constantly exposed to airborne pathogens, including LPS-containing gram-negative bacteria (Hayes et al., 2013), and we have shown that LPS, a signature molecule in gram-negative bacteria, in conjunction with Vorinostat, can activate the latent HIV-provirus in HIV-infected airway epithelial cells. Given that airway epithelial cells are very long-lived (Rawlins and Hogan, 2008), in the presence of cART, these cells are likely to make good

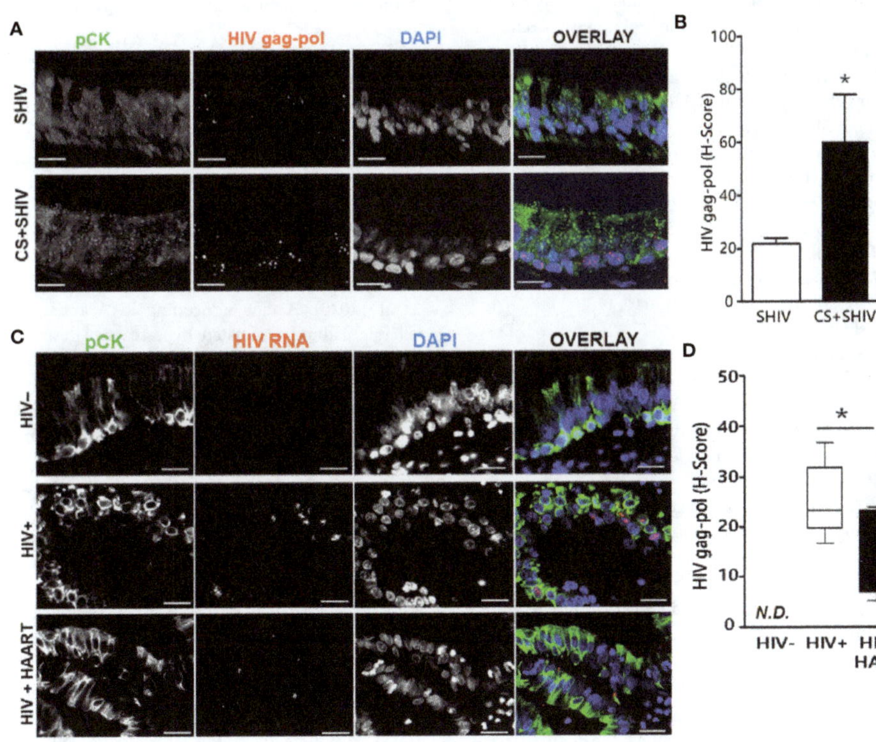

FIGURE 4 | Expression of HIV-gag-pol RNAs in the lung epithelial cells of SHIV-infected macaques and HIV-infected human subjects treated with antiretrovirals. Archived 5 μm FFPE lung tissue sections were used for HIV-1-gag-pol RNA detection using RNAscope® and immunostained for the epithelial cell marker, pan-cytokeratin (pCK). **(A)** Representative micrographs of bronchial epithelial cells showing pan-cytokeratin, pCK (green), and HIV-gag-pol (red) colocalization along with the DAPI-stained nuclei (blue) from SHIV- and CS+SHIV-infected groups; CS, cigarette smoke, Scale—5μ. **(B)** Quantification of epithelial HIV-gag-pol expression denoted as H-score, see *Materials and Methods* for details; *p < 0.05. **(C)** Representative micrographs of bronchial epithelial cells showing pCK (green) and HIV-gag-pol (red) colocalization along with the DAPI-stained nuclei (blue) in archived lung tissues from HIV-negative controls (HIV–), and from HIV-infected (HIV+) subjects and HIV+ subjects on HAART treatment (HIV+HAART). Scale—5μ. **(D)** Quantification of HIV-gag-pol expression in bronchial epithelial cells (denoted as H-score). N.D., Not detected. Data are shown as mean ± SEM; n = 4/group; *p < 0.05.

targets for latent HIV infections and may significantly contribute to the HIV-1-reservoir function of the lung.

ETHICS STATEMENT

All experimental protocols carried out on cynomologus macaques were approved by the Institutional Animal Care and Use Committee of Lovelace Respiratory Research Institute, Albuquerque, NM in accordance with the Guidelines from the Association for the Assessment and Accreditation for Laboratory Animal Care International as reported recently (Chand et al., 2018).

AUTHOR CONTRIBUTIONS

DD and SS performed the sample analysis, analyzed the data, and wrote the manuscript. AA, KD, PP, MM, NM, and CT performed the sample analysis and analyzed the data. SR, SAB, SNB, and SB analyzed the data. HSC and MS designed the studies, analyzed the data, and wrote the manuscript. All authors reviewed the manuscript. All authors contributed to the article and approved the submitted version.

ACKNOWLEDGMENTS

The authors acknowledge the help from the Inhalation and Necropsy Cores of Lovelace Respiratory Research Institute and thank Gilead Sciences, Inc. CA for the gift of antiretroviral drugs Tenofovir and emtricitabine. We also appreciate the technical support provided by Ruben Castro.

REFERENCES

Aiyar, A. (2000). The use of CLUSTAL W and CLUSTAL X for multiple sequence alignment. *Methods Mol. Biol.* 132, 221–241. doi: 10.1385/1-59259-192-2:221

Almodovar, S., Wade, B. E., Porter, K. M., Smith, J. M., Lopez-Astacio, R. A., Bijli, K., et al. (2020). HIV X4 Variants Increase Arachidonate 5-Lipoxygenase in the Pulmonary Microenvironment and are associated with Pulmonary Arterial Hypertension. *Sci. Rep.* 10, 11696. doi: 10.1038/s41598-020-68060-9

Almodovar, S. (2014). The complexity of HIV persistence and pathogenesis in the lung under antiretroviral therapy: challenges beyond AIDS. *Viral Immunol.* 27, 186–199. doi: 10.1089/vim.2013.0130

Alvarez-Carbonell, D., Garcia-Mesa, Y., Milne, S., Das, B., Dobrowolski, C., and Karn, J. (2017). Toll-like receptor 3 activation selectively reverses HIV latency in microglial cells. *Retrovirology* 14, 9. doi: 10.1186/s12977-017-0335-8

Andrade, V. M., Mavian, C., Babic, D., Cordeiro, T., Sharkey, M., Barrios, L., et al. (2020). A minor population of macrophage-tropic HIV-1 variants is identified in recrudescing viremia following analytic treatment interruption. *Proc. Natl. Acad. Sci. U.S.A.* 117, 9981–9990. doi: 10.1073/pnas.1917034117

Archin, N. M., Liberty, A. L., Kashuba, A. D., Choudhary, S. K., Kuruc, J. D., Crooks, A. M., et al. (2012). Administration of vorinostat disrupts HIV-1 latency in patients on antiretroviral therapy. *Nature* 487, 482–485. doi: 10.1038/nature11286

Baron, S., Poast, J., and Cloyd, M. W. (1999). Why is HIV rarely transmitted by oral secretions? Saliva can disrupt orally shed, infected leukocytes. *Arch. Intern. Med.* 159, 303–310. doi: 10.1001/archinte.159.3.303

Brelot, A., and Chakrabarti, L. A. (2018). CCR5 Revisited: How Mechanisms of HIV Entry Govern AIDS Pathogenesis. *J. Mol. Biol.* 430, 2557–2589. doi: 10.1016/j.jmb.2018.06.027

Brune, K. A., Ferreira, F., Mandke, P., Chau, E., Aggarwal, N. R., D'Alessio, F. R., et al. (2016). HIV Impairs Lung Epithelial Integrity and Enters the Epithelium to Promote Chronic Lung Inflammation. *PloS One* 11, e0149679. doi: 10.1371/journal.pone.0149679

Chand, H. S., Mebratu, Y. A., Kuehl, P. J., and Tesfaigzi, Y. (2017). Blocking Bcl-2 resolves IL-13-mediated mucous cell hyperplasia in a Bik-dependent manner. *J. Allergy Clin. Immunol.* 140, 1456–1459.e9. doi: 10.1016/j.jaci.2017.05.038

Chand, H. S., Vazquez-Guillamet, R., Royer, C., Rudolph, K., Mishra, N., Singh, S. P., et al. (2018). Cigarette smoke and HIV synergistically affect lung pathology in cynomolgus macaques. *J. Clin. Invest.* 128, 5428–5433. doi: 10.1172/JCI121935

Chinnapaiyan, S., Parira, T., Dutta, R., Agudelo, M., Morris, A., Nair, M., et al. (2017). HIV Infects Bronchial Epithelium and Suppresses Components of the Mucociliary Clearance Apparatus. *PloS One* 12, e0169161. doi: 10.1371/journal.pone.0169161

Chun, T. W., Carruth, L., Finzi, D., Shen, X., DiGiuseppe, J. A., Taylor, H., et al. (1997). Quantification of latent tissue reservoirs and total body viral load in HIV-1 infection. *Nature* 387, 183–188. doi: 10.1038/387183a0

Cooper, A., Garcia, M., Petrovas, C., Yamamoto, T., Koup, R. A., and Nabel, G. J. (2013). HIV-1 causes CD4 cell death through DNA-dependent protein kinase during viral integration. *Nature* 498, 376–379. doi: 10.1038/nature12274

Costiniuk, C. T., Salahuddin, S., Farnos, O., Olivenstein, R., Pagliuzza, A., Orlova, M., et al. (2018). HIV persistence in mucosal CD4+ T cells within the lungs of adults receiving long-term suppressive antiretroviral therapy. *AIDS* 32, 2279–2289. doi: 10.1097/QAD.0000000000001962

Craigie, R., and Bushman, F. D. (2012). HIV DNA integration. *Cold Spring Harb. Perspect. Med.* 2, a006890. doi: 10.1101/cshperspect.a006890

Dahabieh, M. S., Battivelli, E., and Verdin, E. (2015). Understanding HIV latency: the road to an HIV cure. *Annu. Rev. Med.* 66, 407–421. doi: 10.1146/annurev-med-092112-152941

Devadoss, D., Daly, G., Manevski, M., Houserova, D., Hussain, S. S., Baumlin, N., et al. (2020). A long noncoding RNA antisense to ICAM-1 is involved in allergic asthma associated hyperreactive response of airway epithelial cells. *Mucosal Immunol.* doi: 10.1038/s41385-020-00352-9

Eddleston, J., Christiansen, S. C., and Zuraw, B. L. (2002). Functional expression of the C-X-C chemokine receptor CXCR4 by human bronchial epithelial cells: regulation by proinflammatory mediators. *J. Immunol.* 169, 6445–6451. doi: 10.4049/jimmunol.169.11.6445

Ferrer, P., Tello, M., Montecinos, L., Tordecilla, R., Rodriguez, C., Beltran, C., et al. (2014). Prevalence of R5 and X4 HIV variants in antiretroviral treatment experienced patients with virologic failure. *J. Clin. Virol.* 60, 290–294. doi: 10.1016/j.jcv.2014.04.004

Gundavarapu, S., Mishra, N. C., Singh, S. P., Langley, R. J., Saeed, A. I., Feghali-Bostwick, C. A., et al. (2013). HIV gp120 induces mucus formation in human bronchial epithelial cells through CXCR4/alpha7-nicotinic acetylcholine receptors. *PloS One* 8, e77160. doi: 10.1371/journal.pone.0077160

Hansbro, P. M., Starkey, M. R., Mattes, J., and Horvat, J. C. (2014). Pulmonary immunity during respiratory infections in early life and the development of severe asthma. *Ann. Am. Thorac. Soc.* 11 Suppl 5, S297–S302. doi: 10.1513/AnnalsATS.201402-086AW

Hayes, D. Jr., Weiland, A., Kirkby, S., Galantowicz, M., McConnell, P. I., and Tobias, J. D. (2013). Gram-negative infection and bronchiectasis in lung transplant recipients with bronchiolitis obliterans syndrome. *Thorac. Cardiovasc. Surg.* 61, 240–245. doi: 10.1055/s-0032-1322619

Hussain, S. S., George, S., Singh, S., Jayant, R., Hu, C. A., Sopori, M., et al. (2018). A Small Molecule BH3-mimetic Suppresses Cigarette Smoke-Induced Mucous Expression in Airway Epithelial Cells. *Sci. Rep.* 8, 13796. doi: 10.1038/s41598-018-32114-w

Jiao, X., Nawab, O., Patel, T., Kossenkov, A. V., Halama, N., Jaeger, D., et al. (2019). Recent Advances Targeting CCR5 for Cancer and Its Role in Immuno-Oncology. *Cancer Res.* 79, 4801–4807. doi: 10.1158/0008-5472.CAN-19-1167

Khoja, S., Ojwang, P., Khan, S., Okinda, N., Harania, R., and Ali, S. (2008). Genetic analysis of HIV-1 subtypes in Nairobi, Kenya. *PloS One* 3, e3191. doi: 10.1371/journal.pone.0003191

Liszewski, M. K., Yu, J. J., and O'Doherty, U. (2009). Detecting HIV-1 integration by repetitive-sampling Alu-gag PCR. *Methods (San Diego Calif.)* 47, 254–260. doi: 10.1016/j.ymeth.2009.01.002

Liu, A., Yang, Y., Liu, L., Meng, Z., Li, L., Qiu, C., et al. (2014). Differential compartmentalization of HIV-targeting immune cells in inner and outer foreskin tissue. *PloS One* 9, e85176. doi: 10.1371/journal.pone.0085176

Ma, B., Liu, W., Homer, R. J., Lee, P. J., Coyle, A. J., Lora, J. M., et al. (2006). Role of CCR5 in the pathogenesis of IL-13-induced inflammation and remodeling. *J. Immunol.* 176, 4968–4978. doi: 10.4049/jimmunol.176.8.4968

Maitre, T., Cottenet, J., Beltramo, G., Georges, M., Blot, M., Piroth, L., et al. (2018). Increasing burden of noninfectious lung disease in persons living with HIV: a 7-year study using the French nationwide hospital administrative database. *Eur. Respir. J.* 52, 1800359. doi: 10.1183/13993003.00359-2018

Margolis, D. M., and Archin, N. M. (2017). Proviral Latency, Persistent Human Immunodeficiency Virus Infection, and the Development of Latency Reversing Agents. *J. Infect. Dis.* 215, S111–S118. doi: 10.1093/infdis/jiw618

Pasternak, A. O., Adema, K. W., Bakker, M., Jurriaans, S., Berkhout, B., Cornelissen, M., et al. (2008). Highly sensitive methods based on seminested real-time reverse transcription-PCR for quantitation of human immunodeficiency virus type 1 unspliced and multiply spliced RNA and proviral DNA. *J. Clin. Microbiol.* 46, 2206–2211. doi: 10.1128/JCM.00055-08

Poon, A. F., Swenson, L. C., Bunnik, E. M., Edo-Matas, D., Schuitemaker, H., van 't Wout, A. B., et al. (2012). Reconstructing the dynamics of HIV evolution within hosts from serial deep sequence data. *PloS Comput. Biol.* 8, e1002753. doi: 10.1371/journal.pcbi.1002753

Quentin, Y., and Fichant, G. A. (1994). Fast identification of repetitive elements in biological sequences. *J. Theor. Biol.* 166, 51–61. doi: 10.1006/jtbi.1994.1004

Rawlins, E. L., and Hogan, B. L. (2008). Ciliated epithelial cell lifespan in the mouse trachea and lung. *Am. J. Physiol. Lung Cell Mol. Physiol.* 295, L231–L234. doi: 10.1152/ajplung.90209.2008

Richman, D. D., Margolis, D. M., Delaney, M., Greene, W. C., Hazuda, D., and Pomerantz, R. J. (2009). The challenge of finding a cure for HIV infection. *Science* 323, 1304–1307. doi: 10.1126/science.1165706

Schmid, C. W. (1996). Alu: structure, origin, evolution, significance and function of one-tenth of human DNA. *Prog. Nucleic Acid Res. Mol. Biol.* 53, 283–319. doi: 10.1016/S0079-6603(08)60148-8

Sengupta, S., and Siliciano, R. F. (2018). Targeting the Latent Reservoir for HIV-1. *Immunity* 48, 872–895. doi: 10.1016/j.immuni.2018.04.030

Shugars, D. C., Smith, M. S., Glueck, D. H., Nantermet, P. V., Seillier-Moiseiwitsch, F., and Swanstrom, R. (1993). Analysis of human immunodeficiency virus type 1 nef gene sequences present in vivo. *J. Virol.* 67, 4639–4650. doi: 10.1128/JVI.67.8.4639-4650.1993

Singhvi, D., Bon, J., and Morris, A. (2019). Obstructive Lung Disease in HIV-Phenotypes and Pathogenesis. *Curr. HIV/AIDS Rep.* 16, 359–369. doi: 10.1007/s11904-019-00456-3

Takahama, S., and Yamamoto, T. (2020). Pattern Recognition Receptor Ligands as an Emerging Therapeutic Agent for Latent HIV-1 Infection. *Front. Cell Infect. Microbiol.* 10, 216. doi: 10.3389/fcimb.2020.00216

Vanhamel, J., Bruggemans, A., and Debyser, Z. (2019). Establishment of latent HIV-1 reservoirs: what do we really know? *J. Virus Erad.* 5, 3–9. doi: 10.1016/S2055-6640(20)30275-2

Wu, Q., Jiang, D., Minor, M. N., Martin, R. J., and Chu, H. W. (2011). In vivo function of airway epithelial TLR2 in host defense against bacterial infection. *Am. J. Physiol. Lung Cell Mol. Physiol.* 300, L579–L586. doi: 10.1152/ajplung.00336.2010

Yasen, A., Herrera, R., Rosbe, K., Lien, K., and Tugizov, S. M. (2017). Release of HIV-1 sequestered in the vesicles of oral and genital mucosal epithelial cells by epithelial-lymphocyte interaction. *PloS Pathog.* 13, e1006247. doi: 10.1371/journal.ppat.1006247

16

The Interplay of HIV and Autophagy in Early Infection

Romina Cabrera-Rodríguez[1], Silvia Pérez-Yanes[1], Judith Estévez-Herrera[1], Daniel Márquez-Arce[1], Cecilia Cabrera[2], Lucile Espert[3], Julià Blanco[2,4] and Agustín Valenzuela-Fernández[1]*

[1] Laboratorio de Inmunología Celular y Viral, Unidad de Farmacología, Sección de Medicina, Facultad de Ciencias de la Salud, e IUETSPC de la Universidad de La Laguna, Campus de Ofra s/n, Tenerife, Spain, [2] AIDS Research Institute IrsiCaixa, Institut de Recerca en Ciències de la Salut Germans Trias i Pujol (IGTP), Barcelona, Spain, [3] Institut de Recherche en Infectiologie de Montpellier, Université de Montpellier, CNRS, Montpellier, France, [4] Universitat de Vic-Central de Catalunya (UVIC-UCC), Catalonia, Spain

Correspondence:
Agustín Valenzuela-Fernández
avalenzu@ull.edu.es

HIV/AIDS is still a global threat despite the notable efforts made by the scientific and health communities to understand viral infection, to design new drugs or to improve existing ones, as well as to develop advanced therapies and vaccine designs for functional cure and viral eradication. The identification and analysis of HIV-1 positive individuals that naturally control viral replication in the absence of antiretroviral treatment has provided clues about cellular processes that could interact with viral proteins and RNA and define subsequent viral replication and clinical progression. This is the case of autophagy, a degradative process that not only maintains cell homeostasis by recycling misfolded/old cellular elements to obtain nutrients, but is also relevant in the innate and adaptive immunity against viruses, such as HIV-1. Several studies suggest that early steps of HIV-1 infection, such as virus binding to CD4 or membrane fusion, allow the virus to modulate autophagy pathways preparing cells to be permissive for viral infection. Confirming this interplay, strategies based on autophagy modulation are able to inhibit early steps of HIV-1 infection. Moreover, autophagy dysregulation in late steps of the HIV-1 replication cycle may promote autophagic cell-death of $CD4^+$ T cells or control of HIV-1 latency, likely contributing to disease progression and HIV persistence in infected individuals. In this scenario, understanding the molecular mechanisms underlying HIV/autophagy interplay may contribute to the development of new strategies to control HIV-1 replication. Therefore, the aim of this review is to summarize the knowledge of the interplay between autophagy and the early events of HIV-1 infection, and how autophagy modulation could impair or benefit HIV-1 infection and persistence, impacting viral pathogenesis, immune control of viral replication, and clinical progression of HIV-1 infected patients.

Keywords: HIV-1, autophagy, Env signaling, early infection, cell-death

INTRODUCTION

A General Overview of HIV: Factors Related to the Control of the Infection and Pathogenesis

According to the Global Human Immunodeficiency Virus (HIV) and Acquired Immune Deficiency Syndrome (AIDS) statistics report published in 2020 by UNAIDS (2020), there were around 38 million people living with HIV and 1.7 million new cases in 2019, and about 26 million people had access to the antiretroviral therapy (ART) at the end of June 2020. Most new infections and deaths are caused by HIV-1 subtype. Advances in science, accumulated experience in the field, along with active community and political commitment, mean that the public health threat of the HIV pandemic could be over by 2030, but there are still many social, economic and healthcare obstacles and inequalities to overcome (Colvin, 2011; UNAIDS, 2015; Poku, 2016). Due to active ART and associated medical achievements, the scientific community considers HIV/AIDS a chronic disease, mainly when access to effective care is assured (Forsyth and Valdiserri, 2012; McGrath et al., 2014).

Regardless of the above-mentioned achievements, ART does not eliminate the virus from latent reservoirs (Chun et al., 1997, 1998; Finzi et al., 1997; Perelson et al., 1997; Wong et al., 1997; Chun and Fauci, 1999; Davey et al., 1999; Hermankova et al., 2003; Siliciano and Greene, 2011; Rosenbloom et al., 2017), such as lymph nodes, gut associated lymphoid tissue (GALT), the central nervous system (CNS) or the most recent discovery of persistence in adipose tissue (Couturier and Lewis, 2018; van Marle et al., 2018). Latent reservoirs favor the emergence of new drug resistances which affect treatment adherence. Moreover, as HIV patients need long-term medication, metabolic concerns, tissue damage and associated aging emerge as a challenge for new drugs and ART regimes (Chawla et al., 2018; Gu et al., 2020). Thus, promising results have been obtained with pre-exposure prophylaxis (PrEP) strategies, which aim to prevent both HIV-1 infection and transmission and are highly dependent on patient adherence (Straubinger et al., 2019), or by using broadly neutralizing antibodies (bnAbs) that could achieve prolonged viral suppression by directly targeting different epitopes from key viral proteins and activating the immune response in order to remove Ab-targeted infected cells (Carrillo et al., 2018; Kumar et al., 2018; Grobben et al., 2019).

HIV-1 entry and early infection is mediated when the virus interacts with a main receptor in target cells, CD4, and a co-receptor, mainly CCR5 or CXCR4 which are involved in HIV-1 pathogenesis (Dalgleish et al., 1984; McDougal et al., 1985, 1986; Cocchi et al., 1995, 1996; Alkhatib et al., 1996; Bleul et al., 1996; Choe et al., 1996; Deng et al., 1996; Doranz et al., 1996, 1999; Dragic et al., 1996; Liu et al., 1996; Samson et al., 1996; Aramori et al., 1997; Davis et al., 1997; Farzan et al., 1997; Weissman et al., 1997; Blanco et al., 2000; Brelot et al., 2000; Clapham and McKnight, 2001; Chanel et al., 2002; Moore et al., 2004; Tuttle et al., 2004; Cavarelli et al., 2008; Cavarelli and Scarlatti, 2011; Gorry and Ancuta, 2011; Wilen et al., 2012; Melikyan, 2014). It should be mentioned that an effective cure for HIV-1 infection has been reported in two patients by *CCR5Δ32/Δ32*-hematopoietic stem cells (HSCs) transplantation, observing that latently infected cells were eliminated and replaced with HIV-1 resistant donor CCR5$^{-/-}$ cells (Hütter et al., 2009; Gupta et al., 2019). Although it is not possible to universally apply this method (Kordelas et al., 2014), it shows that HIV-1 can be eradicated from the organism (Hütter et al., 2009; Allers et al., 2011; Allers and Schneider, 2015; Haworth et al., 2017; Ambinder et al., 2020). In addition, a plethora of different strategies to keep the latent reservoir under control have been developed, from gene therapy to therapeutic vaccines (Rerks-Ngarm et al., 2009; Elliott et al., 2014; Henrich et al., 2014, 2017; Rasmussen et al., 2014; Luzuriaga et al., 2015; Søgaard et al., 2015; Zhu et al., 2015; Bar et al., 2016; Kaminski et al., 2016a,b; Kuritzkes, 2016; Scheid et al., 2016; Wang et al., 2016; Colby et al., 2018; Davenport et al., 2019).

The relationship between CCR5 or more precisely the lack of CCR5 expression and autophagy in the context of HIV-1 infection is not clear enough. It has been reported that HIV-1 envelope (Env) complex of proteins that targets cells through the cell-surface CCR5 receptor (i.e., R5-tropic Envs) triggers autophagy and cell death in bystander uninfected CD4$^+$ T cells, after long-term virus-cell contacts (Blanco et al., 2004; Espert et al., 2009). However, this autophagy cell death process is triggered by gp41-induced membrane fusion, and is independent of the co-receptor usage (Espert et al., 2009). Additionally, the role of CCR5 seems to differ in CD4$^+$ T cells and monocyte-differentiated macrophages (MDMs). CD4$^+$ T cells are susceptible to cell death induced by CXCR4 and CCR5 using viral strains and MDMs infected by CCR5-using viruses show weak autophagy activation and increased viral replication compared to MDMs infected with viral strains that use CXCR4 (Espert et al., 2009). This is consistent with the fact that CCR5-tropic viral strains are more infectious than CXCX4-tropic viral strains in MDMs (Schweighardt et al., 2004; Willey et al., 2005; Petrov et al., 2013; Wang et al., 2015; Bolduc et al., 2017; Quitadamo et al., 2018; Borrajo et al., 2019), and with the *in vivo* prevalence of viruses that utilize CCR5 in the majority of infected individuals (De Jong et al., 1992; Roos et al., 1992; Schuitemaker et al., 1992; Connor et al., 1993; Zhu et al., 1993; van't Wout et al., 1994; Cornelissen et al., 1995; Spijkerman et al., 1995; Huang et al., 1996; Reece et al., 1998; Keele and Derdeyn, 2009; Salazar-Gonzalez et al., 2009). Likewise, functional CCR5 reduced the expression of autophagy genes, such as *BECN1*, *ATG5* and *microtubule associated protein 1 light chain 3 (LC3) alpha* (*MAP1LC3A*), and promoted inflammation in an experimental asthmatic mouse model (Liu et al., 2021). Hence, an antagonist peptide of CCR5 enhances the mRNA levels of *BECN1*, *ATG5*, and *MAP1LC3A* and their proteins level, as well as double-membrane autophagic vesicles or vacuoles (AVs), thereby decreasing inflammation (Liu et al., 2021). These AVs are considered hallmarks of autophagy (Arstila and Trump, 1968; Punnonen et al., 1989; Dunn, 1990a,b; Liou et al., 1997; Mizushima et al., 2002; Zhou et al., 2016), the autophagosomes. Therefore, it is plausible that the lack of CCR5 expression could be associated with a fully active autophagy process presenting a protective phenotype against X4-tropic viral strains. Thus, functional CCR5 appears to be involved in autophagy inhibition during HIV infection with R5-tropic strains. However, HIV-1 mediated cell-death autophagy by long-term non-infectious HIV-1 Env/cell contacts is independent of CCR5 (Espert et al., 2009). Therefore, the CCR5/HIV-1/autophagy interplay and its role in viral life cycle is a complex and active subject of research (reviewed in Espert et al., 2008).

One noteworthy discovery in the HIV-1 pandemic history is the existence of infected individuals that naturally control the viral replication for longer than 10 years in the absence of ART, known as long-term non-progressors (LTNP; Lambotte et al., 2005). Briefly, depending on the clinical progression of the disease, there are different groups of LTNP HIV$^+$ individuals: the elite controllers (LTNP-EC), with HIV-1 RNA plasma levels below the level of detection (less than 50 copies of HIV-1 RNA/mL), viremic controllers (LTNP-VC) with HIV-1 RNA levels equal to or below 2,000 copies/mL, non-controllers (LTNP-NC) with levels above 2,000 copies/mL and viremic non-progressors (VNP) with more than 10,000 copies/mL and normal levels of CD4$^+$ T lymphocytes (Lambotte et al., 2005; Diop et al., 2006; Deeks and Walker, 2007; Canducci et al., 2009; Grabar et al., 2009; Lajoie et al., 2009; Limou et al., 2009; Okulicz et al., 2009; Casado et al., 2010, 2018; Rotger et al., 2010; Zhang et al., 2010; Gurdasani et al., 2014; Cabrera-Rodriguez et al., 2019). Nevertheless, despite being controllers, there is evidence of ongoing viral replication in LTNP-EC (Blankson et al., 2007; Lamine et al., 2007; Dinoso et al., 2008; Migueles et al., 2008; Pereyra et al., 2008, 2009; Hatano et al., 2009; Julg et al., 2010; Mens et al., 2010; O'Connell et al., 2010; Salgado et al., 2010; Zaunders et al., 2011; Noel et al., 2016; Ali et al., 2018; Casado et al., 2018; Woldemeskel et al., 2020), and this endorses the importance of periodically monitoring these patients. The causes of this viral replication control are diverse and may be due to both host and viral factors, thereby making it difficult to establish a precise cause for the natural control of HIV. The viral factors include replicative capacity, infectivity, tropism, virulence, mutation rate, viral load or genetic variants in different genes. This is the case of the Australian cohort characterized by invalidating alterations in the *nef* gene or the Spanish LTNP-C cluster with a heritable conserved non-functional *env* gene, which is responsible for the low binding of the viral Env complex to CD4, inefficient cell-signaling and subsequent impaired fusion, infection and viral transmission capacities (Zaunders et al., 2011; Casado et al., 2018; Lopez-Galindez et al., 2019; López-Galíndez, 2019). Likewise, LTNP phenotypes are usually associated with genetic factors in the host related to immune control in viral replication and reservoir generation (Pereyra et al., 2010; Poropatich and Sullivan, 2011; Whittall et al., 2011; Buckheit et al., 2012; Bullen et al., 2014; Colomer-Lluch et al., 2018; Goulder and Deeks, 2018; Lopez-Galindez et al., 2019). HLA alleles are well known genetic markers associated with protection or progressive disease, but *CCR5-Δ32* allelic deletions or forkhead box O3a (FOXO3) mutations are also linked with the survival of memory CD4$^+$ T cells (de Roda Husman et al., 1997; Eugen-Olsen et al., 1997; Pasi et al., 2000; Dabrowska et al., 2008; van Grevenynghe et al., 2008; Casado et al., 2010; López-Galíndez, 2019). Cell antiviral restriction factors are a first line of defense against viral infection, replication and spreading, such as the tripartite motif-containing protein 5 alpha isoform (TRIM5α), SAM and HD domain containing deoxynucleoside triphosphate triphosphohydrolase 1 (SAMHD1), tetherin or BST2 (bone marrow stromal cell antigen 2), apolipoprotein B mRNA editing enzyme, catalytic polypeptide-like (APOBEC) proteins or histone deacetylase 6 (HDAC6; Valenzuela-Fernandez et al., 2005; Valera et al., 2015; Soliman et al., 2017; Marrero-Hernández et al., 2019). In this regard, proautophagic HDAC6 has recently been reported to be closely linked to HIV-1 control (Valenzuela-Fernandez et al., 2005, 2008; Valera et al., 2015; Casado et al., 2018; Marrero-Hernández et al., 2019), similar to other proteins implicated in the autophagy process (Rotger et al., 2011; Nardacci et al., 2014, 2017), opening up a new pathway to control HIV-1 infection. Thus, recent data are addressed below that indicate that non-functional *env*-gene of viruses from LTNP-EC individuals is responsible for a defect in Env-mediated productive signaling to overcome the barrier of HDAC6, an autophagy-related factor which blocks HIV-1 fusion, transmission and early infection (Casado et al., 2018). Therefore, the capacity of primary viral Env to signal and overcome this proautophagic restriction factor, at the early stage of the viral life cycle, is related to the progressor phenotype of HIV$^+$ patients (Casado et al., 2018; Cabrera-Rodriguez et al., 2019), whereas non-functional viral Envs are associated with viruses of HIV$^+$ individuals presenting the LTNP-EC phenotype (Casado et al., 2018).

Autophagy and HIV

Autophagy is a complex and orchestrated degradative process that maintains cell homeostasis, eliminating misfolded/old elements and recycling them to obtain nutrients, and is also relevant in the innate and adaptive immunity against pathogen infection, including viruses (Liang et al., 1998, 2014; Meléndez et al., 2003; Pinan-Lucarré et al., 2003; Gutierrez et al., 2004; Nakagawa et al., 2004; Dengjel et al., 2005; Ogawa et al., 2005; Paludan et al., 2005; Birmingham et al., 2006; Hara et al., 2006; Komatsu et al., 2006, 2007; Jounai et al., 2007; Kohda et al., 2007; Lee et al., 2007; Nakai et al., 2007; Nishiyama et al., 2007; Py et al., 2007; Nedjic et al., 2008; Dupont et al., 2009; English et al., 2009; Fujita et al., 2009; Masiero et al., 2009; Yamaguchi et al., 2009; Zhang et al., 2009b; Lee H.K. et al., 2010; Liu et al., 2010; Orvedahl et al., 2010; Ponpuak et al., 2010; Travassos et al., 2010; Levine et al., 2011; Benjamin et al., 2013; Randow and Youle, 2014; Sagnier et al., 2015; Valera et al., 2015; Dasari et al., 2016; Hu et al., 2016; Paul and Münz, 2016; Staring et al., 2017; Viret et al., 2018; Oh and Lee, 2019; Dong et al., 2021).

In mammalian cells autophagosome formation is initiated by signals that activate the mammalian autophagy-related 1 (ATG1) homologs, unc-51 like autophagy activating kinase 1 (ULK1) and ULK2 (Kuroyanagi et al., 1998; Yan et al., 1998, 1999; Tomoda et al., 1999; Young et al., 2006; Chan et al., 2007; Kundu et al., 2008; Egan et al., 2011; Chan, 2012). The mammalian ULK complex is formed by the serin/threonin protein kinase ULK1 and ULK2, ATG13, ATG101, and RB1CC1 (RB1-inducible coiled-coil protein 1) (named FIP200, focal adhesion kinase family interacting protein of 200 kDa) (Hosokawa et al., 2009; Jung et al., 2009; Mercer et al., 2009; Noda and Fujioka,

2015; Qi et al., 2015). This complex initiates the formation of the phagophore, a shaped double membrane structure, which elongates to engulf cytoplasmic components, and finally closes to form an autophagosome (Hara et al., 2008; Chan, 2009; Nakatogawa et al., 2009; Yang and Klionsky, 2010; Weidberg et al., 2011b). The ULK complex is then located in phagophores (Hara et al., 2008) where it regulates the initial events of autophagosome formation together with the class III phosphatidylinositol 3-kinase catalytic subunit type 3 (PIK3C3) complex, consisting of BECN1 (named beclin 1 or ATG6), ATG14 (also named ATG14L), PIK3C3 (named VPS34), and PIK3R4 (phosphoinositide-3-kinase regulatory subunit 4) (named VPS15) (Hara et al., 2008; Itakura et al., 2008; Liang et al., 2008; Ganley et al., 2009; Hosokawa et al., 2009; Jung et al., 2009; Matsunaga et al., 2009; Mercer et al., 2009; Zhong et al., 2009; Yang and Klionsky, 2010). Of note, the ULK complex is negatively regulated by the mechanistic target of rapamycin complex 1 or mammalian target of rapamycin complex 1 (MTORC1, named mTORC1)-mediated phosphorylation of ULK1, ULK2, and ATG13 (Ganley et al., 2009; Hosokawa et al., 2009; Jung et al., 2009), whereas the activity of the BECN1-PIK3C3 complex could be regulated by its interaction with several cofactors, such as UVRAG (UV radiation resistance associated), ATG14 and AMBRA1 (autophagy and beclin 1 regulator 1) (Matsunaga et al., 2009; Zhong et al., 2009; Di Bartolomeo et al., 2010; Mizushima et al., 2011). The elongation of the phagophore needs the recruitment of different factors, such as the WD-repeat protein interacting with phosphoinositides (WIPI) family proteins (yeast ATG18 homologs), ATG2 and the transmembrane protein ATG9 (Lang et al., 2000; Jeffries et al., 2004; Proikas-Cezanne et al., 2004; Young et al., 2006; Obara et al., 2008; Longatti and Tooze, 2009; Polson et al., 2010; Mauthe et al., 2011; Dooley et al., 2014; Grimmel et al., 2015; Gómez-Sánchez et al., 2018; Osawa et al., 2019; Tang et al., 2019; Bozic et al., 2020; Matoba et al., 2020; Sawa-Makarska et al., 2020). The ubiquitin-like (Ubl) conjugation reaction is also required for elongation of the phagophore and involves the conjugation of ATG12 to ATG5 which recruits autophagy related 16 like 1 (ATG16L1) (previous name ATG16L) (Mizushima et al., 1999, 2003; Kuma et al., 2002; Hanada et al., 2007; Walczak and Martens, 2013; Fahmy and Labonté, 2017; Harada et al., 2019; Karow et al., 2020). Furthermore, this complex is able to associate with ATG8 family proteins, thereby allowing ATG8 proteins to conjugate to phosphatidylethanolamine on the phagophore membrane (Nakatogawa et al., 2007). In mammals, there are at least seven ATG8 family members, such as MAP1LC3A and MAP1LC3B, with two isoforms of MAP1LC3B: gamma-aminobutyric acid receptor-associated protein (GABARAP) and GABARAP like 1 and 2 (GABARAPL1 and GABARAPL2) (Xin et al., 2001; He et al., 2003; Weidberg et al., 2010, 2011a; Shpilka et al., 2011; Shvets et al., 2011). Both MAP1LC3A/B and GABARAP subfamily members are conjugated to the phagophore (Kabeya et al., 2000, 2004) and required for the formation of the autophagosome (Weidberg et al., 2010). Additionally, ULK1, ATG13, and RB1CC1 (members of the UKL1 complex) have been reported to interact with members of the MAP1LC3A/B family of proteins (Alemu et al., 2012; Suzuki et al., 2014). Then, phosphorylation of several of these factors by ULK1 initiates the nucleation process and autophagosome biogenesis (Ganley et al., 2009; Hosokawa et al., 2009; Jung et al., 2009). The outer membrane of autophagosomes then fuses with a lysosome allowing lysosomal hydrolytic enzymes to degrade the intra-autophagosomal components together with the inner membrane. Finally, selective autophagy clearance of different cargos is driven by their association with several factors that are recruited to the inner surface of the phagophore via their LC3-interacting region (LIR) motifs, such as sequestosome 1 (SQSTM1)/p62, NBR1 [neighbor of breast cancer 1 (NBR1) autophagy cargo receptor; also named neighbor of BRCA1 gene 1] and OPTN (optineurin) (Pankiv et al., 2007; Ichimura et al., 2008; Kirkin et al., 2009; Wild et al., 2011).

Furthermore, as introduced above, autophagy could act as a first innate immune barrier against invading viruses, clearing them, and also being part of the immune response by means of antigen presentation by major histocompatibility complex (MHC) or human leukocyte antigen (HLA) class I and class II molecules (Brazil et al., 1997; Nimmerjahn et al., 2003; Dengjel et al., 2005; Dörfel et al., 2005; Paludan et al., 2005; Zhou et al., 2005; Zwart et al., 2005; Schmid et al., 2007; Li et al., 2008; Gannage and Münz, 2010; Tey and Khanna, 2012; Bell et al., 2013; Valečka et al., 2018). In this respect, different research studies have tried to develop vaccines in order to promote immune presentation of viral proteins through the autophagy degradation pathway (Andersen et al., 2016). However, autophagy/virus interplay is complex as pathogens have evolved strategies to inhibit or use autophagy to their own benefit. Thus, this process can be either favoring or blocking viral replication (Lee et al., 2007; Denizot et al., 2008; Zhou and Spector, 2008; Espert et al., 2009; Joubert et al., 2009; Kyei et al., 2009; Blanchet et al., 2010; Grégoire et al., 2011, 2012; Levine et al., 2011; Bhatt and Damania, 2012; Chaumorcel et al., 2012; Campbell and Spector, 2013; Liang et al., 2013; Richetta et al., 2013; Jackson, 2015; Valera et al., 2015; Mailler et al., 2019; Mao et al., 2019; Marrero-Hernández et al., 2019; Chen et al., 2020).

Autophagy has become relevant in HIV-1 infection, since it is clearly involved in the late stages of the viral life cycle (i.e., replication and viral egress), preventingviral infection in CD4^{+} T cells and favoring viral replication in macrophages (Zhou and Spector, 2008; Espert et al., 2009; Kyei et al., 2009; Valera et al., 2015; Mailler et al., 2019; Marrero-Hernández et al., 2019; Chen et al., 2020).

The sections below describe scientific data concerning the role of autophagy in the first steps of HIV-1 infection, presented from two points of view: (i) the ability of the virus to modulate autophagy during viral entry and infection and (ii) the consequences of autophagy modulation, in target cells, for early HIV-1 infection.

THE ROLE OF AUTOPHAGY IN THE EARLY STEPS OF HIV-1 INFECTION

The HIV-1 life cycle could be divided into early and late stages, defined by the integration of viral genome into host cells. The early (pre-integration) steps of the infection begin with the attachment of the virion at the cell-surface and end with the integration of the proviral DNA into the host genome (Arhel, 2010; Campbell and Hope, 2015; Deeks et al., 2015; Goodsell, 2015). The late stages (post-integration) initiate with proviral transcription, assembly of viral components at cell-surface, viral egress, and maturation (Stevenson, 2003; Sutton et al., 2013; Deeks et al., 2015; Freed, 2015; Goodsell, 2015; Mailler et al., 2016). The HIV life cycle could end with cell death of infected cells or by HIV-1 Env-mediated cell death of uninfected bystander cells (Mohammadi et al., 2013; Cummins and Badley, 2014; Doitsh and Greene, 2016; Li et al., 2020) which occurs during early infection (Espert et al., 2008, 2009). Hence, one of the most relevant HIV-1 modulators of cell death is the Env glycoprotein (Krüger et al., 1996; Blanco et al., 2001; Vlahakis et al., 2001; Garg and Blumenthal, 2006, 2008; Varbanov et al., 2006; Garg et al., 2009; Sivaraman et al., 2009; Gorry and Ancuta, 2011; Cicala et al., 2016; Joshi et al., 2016; Tsao et al., 2016; Evering, 2018; Daussy et al., 2020).

The HIV-1 *env*-gene encodes the Env glycoprotein precursor (gp160), which, upon cleavage by the furin cellular protease, results in the generation of the gp120 surface and the gp41 transmembrane glycoproteins that assemble in trimer to form the active Env complex (Decroly et al., 1994, 1997; Moulard et al., 1999; Staropoli et al., 2000; Checkley et al., 2011; Wilen et al., 2012; Chung et al., 2014; Melikyan, 2014; Ward and Wilson, 2017; Schneck et al., 2020). During HIV-1 entry, the viral surface gp120 subunit of the Env binds to CD4 and CCR5 or CXCR4 key co-receptor (Dalgleish et al., 1984; McDougal et al., 1985, 1986; Cocchi et al., 1995, 1996; Alkhatib et al., 1996; Bleul et al., 1996; Choe et al., 1996; Deng et al., 1996; Doranz et al., 1996, 1999; Dragic et al., 1996; Liu et al., 1996; Samson et al., 1996; Aramori et al., 1997; Davis et al., 1997; Farzan et al., 1997; Weissman et al., 1997; Blanco et al., 2000; Brelot et al., 2000; Clapham and McKnight, 2001; Chanel et al., 2002; Moore et al., 2004; Tuttle et al., 2004; Cavarelli et al., 2008; Cavarelli and Scarlatti, 2011; Gorry and Ancuta, 2011; Wilen et al., 2012; Colin et al., 2013, 2018; Melikyan, 2014; Shaik et al., 2019). Hence, HIV-1 Env is responsible for virus attachment to target cells, membrane fusion and subsequent genome-bearing capsid entry into the cytoplasm, thereby initiating the productive infection process (Markosyan et al., 2003; Chang et al., 2005; Dobrowsky et al., 2008; Wilen et al., 2012; Melikyan, 2014; Sood et al., 2017; Stultz et al., 2017; Iliopoulou et al., 2018; Chen, 2019). During these steps, HIV-1 Env-mediated signals prepare cells to be efficiently infected, where membrane dynamics and intracellular organelles and cytoskeleton reorganization could account for permissive control in early infection (Blanco et al., 2003; Jolly and Sattentau, 2004; Jolly et al., 2004; Valenzuela-Fernandez et al., 2005; Jimenez-Baranda et al., 2007; Barrero-Villar et al., 2008, 2009; Yoder et al., 2008; Liu et al., 2009; Puigdomenech et al., 2009; Garcia-Exposito et al., 2011, 2013; Stolp and Fackler, 2011; Vorster et al., 2011; de Armas-Rillo et al., 2016; Casado et al., 2018; Cabrera-Rodriguez et al., 2019). HIV-1 Env-induced autophagy would therefore be a good way to regulate early steps of the viral life cycle.

The interplay between early HIV-1 infection and autophagy is presented below by mainly focusing on the effects driven by the viral Env, and considering different studies performed in permissive cell types and/or tissues, such as T lymphocytes, peripheral blood mononuclear cells (PBMCs), macrophages and dendritic cells (DCs), and in the central nervous system (CNS).

HIV-1 Env-Mediated Regulation of Autophagy and Related Factors During Early Infection in T Lymphocytes

Although HIV-1 induction of apoptosis in bystander CD4$^+$ T cells was reported to be driven by Env glycoproteins, gp120 and gp41 (Blanco et al., 2003), Env-mediated autophagy during HIV-1 early infection was first described in 2006 (Espert et al., 2006). It was reported that Env-transfected or HIV-infected cells expressing the viral Env complex at the cell-surface induced autophagy and accumulation of BECN1 in uninfected CD4$^+$ T lymphocytes via CXCR4 (Espert et al., 2006), where these autophagy events induce apoptosis in bystander CD4$^+$ cells (Espert et al., 2006). The autophagic machinery is activated after long-lasting interaction of uninfected CD4$^+$ T lymphocytes with Env expressed at the cell-surface of X4-tropic HIV-1 infected cells, thus accumulating the BECN1/ATG6 protein which regulates the mechanism interacting with PIK3 class III (Espert et al., 2006, 2007). These reports further highlighted that CD4 signaling and tyrosine-protein kinase Lck (LCK; named LCK proto-oncogene, Src family tyrosine kinase or p56^{lck}) were not required and that autophagy was necessary for apoptosis to be induced. Moreover, CXCR4 or CCR5 signaling does not seem to be involved in HIV-1 Env-induced autophagy, which is dependent on the gp41 fusion capacity (Blanco et al., 2003; Denizot et al., 2008). These results suggest that HIV-mediated autophagic cell-death of bystander CD4$^+$ T lymphocytes is a mechanism that could contribute to immunodeficiency.

It should also be mentioned that autophagy can be also induced by R5-tropic HIV-1 Env upon binding to bystander, uninfected CCR5$^+$/CD4$^+$ T cells, whereas it is inhibited in CD4$^+$ T cells that are infected either by X4-tropic or R5-tropic viral strains (Molina et al., 2007).

Furthermore, after contact between CD4$^+$ T lymphocytes and Env-expressing cells, reactive oxygen species (ROS) are accumulated and its production is known to be involved in autophagy (Molina et al., 2007; Borel et al., 2012). It has recently been reported that peroxisomes, organelles involved in the control of oxidative stress, are targeted by Env-mediated autophagy, inducing oxidative stress and this leads to uninfected CD4$^+$ T cells death (Daussy et al., 2020).

Another aspect of HIV-1 infection and autophagy is that this retrovirus is also able to manipulate the process in order to survive. A new study in CD4$^+$ T lymphocytes has shown that autophagy is rapidly controlled after HIV-1 entry by the viral protein R (Vpr) which reduces the amount of essential autophagy ATG proteins, such as MAP1LC3 and BECN1, and the autophagy-related protein BNIP3 (BCL2 interacting protein 3) and their mRNA, and is further implicated in the degradation of a transcription factor FOXO3 (Alfaisal et al., 2019).

HIV-1 Env Modulates Autophagy and Related Factors Associated With Membrane and Cytoskeleton Dynamics, Key Events for Productive Early Infection

Autophagy is a paradigm of the cellular membrane dynamics driven by cytoskeleton components and other associated factors (Aplin et al., 1992; Fass et al., 2006; Axe et al., 2008; Nakatogawa et al., 2009; Hailey et al., 2010; Lee J.Y. et al., 2010; Mari et al., 2010; Ravikumar et al., 2010; Aguilera et al., 2012; Longatti and Tooze, 2012; Yamamoto et al., 2012; Ge et al., 2013; Knævelsrud et al., 2013; Puri et al., 2013; Zhuo et al., 2013; Coutts and La Thangue, 2015; Kast and Dominguez, 2015; Kast et al., 2015; Mi et al., 2015; de Armas-Rillo et al., 2016; Galluzzi et al., 2017a; Morel, 2020). Similarly, there are data that point to membrane dynamics being essential for successful HIV-1 entry and infection, but the mechanisms behind these events are complex and likely involve several factors. Thus, phosphatidylinositol (4,5)-bisphosphate (PIP_2) is a second messenger that has been demonstrated to be important not only in the HIV-1 viral egress but also in the entry, synthetized by phosphatidylinositol-4-phosphate 5-kinase type Iα (PIP5K1A), after Env-gp120 interaction with $CD4^+$ T lymphocyte (Barrero-Villar et al., 2008). Another cell factor that works in membrane dynamics is ADP ribosylation factor 6 (ARF6; Radhakrishna and Donaldson, 1997; Franco et al., 1999; Donaldson, 2003; Naslavsky et al., 2003; Aikawa and Martin, 2005; Donaldson and Honda, 2005), a GTPase which plays a role in the PIP_2 generation (Honda et al., 1999; Toda et al., 1999; Brown et al., 2001; Santy and Casanova, 2001; Powner and Wakelam, 2002; Aikawa and Martin, 2005; Bach et al., 2010). ARF6 promotes autophagosome biogenesis, since it works favoring endocytic uptake of the plasma membrane into autophagosome precursors (Moreau et al., 2012), exerting a vital function for effective and productive viral entry (Garcia-Exposito et al., 2011).

In the context of cytoskeleton dynamics, actin adaptors and enzymes that reorganize, stabilize and sever cortical F-actin, such as MSN (moesin), FLNA (filamin A), and GSN (gelsolin) have been involved in early infection, and are responsible for pore fusion and viral entry (Jimenez-Baranda et al., 2007; Barrero-Villar et al., 2009; Garcia-Exposito et al., 2013). Tubulin cytoskeleton and associated factors also play a crucial role in driving membrane dynamics, as reported for cytoplasmic tubulin-deacetylase HDAC6 that controls pore fusion formation and viral entry (Valenzuela-Fernandez et al., 2005, 2008). Viral Env mediates acetylation of α-tubulin in order to allow a reorganization of the tubulin cytoskeleton and efficient pore fusion formation (Valenzuela-Fernandez et al., 2005; Casado et al., 2018). On the contrary, over-expression of HDAC6, which is located in the cytoplasm and regulates deacetylation of α-tubulin in stable microtubules (Hubbert et al., 2002; Valenzuela-Fernandez et al., 2008), inhibits HIV-1 Env-mediated tubulin acetylation, thereby preventing HIV-1 Env-dependent cell fusion and infection (Valenzuela-Fernandez et al., 2005).

Moreover, HDAC6 plays an important role in clearing accumulated protein aggregates, potentially toxic for cells by autophagy (Kawaguchi et al., 2003; Kopito, 2003). The C-terminal ubiquitin-binding ZnF-UBP zinc finger domain (ZnF-UBP or BUZ domain) of HDAC6 binds free ubiquitin as well as mono- and polyubiquitinated proteins with high affinity (Seigneurin-Berny et al., 2001; Hook et al., 2002; Kawaguchi et al., 2003; Boyault et al., 2006), facilitating the transport of ubiquitinated misfolded proteins to form an aggresome in a microtubule network dependent manner (Kawaguchi et al., 2003). In addition, HDAC6 is directly involved in autophagy by promoting the removal of aggresomes (Kawaguchi et al., 2003; Iwata et al., 2005; Pandey et al., 2007; Lee J.Y. et al., 2010). In fact, HDAC6 controls the fusion of autophagosomes and lysosomes by recruiting cortactin, and other key components for actin reorganization, thereby triggering clearance of autophagic substrates (Lee J.Y. et al., 2010). In an HIV-1 context, HDAC6 regulates infectivity of nascent HIV-1 virions by interacting with APOBEC subunit 3G (APOBEC3G; named A3G), stabilizing it and promoting the autophagic degradation of the HIV-1 infectivity factor Vif, thereby impairing the incorporation of Vif in nascent viral particles (Valera et al., 2015; Marrero-Hernández et al., 2019). Moreover, HDAC6 acts as a restriction factor, limiting viral production and infection by driving $Pr55^{Gag}$ and Vif viral proteins to degradation through an aggresome/autophagy route (Marrero-Hernández et al., 2019). Thus, for HIV-1, targeting HDAC6 appears to be critical for assuring viral production and virus infectivity, and this could be a key proinfective function of Nef. Hence, HDAC6 is counteracted by functional Nef which drives its clearance by an acidic, endocytic/lysosomal pathway. In this regard, Nef assures viral production and infection by targeting HDAC6, stabilizing $Pr55^{Gag}$ and Vif, thereby facilitating $Pr55^{Gag}$ location and aggregation at the plasma membrane and subsequent virus production and infection capacity (Marrero-Hernández et al., 2019).

Therefore, the interplay between Nef and HDAC6 may be important to determine the course of HIV-1 infection and pathogenesis in infected individuals, and may contribute to the development of new strategies against HIV.

The Ability of HIV-1 Env of Virus From Infected Individuals to Subvert or Not Autophagy-Associated Factors Is Related to the Patient Phenotype

It has recently been shown that inefficient HIV-1 Env functions and signaling may contribute to the low viral replication capacity and transmissibility of the viruses from natural controllers (LTNP-ECs) (Casado et al., 2013). Furthermore, the contribution of common viral features to the clinical LTNP-EC phenotype and a functional characterization of the initial events of the viral infection demonstrated that Envs from virus of LTNP-EC individuals were ineffective in the binding to CD4 and in the key triggering of actin/tubulin-cytoskeleton modifications, compared to Envs from viruses of $HIV-1^+$ chronic patients (Casado et al., 2018). The viral properties of the cluster viruses result in defective viral fusion, entry, and infection, and these properties were inherited by every virus in the cluster (Casado et al., 2018). Along the same lines, another study that compared Env clones from virus of VNP patients with those from rapid progressors (RPs), revealed that both groups of primary viral Envs induced autophagy in bystander uninfected CD4$^+$ T cells after 3 days of co-culture (Cabrera-Rodriguez et al., 2019). These results were demonstrated after long-lasting cell-to-cell experiments, and were entirely different to first HIV-1-cell contact and signaling to productive early infection (Casado et al., 2018), as this type of late transmission activates different mechanisms such as apoptosis and linked autophagy, leading to an increase in MAP1LC3 and cell-death (Espert et al., 2007; Cabrera-Rodriguez et al., 2019).

Related to the above deadly autophagy activation by HIV-1 Env, it has been reported that viral Env activates peroxisome degradation with a concomitant decrease in the expression of peroxisomal proteins [i.e., CAT (catalase) and PEX14 (peroxisomal biogenesis factor 14; also named peroxin 14)], which appears to be autophagy dependent, since down-regulation of BECN1 and SQSTM1/p62 restores their expression levels (Daussy et al., 2020). It is noteworthy that late autophagy occurrence is reported to be independent of the HIV-1 infected phenotype, VNP or RP, but it strongly correlated with the fusogenic capacity of viral Envs (Cabrera-Rodriguez et al., 2019). This means that functional viral Envs promote deadly late autophagy, under these experimental conditions, regardless of the HIV-1$^+$ patients' phenotype, and is directly related to the infectious capacity of the HIV-1 Envs. In this regard, inefficient primary HIV-1 Envs from LTNP-EC individuals are not able to signal and surpass the blockade exerted by the proautophagic, tubulin-deacetylase HDAC6 function. However, functional HIV-1 Envs from VNP or RP patients manage to signalize, overcoming the tubulin-deacetylase HDAC6 protective barrier and infect (Casado et al., 2018; Cabrera-Rodriguez et al., 2019). Therefore, this is the first evidence that a defect of the viral Env from HIV-1$^+$ natural controllers to signal and neutralize the proautophagic factor HDAC6 is related to a defect in infection, virus variability and the LTNP-EC phenotype.

Regarding the above-mentioned ideas, the association between autophagy events, viremic control in HIV$^+$ individuals and the progression of the disease suggests a new clinical perspective for HIV/AIDS. In this regard, it has been reported that LTNP and LTNP-EC phenotypes have PBMCs with a higher amount of AVs together with an increased expression of autophagic factors with respect to normal progressors (Nardacci et al., 2014). Additionally, this work shows that treatment of PBMC isolated from LTNP-EC individuals with rapamycin, an inhibitor of the MTOR, promotes autophagy, resulting in the impairment of viral production (Nardacci et al., 2014). Of note, in humanized mouse models, pan-inhibitors of the MTORC1 inhibit HIV-1 infection by interfering with virus entry, reducing CCR5 levels, and with transcription (Heredia et al., 2015). These data suggest that autophagy could contribute to the control of viral pathogenesis in HIV-1 viremic controllers (LTNP and LTNP-EC) and interfere with CCR5-mediated virus transmission, thereby constituting a potential target to drive the development of new therapies (Nardacci et al., 2014).

Autophagy and Early HIV-1 Infection in Macrophages and Dendritic Cells

It is noteworthy that autophagy-associated cell-death is not similarly induced in uninfected macrophages, following exposure to viral particles (van Grol et al., 2010), despite being positive for the presence of autophagosomes (Espert et al., 2009), suggesting that Env-mediated autophagy is a cell-dependent process. However, it is important to bear in mind that during macrophage entry of the virus, other molecules are involved in the reorganization of membrane proteins necessary for HIV-1 entry, such as ceramides, integrins and heparan sulfate proteoglycan, with a demonstrated role of ceramides as inducers of autophagy that could eclipse the pro-autophagic functions of the HIV-1 Env/main receptor interplay (Finnegan et al., 2004; Borel et al., 2012). Furthermore, blockade of macrophage-autophagy appears to be a barrier for HIV-1, since viral replication is favored by inducing autophagy in infected macrophages (Kyei et al., 2009) and autophagy inhibition in infected macrophages abrogates viral replication (Espert et al., 2009; Kyei et al., 2009).

In DCs, HIV-1 induces a rapid shutdown of autophagy as HIV-1 Env activates the MTOR pathways, increasing cell-associated HIV-1 and transfer of the virus to CD4$^+$ T cells and, thus, altering autophagy initiation leading to progressive autophagy exhaustion (Blanchet et al., 2010). In this regard, it has been demonstrated that fusion between endosomes and autophagosomes is inhibited during early HIV-1 infection by activation of MTOR, which is a negative regulator of autophagy (Altfeld et al., 2011). HIV-1 Env can activate the MTORC1 complex resulting in efficient viral replication and viral production. In fact, HIV-1 infection increases MTORC1 activity in both productively infected and bystander cells (Akbay et al., 2020).

On the contrary, it has been reported that autophagy is activated during HIV-1 infection in DCs. HIV-1 enters these cells by using C-type lectins as a receptor, and once inside the cell its RNA is recognized by toll-like receptors (TLRs), inducing the immune response and the beginning of the autophagy process. Although these events are under discussion, there is a clear-cut relationship between this viral recognition and the activation of the immune response together with the antiviral autophagy (Lee et al., 2007; Delgado et al., 2008; Shi and Kehrl, 2008; Blanchet et al., 2010; Altfeld et al., 2011; Nakamoto et al., 2012).

Autophagy and HIV-1 Infection in the Central Nervous System

The CNS is also attacked by HIV-1 and, even under ART, at least half of HIV-1 positive individuals present associated neurocognitive disorders (HAND) with progressive neurotoxicity, neurodegeneration, and a chronic activation of the inflammatory response, but it is difficult to study and is a matter of controversy how HIV-1 manages to reach the CNS and how it infects different cell types (reviewed in Rojas-Celis et al., 2019). Autophagy is involved in both neuroprotection and neurodegeneration, but some research data support the hypothesis that the dysregulation of autophagy during HIV-1 infection is important in the pathogenesis of the neuropathology associated with AIDS.

At a more physiologically relevant level, it has been reported that the levels of several key autophagy factors, such as BECN1, ATG5, ATG7 and the membrane-associated MAP1LC3-phosphatidylethanolamine conjugate (named LC3-II) were higher in postmortem brains presenting HIV-1 encephalitis, compared with HIV-1 patients without encephalitis (Zhou et al., 2011). Additionally, these authors confirmed that overexpression of both X4- or R5-tropic gp120 increased the presence of these autophagy markers. The study further suggests that HIV-1 gp120 induces autophagy in neuron cells, and that the induction of autophagy might be related to the pathogenesis of neuroAIDS (Zhou et al., 2011).

Furthermore, a study carried out on primary human fetal astrocytes revealed that the HIV-1 Env subunit gp120 induced the expression of interleukin 6 (IL6) [named IFNB2 (interferon, beta 2)] through nuclear factor-kappa B (NFKB; named NF-κB) (Shah et al., 2011). This NFKB1-associated signal triggered the expression of some autophagy genes, such as *BECN1*, *ATG5*, and *MAP1LC3* whose proteins translocate from cytoplasm to the nucleus, and induce the phosphorylation of the inhibitory kappa B (IκB) factor (NFKB inhibitor), which promotes the autophagy degradative pathway (Copetti et al., 2009; Nivon et al., 2009, 2012; Zhang et al., 2009a; Romano et al., 2010; Jiang et al., 2011; Meng and Cai, 2011; Shah et al., 2011; Bhatnagar et al., 2012; Verzella et al., 2020). This event has also been reported in astrocytes, where HIV-1 gp120 increases CXCL8 (named IL8) production involving NFKB (Shah and Kumar, 2010). There have also been some works implicating HIV-1 gp120 in an increase of autophagy proteins, such as the MAP1LC3-phosphatidylethanolamine conjugate, ATG5, ATG7 and a downregulation of *MTOR*, whose phosphorylated form suppresses autophagy in the astrocyte cell line or in human fetal astrocytes (Cao et al., 2016). A recent study showed that the V3 loop region of HIV-1 gp120 is responsible for inducing autophagy in primary rat hippocampal neurons in a PRKA (protein kinase AMP-activated; named AMPK)/MTOR-dependent pathway (Liu et al., 2019). Moreover, if the autophagy induction is short term, it could inhibit apoptosis. On the contrary, if it lasts for a long time, it could play a detrimental role (Liu et al., 2019).

The relationship between HIV-1 Env and autophagy in the CNS seems to be highly important but little is known about the mechanisms behind the early phases of HIV-1 infection and more studies are needed to elucidate these questions (Rojas-Celis et al., 2019).

Therefore, autophagy is able to play a role as a modulator of HIV-1 infection at the early stages of its viral life cycle (summarized in **Table 1** and **Figure 1**), but all these ideas and conclusions should be appropriately contextualized, since the use of a particular cell model or experimental procedure could condition the results obtained and conclusions drawn (reviewed in Killian, 2012; Leymarie et al., 2017). Taken together, HIV-1-mediated autophagy events could explain, at least in part, the pathophysiology of the viral disease.

THE EFFECT OF AUTOPHAGY MODULATION IN THE EARLY STEPS OF HIV-1 INFECTION

There are other strategies that have shed some light on the involvement of autophagy in HIV-1 early infection, such as the use of autophagy-chemical inhibitors, targeting the expression of autophagy-associated proteins by RNA interference (RNAi) or over-expressing its mutants, or by using the new clustered regularly interspaced short palindromic repeats (CRISPR)/Cas9 technology to abrogate their functions. The CRISPR/Cas system is the most recent genome-edition toolbox of much interest because of its ability to manipulate genomic sequences, enabling the creation of cell lines and animal models for the study of human diseases with promising clinical therapeutic applications, as well as in science and biotechnology (reviewed in Horvath and Barrangou, 2010; Marraffini and Sontheimer, 2010; Zhang et al., 2014; Hille et al., 2018; Leonova and Gainetdinov, 2020).

The inhibition of autophagy during active HIV-1 infection has been considered as a potential supplementary treatment to effective ART for controlling HIV-1 infection (Li et al., 2020).

There are diverse pharmacological ways to inhibit the autophagy process (Vakifahmetoglu-Norberg et al., 2015; Galluzzi et al., 2017b) and some of these have been assayed on HIV-1 infection. The chemical autophagy inhibitor 3-methyladenine (3-MA) that interferes with the PIK3 class III activity to impair autophagosome formation (Seglen and Gordon, 1982; Liang et al., 1999; Klionsky et al., 2008), prevents apoptosis in target $CD4^+$ T cells exposed to Env-expressing effector cells, and monocyte-derived macrophage infection (Espert et al., 2009). Moreover, HDAC6-mediated pro-autophagic and anti-HIV-1 activity is abrogated by 3-MA, thereby stabilizing viral $Pr55^{Gag}$ and Vif, assuring efficient viral production and infectiveness, respectively (Valera et al., 2015; Marrero-Hernández et al., 2019). This fact has been confirmed by using dead-mutants of HDAC6, neutralized in the deacetylase activity of the enzyme and deleted in the proautophagic BUZ C-terminal domain, which are both unable to promote autophagy degradation of these key viral proteins (Valenzuela-Fernandez et al., 2005; Valera et al., 2015; Marrero-Hernández et al., 2019).

The use of constructs that directly encode mutants of proteins, as previously seen with MAP1LC3 (Borel et al., 2015), or indirectly implicated in autophagy membrane dynamics provides some indicators for developing possible strategies against HIV-1 infection. For example, and taking together some of the ideas described above, the expression of kinase-dead mutant D227A (D/A)-PIP5K1A, reduces PIP_2 production during first virus-cell contacts impairing HIV-1 infection (Barrero-Villar et al., 2008), and perturbing ARF6/PIP_2-plasma membrane bio-regeneration, by using non-functional ARF6 mutants, abrogates HIV-1 Env/CD4-driven viral entry and infection (Garcia-Exposito et al., 2011). An interesting strategy to control autophagy and affect

TABLE 1 | Summary of the HIV-1 effect on autophagy or associated factors.

	HIV-1 effect on autophagy or associated factors	
	Inhibition	**Activation**
Productive early infection	MTOR[2], HDAC6, APOBEC3G, *SQSTM1/p62*, ATG5, ATG7, MAP1LC3-phosphatidylethanolamine conjugate, *BECN1*, BNIP3	ARF6
Bystander cell death (Late autophagy and cell death)		Class III PIK3s, ceramides[1], ROS, peroxisomes proteins (CAT or PEX14), BECN1, ATG5, ATG7, MAP1LC3-phosphatidylethanolamine conjugate
Infected cells/tissue		TLR[2], BECN1 [3,A,B,C] ATG5[3,A,B,C], ATG7[3,A,B], MAP1LC3-phosphatidylethanolamine conjugate[3,A,B,C], MTOR[3,D], NFKB[3,D]

This table summarizes the effect of HIV-1 on autophagy and associated factors in different HIV-1 scenarios (indicated in left column): (i) during productive infection; (ii) by Env-mediated virus or infected cells contact with bystander target $CD4^+$ cells; and (iii) in persistent infected cells and tissues. The modulatory effect of HIV-1 on autophagy or associated factors that are indicated refer to results obtained in $CD4^+$ T lymphocytes, and when data have also been reported in other cell types and tissues, they are indicated as follows: [1]Macrophages; [2]DCs; [3]studies in CNS. Regarding the latter, the data are indicated in terms of the studied cell/tissue as follows: [A]Neuroblastoma cells, [B]human brain tissue, [C]human astrocytes and [D]rat hippocampal neurons. This information is illustrated in ***Figure 1***.

HIV-1 infection has been developed by using Tat-Beclin 1 construct, which is able to interact with the auxiliary viral factor Nef, that inhibits HIV-1 replication in primary human macrophages (Shoji-Kawata et al., 2013).

Bafilomycin A1 (Baf A1) is another candidate to analyze the effect of autophagy inhibition on HIV-1 infection. Baf A1 is an inhibitor of vacuolar H^+ ATPases [V-type ATPases (ATP6V)] that blocks acidification of the lysosome and its fusion with autophagosomes, thus inhibiting autophagic degradation (Yamamoto et al., 1998; Klionsky et al., 2012). It has been reported that Baf A1 prevents HDAC6-mediated autophagy degradation of viral $Pr55^{Gag}$ and Vif proteins and stabilizes SQSTM1/p62 protein (Marrero-Hernández et al., 2019), which is a key autophagic factor that fades during active autophagy (Ichimura et al., 2008; Knaevelsrud and Simonsen, 2010; Komatsu and Ichimura, 2010; Rogov et al., 2014; Katsuragi et al., 2015; Valera et al., 2015; Marrero-Hernández et al., 2019).

Infection of macrophages with purified HIV-1 leads to a decrease in SQSTM1/p62, meaning that the autophagy flux is working during the first stages of the infection, and the lysosomal protease inhibitor pepstatin A reverts this situation (Campbell et al., 2015). This study was carried out in MDMs generated from blood of HIV seronegative donors. Another drug, LY 294002 that inhibits PIK3 class I as well as MTORC1, suppresses viral infection of macrophages in post-entry and post-reverse transcription steps prior to HIV-1 gene expression (François and Klotman, 2003). Pan-inhibitors of MTORC1 neutralize HIV-1 infection by interfering with viral entry in humanized mouse *in vivo* models, since these inhibitors decrease CCR5 levels at the cell-surface of target cells, and also act during viral transcription (Heredia et al., 2015; Akbay et al., 2020). Likewise, other research showed that HIV-1 gp41-induced apoptosis is mediated by caspase-3-dependent mitochondrial production of ROS (Garg and Blumenthal, 2006), which acts as a stimulus to sustain the autophagy process (Levonen et al., 2014; Filomeni et al., 2015). This phenomenon is inhibited by the HIV-1 protease inhibitor nelfinavir (Garg and Blumenthal, 2006).

Trehalose, a natural sugar that inhibits the cellular import of glucose and fructose, with concomitant stimulation of autophagy (Sarkar et al., 2007; Castillo et al., 2013; DeBosch et al., 2016; Mardones et al., 2016) has been found to be involved in controlling early HIV-1 infection (Rawat et al., 2020). Although its action on autophagy is not well elucidated (Yoon et al., 2017), it appears that knockdown of the autophagic *ATG5* gene reduces the anti-HIV-1 effect of trehalose in primary human macrophages (Rawat et al., 2020). Likewise, trehalose promotes viral material degradation by MTOR-independent autophagy soon after viral entry. It is noteworthy that trehalose also affects viral entry by down-regulating viral receptors CCR5 and CD4 in $CD4^+$ T cells and macrophages (Rawat et al., 2020).

On the other hand, the ability of HIV-1 Env-early signal to promote autophagy has been confirmed by specific small interfering RNA (siRNA) silencing of *BECN1* and *ATG7* in $CD4^+$ T lymphocytes, which induce a marked decrease in the Env-mediated cell death (Espert et al., 2006). Similar data have been reported in macrophages and microglia (Kyei et al., 2009; El-Hage et al., 2015). Of note, microglia are the only true CNS parenchymal macrophages and it is thought that they constitute 5-10% of total brain cells (Aguzzi et al., 2013; Li and Barres, 2018). Autophagy inhibition by *BECN1* silencing has also been proposed to mitigate neurodegenerative effects mediated by HIV-1 induced inflammation (El-Hage et al., 2015). In this line of action and by using large-scale RNAi screening, several autophagy- and lysosome-related genes have been found to be involved in HIV-1 replication, such as *ATG7*, *ATG12*, *ATG16L2 (autophagy related 16 like 2)*, *MAP1LC3B*, and *LAPTM5 (lysosomal protein transmembrane 5)* and *CLN3 (CLN3 lysosomal/endosomal transmembrane protein, battenin)*, respectively (Brass et al., 2008; Eekels et al., 2012), as well as *PIK3R4 (phosphoinositide-3-kinase regulatory subunit 4)*, *ATG4A (autophagy related 4A cysteine peptidase)*, *ATG5*, *ATG7* and *BECN1*, in cell lines or in cells isolated from blood samples (Kyei et al., 2009; Campbell and Spector, 2011, 2012a,b; Eekels et al., 2012). The importance of HIV-1 Env-mediated autophagy has also been identified in HIV-1 infection of $CD4^+$ T cells as

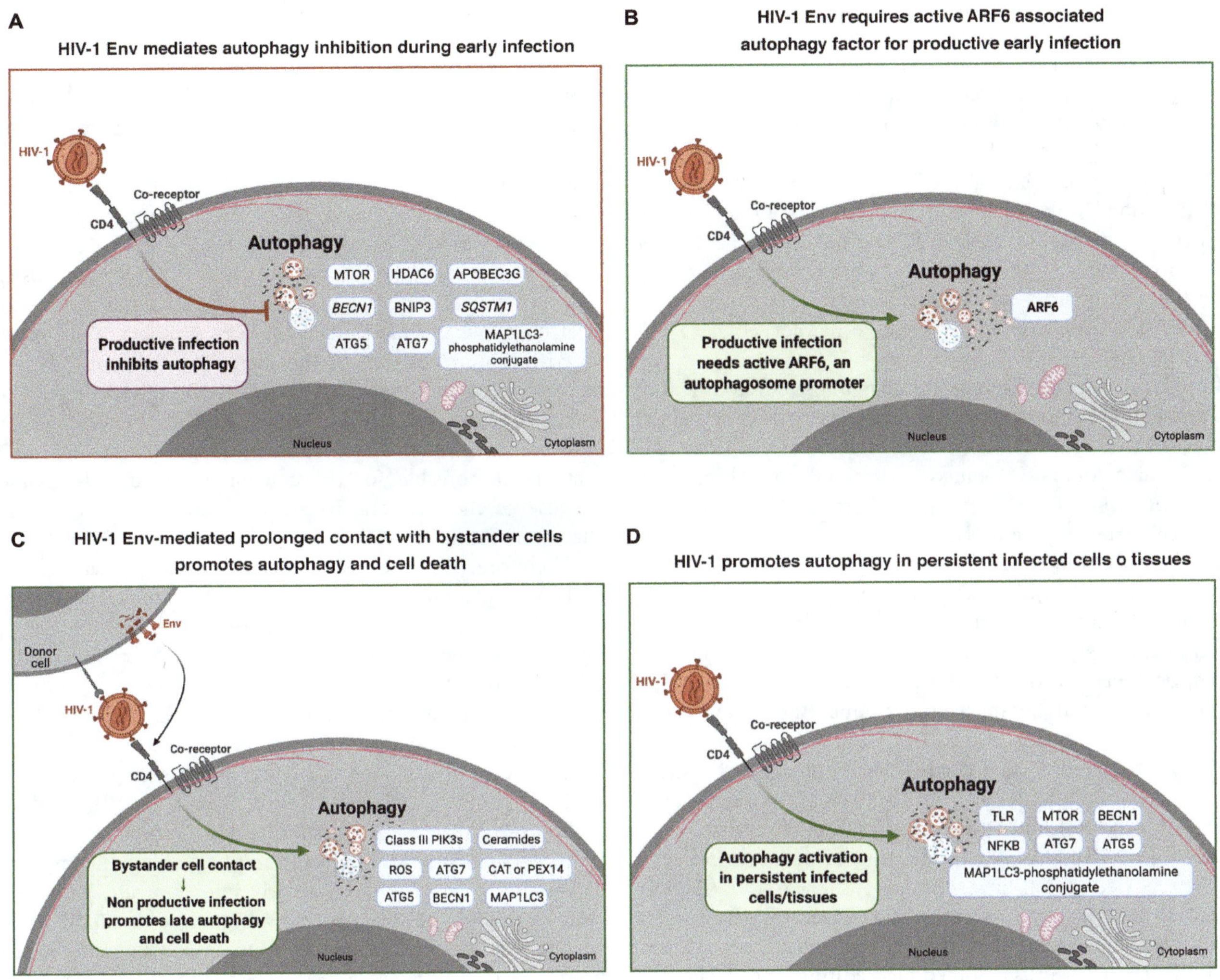

FIGURE 1 | HIV-1 modulation of autophagy during early infection and viral non-productive bystander cell contact, and in persistent infected cells/tissues. Cell scheme summarizing the effect of HIV-1 on autophagy and associated factors in different HIV-1 scenarios. **(A)** HIV-1 Env mediates autophagy inhibition during early infection in CD4$^+$ T cells. Autophagy associated factors affected by HIV-1 Env signaling are shown in blue boxes. **(B)** This scheme shows that HIV-1 Env requires active ARF6 associated autophagy factor for productive infection in CD4$^+$ T cells. **(C)** This panel shows autophagy associated factors (blue boxes) that are activated during non-productive virus-bystander cell contacts. This HIV-1 Env-triggered late autophagy activation leads to CD4$^+$ cell death. **(D)** This panel shows autophagy associated factors (in blue boxes) that are activated by HIV-1 infection in persistent infected cells and/or tissues. Arrow colors represent the reported positive (green) and negative (red) effects on the different steps of the viral life cycle, with dotted arrows signaling the HIV-1 activation pathway. This figure supports the information summarized in **Table 1**. Cell schemes were created with BioRender.com.

this process can selectively degrade the viral transactivator Tat, thus acting as an antiviral process. However, HIV-1 has evolved strategies to inhibit Env-induced autophagy in infected CD4$^+$ T cells, thereby preventing Tat degradation and ensuring viral replication (Sagnier et al., 2015).

A recent study using cell lines suggests that ATG9 is required for HIV-1 infectivity in an Env-dependent way, as the knockout of *ATG9* gene does not affect Env incorporation into nascent virions, but it does have an effect on the infectivity, may be because ATG9 is thought to be a lipid transporter and perhaps promotes Env fusion with the host cell (Mailler et al., 2019). Similarly, HIV-1 Env induces a rapid shutdown of autophagy and immunoamphisomes in DCs, and is thus related to an increase in cell-associated HIV-1 and virus transfer to CD4$^+$ T cells (Blanchet et al., 2010). This work reports that downregulation of autophagy by siRNA knock-down of *BECN1*, *ATG5*, and *MAP1LC3*, or by using 3-MA or chloroquine chemical inhibitors does not negatively affect the HIV-1 viral life cycle in cell lines. However, these treatments impede the innate and adaptive immune responses mediated by immunoamphisomes, in a similar way as HIV-1 does during HIV-1 infection in DCs isolated from donors or cell lines (Blanchet et al., 2010).

RNA silencing of the PIP_2-membrane recycling driver, ARF6, or the use of mutant constructs of this protein inhibited HIV-1 Env-induced virus-cell membrane fusion, entry in and infection of CD4$^+$ T cells, regardless of viral tropism, highlighting the importance of ARF6 in the regulation of HIV-1 infection (Barrero-Villar et al., 2008; Garcia-Exposito et al., 2011). Furthermore, inhibition of the actin-severing protein gelsolin results in HIV-1 gp120-mediated aberrant pseudopodia formation, a membrane dynamics process regulated by actin cytoskeleton reorganization, with aberrant viral receptors clustering at cell-surface that inhibit early HIV-1 infection (Garcia-Exposito et al., 2013). Other studies demonstrate that specific siRNA inhibition of *HDAC6* increases HIV-1 entry due to the increased amount of acetylated α-tubulin that favors virus-cell membrane fusion (i.e., pore fusion formation) and infection (Valenzuela-Fernandez et al., 2005; Valera et al., 2015).

CRISPR/Cas9, a promising technology in the development of strategies against different pathologies, has emerged as a potential anti-HIV-1 tool. One of the first factors targeted by this strategy is *TRIM5α*, which could be modified to restrict retroviral infection by promoting autophagy against HIV-1, soon after viral entry into the cell (Hatziioannou et al., 2004; Stremlau et al., 2004; Mandell et al., 2014a,b; Richardson et al., 2014; Ribeiro et al., 2016; Saha et al., 2020). Thus, it has been proposed that HSCs harvested from an HIV-positive patient could be transduced with an adeno-associated virus (AAV) vector bearing the Cas9 enzyme together with the single guide RNA (sgRNA) targeting *TRIM5α* and a repair template to introduce the mutations to target HIV-1 (Weatherley et al., 2017). These transgenic HSCs bearing the mutated *TRIM5α* would be implanted to achieve long-term cell repopulation in order to generate a durable subset of $CD4^+$ T cells resistant to HIV-1 infection as reported with the *CCR5* gene (Xu et al., 2017). Editing of the *TRIM5α* gene was first reported in cell lines with suboptimal results (Dufour et al., 2018). However, this study suggested that the editing of the *TRIM5α* gene could be feasible in human cells. In this regard, biallelic CRISPR/Cas9-mediated editing of the *TRIM5α* gene has recently been associated with the protection of human T lymphocytic cells against infection by HIV-1 (Désaulniers et al., 2020). Furthermore, a link between TRIM5α and several autophagy factors, such as *BECN1*, *ATG7* and *ULK1*, has been observed by targeting these genes with the CRISPR/Cas9 editing machinery (Saha et al., 2020). This genetic depletion strategy inhibits the anti-HIV-1 proinflammatory function of TRIM5α impairing its capacity to activate adaptor related protein complex 1 (AP1) and NFKB factors that results in the inhibition of the production of the antiviral IFNB1 (named IFN-β) (Saha et al., 2020). All these data are indicative of the importance of the interplay between TRIM5α and autophagy during HIV-1 infection (Saha et al., 2020).

Taken together, all the above studies (summarized in **Table 2** and **Figure 2**), clearly show that autophagy is a potential therapeutic target to control HIV-1 infection and associated pathogenesis.

CONCLUDING REMARKS

One way to block HIV-1 transmission is to inhibit viral spreading into the immune host cells by acting on the viral machinery rather than targeting the intracellular enzymes. However, this is a complex goal, due to viral latency and because viral proteins are highly variable if one only considers the virus as a potential long-term drug-resistant quasi-species (Chun et al., 1998; Schuurman et al., 2002; Zhu et al., 2002; Korn et al., 2003; Belmonte et al., 2007; Buzon et al., 2014; Raymond et al., 2014; Ananworanich et al., 2016; Lorenzo-Redondo et al., 2016; Brenner et al., 2017; Malet et al., 2017; Bandera et al., 2019; Monaco et al., 2020). This is why many of the efforts in basic and clinical research have been aimed at developing strategies to block the virus entry into target cells. Most of the current approaches are based on pharmacological inhibition of the Env proteins, main receptor or co-receptors, as well as the membrane-hemifusion process before viral entry (reviewed in Mostashari Rad et al., 2018). The discovery of LTNP patients (Lambotte et al., 2005) may help to shed some light on identifying cellular mechanisms that are responsible for the control of the disease, not only because of their genetic background but also because of the characteristics of the virus.

Therefore, it is necessary to study the cellular events triggered by HIV-1 infection and to identify the factors implicated in the control of early HIV-1 infection in order to design valid therapies or vaccines. Hence, HIV-1 Env-mediated signals triggered in the cells susceptible to infection become a target of interest, since they induce cellular mechanisms involved in immune response (both innate and adaptive) (Blanco et al., 2003; Altfeld and Gale, 2015) among which is the autophagy process (Espert et al., 2006, 2007; Rotger et al., 2011; Nardacci et al., 2014, 2017). In addition, the recent discovery that functional Env from virus of VNP and RP individuals similarly triggers autophagy shows the importance of this mechanism in HIV-1 early infection and pathogenesis (Nardacci et al., 2014; Cabrera-Rodriguez et al., 2019), and this is supported by the fact that non-functional, signaling-defective primary HIV-1 Envs are associated with the LTNP-EC phenotype (Casado et al., 2018).

The duration of the HIV-1 Env-mediated signals on target cells differentially acts on autophagy functions, having distinct functional roles in HIV-1 infection and pathogenesis. Productive early HIV-1 infection requires the inhibition of autophagy and its related machinery, whereas non-productive signaling in bystander target cells promotes late autophagy and subsequent cell death (Blanco et al., 2003; Valenzuela-Fernandez et al., 2005; Espert et al., 2009; Casado et al., 2018; Cabrera-Rodriguez et al., 2019). In this respect, pro-autophagic and tubulin-deacetylase HDAC6 functions play a crucial role in limiting early HIV-1 entry and infection (Valenzuela-Fernandez et al., 2005, 2008; Valera et al., 2015), which is indicative of the relevance for HIV-1 of abrogating autophagy and factors related to allowing productive infection from the very beginning of HIV-1 fusion and entry. Other studies have analyzed the importance of autophagy after infection or in non-infected bystander cells in long contact with infected Env-expressing cells (Espert et al., 2006, 2007; Denizot et al., 2008; Shah et al., 2011), again confirming an interplay between autophagy and HIV-1 which is key for viral replication achievement and pathogenesis. It should be mentioned that some conclusions may depend on viral and cellular models used to look for

TABLE 2 | Summary of the effect of autophagy modulation in the early steps of HIV-1 infection.

	Effect of autophagy modulation by chemical inhibitors* on HIV-1 viral cycle		Effect of autophagy-gene modification (mutants, RNAi or CRISPR/Cas) on HIV-1 viral cycle	
Effect on HIV-1	**Viral entry and Infection**	**Viral replication**	**Viral entry and Infection**	**Viral replication**
+	3-MA[B], Bafilomycin A	3-MA, Bafilomycin A	*HDAC6*[2], *ATG5*[2], *ATG7*[A,2,3], *BECN1*[A,2,3], *MAP1LC3*, *TRIM5α*[3], *ULK1*[3]	HDAC6[1], *ATG7*[2], *ATG12*[2], *ATG16L2*[2], *MAP1LC3B*[2], *LAPTM5*[2], *CLN3*[2], *PIK3R4*[2], *ATG4A*[2], *ATG5*[2], *ATG7*[2], *BECN1*[2]
-	Pepstatin A[A], LY 294002[A], Pan-inhibitors of MTORC1, nelfinavir		PIP5K1A[1,2], ARF6[1,2], Trehalose[A], ATG9[B]	Tat-Beclin 1 construct[A]

*The table summarizes the autophagy modulatory effect on HIV-1 viral cycle (viral entry and infection or viral replication) exerted either by chemical inhibitors acting on autophagy-associated factors, *which could activate or prevent autophagy, or by acting on autophagy-associated genes by using related mutants, specific RNA interference or CRISPR/Cas editing, as follows: [1] Dead mutant or modified protein; [2] RNAi; [3] CRISPR/Cas9. Left column groups the reported positive* **(+)** *and negative (–) effects on the viral cycle. In general, all these data refer to results obtained in CD4$^+$ T lymphocytes, and when data have also been reported in other cell types and tissues, they are indicated as follows: [A]Macrophages, [B]DCs and [C]studies in CNS (microglia). This information is illustrated in* ***Figure 2****.*

this interplay that might bias the reported pro- or anti-autophagy mechanisms.

Moreover, viral factors that could impair or block the autophagy response to infection have also been looked for. In addition, it has been reported that Vif interacts with APOBEC3G promoting its degradation by the proteasome, thus eluding antiviral APOBEC3G activity (Valera et al., 2015). Vif exerts an anti-autophagy role, due to its interaction with MAP1LC3, and that the blockade of the degradative process by Vif is independent of its association with APOBEC3G (Borel et al., 2015). It has recently been demonstrated that Vpr is able to block HIV-1-mediated autophagy soon after its entry into CD4$^+$ T cells (Alfaisal et al., 2019). Vpr down-regulates the expression of essential proteins, such as BECN1 or MAP1LC3, by inducing the proteasomal degradation of the transcription factor FOXO3 which control these autophagy genes. The power of Vpr in controlling autophagy is so strong that even in the presence of autophagy inducers, such as rapamycin or Torin 1, it is still able to block autophagy (Alfaisal et al., 2019).

All the aforementioned autophagy events in favor of and against early HIV-1 infection have led to a longstanding debate about the so-called "dual role" of autophagy in HIV infection. On the one hand, HIV-1 Env produces different signals that promote autophagy events which play a nullifying role in the virus life cycle but, on the other hand, other authors argue that the virus is able to activate or inactivate autophagy for its survival (reviewed in Espert et al., 2008; Killian, 2012; Leymarie et al., 2017). The results need to be carefully interpreted and different conclusions are reached because different strategies have been used, since the use of a construct of a protein, a virus or an Env expressed on a pseudovirus or at the cell-surface may not have the same effect on target cells, as the latter could also differ between independent studies. The case of what happens in the CNS of HIV-1 infected individuals is even more complicated as tissue can only be obtained post-mortem (Zhou et al., 2011; Dever et al., 2015) and the changes observed postmortem might not be present during life.

In summary, it is clear that autophagy has a highly important role in the early stages of HIV-1 infection, and deep characterization of its interplay with HIV-1 Env-triggered functions could play a major role in paving the way for HIV-1 eradication. Thus, more research is needed to address some important questions regarding the relevance of autophagy modulation (i.e., inhibition or activation) by the HIV-1 Env-mediated signaling during the early steps of the viral productive infection or in a context of long virus-target cell contact without productive infection but resulting in bystander cell death (i.e., a critical process that could favor immunodeficiency) (Espert et al., 2006, 2007, 2008, 2009). Elucidating the relationship between HIV-1 Env-mediated signals and autophagy is a priority, after observing that LTNP-EC phenotype is associated with non-functional Env unable to overcome the barrier of autophagy associated factors, such as HDAC6 restriction factor (Valenzuela-Fernandez et al., 2005; Casado et al., 2018; Cabrera-Rodriguez et al., 2019).

Similarly, controlled clinical trials are needed to determine whether addition of autophagy inducers together with ART in HIV-infected individuals may impact HIV-1 reservoirs *in vivo*. Hence, it is important to analyze the potential universal therapeutic modulation of autophagy in different HIV$^+$ patients, considering factors such as age, coinfections and pharmacological interaction of autophagy drugs with ART. Likewise, there is a growing interest in understanding the complex relationship existing between autophagy functions and HIV-1 pathogenesis in treated patients co-exposed to illicit drugs (Cao et al., 2017). It seems that autophagy is targeted by the use of drugs in HIV$^+$ patients. Thus, the abuse of drugs could favor viral replication not only by increasing inflammation, oxidative and ER stress, but also acting on autophagy (Qi et al., 2011; Dever et al., 2015; El-Hage et al., 2015), thereby affecting the efficiency of ART. On the other hand, autophagy inhibitors could also favor HIV-1 pathogenesis in this scenario, since it has been reported that autophagy inhibitors exacerbated HIV-1 Env/methamphetamine-mediated cell death (Cao et al., 2016). Hence, these data suggest a protective role of autophagy in astrocyte death. Moreover, the use of the autophagy process as a target for HIV-1 therapy should be carefully and deeply studied as this cellular mechanism is implicated in the development of pathogenic reactions, such as

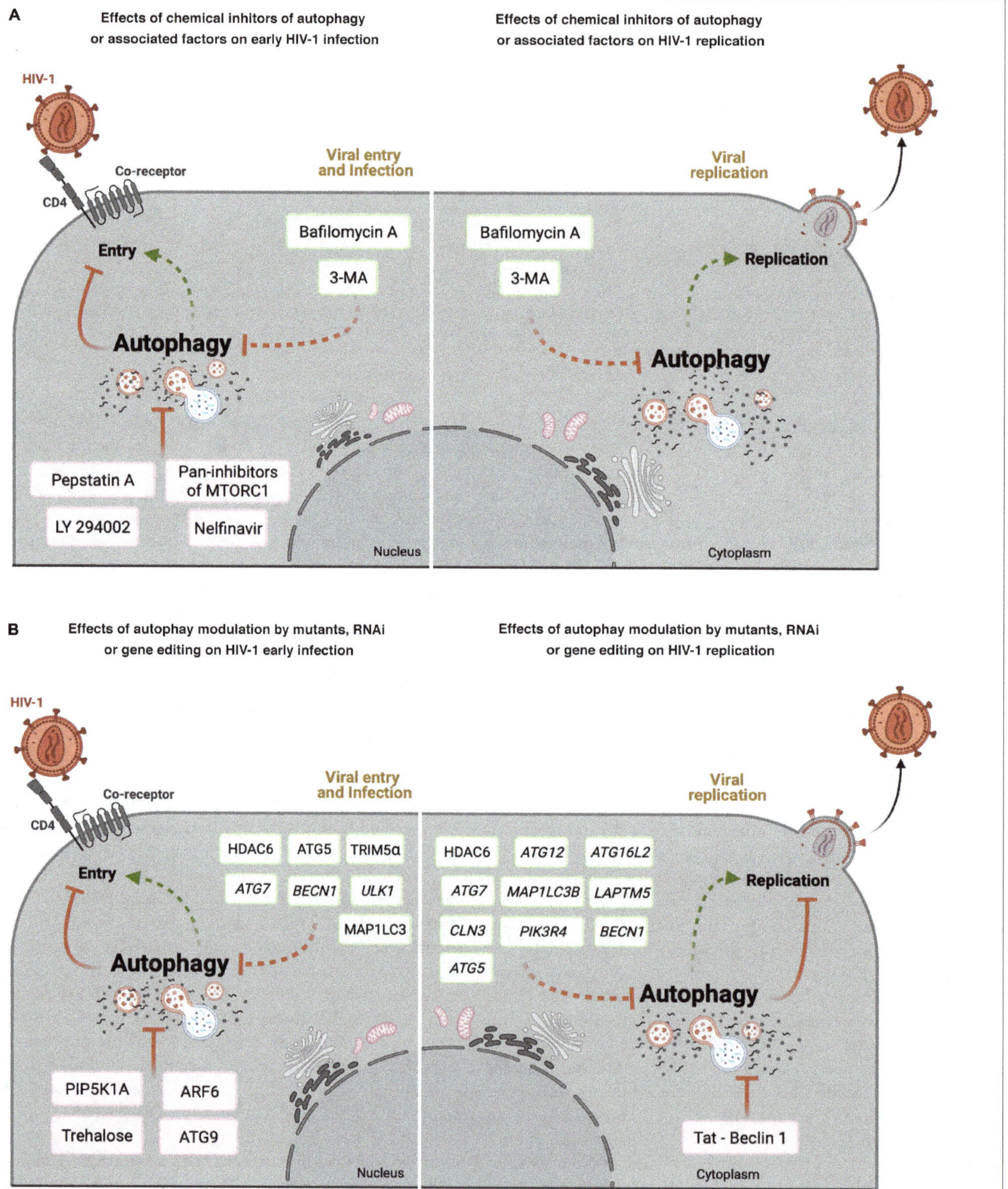

FIGURE 2 | Effect of autophagy modulation on HIV-1 infection. Cell scheme summarizing the autophagy modulatory effect on HIV-1 viral life cycle (early steps: viral entry and infection; late steps: viral replication). **(A)** This panel shows that chemical inhibitors of autophagy and associated factors could activate (factors indicated in green boxes) or prevent (factors indicated in pink boxes) early HIV- 1 infection **(left)**, or promote viral replication **(right)**. **(B)** This panel shows the effect of mutants of autophagy associated factors, or specific RNAi or CRISPR/Cas editing acting on autophagy-associated genes in HIV-1 early infection or viral replication. Autophagic factors that activate HIV-1 infection or replication are indicated in green boxes, whereas factors inhibiting HIV-1 are indicated in pink boxes. Arrow colors represent the reported positive (green) and negative (red) effects on the different steps of the viral life cycle, with dotted arrows signaling the HIV-1 activation pathway. This figure supports the information summarized in **Table 2**. Cell schemes were created with BioRender.com.

cancer or CNS disorders (Aita et al., 1999; Qu et al., 2003; Yue et al., 2003; Ravikumar et al., 2004; Iwata et al., 2005; Hara et al., 2006; Komatsu et al., 2006, 2010; Sarkar et al., 2007; Cherra and Chu, 2008; Koike et al., 2008; Pickford et al., 2008; Martinet et al., 2009; Guo et al., 2011, 2013; Yang et al., 2011, 2014; White, 2012; Levy et al., 2014; Vogl et al., 2014; Wei et al., 2014; Perera et al., 2015; Rohatgi et al., 2015; Tang et al., 2015; Bar-Yosef et al., 2019).

Therefore, it is important to understand how the interplay between autophagy and HIV-1 Env-mediated signal and infection could determine the clinical outcome of HIV-1 patients (i.e., comparing long-term non-progressors that control viremia with progressors) (Espert et al., 2006, 2007, 2008, 2009; Valenzuela-Fernandez et al., 2008; van Grol et al., 2010; Valera et al., 2015; Casado et al., 2018, 2020; Cabrera-Rodriguez et al., 2019) and pathogenesis. In sum, determining the mechanisms underlying HIV/autophagy interplay is probably key to developing novel drug candidates in the challenge of preventing HIV infection and related pathology, thereby offering new insights into HIV-1 functional cure and/or eradication.

AUTHOR CONTRIBUTIONS

A-VF and R-CR drafted and wrote the manuscript. All authors read, edited, supervised the scientific content and approved the final manuscript.

Conocimiento y Empleo, Gobierno de Canarias"), UNLL10-3E-783 (ERDF and "Fundación CajaCanarias"), and by the Spanish AIDS network "Red Temática Cooperativa de Investigación en SIDA" RD12/0017/0034 as part of the Plan Nacional R + D + I and co-funded by the Spanish "Instituto de Salud Carlos III (ISCIII)-Subdirección General de Evaluación y el Fondo Europeo de Desarrollo Regional (FEDER)". RC-R., SP-Y, and DM-A were funded by RD12/0017/0034, M-ULL Ph.D.-training contract ("Contratos predoctorales M-ULL para la Formación de Doctores, Convocatoria 2019, Universidad de La Laguna and Ministerio de Ciencia, Innovación y Universidades", Spain), "Fundación Doctor Manuel Morales" and "TESIS2017010116" ("Programa Predoctoral de Formación del Personal Investigador, Agencia Canaria de Investigación, Innovación y Sociedad de la Información" and European Social Fund-fellowships). JE-H was funded by the Cabildo of Tenerife "Agustin de Betancourt" 2017 Program. JB and CC are researchers from the Fundació Institut de Recerca en Ciències de la Salut Germans Trias i Pujol supported by the CERCA Programme and the Health Department of the Catalan Government/Generalitat de Catalunya and ISCIII grant numbers PI17/0151 and PI20/00093 (to JB) and PI18/01226 (to CC). LE was supported by institutional funds from the Centre National de la Recherche Scientifique (CNRS) and the Montpellier University and grants from the "Agence Nationale de Recherches sur le SIDA et les Hépatites Virales" (ANRS) and Sidaction. The funders had no role in the study design, data collection and analysis, decision to publish or preparation of the manuscript.

ACKNOWLEDGMENTS

We would like to thank Patrick Dennis for his support. The manuscript was English language edited by Patrick Dennis, an experienced English language editor of scientific manuscripts for international publications.

REFERENCES

Aguilera, M. O., Berón, W., and Colombo, M. I. (2012). The actin cytoskeleton participates in the early events of autophagosome formation upon starvation induced autophagy. *Autophagy* 8, 1590–1603. doi: 10.4161/auto.21459

Aguzzi, A., Barres, B. A., and Bennett, M. L. (2013). Microglia: scapegoat, saboteur, or something else? *Science* 339, 156–161. doi: 10.1126/science.1227901

Aikawa, Y., and Martin, T. F. (2005). ADP-ribosylation factor 6 regulation of phosphatidylinositol-4,5-bisphosphate synthesis, endocytosis, and exocytosis. *Methods Enzymol.* 404, 422–431. doi: 10.1016/s0076-6879(05)04037-1

Aita, V. M., Liang, X. H., Murty, V. V., Pincus, D. L., Yu, W., Cayanis, E., et al. (1999). Cloning and genomic organization of beclin 1, a candidate tumor suppressor gene on chromosome 17q21. *Genomics* 59, 59–65. doi: 10.1006/geno.1999.5851

Akbay, B., Shmakova, A., Vassetzky, Y., and Dokudovskaya, S. (2020). Modulation of mTORC1 signaling pathway by HIV-1. *Cells* 9:1090. doi: 10.3390/cells9051090

Alemu, E. A., Lamark, T., Torgersen, K. M., Birgisdottir, A. B., Larsen, K. B., Jain, A., et al. (2012). ATG8 family proteins act as scaffolds for assembly of the ULK complex: sequence requirements for LC3-interacting region (LIR) motifs. *J. Biol. Chem.* 287, 39275–39290. doi: 10.1074/jbc.m112.378109

Alfaisal, J., Machado, A., Galais, M., Robert-Hebmann, V., Arnauné-Pelloquin, L., Espert, L., et al. (2019). HIV-1 Vpr inhibits autophagy during the early steps of infection of CD4 T cells. *Biol. Cell* 111, 308–318. doi: 10.1111/boc.201900071

Ali, A., Ng, H. L., Blankson, J. N., Burton, D. R., Buckheit, R. W. III, Moldt, B., et al. (2018). Highly attenuated infection with a Vpr-deleted molecular clone of human immunodeficiency virus-1. *J. Infect. Dis.* 218, 1447–1452. doi: 10.1093/infdis/jiy346

Alkhatib, G., Combadiere, C., Broder, C. C., Feng, Y., Kennedy, P. E., Murphy, P. M., et al. (1996). CC CKR5: a RANTES, MIP-1alpha, MIP-1beta receptor as a fusion cofactor for macrophage-tropic HIV-1. *Science* 272, 1955–1958. doi: 10.1126/science.272.5270.1955

Allers, K., Hütter, G., Hofmann, J., Loddenkemper, C., Rieger, K., Thiel, E., et al. (2011). Evidence for the cure of HIV infection by CCR5Δ32/Δ32 stem cell transplantation. *Blood* 117, 2791–2799.

Allers, K., and Schneider, T. (2015). CCR5Δ32 mutation and HIV infection: basis for curative HIV therapy. *Curr. Opin. Virol.* 14, 24–29. doi: 10.1016/j.coviro.2015.06.007

Altfeld, M., Fadda, L., Frleta, D., and Bhardwaj, N. (2011). DCs and NK cells: critical effectors in the immune response to HIV-1. *Nat. Rev. Immunol.* 11, 176–186. doi: 10.1038/nri2935

Altfeld, M., and Gale, M. Jr. (2015). Innate immunity against HIV-1 infection. *Nat. Immunol.* 16, 554–562. doi: 10.1038/ni.3157

Ambinder, R. F., Capoferri, A. A., and Durand, C. M. (2020). Haemopoietic cell transplantation in patients living with HIV. *Lancet HIV* 7, e652–e660.

Ananworanich, J., Chomont, N., Eller, L. A., Kroon, E., Tovanabutra, S., Bose, M., et al. (2016). HIV DNA set point is rapidly established in acute HIV infection and dramatically reduced by early ART. *EBioMedicine* 11, 68–72. doi: 10.1016/j.ebiom.2016.07.024

Andersen, A. N., Landsverk, O. J., Simonsen, A., Bogen, B., Corthay, A., and Øynebråten, I. (2016). Coupling of HIV-1 antigen to the selective autophagy receptor SQSTM1/p62 promotes T-Cell-mediated immunity. *Front. Immunol.* 7:167.

Aplin, A., Jasionowski, T., Tuttle, D. L., Lenk, S. E., and Dunn, W. A. Jr. (1992). Cytoskeletal elements are required for the formation and maturation of autophagic vacuoles. *J. Cell. Physiol.* 152, 458–466. doi: 10.1002/jcp.1041520304

Aramori, I., Ferguson, S. S., Bieniasz, P. D., Zhang, J., Cullen, B., and Cullen, M. G. (1997). Molecular mechanism of desensitization of the chemokine receptor CCR-5: receptor signaling and internalization are dissociable from its role as an HIV-1 co-receptor. *EMBO J.* 16, 4606–4616. doi: 10.1093/emboj/16.15.4606

Arhel, N. (2010). Revisiting HIV-1 uncoating. *Retrovirology* 7:96.

Arstila, A. U., and Trump, B. F. (1968). Studies on cellular autophagocytosis. The formation of autophagic vacuoles in the liver after glucagon administration. *Am. J. Pathol.* 53, 687–733.

Axe, E. L., Walker, S. A., Manifava, M., Chandra, P., Roderick, H. L., Habermann, A., et al. (2008). Autophagosome formation from membrane compartments enriched in phosphatidylinositol 3-phosphate and dynamically connected to the endoplasmic reticulum. *J. Cell Biol.* 182, 685–701. doi: 10.1083/jcb.200803137

Bach, A. S., Enjalbert, S., Comunale, F., Bodin, S., Vitale, N., Charrasse, S., et al. (2010). ADP-ribosylation factor 6 regulates mammalian myoblast fusion through phospholipase D1 and phosphatidylinositol 4,5-bisphosphate signaling pathways. *Mol. Biol. Cell* 21, 2412–2424. doi: 10.1091/mbc.e09-12-1063

Bandera, A., Gori, A., Clerici, M., and Sironi, M. (2019). Phylogenies in ART: HIV reservoirs, HIV latency and drug resistance. *Curr. Opin. Pharmacol.* 48, 24–32. doi: 10.1016/j.coph.2019.03.003

Bar, K. J., Sneller, M. C., Harrison, L. J., Justement, J. S., Overton, E. T., Petrone, M. E., et al. (2016). Effect of HIV Antibody VRC01 on Viral Rebound after Treatment Interruption. *N. Engl. J. Med.* 375, 2037–2050.

Barrero-Villar, M., Barroso-Gonzalez, J., Cabrero, J. R., Gordon-Alonso, M., Alvarez-Losada, S., Munoz-Fernandez, M. A., et al. (2008). PI4P5-kinase Ialpha is required for efficient HIV-1 entry and infection of T cells. *J. Immunol.* 181, 6882–6888. doi: 10.4049/jimmunol.181.10.6882

Barrero-Villar, M., Cabrero, J. R., Gordon-Alonso, M., Barroso-Gonzalez, J., Alvarez-Losada, S., Munoz-Fernandez, M. A., et al. (2009). Moesin is required for HIV-1-induced CD4-CXCR4 interaction, F-actin redistribution, membrane fusion and viral infection in lymphocytes. *J. Cell Sci.* 122, 103–113. doi: 10.1242/jcs.035873

Bar-Yosef, T., Damri, O., and Agam, G. (2019). Dual role of autophagy in diseases of the central nervous system. *Front. Cell Neurosci.* 13:196.

Bell, C., English, L., Boulais, J., Chemali, M., Caron-Lizotte, O., Desjardins, M., et al. (2013). Quantitative proteomics reveals the induction of mitophagy in tumor necrosis factor-α-activated (TNFα) macrophages. *Mol. Cell. Proteomics* 12, 2394–2407. doi: 10.1074/mcp.m112.025775

Belmonte, L., Olmos, M., Fanin, A., Parodi, C., Baré, P., Concetti, H., et al. (2007). The intestinal mucosa as a reservoir of HIV-1 infection after successful HAART. *Aids* 21, 2106–2108. doi: 10.1097/qad.0b013e3282efb74b

Benjamin, J. L., Sumpter, R. Jr., Levine, B., and Hooper, L. V. (2013). Intestinal epithelial autophagy is essential for host defense against invasive bacteria. *Cell Host Microbe* 13, 723–734. doi: 10.1016/j.chom.2013.05.004

Bhatnagar, S., Mittal, A., Gupta, S. K., and Kumar, A. (2012). TWEAK causes myotube atrophy through coordinated activation of ubiquitin-proteasome system, autophagy, and caspases. *J. Cell. Physiol.* 227, 1042–1051. doi: 10.1002/jcp.22821

Bhatt, A. P., and Damania, B. (2012). AKTivation of PI3K/AKT/mTOR signaling pathway by KSHV. *Front. Immunol.* 3:401.

Birmingham, C. L., Smith, A. C., Bakowski, M. A., Yoshimori, T., and Brumell, J. H. (2006). Autophagy controls *Salmonella* infection in response to damage to the *Salmonella*-containing vacuole. *J. Biol. Chem.* 281, 11374–11383. doi: 10.1074/jbc.m509157200

Blanchet, F. P., Moris, A., Nikolic, D. S., Lehmann, M., Cardinaud, S., Stalder, R., et al. (2010). Human immunodeficiency virus-1 inhibition of immunoamphisomes in dendritic cells impairs early innate and adaptive immune responses. *Immunity* 32, 654–669. doi: 10.1016/j.immuni.2010.04.011

Blanco, J., Barretina, J., Cabrera, C., Gutiérrez, A., Clotet, B., and Esté, J. A. (2001). CD4(+) and CD8(+) T cell death during human immunodeficiency virus infection in vitro. *Virology* 285, 356–365. doi: 10.1006/viro.2001.0969

Blanco, J., Barretina, J., Clotet, B., and Esté, J. A. (2004). R5 HIV gp120-mediated cellular contacts induce the death of single CCR5-expressing CD4 T cells by a gp41-dependent mechanism. *J. Leukoc. Biol.* 76, 804–811. doi: 10.1189/jlb.0204100

Blanco, J., Barretina, J., Ferri, K. F., Jacotot, E., Gutiérrez, A., Armand-Ugón, M., et al. (2003). Cell-surface-expressed HIV-1 envelope induces the death of CD4 T cells during GP41-mediated hemifusion-like events. *Virology* 305, 318–329. doi: 10.1006/viro.2002.1764

Blanco, J., Valenzuela, A., Herrera, C., Lluis, C., Hovanessian, A. G., and Franco, R. (2000). The HIV-1 gp120 inhibits the binding of adenosine deaminase to CD26 by a mechanism modulated by CD4 and CXCR4 expression. *FEBS Lett.* 477, 123–128. doi: 10.1016/s0014-5793(00)01751-8

Blankson, J. N., Bailey, J. R., Thayil, S., Yang, H. C., Lassen, K., Lai, J., et al. (2007). Isolation and characterization of replication-competent human immunodeficiency virus type 1 from a subset of elite suppressors. *J. Virol.* 81, 2508–2518. doi: 10.1128/jvi.02165-06

Bleul, C. C., Farzan, M., Choe, H., Parolin, C., Clark-Lewis, I., Sodroski, J., et al. (1996). The lymphocyte chemoattractant SDF-1 is a ligand for LESTR/fusin and blocks HIV-1 entry. *Nature* 382, 829–833. doi: 10.1038/382829a0

Bolduc, J. F., Ouellet, M., Hany, L., and Tremblay, M. J. (2017). Toll-like receptor 2 ligation enhances HIV-1 replication in activated CCR6+ CD4+ T cells by increasing virus entry and establishing a more permissive environment to infection. *J. Virol.* 91:e01402-16.

Borel, S., Espert, L., and Biard-Piechaczyk, M. (2012). Macroautophagy regulation during HIV-1 infection of CD4+ T cells and macrophages. *Front. Immunol.* 3:97.

Borel, S., Robert-Hebmann, V., Alfaisal, J., Jain, A., Faure, M., Espert, L., et al. (2015). HIV-1 viral infectivity factor interacts with microtubule-associated protein light chain 3 and inhibits autophagy. *Aids* 29, 275–286. doi: 10.1097/qad.0000000000000554

Borrajo, A., Ranazzi, A., Pollicita, M., Bellocchi, M. C., Salpini, R., Mauro, M. V., et al. (2019). Different patterns of HIV-1 replication in MACROPHAGES is Led by Co-receptor usage. *Medicina* 55:297. doi: 10.3390/medicina55060297

Boyault, C., Gilquin, B., Zhang, Y., Rybin, V., Garman, E., Meyer-Klaucke, W., et al. (2006). HDAC6-p97/VCP controlled polyubiquitin chain turnover. *EMBO J.* 25, 3357–3366. doi: 10.1038/sj.emboj.7601210

Bozic, M., van Den Bekerom, L., Milne, B. A., Goodman, N., Roberston, L., Prescott, A. R., et al. (2020). A conserved ATG2-GABARAP family interaction is critical for phagophore formation. *EMBO Rep.* 21:e48412.

Brass, A. L., Dykxhoorn, D. M., Benita, Y., Yan, N., Engelman, A., Xavier, R. J., et al. (2008). Identification of host proteins required for HIV infection through a functional genomic screen. *Science* 319, 921–926. doi: 10.1126/science.1152725

Brazil, M. I., Weiss, S., and Stockinger, B. (1997). Excessive degradation of intracellular protein in macrophages prevents presentation in the context of major histocompatibility complex class II molecules. *Eur. J. Immunol.* 27, 1506–1514. doi: 10.1002/eji.1830270629

Brelot, A., Heveker, N., Montes, M., and Alizon, M. (2000). Identification of residues of CXCR4 critical for human immunodeficiency virus coreceptor and chemokine receptor activities. *J. Biol. Chem.* 275, 23736–23744. doi: 10.1074/jbc.m000776200

Brenner, B. G., Ibanescu, R. I., Oliveira, M., Roger, M., Hardy, I., Routy, J. P., et al. (2017). HIV-1 strains belonging to large phylogenetic clusters show accelerated escape from integrase inhibitors in cell culture compared with viral isolates from singleton/small clusters. *J. Antimicrob. Chemother.* 72, 2171–2183. doi: 10.1093/jac/dkx118

Brown, F. D., Rozelle, A. L., Yin, H. L., Balla, T., and Donaldson, J. G. (2001). Phosphatidylinositol 4,5-bisphosphate and Arf6-regulated membrane traffic. *J. Cell Biol.* 154, 1007–1017. doi: 10.1083/jcb.200103107

Buckheit, R. W. III, Allen, T. G., Alme, A., Salgado, M., O'Connell, K. A., Huculak, S., et al. (2012). Host factors dictate control of viral replication in two HIV-1 controller/chronic progressor transmission pairs. *Nat. Commun.* 3:716.

Bullen, C. K., Laird, G. M., Durand, C. M., Siliciano, J. D., and Siliciano, R. F. (2014). New ex vivo approaches distinguish effective and ineffective single agents for reversing HIV-1 latency in vivo. *Nat. Med.* 20, 425–429. doi: 10.1038/nm.3489

Buzon, M. J., Sun, H., Li, C., Shaw, A., Seiss, K., Ouyang, Z., et al. (2014). HIV-1 persistence in CD4+ T cells with stem cell-like properties. *Nat. Med.* 20, 139–142.

Cabrera-Rodriguez, R., Hebmann, V., Marfil, S., Pernas, M., Marrero-Hernandez, S., Cabrera, C., et al. (2019). HIV-1 envelope glycoproteins isolated from Viremic Non-Progressor individuals are fully functional and cytopathic. *Sci. Rep.* 9:5544.

Campbell, E. M., and Hope, T. J. (2015). HIV-1 capsid: the multifaceted key player in HIV-1 infection. *Nat. Rev. Microbiol.* 13, 471–483. doi: 10.1038/nrmicro3503

Campbell, G. R., Rawat, P., Bruckman, R. S., and Spector, S. A. (2015). Human immunodeficiency virus type 1 Nef inhibits autophagy through transcription factor EB sequestration. *PLoS Pathog.* 11:e1005018. doi: 10.1371/journal.ppat.1005018

Campbell, G. R., and Spector, S. A. (2011). Hormonally active vitamin D3 (1alpha,25-dihydroxycholecalciferol) triggers autophagy in human macrophages that inhibits HIV-1 infection. *J. Biol. Chem.* 286, 18890–18902. doi: 10.1074/jbc.m110.206110

Campbell, G. R., and Spector, S. A. (2012a). Toll-like receptor 8 ligands activate a vitamin D mediated autophagic response that inhibits human immunodeficiency virus type 1. *PLoS Pathog.* 8:e1003017. doi: 10.1371/journal.ppat.1003017

Campbell, G. R., and Spector, S. A. (2012b). Vitamin D inhibits human immunodeficiency virus type 1 and Mycobacterium tuberculosis infection in macrophages through the induction of autophagy. *PLoS Pathog.* 8:e1002689. doi: 10.1371/journal.ppat.1002689

Campbell, G. R., and Spector, S. A. (2013). Inhibition of human immunodeficiency virus type-1 through autophagy. *Curr. Opin. Microbiol.* 16, 349–354. doi: 10.1016/j.mib.2013.05.006

Canducci, F., Marinozzi, M. C., Sampaolo, M., Berrè, S., Bagnarelli, P., Degano, M., et al. (2009). Dynamic features of the selective pressure on the human immunodeficiency virus type 1 (HIV-1) gp120 CD4-binding site in a group of long term non progressor (LTNP) subjects. *Retrovirology* 6:4.

Cao, L., Fu, M., Kumar, S., and Kumar, A. (2016). Methamphetamine potentiates HIV-1 gp120-mediated autophagy via Beclin-1 and Atg5/7 as a pro-survival response in astrocytes. *Cell Death Dis.* 7:e2425. doi: 10.1038/cddis.2016.317

Cao, L., Glazyrin, A., Kumar, S., and Kumar, A. (2017). Role of autophagy in HIV pathogenesis and drug abuse. *Mol. Neurobiol.* 54, 5855–5867. doi: 10.1007/s12035-016-0118-6

Carrillo, J., Clotet, B., and Blanco, J. (2018). Antibodies and antibody derivatives: new partners in HIV eradication strategies. *Front. Immunol.* 9:2429.

Casado, C., Colombo, S., Rauch, A., Martínez, R., Günthard, H. F., Garcia, S., et al. (2010). Host and viral genetic correlates of clinical definitions of HIV-1 disease progression. *PLoS One* 5:e11079. doi: 10.1371/journal.pone.0011079

Casado, C., Galvez, C., Pernas, M., Tarancon-Diez, L., Rodriguez, C., Sanchez-Merino, V., et al. (2020). Permanent control of HIV-1 pathogenesis in exceptional elite controllers: a model of spontaneous cure. *Sci. Rep.* 10:1902.

Casado, C., Marrero-Hernandez, S., Marquez-Arce, D., Pernas, M., Marfil, S., Borras-Granana, F., et al. (2018). Viral characteristics associated with the clinical nonprogressor phenotype are inherited by viruses from a cluster of HIV-1 elite controllers. *mBio* 9:e02338-17.

Casado, C., Pernas, M., Sandonis, V., Alvaro-Cifuentes, T., Olivares, I., Fuentes, R., et al. (2013). Identification of a cluster of HIV-1 controllers infected with low replicating viruses. *PLoS One* 8:e77663. doi: 10.1371/journal.pone.0077663

Castillo, K., Nassif, M., Valenzuela, V., Rojas, F., Matus, S., Mercado, G., et al. (2013). Trehalose delays the progression of amyotrophic lateral sclerosis by enhancing autophagy in motoneurons. *Autophagy* 9, 1308–1320. doi: 10.4161/auto.25188

Cavarelli, M., Karlsson, I., Zanchetta, M., Antonsson, L., Plebani, A., Giaquinto, C., et al. (2008). HIV-1 with multiple CCR5/CXCR4 chimeric receptor use is predictive of immunological failure in infected children. *PLoS One* 3:e3292. doi: 10.1371/journal.pone.0003292

Cavarelli, M., and Scarlatti, G. (2011). HIV-1 co-receptor usage: influence on mother-to-child transmission and pediatric infection. *J. Transl. Med.* 9(Suppl. 1), S10.

Chan, E. Y. (2009). mTORC1 phosphorylates the ULK1-mAtg13-FIP200 autophagy regulatory complex. *Sci. Signal.* 2:e51.

Chan, E. Y. (2012). Regulation and function of uncoordinated-51 like kinase proteins. *Antioxid. Redox. Signal.* 17, 775–785. doi: 10.1089/ars.2011.4396

Chan, E. Y., Kir, S., and Tooze, S. A. (2007). siRNA screening of the kinome identifies ULK1 as a multidomain modulator of autophagy. *J. Biol. Chem.* 282, 25464–25474. doi: 10.1074/jbc.m703663200

Chanel, C., Staropoli, I., Baleux, F., Amara, A., Valenzuela-Fernandez, A., Virelizier, J. L., et al. (2002). Low levels of co-receptor CCR5 are sufficient to permit HIV envelope-mediated fusion with resting CD4 T cells. *Aids* 16, 2337–2340. doi: 10.1097/00002030-200211220-00016

Chang, M. I., Panorchan, P., Dobrowsky, T. M., Tseng, Y., and Wirtz, D. (2005). Single-molecule analysis of human immunodeficiency virus type 1 gp120-receptor interactions in living cells. *J. Virol.* 79, 14748–14755. doi: 10.1128/jvi.79.23.14748-14755.2005

Chaumorcel, M., Lussignol, M., Mouna, L., Cavignac, Y., Fahie, K., Cotte-Laffitte, J., et al. (2012). The human cytomegalovirus protein TRS1 inhibits autophagy via its interaction with Beclin 1. *J. Virol.* 86, 2571–2584. doi: 10.1128/jvi.05746-11

Chawla, A., Wang, C., Patton, C., Murray, M., Punekar, Y., De Ruiter, A., et al. (2018). A review of long-term toxicity of antiretroviral treatment regimens and implications for an aging population. *Infect. Dis. Ther.* 7, 183–195. doi: 10.1007/s40121-018-0201-6

Checkley, M. A., Luttge, B. G., and Freed, E. O. (2011). HIV-1 envelope glycoprotein biosynthesis, trafficking, and incorporation. *J. Mol. Biol.* 410, 582–608. doi: 10.1016/j.jmb.2011.04.042

Chen, B. (2019). Molecular mechanism of HIV-1 entry. *Trends Microbiol.* 27, 878–891. doi: 10.1016/j.tim.2019.06.002

Chen, X., Zhang, T., and Zhang, Y. (2020). Endoplasmic reticulum stress and autophagy in HIV-1-associated neurocognitive disorders. *J. Neurovirol.* 26, 824–833. doi: 10.1007/s13365-020-00906-4

Cherra, S. J. III, and Chu, C. T. (2008). Autophagy in neuroprotection and neurodegeneration: a question of balance. *Future Neurol.* 3, 309–323.

Choe, H., Farzan, M., Sun, Y., Sullivan, N., Rollins, B., Ponath, P. D., et al. (1996). The beta-chemokine receptors CCR3 and CCR5 facilitate infection by primary HIV-1 isolates. *Cell* 85, 1135–1148. doi: 10.1016/s0092-8674(00)81313-6

Chun, T. W., Engel, D., Berrey, M. M., Shea, T., Corey, L., and Fauci, A. S. (1998). Early establishment of a pool of latently infected, resting CD4(+) T cells during primary HIV-1 infection. *Proc. Natl. Acad. Sci. U.S.A.* 95, 8869–8873. doi: 10.1073/pnas.95.15.8869

Chun, T. W., and Fauci, A. S. (1999). Latent reservoirs of HIV: obstacles to the eradication of virus. *Proc. Natl. Acad. Sci. U.S.A.* 96, 10958–10961. doi: 10.1073/pnas.96.20.10958

Chun, T. W., Stuyver, L., Mizell, S. B., Ehler, L. A., Mican, J. A., Baseler, M., et al. (1997). Presence of an inducible HIV-1 latent reservoir during highly active antiretroviral therapy. *Proc. Natl. Acad. Sci. U.S.A.* 94, 13193–13197. doi: 10.1073/pnas.94.24.13193

Chung, N. P., Matthews, K., Kim, H. J., Ketas, T. J., Golabek, M., De Los Reyes, K., et al. (2014). Stable 293 T and CHO cell lines expressing cleaved, stable HIV-1 envelope glycoprotein trimers for structural and vaccine studies. *Retrovirology* 11:33. doi: 10.1186/1742-4690-11-33

Cicala, C., Nawaz, F., Jelicic, K., Arthos, J., and Fauci, A. S. (2016). HIV-1 gp120: a target for therapeutics and vaccine design. *Curr. Drug Targets* 17, 122–135. doi: 10.2174/1389450116666150825120735

Clapham, P. R., and McKnight, A. (2001). HIV-1 receptors and cell tropism. *Br. Med. Bull.* 58, 43–59. doi: 10.1093/bmb/58.1.43

Cocchi, F., Devico, A. L., Garzino-Demo, A., Arya, S. K., Gallo, R. C., and Lusso, P. (1995). Identification of RANTES, MIP-1 alpha, and MIP-1 beta as the major HIV-suppressive factors produced by CD8+ T cells. *Science* 270, 1811–1815. doi: 10.1126/science.270.5243.1811

Cocchi, F., Devico, A. L., Garzino-Demo, A., Cara, A., Gallo, R. C., and Lusso, P. (1996). The V3 domain of the HIV-1 gp120 envelope glycoprotein is critical for chemokine-mediated blockade of infection. *Nat. Med.* 2, 1244–1247. doi: 10.1038/nm1196-1244

Colby, D. J., Trautmann, L., Pinyakorn, S., Leyre, L., Pagliuzza, A., Kroon, E., et al. (2018). Rapid HIV RNA rebound after antiretroviral treatment interruption in persons durably suppressed in Fiebig I acute HIV infection. *Nat. Med.* 24, 923–926. doi: 10.1038/s41591-018-0026-6

Colin, P., Bénureau, Y., Staropoli, I., Wang, Y., Gonzalez, N., Alcami, J., et al. (2013). HIV-1 exploits CCR5 conformational heterogeneity to escape inhibition by chemokines. *Proc. Natl. Acad. Sci. U.S.A.* 110, 9475–9480. doi: 10.1073/pnas.1222205110

Colin, P., Zhou, Z., Staropoli, I., Garcia-Perez, J., Gasser, R., Armani-Tourret, M., et al. (2018). CCR5 structural plasticity shapes HIV-1 phenotypic properties. *PLoS Pathog.* 14:e1007432. doi: 10.1371/journal.ppat.1007432

Colomer-Lluch, M., Ruiz, A., Moris, A., and Prado, J. G. (2018). Restriction factors: from intrinsic viral restriction to shaping cellular immunity against HIV-1. *Front. Immunol.* 9:2876.

Colvin, C. J. (2011). HIV/AIDS, chronic diseases and globalisation. *Global Health* 7:31. doi: 10.1186/1744-8603-7-31

Connor, R. I., Mohri, H., Cao, Y., and Ho, D. D. (1993). Increased viral burden and cytopathicity correlate temporally with CD4+ T-lymphocyte decline and clinical progression in human immunodeficiency virus type 1-infected individuals. *J. Virol.* 67, 1772–1777. doi: 10.1128/jvi.67.4.1772-1777.1993

Copetti, T., Bertoli, C., Dalla, E., Demarchi, F., and Schneider, C. (2009). p65/RelA modulates BECN1 transcription and autophagy. *Mol. Cell. Biol.* 29, 2594–2608. doi: 10.1128/mcb.01396-08

Cornelissen, M., Mulder-Kampinga, G., Veenstra, J., Zorgdrager, F., Kuiken, C., Hartman, S., et al. (1995). Syncytium-inducing (SI) phenotype suppression at seroconversion after intramuscular inoculation of a non-syncytium-inducing/SI phenotypically mixed human immunodeficiency virus population. *J. Virol.* 69, 1810–1818. doi: 10.1128/jvi.69.3.1810-1818.1995

Coutts, A. S., and La Thangue, N. B. (2015). Actin nucleation by WH2 domains at the autophagosome. *Nat. Commun.* 6:7888.

Couturier, J., and Lewis, D. E. (2018). HIV persistence in adipose tissue reservoirs. *Curr. HIV/AIDS Rep.* 15, 60–71. doi: 10.1007/s11904-018-0378-z

Cummins, N. W., and Badley, A. D. (2014). Making sense of how HIV kills infected CD4 T cells: implications for HIV cure. *Mol. Cell. Ther.* 2:20. doi: 10.1186/2052-8426-2-20

Dabrowska, A., Kim, N., and Aldovini, A. (2008). Tat-induced FOXO3a is a key mediator of apoptosis in HIV-1-infected human CD4+ T lymphocytes. *J. Immunol.* 181, 8460–8477. doi: 10.4049/jimmunol.181.12.8460

Dalgleish, A. G., Beverley, P. C., Clapham, P. R., Crawford, D. H., Greaves, M. F., and Weiss, R. A. (1984). The CD4 (T4) antigen is an essential component of the receptor for the AIDS retrovirus. *Nature* 312, 763–767. doi: 10.1038/312763a0

Dasari, V., Rehan, S., Tey, S. K., Smyth, M. J., Smith, C., and Khanna, R. (2016). Autophagy and proteasome interconnect to coordinate cross-presentation through MHC class I pathway in B cells. *Immunol. Cell Biol.* 94, 964–974. doi: 10.1038/icb.2016.59

Daussy, C. F., Galais, M., Pradel, B., Robert-Hebmann, V., Sagnier, S., Pattingre, S., et al. (2020). HIV-1 Env induces pexophagy and an oxidative stress leading to uninfected CD4(+) T cell death. *Autophagy* [Epub ahead of print].

Davenport, M. P., Khoury, D. S., Cromer, D., Lewin, S. R., Kelleher, A. D., and Kent, S. J. (2019). Functional cure of HIV: the scale of the challenge. *Nat. Rev. Immunol.* 19, 45–54. doi: 10.1038/s41577-018-0085-4

Davey, R. T. Jr., Bhat, N., Yoder, C., Chun, T. W., Metcalf, J. A., Dewar, R., et al. (1999). HIV-1 and T cell dynamics after interruption of highly active antiretroviral therapy (HAART) in patients with a history of sustained viral suppression. *Proc. Natl. Acad. Sci. U.S.A.* 96, 15109–15114. doi: 10.1073/pnas.96.26.15109

Davis, C. B., Dikic, I., Unutmaz, D., Hill, C. M., Arthos, J., Siani, M. A., et al. (1997). Signal transduction due to HIV-1 envelope interactions with chemokine receptors CXCR4 or CCR5. *J. Exp. Med.* 186, 1793–1798. doi: 10.1084/jem.186.10.1793

de Armas-Rillo, L., Valera, M. S., Marrero-Hernández, S., and Valenzuela-Fernández, A. (2016). Membrane dynamics associated with viral infection. *Rev. Med. Virol.* 26, 146–160. doi: 10.1002/rmv.1872

De Jong, J. J., De Ronde, A., Keulen, W., Tersmette, M., and Goudsmit, J. (1992). Minimal requirements for the human immunodeficiency virus type 1 V3 domain to support the syncytium-inducing phenotype: analysis by single amino acid substitution. *J. Virol.* 66, 6777–6780. doi: 10.1128/jvi.66.11.6777-6780.1992

de Roda Husman, A. M., Koot, M., Cornelissen, M., Keet, I. P., Brouwer, M., Broersen, S. M., et al. (1997). Association between CCR5 genotype and the clinical course of HIV-1 infection. *Ann. Intern. Med.* 127, 882–890. doi: 10.7326/0003-4819-127-10-199711150-00004

DeBosch, B. J., Heitmeier, M. R., Mayer, A. L., Higgins, C. B., Crowley, J. R., Kraft, T. E., et al. (2016). Trehalose inhibits solute carrier 2A (SLC2A) proteins to induce autophagy and prevent hepatic steatosis. *Sci. Signal.* 9:ra21. doi: 10.1126/scisignal.aac5472

Decroly, E., Benjannet, S., Savaria, D., and Seidah, N. G. (1997). Comparative functional role of PC7 and furin in the processing of the HIV envelope glycoprotein gp160. *FEBS Lett.* 405, 68–72. doi: 10.1016/s0014-5793(97)00156-7

Decroly, E., Vandenbranden, M., Ruysschaert, J. M., Cogniaux, J., Jacob, G. S., Howard, S. C., et al. (1994). The convertases furin and PC1 can both cleave the human immunodeficiency virus (HIV)-1 envelope glycoprotein gp160 into gp120 (HIV-1 SU) and gp41 (HIV-I TM). *J. Biol. Chem.* 269, 12240–12247. doi: 10.1016/s0021-9258(17)32707-2

Deeks, S. G., Overbaugh, J., Phillips, A., and Buchbinder, S. (2015). HIV infection. *Nat. Rev. Dis. Primers* 1:15035.

Deeks, S. G., and Walker, B. D. (2007). Human immunodeficiency virus controllers: mechanisms of durable virus control in the absence of antiretroviral therapy. *Immunity* 27, 406–416. doi: 10.1016/j.immuni.2007.08.010

Delgado, M. A., Elmaoued, R. A., Davis, A. S., Kyei, G., and Deretic, V. (2008). Toll-like receptors control autophagy. *EMBO J.* 27, 1110–1121.

Deng, H., Liu, R., Ellmeier, W., Choe, S., Unutmaz, D., Burkhart, M., et al. (1996). Identification of a major co-receptor for primary isolates of HIV-1. *Nature* 381, 661–666. doi: 10.1038/381661a0

Dengjel, J., Schoor, O., Fischer, R., Reich, M., Kraus, M., Müller, M., et al. (2005). Autophagy promotes MHC class II presentation of peptides from intracellular source proteins. *Proc. Natl. Acad. Sci. U.S.A.* 102, 7922–7927. doi: 10.1073/pnas.0501190102

Denizot, M., Varbanov, M., Espert, L., Robert-Hebmann, V., Sagnier, S., Garcia, E., et al. (2008). HIV-1 gp41 fusogenic function triggers autophagy in uninfected cells. *Autophagy* 4, 998–1008. doi: 10.4161/auto.6880

Désaulniers, K., Ortiz, L., Dufour, C., Claudel, A., Plourde, M. B., Merindol, N., et al. (2020). Editing of the TRIM5 gene decreases the permissiveness of human T lymphocytic cells to HIV-1. *Viruses* 13:24. doi: 10.3390/v13010024

Dever, S. M., Rodriguez, M., Lapierre, J., Costin, B. N., and El-Hage, N. (2015). Differing roles of autophagy in HIV-associated neurocognitive impairment and encephalitis with implications for morphine co-exposure. *Front. Microbiol.* 6:653.

Di Bartolomeo, S., Corazzari, M., Nazio, F., Oliverio, S., Lisi, G., Antonioli, M., et al. (2010). The dynamic interaction of AMBRA1 with the dynein motor complex regulates mammalian autophagy. *J. Cell Biol.* 191, 155–168. doi: 10.1083/jcb.201002100

Dinoso, J. B., Kim, S. Y., Siliciano, R. F., and Blankson, J. N. (2008). A comparison of viral loads between HIV-1-infected elite suppressors and individuals who receive suppressive highly active antiretroviral therapy. *Clin. Infect. Dis.* 47, 102–104. doi: 10.1086/588791

Diop, G., Hirtzig, T., Do, H., Coulonges, C., Vasilescu, A., Labib, T., et al. (2006). Exhaustive genotyping of the interferon alpha receptor 1 (IFNAR1) gene and association of an IFNAR1 protein variant with AIDS progression or susceptibility to HIV-1 infection in a French AIDS cohort. *Biomed. Pharmacother.* 60, 569–577. doi: 10.1016/j.biopha.2006.08.002

Dobrowsky, T. M., Zhou, Y., Sun, S. X., Siliciano, R. F., and Wirtz, D. (2008). Monitoring early fusion dynamics of human immunodeficiency virus type 1 at single-molecule resolution. *J. Virol.* 82, 7022–7033. doi: 10.1128/jvi.00053-08

Doitsh, G., and Greene, W. C. (2016). Dissecting how CD4 T cells are lost during HIV infection. *Cell Host Microbe* 19, 280–291. doi: 10.1016/j.chom.2016.02.012

Donaldson, J. G. (2003). Multiple roles for Arf6: sorting, structuring, and signaling at the plasma membrane. *J. Biol. Chem.* 278, 41573–41576. doi: 10.1074/jbc.r300026200

Donaldson, J. G., and Honda, A. (2005). Localization and function of Arf family GTPases. *Biochem. Soc. Trans.* 33, 639–642. doi: 10.1042/bst0330639

Dong, X., Yang, Y., Zou, Z., Zhao, Y., Ci, B., Zhong, L., et al. (2021). Sorting nexin 5 mediates virus-induced autophagy and immunity. *Nature* 589, 456–461. doi: 10.1038/s41586-020-03056-z

Dooley, H. C., Razi, M., Polson, H. E., Girardin, S. E., Wilson, M. I., and Tooze, S. A. (2014). WIPI2 links LC3 conjugation with PI3P, autophagosome formation, and pathogen clearance by recruiting Atg12-5-16L1. *Mol. Cell.* 55, 238–252. doi: 10.1016/j.molcel.2014.05.021

Doranz, B. J., Orsini, M. J., Turner, J. D., Hoffman, T. L., Berson, J. F., Hoxie, J. A., et al. (1999). Identification of CXCR4 domains that support coreceptor and chemokine receptor functions. *J. Virol.* 73, 2752–2761. doi: 10.1128/jvi.73.4.2752-2761.1999

Doranz, B. J., Rucker, J., Yi, Y., Smyth, R. J., Samson, M., Peiper, S. C., et al. (1996). A dual-tropic primary HIV-1 isolate that uses fusin and the beta-chemokine receptors CKR-5, CKR-3, and CKR-2b as fusion cofactors. *Cell* 85, 1149–1158. doi: 10.1016/s0092-8674(00)81314-8

Dörfel, D., Appel, S., Grünebach, F., Weck, M. M., Müller, M. R., Heine, A., et al. (2005). Processing and presentation of HLA class I and II epitopes by dendritic cells after transfection with in vitro-transcribed MUC1 RNA. *Blood* 105, 3199–3205. doi: 10.1182/blood-2004-09-3556

Dragic, T., Litwin, V., Allaway, G. P., Martin, S. R., Huang, Y., Nagashima, K. A., et al. (1996). HIV-1 entry into CD4+ cells is mediated by the chemokine receptor CC-CKR-5. *Nature* 381, 667–673. doi: 10.1038/381667a0

Dufour, C., Claudel, A., Joubarne, N., Merindol, N., Maisonnet, T., Masroori, N., et al. (2018). Editing of the human TRIM5 gene to introduce mutations with the potential to inhibit HIV-1. *PLoS One* 13:e0191709. doi: 10.1371/journal.pone.0191709

Dunn, W. A. Jr. (1990a). Studies on the mechanisms of autophagy: formation of the autophagic vacuole. *J. Cell Biol.* 110, 1923—-1933.

Dunn, W. A. Jr. (1990b). Studies on the mechanisms of autophagy: maturation of the autophagic vacuole. *J. Cell Biol.* 110, 1935–1945. doi: 10.1083/jcb.110.6.1935

Dupont, N., Lacas-Gervais, S., Bertout, J., Paz, I., Freche, B., van Nhieu, G. T., et al. (2009). *Shigella* phagocytic vacuolar membrane remnants participate in the cellular response to pathogen invasion and are regulated by autophagy. *Cell Host Microbe* 6, 137–149. doi: 10.1016/j.chom.2009.07.005

Eekels, J. J., Sagnier, S., Geerts, D., Jeeninga, R. E., Biard-Piechaczyk, M., and Berkhout, B. (2012). Inhibition of HIV-1 replication with stable RNAi-mediated knockdown of autophagy factors. *Virol. J.* 9:69. doi: 10.1186/1743-422x-9-69

Egan, D. F., Shackelford, D. B., Mihaylova, M. M., Gelino, S., Kohnz, R. A., Mair, W., et al. (2011). Phosphorylation of ULK1 (hATG1) by AMP-activated protein kinase connects energy sensing to mitophagy. *Science* 331, 456–461. doi: 10.1126/science.1196371

El-Hage, N., Rodriguez, M., Dever, S. M., Masvekar, R. R., Gewirtz, D. A., and Shacka, J. J. (2015). HIV-1 and morphine regulation of autophagy in microglia: limited interactions in the context of HIV-1 infection and opioid abuse. *J. Virol.* 89, 1024–1035. doi: 10.1128/jvi.02022-14

Elliott, J. H., Wightman, F., Solomon, A., Ghneim, K., Ahlers, J., Cameron, M. J., et al. (2014). Activation of HIV transcription with short-course vorinostat in HIV-infected patients on suppressive antiretroviral therapy. *PLoS Pathog.* 10:e1004473. doi: 10.1371/journal.ppat.1004473

English, L., Chemali, M., Duron, J., Rondeau, C., Laplante, A., Gingras, D., et al. (2009). Autophagy enhances the presentation of endogenous viral antigens on MHC class I molecules during HSV-1 infection. *Nat. Immunol.* 10, 480–487. doi: 10.1038/ni.1720

Espert, L., Codogno, P., and Biard-Piechaczyk, M. (2008). What is the role of autophagy in HIV-1 infection? *Autophagy* 4, 273–275. doi: 10.4161/auto.5211

Espert, L., Denizot, M., Grimaldi, M., Robert-Hebmann, V., Gay, B., Varbanov, M., et al. (2006). Autophagy is involved in T cell death after binding of HIV-1 envelope proteins to CXCR4. *J. Clin. Invest.* 116, 2161–2172. doi: 10.1172/jci26185

Espert, L., Denizot, M., Grimaldi, M., Robert-Hebmann, V., Gay, B., Varbanov, M., et al. (2007). Autophagy and CD4+ T lymphocyte destruction by HIV-1. *Autophagy* 3, 32–34. doi: 10.4161/auto.3275

Espert, L., Varbanov, M., Robert-Hebmann, V., Sagnier, S., Robbins, I., Sanchez, F., et al. (2009). Differential role of autophagy in CD4 T cells and macrophages during X4 and R5 HIV-1 infection. *PLoS One* 4:e5787. doi: 10.1371/journal.pone.0005787

Eugen-Olsen, J., Iversen, A. K., Garred, P., Koppelhus, U., Pedersen, C., Benfield, T. L., et al. (1997). Heterozygosity for a deletion in the CKR-5 gene leads to prolonged AIDS-free survival and slower CD4 T-cell decline in a cohort of HIV-seropositive individuals. *Aids* 11, 305–310. doi: 10.1097/00002030-199703110-00007

Evering, T. H. (2018). Molecular signatures of HIV-1 envelope associated with HIV-associated neurocognitive disorders. *Curr. HIV/AIDS Rep.* 15, 72–83. doi: 10.1007/s11904-018-0374-3

Fahmy, A. M., and Labonté, P. (2017). The autophagy elongation complex (ATG5-12/16L1) positively regulates HCV replication and is required for wild-type membranous web formation. *Sci. Rep.* 7:40351.

Farzan, M., Choe, H., Martin, K. A., Sun, Y., Sidelko, M., Mackay, C. R., et al. (1997). HIV-1 entry and macrophage inflammatory protein-1beta-mediated signaling are independent functions of the chemokine receptor CCR5. *J. Biol. Chem.* 272, 6854–6857. doi: 10.1074/jbc.272.11.6854

Fass, E., Shvets, E., Degani, I., Hirschberg, K., and Elazar, Z. (2006). Microtubules support production of starvation-induced autophagosomes but not their targeting and fusion with lysosomes. *J. Biol. Chem.* 281, 36303–36316. doi: 10.1074/jbc.m607031200

Filomeni, G., De Zio, D., and Cecconi, F. (2015). Oxidative stress and autophagy: the clash between damage and metabolic needs. *Cell Death Differ.* 22, 377–388. doi: 10.1038/cdd.2014.150

Finnegan, C. M., Rawat, S. S., Puri, A., Wang, J. M., Ruscetti, F. W., and Blumenthal, R. (2004). Ceramide, a target for antiretroviral therapy. *Proc. Natl. Acad. Sci. U.S.A.* 101, 15452–15457. doi: 10.1073/pnas.0402874101

Finzi, D., Hermankova, M., Pierson, T., Carruth, L. M., Buck, C., Chaisson, R. E., et al. (1997). Identification of a reservoir for HIV-1 in patients on highly active antiretroviral therapy. *Science* 278, 1295–1300. doi: 10.1126/science.278.5341.1295

Forsyth, A. D., and Valdiserri, R. O. (2012). Reaping the prevention benefits of highly active antiretroviral treatment: policy implications of HIV prevention trials network 052. *Curr. Opin. HIV AIDS* 7, 111–116. doi: 10.1097/coh.0b013e32834fcff6

Franco, M., Peters, P. J., Boretto, J., van Donselaar, E., Neri, A., D'souza-Schorey, C., et al. (1999). EFA6, a sec7 domain-containing exchange factor for ARF6, coordinates membrane recycling and actin cytoskeleton organization. *EMBO J.* 18, 1480–1491. doi: 10.1093/emboj/18.6.1480

François, F., and Klotman, M. E. (2003). Phosphatidylinositol 3-kinase regulates human immunodeficiency virus type 1 replication following viral entry in primary CD4+ T lymphocytes and macrophages. *J. Virol.* 77, 2539–2549. doi: 10.1128/jvi.77.4.2539-2549.2003

Freed, E. O. (2015). HIV-1 assembly, release and maturation. *Nat. Rev. Microbiol.* 13, 484–496. doi: 10.1038/nrmicro3490

Fujita, N., Saitoh, T., Kageyama, S., Akira, S., Noda, T., and Yoshimori, T. (2009). Differential involvement of Atg16L1 in Crohn disease and canonical autophagy: analysis of the organization of the Atg16L1 complex in fibroblasts. *J. Biol. Chem.* 284, 32602–32609. doi: 10.1074/jbc.m109.037671

Galluzzi, L., Baehrecke, E. H., Ballabio, A., Boya, P., Bravo-San Pedro, J. M., Cecconi, F., et al. (2017a). Molecular definitions of autophagy and related processes. *EMBO J.* 36, 1811–1836.

Galluzzi, L., Bravo-San Pedro, J. M., Levine, B., Green, D. R., and Kroemer, G. (2017b). Pharmacological modulation of autophagy: therapeutic potential and persisting obstacles. *Nat. Rev. Drug Discov.* 16, 487–511. doi: 10.1038/nrd.2017.22

Ganley, I. G., Lam Du, H., Wang, J., Ding, X., Chen, S., and Jiang, X. (2009). ULK1.ATG13.FIP200 complex mediates mTOR signaling and is essential for autophagy. *J. Biol. Chem.* 284, 12297–12305. doi: 10.1074/jbc.m900573200

Gannage, M., and Münz, C. (2010). MHC presentation via autophagy and how viruses escape from it. *Semin. Immunopathol.* 32, 373–381. doi: 10.1007/s00281-010-0227-7

Garcia-Exposito, L., Barroso-Gonzalez, J., Puigdomenech, I., Machado, J. D., Blanco, J., and Valenzuela-Fernandez, A. (2011). HIV-1 requires Arf6-mediated membrane dynamics to efficiently enter and infect T lymphocytes. *Mol. Biol. Cell* 22, 1148–1166. doi: 10.1091/mbc.e10-08-0722

Garcia-Exposito, L., Ziglio, S., Barroso-Gonzalez, J., de Armas-Rillo, L., Valera, M. S., Zipeto, D., et al. (2013). Gelsolin activity controls efficient early HIV-1 infection. *Retrovirology* 10:39. doi: 10.1186/1742-4690-10-39

Garg, H., and Blumenthal, R. (2006). HIV gp41-induced apoptosis is mediated by caspase-3-dependent mitochondrial depolarization, which is inhibited by HIV protease inhibitor nelfinavir. *J. Leukoc. Biol.* 79, 351–362. doi: 10.1189/jlb.0805430

Garg, H., and Blumenthal, R. (2008). Role of HIV Gp41 mediated fusion/hemifusion in bystander apoptosis. *Cell Mol. Life Sci.* 65, 3134–3144. doi: 10.1007/s00018-008-8147-6

Garg, H., Joshi, A., and Blumenthal, R. (2009). Altered bystander apoptosis induction and pathogenesis of enfuvirtide-resistant HIV type 1 Env mutants. *AIDS Res. Hum. Retroviruses* 25, 811–817. doi: 10.1089/aid.2009.0010

Ge, L., Melville, D., Zhang, M., and Schekman, R. (2013). The ER-Golgi intermediate compartment is a key membrane source for the LC3 lipidation step of autophagosome biogenesis. *eLife* 2:e00947.

Gómez-Sánchez, R., Rose, J., Guimarães, R., Mari, M., Papinski, D., Rieter, E., et al. (2018). Atg9 establishes Atg2-dependent contact sites between the endoplasmic reticulum and phagophores. *J. Cell Biol.* 217, 2743–2763. doi: 10.1083/jcb.201710116

Goodsell, D. S. (2015). Illustrations of the HIV life cycle. *Curr. Top. Microbiol. Immunol.* 389, 243–252. doi: 10.1007/82_2015_437

Gorry, P. R., and Ancuta, P. (2011). Coreceptors and HIV-1 pathogenesis. *Curr. HIV/AIDS Rep.* 8, 45–53. doi: 10.1007/s11904-010-0069-x

Goulder, P., and Deeks, S. G. (2018). HIV control: is getting there the same as staying there? *PLoS Pathog.* 14:e1007222. doi: 10.1371/journal.ppat.1007222

Grabar, S., Selinger-Leneman, H., Abgrall, S., Pialoux, G., Weiss, L., and Costagliola, D. (2009). Prevalence and comparative characteristics of long-term nonprogressors and HIV controller patients in the french hospital database on HIV. *Aids* 23, 1163–1169. doi: 10.1097/qad.0b013e32832b44c8

Grégoire, I. P., Rabourdin-Combe, C., and Faure, M. (2012). Autophagy and RNA virus interactomes reveal IRGM as a common target. *Autophagy* 8, 1136–1137. doi: 10.4161/auto.20339

Grégoire, I. P., Richetta, C., Meyniel-Schicklin, L., Borel, S., Pradezynski, F., Diaz, O., et al. (2011). IRGM is a common target of RNA viruses that subvert the autophagy network. *PLoS Pathog.* 7:e1002422. doi: 10.1371/journal.ppat.1002422

Grimmel, M., Backhaus, C., and Proikas-Cezanne, T. (2015). WIPI-mediated autophagy and longevity. *Cells* 4, 202–217. doi: 10.3390/cells4020202

Grobben, M., Stuart, R. A., and van Gils, M. J. (2019). The potential of engineered antibodies for HIV-1 therapy and cure. *Curr. Opin. Virol.* 38, 70–80. doi: 10.1016/j.coviro.2019.07.007

Gu, S. X., Zhu, Y. Y., Wang, C., Wang, H. F., Liu, G. Y., Cao, S., et al. (2020). Recent discoveries in HIV-1 reverse transcriptase inhibitors. *Curr. Opin. Pharmacol.* 54, 166–172.

Guo, J. Y., Chen, H. Y., Mathew, R., Fan, J., Strohecker, A. M., Karsli-Uzunbas, G., et al. (2011). Activated Ras requires autophagy to maintain oxidative metabolism and tumorigenesis. *Genes Dev.* 25, 460–470. doi: 10.1101/gad.2016311

Guo, J. Y., Karsli-Uzunbas, G., Mathew, R., Aisner, S. C., Kamphorst, J. J., Strohecker, A. M., et al. (2013). Autophagy suppresses progression of K-ras-induced lung tumors to oncocytomas and maintains lipid homeostasis. *Genes Dev.* 27, 1447–1461. doi: 10.1101/gad.219642.113

Gupta, R. K., Abdul-Jawad, S., Mccoy, L. E., Mok, H. P., Peppa, D., Salgado, M., et al. (2019). HIV-1 remission following CCR5Δ32/Δ32 haematopoietic stem-cell transplantation. *Nature* 568, 244–248.

Gurdasani, D., Iles, L., Dillon, D. G., Young, E. H., Olson, A. D., Naranbhai, V., et al. (2014). A systematic review of definitions of extreme phenotypes of HIV control and progression. *Aids* 28, 149–162. doi: 10.1097/qad.0000000000000049

Gutierrez, M. G., Master, S. S., Singh, S. B., Taylor, G. A., Colombo, M. I., and Deretic, V. (2004). Autophagy is a defense mechanism inhibiting BCG and Mycobacterium tuberculosis survival in infected macrophages. *Cell* 119, 753–766. doi: 10.1016/j.cell.2004.11.038

Hailey, D. W., Rambold, A. S., Satpute-Krishnan, P., Mitra, K., Sougrat, R., Kim, P. K., et al. (2010). Mitochondria supply membranes for autophagosome biogenesis during starvation. *Cell* 141, 656–667. doi: 10.1016/j.cell.2010.04.009

Hanada, T., Noda, N. N., Satomi, Y., Ichimura, Y., Fujioka, Y., Takao, T., et al. (2007). The Atg12-Atg5 conjugate has a novel E3-like activity for protein lipidation in autophagy. *J. Biol. Chem.* 282, 37298–37302. doi: 10.1074/jbc.c700195200

Hara, T., Nakamura, K., Matsui, M., Yamamoto, A., Nakahara, Y., Suzuki-Migishima, R., et al. (2006). Suppression of basal autophagy in neural cells causes neurodegenerative disease in mice. *Nature* 441, 885–889. doi: 10.1038/nature04724

Hara, T., Takamura, A., Kishi, C., Iemura, S., Natsume, T., Guan, J. L., et al. (2008). FIP200, a ULK-interacting protein, is required for autophagosome formation in mammalian cells. *J. Cell Biol.* 181, 497–510. doi: 10.1083/jcb.200712064

Harada, K., Kotani, T., Kirisako, H., Sakoh-Nakatogawa, M., Oikawa, Y., Kimura, Y., et al. (2019). Two distinct mechanisms target the autophagy-related E3 complex to the pre-autophagosomal structure. *eLife* 8:e43088.

Hatano, H., Delwart, E. L., Norris, P. J., Lee, T. H., Dunn-Williams, J., Hunt, P. W., et al. (2009). Evidence for persistent low-level viremia in individuals who control human immunodeficiency virus in the absence of antiretroviral therapy. *J. Virol.* 83, 329–335. doi: 10.1128/jvi.01763-08

Hatziioannou, T., Perez-Caballero, D., Yang, A., Cowan, S., and Bieniasz, P. D. (2004). Retrovirus resistance factors Ref1 and Lv1 are species-specific variants of TRIM5alpha. *Proc. Natl. Acad. Sci. U.S.A.* 101, 10774–10779. doi: 10.1073/pnas.0402361101

Haworth, K. G., Peterson, C. W., and Kiem, H. P. (2017). CCR5-edited gene therapies for HIV cure: closing the door to viral entry. *Cytotherapy* 19, 1325–1338. doi: 10.1016/j.jcyt.2017.05.013

He, H., Dang, Y., Dai, F., Guo, Z., Wu, J., She, X., et al. (2003). Post-translational modifications of three members of the human MAP1LC3 family and detection of a novel type of modification for MAP1LC3B. *J. Biol. Chem.* 278, 29278–29287. doi: 10.1074/jbc.m303800200

Henrich, T. J., Hanhauser, E., Marty, F. M., Sirignano, M. N., Keating, S., Lee, T. H., et al. (2014). Antiretroviral-free HIV-1 remission and viral rebound after allogeneic stem cell transplantation: report of 2 cases. *Ann. Intern. Med.* 161, 319–327. doi: 10.7326/m14-1027

Henrich, T. J., Hatano, H., Bacon, O., Hogan, L. E., Rutishauser, R., Hill, A., et al. (2017). HIV-1 persistence following extremely early initiation of antiretroviral therapy (ART) during acute HIV-1 infection: an observational study. *PLoS Med.* 14:e1002417.

Heredia, A., Le, N., Gartenhaus, R. B., Sausville, E., Medina-Moreno, S., Zapata, J. C., et al. (2015). Targeting of mTOR catalytic site inhibits multiple steps of the HIV-1 lifecycle and suppresses HIV-1 viremia in humanized mice. *Proc. Natl. Acad. Sci. U.S.A.* 112, 9412–9417. doi: 10.1073/pnas.1511144112

Hermankova, M., Siliciano, J. D., Zhou, Y., Monie, D., Chadwick, K., Margolick, J. B., et al. (2003). Analysis of human immunodeficiency virus type 1 gene expression in latently infected resting CD4+ T lymphocytes in vivo. *J. Virol.* 77, 7383–7392. doi: 10.1128/jvi.77.13.7383-7392.2003

Hille, F., Richter, H., Wong, S. P., Bratoviè, M., Ressel, S., and Charpentier, E. (2018). The biology of CRISPR-Cas: backward and forward. *Cell* 172, 1239–1259. doi: 10.1016/j.cell.2017.11.032

Honda, A., Nogami, M., Yokozeki, T., Yamazaki, M., Nakamura, H., Watanabe, H., et al. (1999). Phosphatidylinositol 4-phosphate 5-kinase alpha is a downstream effector of the small G protein ARF6 in membrane ruffle formation. *Cell* 99, 521–532. doi: 10.1016/s0092-8674(00)81540-8

Hook, S. S., Orian, A., Cowley, S. M., and Eisenman, R. N. (2002). Histone deacetylase 6 binds polyubiquitin through its zinc finger (PAZ domain) and copurifies with deubiquitinating enzymes. *Proc. Natl. Acad. Sci. U.S.A.* 99, 13425–13430. doi: 10.1073/pnas.172511699

Horvath, P., and Barrangou, R. (2010). CRISPR/Cas, the immune system of bacteria and archaea. *Science* 327, 167–170. doi: 10.1126/science.1179555

Hosokawa, N., Hara, T., Kaizuka, T., Kishi, C., Takamura, A., Miura, Y., et al. (2009). Nutrient-dependent mTORC1 association with the ULK1-Atg13-FIP200 complex required for autophagy. *Mol. Biol. Cell* 20, 1981–1991. doi: 10.1091/mbc.e08-12-1248

Hu, M. M., Yang, Q., Xie, X. Q., Liao, C. Y., Lin, H., Liu, T. T., et al. (2016). Sumoylation promotes the stability of the DNA sensor cGAS and the adaptor STING to regulate the kinetics of response to DNA virus. *Immunity* 45, 555–569. doi: 10.1016/j.immuni.2016.08.014

Huang, Y., Paxton, W. A., Wolinsky, S. M., Neumann, A. U., Zhang, L., He, T., et al. (1996). The role of a mutant CCR5 allele in HIV-1 transmission and disease progression. *Nat. Med.* 2, 1240–1243. doi: 10.1038/nm1196-1240

Hubbert, C., Guardiola, A., Shao, R., Kawaguchi, Y., Ito, A., Nixon, A., et al. (2002). HDAC6 is a microtubule-associated deacetylase. *Nature* 417, 455–458. doi: 10.1038/417455a

Hütter, G., Nowak, D., Mossner, M., Ganepola, S., Müssig, A., Allers, K., et al. (2009). Long-term control of HIV by CCR5 Delta32/Delta32 stem-cell transplantation. *N. Engl. J. Med.* 360, 692–698. doi: 10.1056/nejmoa0802905

Ichimura, Y., Kumanomidou, T., Sou, Y. S., Mizushima, T., Ezaki, J., Ueno, T., et al. (2008). Structural basis for sorting mechanism of p62 in selective autophagy. *J. Biol. Chem.* 283, 22847–22857. doi: 10.1074/jbc.m802182200

Iliopoulou, M., Nolan, R., Alvarez, L., Watanabe, Y., Coomer, C. A., Jakobsdottir, G. M., et al. (2018). A dynamic three-step mechanism drives the HIV-1 pre-fusion reaction. *Nat. Struct. Mol. Biol.* 25, 814–822. doi: 10.1038/s41594-018-0113-x

Itakura, E., Kishi, C., Inoue, K., and Mizushima, N. (2008). Beclin 1 forms two distinct phosphatidylinositol 3-kinase complexes with mammalian Atg14 and UVRAG. *Mol. Biol. Cell* 19, 5360–5372. doi: 10.1091/mbc.e08-01-0080

Iwata, A., Riley, B. E., Johnston, J. A., and Kopito, R. R. (2005). HDAC6 and microtubules are required for autophagic degradation of aggregated huntingtin. *J. Biol. Chem.* 280, 40282–40292. doi: 10.1074/jbc.m508786200

Jackson, W. T. (2015). Viruses and the autophagy pathway. *Virology* 479-480, 450–456. doi: 10.1016/j.virol.2015.03.042

Jeffries, T. R., Dove, S. K., Michell, R. H., and Parker, P. J. (2004). PtdIns-specific MPR pathway association of a novel WD40 repeat protein, WIPI49. *Mol. Biol. Cell* 15, 2652–2663. doi: 10.1091/mbc.e03-10-0732

Jiang, Q., Wang, Y., Li, T., Shi, K., Li, Z., Ma, Y., et al. (2011). Heat shock protein 90-mediated inactivation of nuclear factor-κB switches autophagy to apoptosis through becn1 transcriptional inhibition in selenite-induced NB4 cells. *Mol. Biol. Cell* 22, 1167–1180. doi: 10.1091/mbc.e10-10-0860

Jimenez-Baranda, S., Gomez-Mouton, C., Rojas, A., Martinez-Prats, L., Mira, E., Ana Lacalle, R., et al. (2007). Filamin-A regulates actin-dependent clustering of HIV receptors. *Nat. Cell Biol.* 9, 838–846. doi: 10.1038/ncb1610

Jolly, C., Kashefi, K., Hollinshead, M., and Sattentau, Q. J. (2004). HIV-1 cell to cell transfer across an Env-induced, actin-dependent synapse. *J. Exp. Med.* 199, 283–293. doi: 10.1084/jem.20030648

Jolly, C., and Sattentau, Q. J. (2004). Retroviral spread by induction of virological synapses. *Traffic* 5, 643–650. doi: 10.1111/j.1600-0854.2004.00209.x

Joshi, A., Sedano, M., Beauchamp, B., Punke, E. B., Mulla, Z. D., Meza, A., et al. (2016). HIV-1 Env glycoprotein phenotype along with immune activation determines CD4 T cell loss in HIV patients. *J. Immunol.* 196, 1768–1779. doi: 10.4049/jimmunol.1501588

Joubert, P. E., Meiffren, G., Grégoire, I. P., Pontini, G., Richetta, C., Flacher, M., et al. (2009). Autophagy induction by the pathogen receptor CD46. *Cell Host Microbe* 6, 354–366. doi: 10.1016/j.chom.2009.09.006

Jounai, N., Takeshita, F., Kobiyama, K., Sawano, A., Miyawaki, A., Xin, K. Q., et al. (2007). The Atg5 Atg12 conjugate associates with innate antiviral immune responses. *Proc. Natl. Acad. Sci. U.S.A.* 104, 14050–14055. doi: 10.1073/pnas.0704014104

Julg, B., Pereyra, F., Buzón, M. J., Piechocka-Trocha, A., Clark, M. J., Baker, B. M., et al. (2010). Infrequent recovery of HIV from but robust exogenous infection of activated CD4(+) T cells in HIV elite controllers. *Clin. Infect. Dis.* 51, 233–238. doi: 10.1086/653677

Jung, C. H., Jun, C. B., Ro, S. H., Kim, Y. M., Otto, N. M., Cao, J., et al. (2009). ULK-Atg13-FIP200 complexes mediate mTOR signaling to the autophagy machinery. *Mol. Biol. Cell* 20, 1992–2003. doi: 10.1091/mbc.e08-12-1249

Kabeya, Y., Mizushima, N., Ueno, T., Yamamoto, A., Kirisako, T., Noda, T., et al. (2000). LC3, a mammalian homologue of yeast Apg8p, is localized in autophagosome membranes after processing. *EMBO J.* 19, 5720–5728. doi: 10.1093/emboj/19.21.5720

Kabeya, Y., Mizushima, N., Yamamoto, A., Oshitani-Okamoto, S., Ohsumi, Y., and Yoshimori, T. (2004). LC3, GABARAP and GATE16 localize to autophagosomal membrane depending on form-II formation. *J. Cell Sci.* 117, 2805–2812. doi: 10.1242/jcs.01131

Kaminski, R., Bella, R., Yin, C., Otte, J., Ferrante, P., Gendelman, H. E., et al. (2016a). Excision of HIV-1 DNA by gene editing: a proof-of-concept in vivo study. *Gene Ther.* 23, 690–695. doi: 10.1038/gt.2016.41

Kaminski, R., Chen, Y., Fischer, T., Tedaldi, E., Napoli, A., Zhang, Y., et al. (2016b). Elimination of HIV-1 genomes from human T-lymphoid cells by CRISPR/Cas9 gene editing. *Sci. Rep.* 6:22555.

Karow, M., Fischer, S., Meßling, S., Konertz, R., Riehl, J., Xiong, Q., et al. (2020). Functional characterisation of the autophagy ATG12~5/16 complex in *Dictyostelium discoideum*. *Cells* 9:1179. doi: 10.3390/cells9051179

Kast, D. J., and Dominguez, R. (2015). WHAMM links actin assembly via the Arp2/3 complex to autophagy. *Autophagy* 11, 1702–1704. doi: 10.1080/15548627.2015.1073434

Kast, D. J., Zajac, A. L., Holzbaur, E. L., Ostap, E. M., and Dominguez, R. (2015). WHAMM directs the Arp2/3 complex to the ER for autophagosome biogenesis through an actin comet tail mechanism. *Curr. Biol.* 25, 1791–1797. doi: 10.1016/j.cub.2015.05.042

Katsuragi, Y., Ichimura, Y., and Komatsu, M. (2015). p62/SQSTM1 functions as a signaling hub and an autophagy adaptor. *FEBS J.* 282, 4672–4678. doi: 10.1111/febs.13540

Kawaguchi, Y., Kovacs, J. J., Mclaurin, A., Vance, J. M., Ito, A., and Yao, T. P. (2003). The deacetylase HDAC6 regulates aggresome formation and cell viability in response to misfolded protein stress. *Cell* 115, 727–738. doi: 10.1016/s0092-8674(03)00939-5

Keele, B. F., and Derdeyn, C. A. (2009). Genetic and antigenic features of the transmitted virus. *Curr. Opin. HIV AIDS* 4, 352–357. doi: 10.1097/coh.0b013e32832d9fef

Killian, M. S. (2012). Dual role of autophagy in HIV-1 replication and pathogenesis. *AIDS Res. Ther.* 9:16. doi: 10.1186/1742-6405-9-16

Kirkin, V., Lamark, T., Sou, Y. S., Bjørkøy, G., Nunn, J. L., Bruun, J. A., et al. (2009). A role for NBR1 in autophagosomal degradation of ubiquitinated substrates. *Mol. Cell.* 33, 505–516. doi: 10.1016/j.molcel.2009.01.020

Klionsky, D. J., Abdalla, F. C., Abeliovich, H., Abraham, R. T., Acevedo-Arozena, A., Adeli, K., et al. (2012). Guidelines for the use and interpretation of assays for monitoring autophagy. *Autophagy* 8, 445–544.

Klionsky, D. J., Abeliovich, H., Agostinis, P., Agrawal, D. K., Aliev, G., Askew, D. S., et al. (2008). Guidelines for the use and interpretation of assays for monitoring autophagy in higher eukaryotes. *Autophagy* 4, 151–175.

Knaevelsrud, H., and Simonsen, A. (2010). Fighting disease by selective autophagy of aggregate-prone proteins. *FEBS Lett.* 584, 2635–2645. doi: 10.1016/j.febslet.2010.04.041

Knævelsrud, H., Søreng, K., Raiborg, C., Håberg, K., Rasmuson, F., Brech, A., et al. (2013). Membrane remodeling by the PX-BAR protein SNX18 promotes autophagosome formation. *J. Cell Biol.* 202, 331–349. doi: 10.1083/jcb.201205129

Kohda, T. A., Tanaka, K., Konomi, M., Sato, M., Osumi, M., and Yamamoto, M. (2007). Fission yeast autophagy induced by nitrogen starvation generates a nitrogen source that drives adaptation processes. *Genes Cells* 12, 155–170. doi: 10.1111/j.1365-2443.2007.01041.x

Koike, M., Shibata, M., Tadakoshi, M., Gotoh, K., Komatsu, M., Waguri, S., et al. (2008). Inhibition of autophagy prevents hippocampal pyramidal neuron death after hypoxic-ischemic injury. *Am. J. Pathol.* 172, 454–469. doi: 10.2353/ajpath.2008.070876

Komatsu, M., and Ichimura, Y. (2010). Physiological significance of selective degradation of p62 by autophagy. *FEBS Lett.* 584, 1374–1378. doi: 10.1016/j.febslet.2010.02.017

Komatsu, M., Kurokawa, H., Waguri, S., Taguchi, K., Kobayashi, A., Ichimura, Y., et al. (2010). The selective autophagy substrate p62 activates the stress responsive transcription factor Nrf2 through inactivation of Keap1. *Nat. Cell Biol.* 12, 213–223. doi: 10.1038/ncb2021

Komatsu, M., Waguri, S., Chiba, T., Murata, S., Iwata, J., Tanida, I., et al. (2006). Loss of autophagy in the central nervous system causes neurodegeneration in mice. *Nature* 441, 880–884. doi: 10.1038/nature04723

Komatsu, M., Wang, Q. J., Holstein, G. R., Friedrich, V. L. Jr., Iwata, J., Kominami, E., et al. (2007). Essential role for autophagy protein Atg7 in the maintenance of axonal homeostasis and the prevention of axonal degeneration. *Proc. Natl. Acad. Sci. U.S.A.* 104, 14489–14494. doi: 10.1073/pnas.0701311104

Kopito, R. R. (2003). The missing linker: an unexpected role for a histone deacetylase. *Mol. Cell.* 12, 1349–1351.

Kordelas, L., Verheyen, J., Beelen, D. W., Horn, P. A., Heinold, A., Kaiser, R., et al. (2014). Shift of HIV tropism in stem-cell transplantation with CCR5 Delta32 mutation. *N. Engl. J. Med.* 371, 880–882. doi: 10.1056/nejmc1405805

Korn, K., Reil, H., Walter, H., and Schmidt, B. (2003). Quality control trial for human immunodeficiency virus type 1 drug resistance testing using clinical samples reveals problems with detecting minority species and interpretation of test results. *J. Clin. Microbiol.* 41, 3559–3565. doi: 10.1128/jcm.41.8.3559-3565.2003

Krüger, U., Pfeiffer, T., and Bosch, V. (1996). Generation of lymphocyte cell lines coexpressing CD4 and wild-type or mutant HIV type 1 glycoproteins: implications for HIV type 1 Env-induced cell lysis. *AIDS Res. Hum. Retroviruses* 12, 783–792. doi: 10.1089/aid.1996.12.783

Kuma, A., Mizushima, N., Ishihara, N., and Ohsumi, Y. (2002). Formation of the approximately 350-kDa Apg12-Apg5.Apg16 multimeric complex, mediated by Apg16 oligomerization, is essential for autophagy in yeast. *J. Biol. Chem.* 277, 18619–18625. doi: 10.1074/jbc.m111889200

Kumar, R., Qureshi, H., Deshpande, S., and Bhattacharya, J. (2018). Broadly neutralizing antibodies in HIV-1 treatment and prevention. *Ther. Adv. Vaccines Immunother.* 6, 61–68. doi: 10.1177/2515135518800689

Kundu, M., Lindsten, T., Yang, C. Y., Wu, J., Zhao, F., Zhang, J., et al. (2008). Ulk1 plays a critical role in the autophagic clearance of mitochondria and ribosomes during reticulocyte maturation. *Blood* 112, 1493–1502. doi: 10.1182/blood-2008-02-137398

Kuritzkes, D. R. (2016). Hematopoietic stem cell transplantation for HIV cure. *J. Clin. Invest.* 126, 432–437. doi: 10.1172/jci80563

Kuroyanagi, H., Yan, J., Seki, N., Yamanouchi, Y., Suzuki, Y., Takano, T., et al. (1998). Human ULK1, a novel serine/threonine kinase related to UNC-51 kinase of Caenorhabditis elegans: cDNA cloning, expression, and chromosomal assignment. *Genomics* 51, 76–85. doi: 10.1006/geno.1998.5340

Kyei, G. B., Dinkins, C., Davis, A. S., Roberts, E., Singh, S. B., Dong, C., et al. (2009). Autophagy pathway intersects with HIV-1 biosynthesis and regulates viral yields in macrophages. *J. Cell Biol.* 186, 255–268. doi: 10.1083/jcb.200903070

Lajoie, J., Fontaine, J., Tremblay, C., Routy, J. P., Poudrier, J., and Roger, M. (2009). Persistence of high levels of blood soluble human leukocyte antigen-G is associated with rapid progression of HIV infection. *Aids* 23, 1437–1440. doi: 10.1097/qad.0b013e32832d0825

Lambotte, O., Boufassa, F., Madec, Y., Nguyen, A., Goujard, C., Meyer, L., et al. (2005). HIV controllers: a homogeneous group of HIV-1-infected patients with spontaneous control of viral replication. *Clin. Infect. Dis.* 41, 1053–1056. doi: 10.1086/433188

Lamine, A., Caumont-Sarcos, A., Chaix, M. L., Saez-Cirion, A., Rouzioux, C., Delfraissy, J. F., et al. (2007). Replication-competent HIV strains infect HIV controllers despite undetectable viremia (ANRS EP36 study). *Aids* 21, 1043–1045. doi: 10.1097/qad.0b013e3280d5a7ac

Lang, T., Reiche, S., Straub, M., Bredschneider, M., and Thumm, M. (2000). Autophagy and the cvt pathway both depend on AUT9. *J. Bacteriol.* 182, 2125–2133. doi: 10.1128/jb.182.8.2125-2133.2000

Lee, H. K., Lund, J. M., Ramanathan, B., Mizushima, N., and Iwasaki, A. (2007). Autophagy-dependent viral recognition by plasmacytoid dendritic cells. *Science* 315, 1398–1401. doi: 10.1126/science.1136880

Lee, H. K., Mattei, L. M., Steinberg, B. E., Alberts, P., Lee, Y. H., Chervonsky, A., et al. (2010). In vivo requirement for Atg5 in antigen presentation by dendritic cells. *Immunity* 32, 227–239. doi: 10.1016/j.immuni.2009.12.006

Lee, J. Y., Koga, H., Kawaguchi, Y., Tang, W., Wong, E., Gao, Y. S., et al. (2010). HDAC6 controls autophagosome maturation essential for ubiquitin-selective quality-control autophagy. *EMBO J.* 29, 969–980. doi: 10.1038/emboj.2009.405

Leonova, E. I., and Gainetdinov, R. R. (2020). CRISPR/Cas9 technology in translational biomedicine. *Cell Physiol. Biochem.* 54, 354–370. doi: 10.33594/000000224

Levine, B., Mizushima, N., and Virgin, H. W. (2011). Autophagy in immunity and inflammation. *Nature* 469, 323–335.

Levonen, A. L., Hill, B. G., Kansanen, E., Zhang, J., and Darley-Usmar, V. M. (2014). Redox regulation of antioxidants, autophagy, and the response to stress: implications for electrophile therapeutics. *Free Radic. Biol. Med.* 71, 196–207. doi: 10.1016/j.freeradbiomed.2014.03.025

Levy, J. M., Thompson, J. C., Griesinger, A. M., Amani, V., Donson, A. M., Birks, D. K., et al. (2014). Autophagy inhibition improves chemosensitivity in BRAF(V600E) brain tumors. *Cancer Discov.* 4, 773–780. doi: 10.1158/2159-8290.cd-14-0049

Leymarie, O., Lepont, L., and Berlioz-Torrent, C. (2017). Canonical and non-canonical autophagy in HIV-1 replication cycle. *Viruses* 9:270. doi: 10.3390/v9100270

Li, M., Liu, W., Bauch, T., Graviss, E. A., Arduino, R. C., Kimata, J. T., et al. (2020). Clearance of HIV infection by selective elimination of host cells capable of producing HIV. *Nat. Commun.* 11:4051.

Li, Q., and Barres, B. A. (2018). Microglia and macrophages in brain homeostasis and disease. *Nat. Rev. Immunol.* 18, 225–242. doi: 10.1038/nri.2017.125

Li, Y., Wang, L. X., Yang, G., Hao, F., Urba, W. J., and Hu, H. M. (2008). Efficient cross-presentation depends on autophagy in tumor cells. *Cancer Res.* 68, 6889–6895. doi: 10.1158/0008-5472.can-08-0161

Liang, C., Lee, J. S., Inn, K. S., Gack, M. U., Li, Q., Roberts, E. A., et al. (2008). Beclin1-binding UVRAG targets the class C Vps complex to coordinate autophagosome maturation and endocytic trafficking. *Nat. Cell Biol.* 10, 776–787. doi: 10.1038/ncb1740

Liang, Q., Chang, B., Brulois, K. F., Castro, K., Min, C. K., Rodgers, M. A., et al. (2013). Kaposi's sarcoma-associated herpesvirus K7 modulates Rubicon-mediated inhibition of autophagosome maturation. *J. Virol.* 87, 12499–12503. doi: 10.1128/jvi.01898-13

Liang, Q., Seo, G. J., Choi, Y. J., Kwak, M. J., Ge, J., Rodgers, M. A., et al. (2014). Crosstalk between the cGAS DNA sensor and Beclin-1 autophagy protein shapes innate antimicrobial immune responses. *Cell Host Microbe* 15, 228–238. doi: 10.1016/j.chom.2014.01.009

Liang, X. H., Jackson, S., Seaman, M., Brown, K., Kempkes, B., Hibshoosh, H., et al. (1999). Induction of autophagy and inhibition of tumorigenesis by beclin 1. *Nature* 402, 672–676. doi: 10.1038/45257

Liang, X. H., Kleeman, L. K., Jiang, H. H., Gordon, G., Goldman, J. E., Berry, G., et al. (1998). Protection against fatal Sindbis virus encephalitis by beclin, a novel Bcl-2-interacting protein. *J. Virol.* 72, 8586–8596. doi: 10.1128/jvi.72.11.8586-8596.1998

Limou, S., Le Clerc, S., Coulonges, C., Carpentier, W., Dina, C., Delaneau, O., et al. (2009). Genomewide association study of an AIDS-nonprogression cohort emphasizes the role played by HLA genes (ANRS genomewide association study 02). *J. Infect. Dis.* 199, 419–426. doi: 10.1086/596067

Liou, W., Geuze, H. J., Geelen, M. J., and Slot, J. W. (1997). The autophagic and endocytic pathways converge at the nascent autophagic vacuoles. *J. Cell Biol.* 136, 61–70. doi: 10.1083/jcb.136.1.61

Liu, F., Lee, J. Y., Wei, H., Tanabe, O., Engel, J. D., Morrison, S. J., et al. (2010). FIP200 is required for the cell-autonomous maintenance of fetal hematopoietic stem cells. *Blood* 116, 4806–4814. doi: 10.1182/blood-2010-06-288589

Liu, J., Liang, R., Huang, H., Zhang, Y., Xie, A., and Zhong, Y. (2021). Effect of an antagonistic peptide of CCR5 on the expression of autophagy-related genes and β-arrestin 2 in lung tissues of asthmatic mice. *Allergy Asthma Immunol. Res.* 13, 106–121. doi: 10.4168/aair.2021.13.1.106

Liu, R., Paxton, W. A., Choe, S., Ceradini, D., Martin, S. R., Horuk, R., et al. (1996). Homozygous defect in HIV-1 coreceptor accounts for resistance of some multiply-exposed individuals to HIV-1 infection. *Cell* 86, 367–377. doi: 10.1016/s0092-8674(00)80110-5

Liu, S., Xing, Y., Wang, J., Pan, R., Li, G., Tang, H., et al. (2019). The dual role of HIV-1 gp120 V3 loop-induced autophagy in the survival and apoptosis of the primary rat hippocampal neurons. *Neurochem. Res.* 44, 1636–1652. doi: 10.1007/s11064-019-02788-3

Liu, Y., Belkina, N. V., and Shaw, S. (2009). HIV infection of T cells: actin-in and actin-out. *Sci. Signal.* 2:e23.

Longatti, A., and Tooze, S. A. (2009). Vesicular trafficking and autophagosome formation. *Cell Death Differ.* 16, 956–965. doi: 10.1038/cdd.2009.39

Longatti, A., and Tooze, S. A. (2012). Recycling endosomes contribute to autophagosome formation. *Autophagy* 8, 1682–1683. doi: 10.4161/auto.21486

López-Galíndez, C. (2019). HIV long-term non-progressors elite controllers: an interplay between host, immune and viral factors. *Future Med.* 14, 287–297. doi: 10.2217/fvl-2018-0207

Lopez-Galindez, C., Pernas, M., Casado, C., Olivares, I., and Lorenzo-Redondo, R. (2019). Elite controllers and lessons learned for HIV-1 cure. *Curr. Opin. Virol.* 38, 31–36. doi: 10.1016/j.coviro.2019.05.010

Lorenzo-Redondo, R., Fryer, H. R., Bedford, T., Kim, E. Y., Archer, J., Pond, S. L. K., et al. (2016). Persistent HIV-1 replication maintains the tissue reservoir during therapy. *Nature* 530, 51–56. doi: 10.1038/nature16933

Luzuriaga, K., Gay, H., Ziemniak, C., Sanborn, K. B., Somasundaran, M., Rainwater-Lovett, K., et al. (2015). Viremic relapse after HIV-1 remission in a perinatally infected child. *N. Engl. J. Med.* 372, 786–788. doi: 10.1056/nejmc1413931

Mailler, E., Bernacchi, S., Marquet, R., Paillart, J. C., Vivet-Boudou, V., and Smyth, R. P. (2016). The life-cycle of the HIV-1 Gag-RNA complex. *Viruses* 8:248. doi: 10.3390/v8090248

Mailler, E., Waheed, A. A., Park, S. Y., Gershlick, D. C., Freed, E. O., and Bonifacino, J. S. (2019). The autophagy protein ATG9A promotes HIV-1 infectivity. *Retrovirology* 16:18.

Malet, I., Subra, F., Charpentier, C., Collin, G., Descamps, D., Calvez, V., et al. (2017). Mutations located outside the integrase gene can confer resistance to HIV-1 integrase strand transfer inhibitors. *mBio* 8:e00922-17.

Mandell, M. A., Jain, A., Arko-Mensah, J., Chauhan, S., Kimura, T., Dinkins, C., et al. (2014a). TRIM proteins regulate autophagy and can target autophagic substrates by direct recognition. *Dev. Cell* 30, 394–409. doi: 10.1016/j.devcel.2014.06.013

Mandell, M. A., Kimura, T., Jain, A., Johansen, T., and Deretic, V. (2014b). TRIM proteins regulate autophagy: TRIM5 is a selective autophagy receptor mediating HIV-1 restriction. *Autophagy* 10, 2387–2388. doi: 10.4161/15548627.2014.984278

Mao, J., Lin, E., He, L., Yu, J., Tan, P., and Zhou, Y. (2019). Autophagy and viral infection. *Adv. Exp. Med. Biol.* 1209, 55–78. doi: 10.1007/978-981-15-0606-2_5

Mardones, P., Rubinsztein, D. C., and Hetz, C. (2016). Mystery solved: trehalose kickstarts autophagy by blocking glucose transport. *Sci. Signal.* 9:fs2. doi: 10.1126/scisignal.aaf1937

Mari, M., Griffith, J., Rieter, E., Krishnappa, L., Klionsky, D. J., and Reggiori, F. (2010). An Atg9-containing compartment that functions in the early steps of autophagosome biogenesis. *J. Cell Biol.* 190, 1005–1022. doi: 10.1083/jcb.200912089

Markosyan, R. M., Cohen, F. S., and Melikyan, G. B. (2003). HIV-1 envelope proteins complete their folding into six-helix bundles immediately after fusion pore formation. *Mol. Biol. Cell* 14, 926–938. doi: 10.1091/mbc.e02-09-0573

Marraffini, L. A., and Sontheimer, E. J. (2010). CRISPR interference: RNA-directed adaptive immunity in bacteria and archaea. *Nat. Rev. Genet.* 11, 181–190. doi: 10.1038/nrg2749

Marrero-Hernández, S., Márquez-Arce, D., Cabrera-Rodríguez, R., Estévez-Herrera, J., Pérez-Yanes, S., Barroso-González, J., et al. (2019). HIV-1 nef targets HDAC6 to assure viral production and virus infection. *Front. Microbiol.* 10:2437.

Martinet, W., Agostinis, P., Vanhoecke, B., Dewaele, M., and De Meyer, G. R. (2009). Autophagy in disease: a double-edged sword with therapeutic potential. *Clin. Sci.* 116, 697–712. doi: 10.1042/cs20080508

Masiero, E., Agatea, L., Mammucari, C., Blaauw, B., Loro, E., Komatsu, M., et al. (2009). Autophagy is required to maintain muscle mass. *Cell Metab.* 10, 507–515. doi: 10.1016/j.cmet.2009.10.008

Matoba, K., Kotani, T., Tsutsumi, A., Tsuji, T., Mori, T., Noshiro, D., et al. (2020). Atg9 is a lipid scramblase that mediates autophagosomal membrane expansion. *Nat. Struct. Mol. Biol.* 27, 1185–1193. doi: 10.1038/s41594-020-00518-w

Matsunaga, K., Saitoh, T., Tabata, K., Omori, H., Satoh, T., Kurotori, N., et al. (2009). Two Beclin 1-binding proteins, Atg14L and Rubicon, reciprocally regulate autophagy at different stages. *Nat. Cell Biol.* 11, 385–396. doi: 10.1038/ncb1846

Mauthe, M., Jacob, A., Freiberger, S., Hentschel, K., Stierhof, Y. D., Codogno, P., et al. (2011). Resveratrol-mediated autophagy requires WIPI-1-regulated LC3 lipidation in the absence of induced phagophore formation. *Autophagy* 7, 1448–1461. doi: 10.4161/auto.7.12.17802

McDougal, J. S., Kennedy, M. S., Sligh, J. M., Cort, S. P., Mawle, A., and Nicholson, J. K. (1986). Binding of HTLV-III/LAV to T4+ T cells by a complex of the 110K viral protein and the T4 molecule. *Science* 231, 382–385. doi: 10.1126/science.3001934

McDougal, J. S., Mawle, A., Cort, S. P., Nicholson, J. K., Cross, G. D., Scheppler-Campbell, J. A., et al. (1985). Cellular tropism of the human retrovirus HTLV-III/LAV. I. Role of T cell activation and expression of the T4 antigen. *J. Immunol.* 135, 3151–3162.

McGrath, J. W., Winchester, M. S., Kaawa-Mafigiri, D., Walakira, E., Namutiibwa, F., Birungi, J., et al. (2014). Challenging the paradigm: anthropological perspectives on HIV as a chronic disease. *Med. Anthropol.* 33, 303–317. doi: 10.1080/01459740.2014.892483

Meléndez, A., Tallóczy, Z., Seaman, M., Eskelinen, E. L., Hall, D. H., and Levine, B. (2003). Autophagy genes are essential for dauer development and life-span extension in *C. elegans*. *Science* 301, 1387–1391. doi: 10.1126/science.1087782

Melikyan, G. B. (2014). HIV entry: a game of hide-and-fuse? *Curr. Opin. Virol.* 4, 1–7. doi: 10.1016/j.coviro.2013.09.004

Meng, Q., and Cai, D. (2011). Defective hypothalamic autophagy directs the central pathogenesis of obesity via the IkappaB kinase beta (IKKbeta)/NF-kappaB pathway. *J. Biol. Chem.* 286, 32324–32332. doi: 10.1074/jbc.m111.254417

Mens, H., Kearney, M., Wiegand, A., Shao, W., Schønning, K., Gerstoft, J., et al. (2010). HIV-1 continues to replicate and evolve in patients with natural control of HIV infection. *J. Virol.* 84, 12971–12981. doi: 10.1128/jvi.00387-10

Mercer, C. A., Kaliappan, A., and Dennis, P. B. (2009). A novel, human Atg13 binding protein, Atg101, interacts with ULK1 and is essential for macroautophagy. *Autophagy* 5, 649–662. doi: 10.4161/auto.5.5.8249

Mi, N., Chen, Y., Wang, S., Chen, M., Zhao, M., Yang, G., et al. (2015). CapZ regulates autophagosomal membrane shaping by promoting actin assembly inside the isolation membrane. *Nat. Cell Biol.* 17, 1112–1123. doi: 10.1038/ncb3215

Migueles, S. A., Osborne, C. M., Royce, C., Compton, A. A., Joshi, R. P., Weeks, K. A., et al. (2008). Lytic granule loading of CD8+ T cells is required for HIV-infected cell elimination associated with immune control. *Immunity* 29, 1009–1021. doi: 10.1016/j.immuni.2008.10.010

Mizushima, N., Kuma, A., Kobayashi, Y., Yamamoto, A., Matsubae, M., Takao, T., et al. (2003). Mouse Apg16L, a novel WD-repeat protein, targets to the autophagic isolation membrane with the Apg12-Apg5 conjugate. *J. Cell Sci.* 116, 1679–1688. doi: 10.1242/jcs.00381

Mizushima, N., Noda, T., and Ohsumi, Y. (1999). Apg16p is required for the function of the Apg12p-Apg5p conjugate in the yeast autophagy pathway. *EMBO J.* 18, 3888–3896. doi: 10.1093/emboj/18.14.3888

Mizushima, N., Ohsumi, Y., and Yoshimori, T. (2002). Autophagosome formation in mammalian cells. *Cell Struct. Funct.* 27, 421–429. doi: 10.1247/csf.27.421

Mizushima, N., Yoshimori, T., and Ohsumi, Y. (2011). The role of Atg proteins in autophagosome formation. *Annu. Rev. Cell Dev. Biol.* 27, 107–132. doi: 10.1146/annurev-cellbio-092910-154005

Mohammadi, P., Desfarges, S., Bartha, I., Joos, B., Zangger, N., Muñ;oz, M., et al. (2013). 24 hours in the life of HIV-1 in a T cell line. *PLoS Pathog.* 9:e1003161. doi: 10.1371/journal.ppat.1003161

Molina, L., Grimaldi, M., Robert-Hebmann, V., Espert, L., Varbanov, M., Devaux, C., et al. (2007). Proteomic analysis of the cellular responses induced in uninfected immune cells by cell-expressed X4 HIV-1 envelope. *Proteomics* 7, 3116–3130. doi: 10.1002/pmic.200700306

Monaco, D. C., Zapata, L., Hunter, E., Salomon, H., and Dilernia, D. A. (2020). Resistance profile of HIV-1 quasispecies in patients under treatment failure using single molecule, real-time sequencing. *Aids* 34, 2201–2210. doi: 10.1097/qad.0000000000002697

Moore, J. P., Kitchen, S. G., Pugach, P., and Zack, J. A. (2004). The CCR5 and CXCR4 coreceptors–central to understanding the transmission and pathogenesis of human immunodeficiency virus type 1 infection. *AIDS Res. Hum. Retroviruses* 20, 111–126. doi: 10.1089/088922204322749567

Moreau, K., Ravikumar, B., Puri, C., and Rubinsztein, D. C. (2012). Arf6 promotes autophagosome formation via effects on phosphatidylinositol 4,5-bisphosphate and phospholipase D. *J. Cell Biol.* 196, 483–496. doi: 10.1083/jcb.201110114

Morel, E. (2020). Endoplasmic reticulum membrane and contact site dynamics in autophagy regulation and stress response. *Front. Cell. Dev. Biol.* 8:343.

Mostashari Rad, T., Saghaie, L., and Fassihi, A. (2018). HIV-1 entry inhibitors: a review of experimental and computational studies. *Chem. Biodivers.* 15:e1800159. doi: 10.1002/cbdv.201800159

Moulard, M., Hallenberger, S., Garten, W., and Klenk, H. D. (1999). Processing and routage of HIV glycoproteins by furin to the cell surface. *Virus Res.* 60, 55–65. doi: 10.1016/s0168-1702(99)00002-7

Nakagawa, I., Amano, A., Mizushima, N., Yamamoto, A., Yamaguchi, H., Kamimoto, T., et al. (2004). Autophagy defends cells against invading group A *Streptococcus*. *Science* 306, 1037–1040. doi: 10.1126/science.1103966

Nakai, A., Yamaguchi, O., Takeda, T., Higuchi, Y., Hikoso, S., Taniike, M., et al. (2007). The role of autophagy in cardiomyocytes in the basal state and in response to hemodynamic stress. *Nat. Med.* 13, 619–624. doi: 10.1038/nm1574

Nakamoto, M., Moy, R. H., Xu, J., Bambina, S., Yasunaga, A., Shelly, S. S., et al. (2012). Virus recognition by Toll-7 activates antiviral autophagy in *Drosophila*. *Immunity* 36, 658–667. doi: 10.1016/j.immuni.2012.03.003

Nakatogawa, H., Ichimura, Y., and Ohsumi, Y. (2007). Atg8, a ubiquitin-like protein required for autophagosome formation, mediates membrane tethering and hemifusion. *Cell* 130, 165–178. doi: 10.1016/j.cell.2007.05.021

Nakatogawa, H., Suzuki, K., Kamada, Y., and Ohsumi, Y. (2009). Dynamics and diversity in autophagy mechanisms: lessons from yeast. *Nat. Rev. Mol. Cell Biol.* 10, 458–467. doi: 10.1038/nrm2708

Nardacci, R., Amendola, A., Ciccosanti, F., Corazzari, M., Esposito, V., Vlassi, C., et al. (2014). Autophagy plays an important role in the containment of HIV-1 in nonprogressor-infected patients. *Autophagy* 10, 1167–1178. doi: 10.4161/auto.28678

Nardacci, R., Ciccosanti, F., Marsella, C., Ippolito, G., Piacentini, M., and Fimia, G. M. (2017). Role of autophagy in HIV infection and pathogenesis. *J. Intern. Med.* 281, 422–432. doi: 10.1111/joim.12596

Naslavsky, N., Weigert, R., and Donaldson, J. G. (2003). Convergence of non-clathrin- and clathrin-derived endosomes involves Arf6 inactivation and changes in phosphoinositides. *Mol. Biol. Cell* 14, 417–431. doi: 10.1091/mbc.02-04-0053

Nedjic, J., Aichinger, M., Emmerich, J., Mizushima, N., and Klein, L. (2008). Autophagy in thymic epithelium shapes the T-cell repertoire and is essential for tolerance. *Nature* 455, 396–400. doi: 10.1038/nature07208

Nimmerjahn, F., Milosevic, S., Behrends, U., Jaffee, E. M., Pardoll, D. M., Bornkamm, G. W., et al. (2003). Major histocompatibility complex class II-restricted presentation of a cytosolic antigen by autophagy. *Eur. J. Immunol.* 33, 1250–1259. doi: 10.1002/eji.200323730

Nishiyama, J., Miura, E., Mizushima, N., Watanabe, M., and Yuzaki, M. (2007). Aberrant membranes and double-membrane structures accumulate in the axons of Atg5-null Purkinje cells before neuronal death. *Autophagy* 3, 591–596. doi: 10.4161/auto.4964

Nivon, M., Abou-Samra, M., Richet, E., Guyot, B., Arrigo, A. P., and Kretz-Remy, C. (2012). NF-κB regulates protein quality control after heat stress through modulation of the BAG3-HspB8 complex. *J. Cell Sci.* 125, 1141–1151. doi: 10.1242/jcs.091041

Nivon, M., Richet, E., Codogno, P., Arrigo, A. P., and Kretz-Remy, C. (2009). Autophagy activation by NFkappaB is essential for cell survival after heat shock. *Autophagy* 5, 766–783. doi: 10.4161/auto.8788

Noda, N. N., and Fujioka, Y. (2015). Atg1 family kinases in autophagy initiation. *Cell Mol. Life Sci.* 72, 3083–3096. doi: 10.1007/s00018-015-1917-z

Noel, N., Peñ;a, R., David, A., Avettand-Fenoel, V., Erkizia, I., Jimenez, E., et al. (2016). Long-term spontaneous control of HIV-1 is related to low frequency of infected cells and inefficient viral reactivation. *J. Virol.* 90, 6148–6158. doi: 10.1128/jvi.00419-16

Obara, K., Sekito, T., Niimi, K., and Ohsumi, Y. (2008). The Atg18-Atg2 complex is recruited to autophagic membranes via phosphatidylinositol 3-phosphate and exerts an essential function. *J. Biol. Chem.* 283, 23972–23980. doi: 10.1074/jbc.m803180200

O'Connell, K. A., Brennan, T. P., Bailey, J. R., Ray, S. C., Siliciano, R. F., and Blankson, J. N. (2010). Control of HIV-1 in elite suppressors despite ongoing replication and evolution in plasma virus. *J. Virol.* 84, 7018–7028. doi: 10.1128/jvi.00548-10

Ogawa, M., Yoshimori, T., Suzuki, T., Sagara, H., Mizushima, N., and Sasakawa, C. (2005). Escape of intracellular *Shigella* from autophagy. *Science* 307, 727–731. doi: 10.1126/science.1106036

Oh, D. S., and Lee, H. K. (2019). Autophagy protein ATG5 regulates CD36 expression and anti-tumor MHC class II antigen presentation in dendritic cells. *Autophagy* 15, 2091–2106. doi: 10.1080/15548627.2019.1596493

Okulicz, J. F., Marconi, V. C., Landrum, M. L., Wegner, S., Weintrob, A., Ganesan, A., et al. (2009). Clinical outcomes of elite controllers, viremic controllers, and long-term nonprogressors in the US Department of Defense HIV natural history study. *J. Infect. Dis.* 200, 1714–1723. doi: 10.1086/646609

Orvedahl, A., Macpherson, S., Sumpter, R. Jr., Tallóczy, Z., Zou, Z., and Levine, B. (2010). Autophagy protects against Sindbis virus infection of the central nervous system. *Cell Host Microbe* 7, 115–127. doi: 10.1016/j.chom.2010.01.007

Osawa, T., Kotani, T., Kawaoka, T., Hirata, E., Suzuki, K., Nakatogawa, H., et al. (2019). Atg2 mediates direct lipid transfer between membranes for autophagosome formation. *Nat. Struct. Mol. Biol.* 26, 281–288. doi: 10.1038/s41594-019-0203-4

Paludan, C., Schmid, D., Landthaler, M., Vockerodt, M., Kube, D., Tuschl, T., et al. (2005). Endogenous MHC class II processing of a viral nuclear antigen after autophagy. *Science* 307, 593–596. doi: 10.1126/science.1104904

Pandey, U. B., Nie, Z., Batlevi, Y., Mccray, B. A., Ritson, G. P., Nedelsky, N. B., et al. (2007). HDAC6 rescues neurodegeneration and provides an essential link between autophagy and the UPS. *Nature* 447, 859–863.

Pankiv, S., Clausen, T. H., Lamark, T., Brech, A., Bruun, J. A., Outzen, H., et al. (2007). p62/SQSTM1 binds directly to Atg8/LC3 to facilitate degradation of ubiquitinated protein aggregates by autophagy. *J. Biol. Chem.* 282, 24131–24145. doi: 10.1074/jbc.m702824200

Pasi, K. J., Sabin, C. A., Jenkins, P. V., Devereux, H. L., Ononye, C., and Lee, C. A. (2000). The effects of the 32-bp CCR-5 deletion on HIV transmission and HIV disease progression in individuals with haemophilia. *Br. J. Haematol.* 111, 136–142. doi: 10.1111/j.1365-2141.2000.02325.x

Paul, P., and Münz, C. (2016). Autophagy and mammalian viruses: roles in immune response, viral replication, and beyond. *Adv. Virus Res.* 95, 149–195.

Perelson, A. S., Essunger, P., and Ho, D. D. (1997). Dynamics of HIV-1 and CD4+ lymphocytes in vivo. *Aids* 11(Suppl. A), S17–S24.

Perera, R. M., Stoykova, S., Nicolay, B. N., Ross, K. N., Fitamant, J., Boukhali, M., et al. (2015). Transcriptional control of autophagy-lysosome function drives pancreatic cancer metabolism. *Nature* 524, 361–365. doi: 10.1038/nature14587

Pereyra, F., Addo, M. M., Kaufmann, D. E., Liu, Y., Miura, T., Rathod, A., et al. (2008). Genetic and immunologic heterogeneity among persons who control HIV infection in the absence of therapy. *J. Infect. Dis.* 197, 563–571. doi: 10.1086/526786

Pereyra, F., Jia, X., Mclaren, P. J., Telenti, A., De Bakker, P. I., Walker, B. D., et al. (2010). The major genetic determinants of HIV-1 control affect HLA class I peptide presentation. *Science* 330, 1551–1557. doi: 10.1126/science.1195271

Pereyra, F., Palmer, S., Miura, T., Block, B. L., Wiegand, A., Rothchild, A. C., et al. (2009). Persistent low-level viremia in HIV-1 elite controllers and relationship to immunologic parameters. *J. Infect. Dis.* 200, 984–990. doi: 10.1086/605446

Petrov, V., Funderburg, N., Weinberg, A., and Sieg, S. (2013). Human β defensin-3 induces chemokines from monocytes and macrophages: diminished activity in cells from HIV-infected persons. *Immunology* 140, 413–420. doi: 10.1111/imm.12148

Pickford, F., Masliah, E., Britschgi, M., Lucin, K., Narasimhan, R., Jaeger, P. A., et al. (2008). The autophagy-related protein beclin 1 shows reduced expression in early Alzheimer disease and regulates amyloid beta accumulation in mice. *J. Clin. Invest.* 118, 2190–2199.

Pinan-Lucarré, B., Paoletti, M., Dementhon, K., Coulary-Salin, B., and Clavé, C. (2003). Autophagy is induced during cell death by incompatibility and is essential for differentiation in the filamentous fungus Podospora anserina. *Mol. Microbiol.* 47, 321–333. doi: 10.1046/j.1365-2958.2003.03208.x

Poku, N. K. (2016). HIV prevention: the key to ending AIDS by 2030. *Open AIDS J.* 10, 65–77. doi: 10.2174/1874613601610010065

Polson, H. E., De Lartigue, J., Rigden, D. J., Reedijk, M., Urbé, S., Clague, M. J., et al. (2010). Mammalian Atg18 (WIPI2) localizes to omegasome-anchored phagophores and positively regulates LC3 lipidation. *Autophagy* 6, 506–522. doi: 10.4161/auto.6.4.11863

Ponpuak, M., Davis, A. S., Roberts, E. A., Delgado, M. A., Dinkins, C., Zhao, Z., et al. (2010). Delivery of cytosolic components by autophagic adaptor protein p62 endows autophagosomes with unique antimicrobial properties. *Immunity* 32, 329–341. doi: 10.1016/j.immuni.2010.02.009

Poropatich, K., and Sullivan, D. J. Jr. (2011). Human immunodeficiency virus type 1 long-term non-progressors: the viral, genetic and immunological basis for disease non-progression. *J. Gen. Virol.* 92, 247–268. doi: 10.1099/vir.0.027102-0

Powner, D. J., and Wakelam, M. J. (2002). The regulation of phospholipase D by inositol phospholipids and small GTPases. *FEBS Lett.* 531, 62–64. doi: 10.1016/s0014-5793(02)03410-5

Proikas-Cezanne, T., Waddell, S., Gaugel, A., Frickey, T., Lupas, A., and Nordheim, A. (2004). WIPI-1alpha (WIPI49), a member of the novel 7-bladed WIPI protein family, is aberrantly expressed in human cancer and is linked to starvation-induced autophagy. *Oncogene* 23, 9314–9325. doi: 10.1038/sj.onc.1208331

Puigdomenech, I., Massanella, M., Cabrera, C., Clotet, B., and Blanco, J. (2009). On the steps of cell-to-cell HIV transmission between CD4 T cells. *Retrovirology* 6:89. doi: 10.1186/1742-4690-6-89

Punnonen, E. L., Pihakaski, K., Mattila, K., Lounatmaa, K., and Hirsimäki, P. (1989). Intramembrane particles and filipin labelling on the membranes of autophagic vacuoles and lysosomes in mouse liver. *Cell Tissue Res.* 258, 269–276.

Puri, C., Renna, M., Bento, C. F., Moreau, K., and Rubinsztein, D. C. (2013). Diverse autophagosome membrane sources coalesce in recycling endosomes. *Cell* 154, 1285–1299. doi: 10.1016/j.cell.2013.08.044

Py, B. F., Lipinski, M. M., and Yuan, J. (2007). Autophagy limits Listeria monocytogenes intracellular growth in the early phase of primary infection. *Autophagy* 3, 117–125. doi: 10.4161/auto.3618

Qi, L., Gang, L., Hang, K. W., Ling, C. H., Xiaofeng, Z., Zhen, L., et al. (2011). Programmed neuronal cell death induced by HIV-1 tat and methamphetamine. *Microsc. Res. Tech.* 74, 1139–1144. doi: 10.1002/jemt.21006

Qi, S., Kim, D. J., Stjepanovic, G., and Hurley, J. H. (2015). Structure of the human Atg13-Atg101 HORMA heterodimer: an interaction hub within the ULK1 complex. *Structure* 23, 1848–1857. doi: 10.1016/j.str.2015.07.011

Qu, X., Yu, J., Bhagat, G., Furuya, N., Hibshoosh, H., Troxel, A., et al. (2003). Promotion of tumorigenesis by heterozygous disruption of the beclin 1 autophagy gene. *J. Clin. Invest.* 112, 1809–1820. doi: 10.1172/jci20039

Quitadamo, B., Peters, P. J., Repik, A., O'Connell, O., Mou, Z., Koch, M., et al. (2018). HIV-1 R5 macrophage-tropic envelope glycoprotein trimers bind CD4 with high affinity, while the CD4 binding site on non-macrophage-tropic, T-tropic R5 envelopes is occluded. *J. Virol.* 92:e00841-17.

Radhakrishna, H., and Donaldson, J. G. (1997). ADP-ribosylation factor 6 regulates a novel plasma membrane recycling pathway. *J. Cell Biol.* 139, 49–61. doi: 10.1083/jcb.139.1.49

Randow, F., and Youle, R. J. (2014). Self and nonself: how autophagy targets mitochondria and bacteria. *Cell Host Microbe* 15, 403–411. doi: 10.1016/j.chom.2014.03.012

Rasmussen, T. A., Tolstrup, M., Brinkmann, C. R., Olesen, R., Erikstrup, C., Solomon, A., et al. (2014). Panobinostat, a histone deacetylase inhibitor, for latent-virus reactivation in HIV-infected patients on suppressive antiretroviral therapy: a phase 1/2, single group, clinical trial. *Lancet HIV* 1, e13–e21.

Ravikumar, B., Moreau, K., Jahreiss, L., Puri, C., and Rubinsztein, D. C. (2010). Plasma membrane contributes to the formation of pre-autophagosomal structures. *Nat. Cell Biol.* 12, 747–757. doi: 10.1038/ncb2078

Ravikumar, B., Vacher, C., Berger, Z., Davies, J. E., Luo, S., Oroz, L. G., et al. (2004). Inhibition of mTOR induces autophagy and reduces toxicity of polyglutamine expansions in fly and mouse models of Huntington disease. *Nat. Genet.* 36, 585–595. doi: 10.1038/ng1362

Rawat, P., Hon, S., Teodorof-Diedrich, C., and Spector, S. A. (2020). Trehalose inhibits human immunodeficiency virus type 1 infection in primary human macrophages and CD4(+) T lymphocytes through two distinct mechanisms. *J. Virol.* 94:e00237-20.

Raymond, S., Saliou, A., Delobel, P., Cazabat, M., Pasquier, C., Jeanne, N., et al. (2014). Evolution of HIV-1 quasispecies and coreceptor use in cell reservoirs of patients on suppressive antiretroviral therapy. *J. Antimicrob. Chemother.* 69, 2527–2530. doi: 10.1093/jac/dku147

Reece, J. C., Handley, A. J., Anstee, E. J., Morrison, W. A., Crowe, S. M., and Cameron, P. U. (1998). HIV-1 selection by epidermal dendritic cells during transmission across human skin. *J. Exp. Med.* 187, 1623–1631. doi: 10.1084/jem.187.10.1623

Rerks-Ngarm, S., Pitisuttithum, P., Nitayaphan, S., Kaewkungwal, J., Chiu, J., Paris, R., et al. (2009). Vaccination with ALVAC and AIDSVAX to prevent HIV-1 infection in Thailand. *N. Engl. J. Med.* 361, 2209–2220.

Ribeiro, C. M., Sarrami-Forooshani, R., Setiawan, L. C., Zijlstra-Willems, E. M., van Hamme, J. L., Tigchelaar, W., et al. (2016). Receptor usage dictates HIV-1 restriction by human TRIM5α in dendritic cell subsets. *Nature* 540, 448–452. doi: 10.1038/nature20567

Richardson, M. W., Guo, L., Xin, F., Yang, X., and Riley, J. L. (2014). Stabilized human TRIM5α protects human T cells from HIV-1 infection. *Mol. Ther.* 22, 1084–1095. doi: 10.1038/mt.2014.52

Richetta, C., Grégoire, I. P., Verlhac, P., Azocar, O., Baguet, J., Flacher, M., et al. (2013). Sustained autophagy contributes to measles virus infectivity. *PLoS Pathog.* 9:e1003599. doi: 10.1371/journal.ppat.1003599

Rogov, V., Dötsch, V., Johansen, T., and Kirkin, V. (2014). Interactions between autophagy receptors and ubiquitin-like proteins form the molecular basis for selective autophagy. *Mol. Cell.* 53, 167–178. doi: 10.1016/j.molcel.2013.12.014

Rohatgi, R. A., Janusis, J., Leonard, D., Bellvé, K. D., Fogarty, K. E., Baehrecke, E. H., et al. (2015). Beclin 1 regulates growth factor receptor signaling in breast cancer. *Oncogene* 34, 5352–5362. doi: 10.1038/onc.2014.454

Rojas-Celis, V., Valiente-Echeverría, F., Soto-Rifo, R., and Toro-Ascuy, D. (2019). New challenges of HIV-1 infection: how HIV-1 attacks and resides in the central nervous system. *Cells* 8:1245. doi: 10.3390/cells8101245

Romano, S., D'angelillo, A., Pacelli, R., Staibano, S., De Luna, E., Bisogni, R., et al. (2010). Role of FK506-binding protein 51 in the control of apoptosis of irradiated melanoma cells. *Cell Death Differ.* 17, 145–157. doi: 10.1038/cdd.2009.115

Roos, M. T., Lange, J. M., De Goede, R. E., Coutinho, R. A., Schellekens, P. T., Miedema, F., et al. (1992). Viral phenotype and immune response in primary human immunodeficiency virus type 1 infection. *J. Infect. Dis.* 165, 427–432. doi: 10.1093/infdis/165.3.427

Rosenbloom, D. I. S., Hill, A. L., Laskey, S. B., and Siliciano, R. F. (2017). Re-evaluating evolution in the HIV reservoir. *Nature* 551, E6–E9.

Rotger, M., Dalmau, J., Rauch, A., Mclaren, P., Bosinger, S. E., Martinez, R., et al. (2011). Comparative transcriptomics of extreme phenotypes of human HIV-1 infection and SIV infection in sooty mangabey and rhesus macaque. *J. Clin. Invest.* 121, 2391–2400. doi: 10.1172/jci45235

Rotger, M., Dang, K. K., Fellay, J., Heinzen, E. L., Feng, S., Descombes, P., et al. (2010). Genome-wide mRNA expression correlates of viral control in CD4+ T-cells from HIV-1-infected individuals. *PLoS Pathog.* 6:e1000781. doi: 10.1371/journal.ppat.1000781

Sagnier, S., Daussy, C. F., Borel, S., Robert-Hebmann, V., Faure, M., Blanchet, F. P., et al. (2015). Autophagy restricts HIV-1 infection by selectively degrading Tat in CD4+ T lymphocytes. *J. Virol.* 89, 615–625. doi: 10.1128/jvi.02174-14

Saha, B., Chisholm, D., Kell, A. M., and Mandell, M. A. (2020). A non-canonical role for the autophagy machinery in anti-retroviral signaling mediated by TRIM5α. *PLoS Pathog.* 16:e1009017. doi: 10.1371/journal.ppat.1009017

Salazar-Gonzalez, J. F., Salazar, M. G., Keele, B. F., Learn, G. H., Giorgi, E. E., Li, H., et al. (2009). Genetic identity, biological phenotype, and evolutionary pathways of transmitted/founder viruses in acute and early HIV-1 infection. *J. Exp. Med.* 206, 1273–1289. doi: 10.1084/jem.20090378

Salgado, M., Brennan, T. P., O'Connell, K. A., Bailey, J. R., Ray, S. C., Siliciano, R. F., et al. (2010). Evolution of the HIV-1 nef gene in HLA-B*57 positive elite suppressors. *Retrovirology* 7:94. doi: 10.1186/1742-4690-7-94

Samson, M., Libert, F., Doranz, B. J., Rucker, J., Liesnard, C., Farber, C. M., et al. (1996). Resistance to HIV-1 infection in caucasian individuals bearing mutant alleles of the CCR-5 chemokine receptor gene. *Nature* 382, 722–725. doi: 10.1038/382722a0

Santy, L. C., and Casanova, J. E. (2001). Activation of ARF6 by ARNO stimulates epithelial cell migration through downstream activation of both Rac1 and phospholipase D. *J. Cell Biol.* 154, 599–610. doi: 10.1083/jcb.200104019

Sarkar, S., Davies, J. E., Huang, Z., Tunnacliffe, A., and Rubinsztein, D. C. (2007). Trehalose, a novel mTOR-independent autophagy enhancer, accelerates the clearance of mutant huntingtin and alpha-synuclein. *J. Biol. Chem.* 282, 5641–5652. doi: 10.1074/jbc.m609532200

Sawa-Makarska, J., Baumann, V., Coudevylle, N., Von Bülow, S., Nogellova, V., Abert, C., et al. (2020). Reconstitution of autophagosome nucleation defines Atg9 vesicles as seeds for membrane formation. *Science* 369:eaaz7714. doi: 10.1126/science.aaz7714

Scheid, J. F., Horwitz, J. A., Bar-On, Y., Kreider, E. F., Lu, C. L., Lorenzi, J. C., et al. (2016). HIV-1 antibody 3BNC117 suppresses viral rebound in humans during treatment interruption. *Nature* 535, 556–560. doi: 10.1038/nature18929

Schmid, D., Pypaert, M., and Münz, C. (2007). Antigen-loading compartments for major histocompatibility complex class II molecules continuously receive input from autophagosomes. *Immunity* 26, 79–92. doi: 10.1016/j.immuni.2006.10.018

Schneck, N. A., Ivleva, V. B., Cai, C. X., Cooper, J. W., and Lei, Q. P. (2020). Characterization of the furin cleavage motif for HIV-1 trimeric envelope glycoprotein by intact LC-MS analysis. *Analyst* 145, 1636–1640. doi: 10.1039/c9an02098e

Schuitemaker, H., Koot, M., Kootstra, N. A., Dercksen, M. W., De Goede, R. E., van Steenwijk, R. P., et al. (1992). Biological phenotype of human immunodeficiency virus type 1 clones at different stages of infection: progression of disease is associated with a shift from monocytotropic to T-cell-tropic virus population. *J. Virol.* 66, 1354–1360. doi: 10.1128/jvi.66.3.1354-1360.1992

Schuurman, R., Brambilla, D., De Groot, T., Huang, D., Land, S., Bremer, J., et al. (2002). Underestimation of HIV type 1 drug resistance mutations: results from the ENVA-2 genotyping proficiency program. *AIDS Res. Hum. Retroviruses* 18, 243–248. doi: 10.1089/088922202753472801

Schweighardt, B., Roy, A. M., Meiklejohn, D. A., Grace, E. J. II, Moretto, W. J., Heymann, J. J., et al. (2004). R5 human immunodeficiency virus type 1 (HIV-1) replicates more efficiently in primary CD4+ T-cell cultures than X4 HIV-1. *J. Virol.* 78, 9164–9173. doi: 10.1128/jvi.78.17.9164-9173.2004

Seglen, P. O., and Gordon, P. B. (1982). 3-Methyladenine: specific inhibitor of autophagic/lysosomal protein degradation in isolated rat hepatocytes. *Proc. Natl. Acad. Sci. U.S.A.* 79, 1889–1892. doi: 10.1073/pnas.79.6.1889

Seigneurin-Berny, D., Verdel, A., Curtet, S., Lemercier, C., Garin, J., Rousseaux, S., et al. (2001). Identification of components of the murine histone deacetylase 6 complex: link between acetylation and ubiquitination signaling pathways. *Mol. Cell. Biol.* 21, 8035–8044. doi: 10.1128/mcb.21.23.8035-8044.2001

Shah, A., and Kumar, A. (2010). HIV-1 gp120-mediated increases in IL-8 production in astrocytes are mediated through the NF-κB pathway and can be silenced by gp120-specific siRNA. *J. Neuroinflammation* 7:96. doi: 10.1186/1742-2094-7-96

Shah, A., Verma, A. S., Patel, K. H., Noel, R., Rivera-Amill, V., Silverstein, P. S., et al. (2011). HIV-1 gp120 induces expression of IL-6 through a nuclear factor-kappa B-dependent mechanism: suppression by gp120 specific small interfering RNA. *PLoS One* 6:e21261. doi: 10.1371/journal.pone.0021261

Shaik, M. M., Peng, H., Lu, J., Rits-Volloch, S., Xu, C., Liao, M., et al. (2019). Structural basis of coreceptor recognition by HIV-1 envelope spike. *Nature* 565, 318–323. doi: 10.1038/s41586-018-0804-9

Shi, C. S., and Kehrl, J. H. (2008). MyD88 and Trif target Beclin 1 to trigger autophagy in macrophages. *J. Biol. Chem.* 283, 33175–33182. doi: 10.1074/jbc.m804478200

Shoji-Kawata, S., Sumpter, R., Leveno, M., Campbell, G. R., Zou, Z., Kinch, L., et al. (2013). Identification of a candidate therapeutic autophagy-inducing peptide. *Nature* 494, 201–206. doi: 10.1038/nature11866

Shpilka, T., Weidberg, H., Pietrokovski, S., and Elazar, Z. (2011). Atg8: an autophagy-related ubiquitin-like protein family. *Genome Biol.* 12:226. doi: 10.1186/gb-2011-12-7-226

Shvets, E., Abada, A., Weidberg, H., and Elazar, Z. (2011). Dissecting the involvement of LC3B and GATE-16 in p62 recruitment into autophagosomes. *Autophagy* 7, 683–688. doi: 10.4161/auto.7.7.15279

Siliciano, R. F., and Greene, W. C. (2011). HIV latency. *Cold Spring Harb. Perspect. Med.* 1:a007096.

Sivaraman, V., Zhang, L., Meissner, E. G., Jeffrey, J. L., and Su, L. (2009). The heptad repeat 2 domain is a major determinant for enhanced human immunodeficiency virus type 1 (HIV-1) fusion and pathogenicity of a highly pathogenic HIV-1 Env. *J. Virol.* 83, 11715–11725. doi: 10.1128/jvi.00649-09

Søgaard, O. S., Graversen, M. E., Leth, S., Olesen, R., Brinkmann, C. R., Nissen, S. K., et al. (2015). The depsipeptide romidepsin reverses HIV-1 latency in vivo. *PLoS Pathog.* 11:e1005142. doi: 10.1371/journal.ppat.1005142

Soliman, M., Srikrishna, G., and Balagopal, A. (2017). Mechanisms of HIV-1 control. *Curr. HIV/AIDS Rep.* 14, 101–109. doi: 10.1007/s11904-017-0357-9

Sood, C., Marin, M., Chande, A., Pizzato, M., and Melikyan, G. B. (2017). SERINC5 protein inhibits HIV-1 fusion pore formation by promoting functional inactivation of envelope glycoproteins. *J. Biol. Chem.* 292, 6014–6026. doi: 10.1074/jbc.m117.777714

Spijkerman, I. J., Koot, M., Prins, M., Keet, I. P., van den Hoek, A. J., Miedema, F., et al. (1995). Lower prevalence and incidence of HIV-1 syncytium-inducing phenotype among injecting drug users compared with homosexual men. *Aids* 9, 1085–1092. doi: 10.1097/00002030-199509000-00016

Staring, J., Von Castelmur, E., Blomen, V. A., van den Hengel, L. G., Brockmann, M., Baggen, J., et al. (2017). PLA2G16 represents a switch between entry and clearance of Picornaviridae. *Nature* 541, 412–416. doi: 10.1038/nature21032

Staropoli, I., Chanel, C., Girard, M., and Altmeyer, R. (2000). Processing, stability, and receptor binding properties of oligomeric envelope glycoprotein from a primary HIV-1 isolate. *J. Biol. Chem.* 275, 35137–35145. doi: 10.1074/jbc.m003868200

Stevenson, M. (2003). HIV-1 pathogenesis. *Nat. Med.* 9, 853–860.

Stolp, B., and Fackler, O. T. (2011). How HIV takes advantage of the cytoskeleton in entry and replication. *Viruses* 3, 293–311. doi: 10.3390/v3040293

Straubinger, T., Kay, K., and Bies, R. (2019). Modeling HIV pre-exposure prophylaxis. *Front. Pharmacol.* 10:1514.

Stremlau, M., Owens, C. M., Perron, M. J., Kiessling, M., Autissier, P., and Sodroski, J. (2004). The cytoplasmic body component TRIM5alpha restricts HIV-1 infection in Old World monkeys. *Nature* 427, 848–853. doi: 10.1038/nature02343

Stultz, R. D., Cenker, J. J., and Mcdonald, D. (2017). Imaging HIV-1 genomic DNA from entry through productive infection. *J. Virol.* 91:e00034-17.

Sutton, J., Dotson, D., and Dong, X. (2013). Molecular events in late stages of HIV-1 replication. *JSM Microbiol.* 1:1004.

Suzuki, H., Tabata, K., Morita, E., Kawasaki, M., Kato, R., Dobson, R. C., et al. (2014). Structural basis of the autophagy-related LC3/Atg13 LIR complex: recognition and interaction mechanism. *Structure* 22, 47–58. doi: 10.1016/j.str.2013.09.023

Tang, H., Sebti, S., Titone, R., Zhou, Y., Isidoro, C., Ross, T. S., et al. (2015). Decreased BECN1 mRNA expression in human breast cancer is associated with estrogen receptor-negative subtypes and poor prognosis. *EBioMedicine* 2, 255–263. doi: 10.1016/j.ebiom.2015.01.008

Tang, Z., Takahashi, Y., and Wang, H. G. (2019). ATG2 regulation of phagophore expansion at mitochondria-associated ER membranes. *Autophagy* 15, 2165–2166. doi: 10.1080/15548627.2019.1666594

Tey, S. K., and Khanna, R. (2012). Autophagy mediates transporter associated with antigen processing-independent presentation of viral epitopes through MHC class I pathway. *Blood* 120, 994–1004. doi: 10.1182/blood-2012-01-402404

Toda, K., Nogami, M., Murakami, K., Kanaho, Y., and Nakayama, K. (1999). Colocalization of phospholipase D1 and GTP-binding-defective mutant of ADP-ribosylation factor 6 to endosomes and lysosomes. *FEBS Lett.* 442, 221–225. doi: 10.1016/s0014-5793(98)01646-9

Tomoda, T., Bhatt, R. S., Kuroyanagi, H., Shirasawa, T., and Hatten, M. E. (1999). A mouse serine/threonine kinase homologous to *C. elegans* UNC51 functions in parallel fiber formation of cerebellar granule neurons. *Neuron* 24, 833–846. doi: 10.1016/s0896-6273(00)81031-4

Travassos, L. H., Carneiro, L. A., Ramjeet, M., Hussey, S., Kim, Y. G., Magalhães, J. G., et al. (2010). Nod1 and Nod2 direct autophagy by recruiting ATG16L1 to the plasma membrane at the site of bacterial entry. *Nat. Immunol.* 11, 55–62. doi: 10.1038/ni.1823

Tsao, L. C., Guo, H., Jeffrey, J., Hoxie, J. A., and Su, L. (2016). CCR5 interaction with HIV-1 Env contributes to Env-induced depletion of CD4 T cells in vitro and in vivo. *Retrovirology* 13:22.

Tuttle, D. L., Coberley, C. R., Xie, X., Kou, Z. C., Sleasman, J. W., and Goodenow, M. M. (2004). Effects of human immunodeficiency virus type 1 infection on CCR5 and CXCR4 coreceptor expression on CD4 T lymphocyte subsets in infants and adolescents. *AIDS Res. Hum. Retroviruses* 20, 305–313. doi: 10.1089/088922204322996545

UNAIDS (2015). *Understanding Fast-Track: Accelerating Action To End the AIDS Epidemic by 2030*. Available online at: https://www.unaids.org/sites/default/files/media_asset/201506_JC2743_Understanding_FastTrack_en.pdf (accesssed June 2015).

UNAIDS (2020). *Global HIV & AIDS Statistics*. Available online at: https://www.unaids.org/en/resources/fact-sheet (accesssed December 2015).

Vakifahmetoglu-Norberg, H., Xia, H. G., and Yuan, J. (2015). Pharmacologic agents targeting autophagy. *J. Clin. Invest.* 125, 5–13. doi: 10.1172/jci73937

Valečka, J., Almeida, C. R., Su, B., Pierre, P., and Gatti, E. (2018). Autophagy and MHC-restricted antigen presentation. *Mol. Immunol.* 99, 163–170. doi: 10.1016/j.molimm.2018.05.009

Valenzuela-Fernandez, A., Alvarez, S., Gordon-Alonso, M., Barrero, M., Ursa, A., Cabrero, J. R., et al. (2005). Histone deacetylase 6 regulates human immunodeficiency virus type 1 infection. *Mol. Biol. Cell* 16, 5445–5454. doi: 10.1091/mbc.e05-04-0354

Valenzuela-Fernandez, A., Cabrero, J. R., Serrador, J. M., and Sanchez-Madrid, F. (2008). HDAC6: a key regulator of cytoskeleton, cell migration and cell-cell interactions. *Trends Cell Biol.* 18, 291–297. doi: 10.1016/j.tcb.2008.04.003

Valera, M. S., de Armas-Rillo, L., Barroso-Gonzalez, J., Ziglio, S., Batisse, J., Dubois, N., et al. (2015). The HDAC6/APOBEC3G complex regulates HIV-1 infectiveness by inducing Vif autophagic degradation. *Retrovirology* 12:53.

van Grevenynghe, J., Procopio, F. A., He, Z., Chomont, N., Riou, C., Zhang, Y., et al. (2008). Transcription factor FOXO3a controls the persistence of memory CD4(+) T cells during HIV infection. *Nat. Med.* 14, 266–274. doi: 10.1038/nm1728

van Grol, J., Subauste, C., Andrade, R. M., Fujinaga, K., Nelson, J., and Subauste, C. S. (2010). HIV-1 inhibits autophagy in bystander macrophage/monocytic cells through Src-Akt and STAT3. *PLoS One* 5:e11733. doi: 10.1371/journal.pone.0011733

van Marle, G., Church, D. L., van der Meer, F., and Gill, M. J. (2018). Combating the HIV reservoirs. *Biotechnol. Genet. Eng. Rev.* 34, 76–89. doi: 10.1080/02648725.2018.1471641

van't Wout, A. B., Kootstra, N. A., Mulder-Kampinga, G. A., Albrecht-van Lent, N., Scherpbier, H. J., Veenstra, J., et al. (1994). Macrophage-tropic variants initiate human immunodeficiency virus type 1 infection after sexual, parenteral, and vertical transmission. *J. Clin. Invest.* 94, 2060–2067. doi: 10.1172/jci117560

Varbanov, M., Espert, L., and Biard-Piechaczyk, M. (2006). Mechanisms of CD4 T-cell depletion triggered by HIV-1 viral proteins. *AIDS Rev.* 8, 221–236.

Verzella, D., Pescatore, A., Capece, D., Vecchiotti, D., Ursini, M. V., Franzoso, G., et al. (2020). Life, death, and autophagy in cancer: NF-κB turns up everywhere. *Cell Death Dis.* 11:210.

Viret, C., Rozières, A., and Faure, M. (2018). Autophagy during early virus-host cell interactions. *J. Mol. Biol.* 430, 1696–1713. doi: 10.1016/j.jmb.2018.04.018

Vlahakis, S. R., Algeciras-Schimnich, A., Bou, G., Heppelmann, C. J., Villasis-Keever, A., Collman, R. G., et al. (2001). Chemokine-receptor activation by env determines the mechanism of death in HIV-infected and uninfected T lymphocytes. *J. Clin. Invest.* 107, 207–215. doi: 10.1172/jci11109

Vogl, D. T., Stadtmauer, E. A., Tan, K. S., Heitjan, D. F., Davis, L. E., Pontiggia, L., et al. (2014). Combined autophagy and proteasome inhibition: a phase 1 trial of hydroxychloroquine and bortezomib in patients with relapsed/refractory myeloma. *Autophagy* 10, 1380–1390. doi: 10.4161/auto.29264

Vorster, P. J., Guo, J., Yoder, A., Wang, W., Zheng, Y., Xu, X., et al. (2011). LIM kinase 1 modulates cortical actin and CXCR4 cycling and is activated by HIV-1 to initiate viral infection. *J. Biol. Chem.* 286, 12554–12564. doi: 10.1074/jbc.m110.182238

Walczak, M., and Martens, S. (2013). Dissecting the role of the Atg12-Atg5-Atg16 complex during autophagosome formation. *Autophagy* 9, 424–425. doi: 10.4161/auto.22931

Wang, G., Zhao, N., Berkhout, B., and Das, A. T. (2016). CRISPR-Cas9 can inhibit HIV-1 replication but NHEJ repair facilitates virus escape. *Mol. Ther.* 24, 522–526. doi: 10.1038/mt.2016.24

Wang, H. W., Zhu, B., Hou, L. J., Lu, G. J., Jiao, L. Y., and Shen, B. S. (2015). An infectious molecular clone in early infection with HIV-1 subtype CRF01_AE strains: construction and biological properties. *Mol. Biol. Rep.* 42, 329–336. doi: 10.1007/s11033-014-3754-9

Ward, A. B., and Wilson, I. A. (2017). The HIV-1 envelope glycoprotein structure: nailing down a moving target. *Immunol. Rev.* 275, 21–32. doi: 10.1111/imr.12507

Weatherley, D. A. V., Boswell, M. T., and Rowland-Jones, S. L. (2017). Targeting TRIM5α in HIV cure strategies for the CRISPR-Cas9 Era. *Front. Immunol.* 8:1616.

Wei, H., Wang, C., Croce, C. M., and Guan, J. L. (2014). p62/SQSTM1 synergizes with autophagy for tumor growth in vivo. *Genes Dev.* 28, 1204–1216. doi: 10.1101/gad.237354.113

Weidberg, H., Shpilka, T., Shvets, E., Abada, A., Shimron, F., and Elazar, Z. (2011a). LC3 and GATE-16 N termini mediate membrane fusion processes required for autophagosome biogenesis. *Dev. Cell* 20, 444–454. doi: 10.1016/j.devcel.2011.02.006

Weidberg, H., Shvets, E., and Elazar, Z. (2011b). Biogenesis and cargo selectivity of autophagosomes. *Annu. Rev. Biochem.* 80, 125–156. doi: 10.1146/annurev-biochem-052709-094552

Weidberg, H., Shvets, E., Shpilka, T., Shimron, F., Shinder, V., and Elazar, Z. (2010). LC3 and GATE-16/GABARAP subfamilies are both essential yet act differently in autophagosome biogenesis. *EMBO J.* 29, 1792–1802. doi: 10.1038/emboj.2010.74

Weissman, D., Rabin, R. L., Arthos, J., Rubbert, A., Dybul, M., Swofford, R., et al. (1997). Macrophage-tropic HIV and SIV envelope proteins induce a signal through the CCR5 chemokine receptor. *Nature* 389, 981–985. doi: 10.1038/40173

White, E. (2012). Deconvoluting the context-dependent role for autophagy in cancer. *Nat. Rev. Cancer* 12, 401–410. doi: 10.1038/nrc3262

Whittall, T., Peters, B., Rahman, D., Kingsley, C. I., Vaughan, R., and Lehner, T. (2011). Immunogenic and tolerogenic signatures in human immunodeficiency virus (HIV)-infected controllers compared with progressors and a conversion strategy of virus control. *Clin. Exp. Immunol.* 166, 208–217. doi: 10.1111/j.1365-2249.2011.04463.x

Wild, P., Farhan, H., Mcewan, D. G., Wagner, S., Rogov, V. V., Brady, N. R., et al. (2011). Phosphorylation of the autophagy receptor optineurin restricts *Salmonella* growth. *Science* 333, 228–233. doi: 10.1126/science.1205405

Wilen, C. B., Tilton, J. C., and Doms, R. W. (2012). HIV: cell binding and entry. *Cold Spring Harb. Perspect. Med.* 2:a006866. doi: 10.1101/cshperspect.a006866

Willey, S., Peters, P. J., Sullivan, W. M., Dorr, P., Perros, M., and Clapham, P. R. (2005). Inhibition of CCR5-mediated infection by diverse R5 and R5X4 HIV and SIV isolates using novel small molecule inhibitors of CCR5: effects of viral diversity, target cell and receptor density. *Antiviral Res.* 68, 96–108. doi: 10.1016/j.antiviral.2005.07.006

Woldemeskel, B. A., Kwaa, A. K., and Blankson, J. N. (2020). Viral reservoirs in elite controllers of HIV-1 infection: implications for HIV cure strategies. *EBioMedicine* 62:103118. doi: 10.1016/j.ebiom.2020.103118

Wong, J. K., Hezareh, M., Günthard, H. F., Havlir, D. V., Ignacio, C. C., Spina, C. A., et al. (1997). Recovery of replication-competent HIV despite prolonged suppression of plasma viremia. *Science* 278, 1291–1295. doi: 10.1126/science.278.5341.1291

Xin, Y., Yu, L., Chen, Z., Zheng, L., Fu, Q., Jiang, J., et al. (2001). Cloning, expression patterns, and chromosome localization of three human and two mouse homologues of GABA(A) receptor-associated protein. *Genomics* 74, 408–413. doi: 10.1006/geno.2001.6555

Xu, L., Yang, H., Gao, Y., Chen, Z., Xie, L., Liu, Y., et al. (2017). CRISPR/Cas9-mediated CCR5 ablation in human hematopoietic stem/progenitor cells confers HIV-1 resistance in vivo. *Mol. Ther.* 25, 1782–1789. doi: 10.1016/j.ymthe.2017.04.027

Yamaguchi, H., Nakagawa, I., Yamamoto, A., Amano, A., Noda, T., and Yoshimori, T. (2009). An initial step of GAS-containing autophagosome-like vacuoles formation requires Rab7. *PLoS Pathog.* 5:e1000670. doi: 10.1371/journal.ppat.1000670

Yamamoto, A., Tagawa, Y., Yoshimori, T., Moriyama, Y., Masaki, R., and Tashiro, Y. (1998). Bafilomycin A1 prevents maturation of autophagic vacuoles by inhibiting fusion between autophagosomes and lysosomes in rat hepatoma cell line, H-4-II-E cells. *Cell Struct. Funct.* 23, 33–42. doi: 10.1247/csf.23.33

Yamamoto, H., Kakuta, S., Watanabe, T. M., Kitamura, A., Sekito, T., Kondo-Kakuta, C., et al. (2012). Atg9 vesicles are an important membrane source during early steps of autophagosome formation. *J. Cell Biol.* 198, 219–233. doi: 10.1083/jcb.201202061

Yan, J., Kuroyanagi, H., Kuroiwa, A., Matsuda, Y., Tokumitsu, H., Tomoda, T., et al. (1998). Identification of mouse ULK1, a novel protein kinase structurally related to *C. elegans* UNC-51. *Biochem. Biophys. Res. Commun.* 246, 222–227. doi: 10.1006/bbrc.1998.8546

Yan, J., Kuroyanagi, H., Tomemori, T., Okazaki, N., Asato, K., Matsuda, Y., et al. (1999). Mouse ULK2, a novel member of the UNC-51-like protein kinases: unique features of functional domains. *Oncogene* 18, 5850–5859. doi: 10.1038/sj.onc.1202988

Yang, A., Rajeshkumar, N. V., Wang, X., Yabuuchi, S., Alexander, B. M., Chu, G. C., et al. (2014). Autophagy is critical for pancreatic tumor growth and progression in tumors with p53 alterations. *Cancer Discov.* 4, 905–913. doi: 10.1158/2159-8290.cd-14-0362

Yang, S., Wang, X., Contino, G., Liesa, M., Sahin, E., Ying, H., et al. (2011). Pancreatic cancers require autophagy for tumor growth. *Genes Dev.* 25, 717–729. doi: 10.1101/gad.2016111

Yang, Z., and Klionsky, D. J. (2010). Mammalian autophagy: core molecular machinery and signaling regulation. *Curr. Opin. Cell Biol.* 22, 124–131. doi: 10.1016/j.ceb.2009.11.014

Yoder, A., Yu, D., Dong, L., Iyer, S. R., Xu, X., Kelly, J., et al. (2008). HIV envelope-CXCR4 signaling activates cofilin to overcome cortical actin restriction in resting CD4 T cells. *Cell* 134, 782–792. doi: 10.1016/j.cell.2008.06.036

Yoon, Y. S., Cho, E. D., Jung Ahn, W., Won Lee, K., Lee, S. J., and Lee, H. J. (2017). Is trehalose an autophagic inducer? Unraveling the roles of non-reducing disaccharides on autophagic flux and alpha-synuclein aggregation. *Cell Death Dis.* 8:e3091. doi: 10.1038/cddis.2017.501

Young, A. R., Chan, E. Y., Hu, X. W., Köchl, R., Crawshaw, S. G., High, S., et al. (2006). Starvation and ULK1-dependent cycling of mammalian Atg9 between the TGN and endosomes. *J. Cell Sci.* 119, 3888–3900. doi: 10.1242/jcs.03172

Yue, Z., Jin, S., Yang, C., Levine, A. J., and Heintz, N. (2003). Beclin 1, an autophagy gene essential for early embryonic development, is a haploinsufficient tumor suppressor. *Proc. Natl. Acad. Sci. U.S.A.* 100, 15077–15082. doi: 10.1073/pnas.2436255100

Zaunders, J., Dyer, W. B., and Churchill, M. (2011). The sydney blood bank cohort: implications for viral fitness as a cause of elite control. *Curr. Opin. HIV AIDS* 6, 151–156. doi: 10.1097/coh.0b013e3283454d5b

Zhang, F., Wen, Y., and Guo, X. (2014). CRISPR/Cas9 for genome editing: progress, implications and challenges. *Hum. Mol. Genet.* 23, R40–R46.

Zhang, Y., Wu, Y., Wu, D., Tashiro, S., Onodera, S., and Ikejima, T. (2009a). NF-kappab facilitates oridonin-induced apoptosis and autophagy in HT1080 cells through a p53-mediated pathway. *Arch. Biochem. Biophys.* 489, 25–33. doi: 10.1016/j.abb.2009.07.017

Zhang, Y., Yan, L., Zhou, Z., Yang, P., Tian, E., Zhang, K., et al. (2009b). SEPA-1 mediates the specific recognition and degradation of P granule components by autophagy in *C. elegans*. *Cell* 136, 308–321. doi: 10.1016/j.cell.2008.12.022

Zhang, Z., Jiang, Y., Zhang, M., Liu, J., Sun, G., Shi, W., et al. (2010). Alterations of CD4(+) CD25(+) Foxp3(+) regulatory T cells in HIV-infected slow progressors of former blood donors in China. *Microbiol. Immunol.* 54, 625–633.

Zhong, Y., Wang, Q. J., Li, X., Yan, Y., Backer, J. M., Chait, B. T., et al. (2009). Distinct regulation of autophagic activity by Atg14L and Rubicon associated with Beclin 1-phosphatidylinositol-3-kinase complex. *Nat. Cell Biol.* 11, 468–476. doi: 10.1038/ncb1854

Zhou, D., Li, P., Lin, Y., Lott, J. M., Hislop, A. D., Canaday, D. H., et al. (2005). Lamp-2a facilitates MHC class II presentation of cytoplasmic antigens. *Immunity* 22, 571–581. doi: 10.1016/j.immuni.2005.03.009

Zhou, D., Masliah, E., and Spector, S. A. (2011). Autophagy is increased in postmortem brains of persons with HIV-1-associated encephalitis. *J. Infect. Dis.* 203, 1647–1657. doi: 10.1093/infdis/jir163

Zhou, D., and Spector, S. A. (2008). Human immunodeficiency virus type-1 infection inhibits autophagy. *Aids* 22, 695–699. doi: 10.1097/qad.0b013e3282f4a836

Zhou, J. S., Zhao, Y., Zhou, H. B., Wang, Y., Wu, Y. F., Li, Z. Y., et al. (2016). Autophagy plays an essential role in cigarette smoke-induced expression of MUC5AC in airway epithelium. *Am. J. Physiol. Lung Cell Mol. Physiol.* 310, L1042–L1052.

Zhu, T., Mo, H., Wang, N., Nam, D. S., Cao, Y., Koup, R. A., et al. (1993). Genotypic and phenotypic characterization of HIV-1 patients with primary infection. *Science* 261, 1179–1181. doi: 10.1126/science.8356453

Zhu, T., Muthui, D., Holte, S., Nickle, D., Feng, F., Brodie, S., et al. (2002). Evidence for human immunodeficiency virus type 1 replication in vivo in CD14(+) monocytes and its potential role as a source of virus in patients on highly active antiretroviral therapy. *J. Virol.* 76, 707–716. doi: 10.1128/jvi.76.2.707-716.2002

Zhu, W., Lei, R., Le Duff, Y., Li, J., Guo, F., Wainberg, M. A., et al. (2015). The CRISPR/Cas9 system inactivates latent HIV-1 proviral DNA. *Retrovirology* 12:22.

Zhuo, C., Ji, Y., Chen, Z., Kitazato, K., Xiang, Y., Zhong, M., et al. (2013). Proteomics analysis of autophagy-deficient Atg7-/- MEFs reveals a close relationship between F-actin and autophagy. *Biochem. Biophys. Res. Commun.* 437, 482–488. doi: 10.1016/j.bbrc.2013.06.111

Zwart, W., Griekspoor, A., Kuijl, C., Marsman, M., van Rheenen, J., Janssen, H., et al. (2005). Spatial separation of HLA-DM/HLA-DR interactions within MIIC and phagosome-induced immune escape. *Immunity* 22, 221–233. doi: 10.1016/j.immuni.2005.01.006

Permissions

All chapters in this book were first published by Frontiers; hereby published with permission under the Creative Commons Attribution License or equivalent. Every chapter published in this book has been scrutinized by our experts. Their significance has been extensively debated. The topics covered herein carry significant findings which will fuel the growth of the discipline. They may even be implemented as practical applications or may be referred to as a beginning point for another development.

The contributors of this book come from diverse backgrounds, making this book a truly international effort. This book will bring forth new frontiers with its revolutionizing research information and detailed analysis of the nascent developments around the world.

We would like to thank all the contributing authors for lending their expertise to make the book truly unique. They have played a crucial role in the development of this book. Without their invaluable contributions this book wouldn't have been possible. They have made vital efforts to compile up to date information on the varied aspects of this subject to make this book a valuable addition to the collection of many professionals and students.

This book was conceptualized with the vision of imparting up-to-date information and advanced data in this field. To ensure the same, a matchless editorial board was set up. Every individual on the board went through rigorous rounds of assessment to prove their worth. After which they invested a large part of their time researching and compiling the most relevant data for our readers.

The editorial board has been involved in producing this book since its inception. They have spent rigorous hours researching and exploring the diverse topics which have resulted in the successful publishing of this book. They have passed on their knowledge of decades through this book. To expedite this challenging task, the publisher supported the team at every step. A small team of assistant editors was also appointed to further simplify the editing procedure and attain best results for the readers.

Apart from the editorial board, the designing team has also invested a significant amount of their time in understanding the subject and creating the most relevant covers. They scrutinized every image to scout for the most suitable representation of the subject and create an appropriate cover for the book.

The publishing team has been an ardent support to the editorial, designing and production team. Their endless efforts to recruit the best for this project, has resulted in the accomplishment of this book. They are a veteran in the field of academics and their pool of knowledge is as vast as their experience in printing. Their expertise and guidance has proved useful at every step. Their uncompromising quality standards have made this book an exceptional effort. Their encouragement from time to time has been an inspiration for everyone.

The publisher and the editorial board hope that this book will prove to be a valuable piece of knowledge for researchers, students, practitioners and scholars across the globe.

List of Contributors

Amina Ait-Ammar, Roxane Verdikt and Carine Van Lint
Service of Molecular Virology, Department of Molecular Virology (DBM), Université Libre de Bruxelles (ULB), Gosselies, Belgium

Anna Kula
Malopolska Centre of Biotechnology, Laboratory of Virology, Jagiellonian University, Krakow, Poland

Gilles Darcis
Laboratory of Experimental Virology, Department of Medical Microbiology, Amsterdam UMC, University of Amsterdam, Amsterdam, Netherlands
Infectious Diseases Department, Liège University Hospital, Liège, Belgium

Stephane De Wit
Service des Maladies Infectieuses, CHU Saint-Pierre, Université Libre de Bruxelles, Bruxelles, Belgium

Virginie Gautier and Patrick W. G. Mallon
UCD Centre for Experimental Pathogen Host Research (CEPHR), School of Medicine, University College Dublin, Dublin, Ireland

Alessandro Marcello
Laboratory of Molecular Virology, International Centre for Genetic Engineering and Biotechnology (ICGEB), Trieste, Italy

Eunok Lee and Sarah Palmer
Centre for Virus Research, The Westmead Institute for Medical Research, Sydney, NSW, Australia
Sydney Medical School, The University of Sydney, Sydney, NSW, Australia

Peter Bacchetti
Department of Epidemiology and Biostatistics, University of California, San Francisco, San Francisco, CA, United States

Jeffery Milush, Teri Liegler, Rebecca Hoh, Steve G. Deeks and Frederick M. Hecht
Department of Medicine, University of California, San Francisco, San Francisco, CA, United States

Wei Shao
Leidos Biomedical Research, Inc., Frederick National Laboratory for Cancer Research, Frederick, MD, United States

Eli Boritz and Daniel Douek
Human Immunology Section, Vaccine Research Center, National Institutes of Allergy and Infectious Diseases, National Institute of Health, Bethesda, MD, United States

Remi Fromentin
Centre de Recherche du CHUM et Département de Microbiologie, Infectiologie et Immunologie, Université de Montreal, Montreal, QC, Canada

Shane D. Falcinelli
UNC HIV Cure Center, The University of North Carolina at Chapel Hill, Chapel Hill, NC, United States
Department of Microbiology and Immunology, The University of North Carolina at Chapel Hill, Chapel Hill, NC, United States

Cristina Ceriani and Nancie M. Archin
UNC HIV Cure Center, The University of North Carolina at Chapel Hill, Chapel Hill, NC, United States
Department of Medicine, The University of North Carolina at Chapel Hill, Chapel Hill, NC, United States

David M. Margolis
UNC HIV Cure Center, The University of North Carolina at Chapel Hill, Chapel Hill, NC, United States
Department of Microbiology and Immunology, The University of North Carolina at Chapel Hill, Chapel Hill, NC, United States
Department of Medicine, The University of North Carolina at Chapel Hill, Chapel Hill, NC, United States

Paul W. Denton
Department of Biology, University of Nebraska Omaha, Omaha, NE, United States

Ole S. Søgaard and Martin Tolstrup
Institute of Clinical Medicine, Aarhus University, Aarhus, Denmark
Department of Infectious Diseases, Aarhus University Hospital, Aarhus, Denmark

Yuwei Zhang, Delphine Planas, Marta Massanella, Huicheng Chen, Vanessa Sue Wacleche, Nicolas Chomont and Petronela Ancuta
Département de microbiologie, infectiologie et immunologie, Faculté de Médecine, Université de Montréal, Montreal, QC, Canada
Centre hospitalier de l'Université de Montréal (CHUM)-Research Centre, Montreal, QC, Canada

Laurence Raymond Marchand and Annie Gosselin
Centre hospitalier de l'Université de Montréal (CHUM)-Research Centre, Montreal, QC, Canada

Jean-Philippe Goulet
Caprion, Montreal, QC, Canada

Mario Filion
Alethia Biotherapeutics, Montreal, QC, Canada

Jean-Pierre Routy
McGill University Health Centre, Montreal, QC, Canada

Sarah E. Beck and Rebecca T. Veenhuis
Department of Molecular and Comparative Pathobiology, Johns Hopkins University School of Medicine, Baltimore, MD, United States

Joel N. Blankson
Department of Molecular and Comparative Pathobiology, Johns Hopkins University School of Medicine, Baltimore, MD, United States
Department of Medicine, Johns Hopkins University School of Medicine, Baltimore, MD, United States

Amanda B. Macedo and Alberto Bosque
Department of Microbiology, Immunology and Tropical Medicine, George Washington University, Washington, DC, United States

Camille L. Novis
Department of Pathology, Division of Microbiology and Immunology, The University of Utah, Salt Lake City, UT, United States

Ben Berkhout and Alexander O. Pasternak
Laboratory of Experimental Virology, Department of Medical Microbiology, Amsterdam UMC, University of Amsterdam, Amsterdam, Netherlands

Zita Kruize and Neeltje A. Kootstra
Laboratory for Viral Immune Pathogenesis, Department of Experimental Immunology, Amsterdam UMC, Amsterdam Infection & Immunity Institute, University of Amsterdam, Amsterdam, Netherlands

Bapi Pahar, Dot Kuebler, Terri Rasmussen, Xiaolei Wang and Ronald S. Veazey
Division of Comparative Pathology, Tulane National Primate Research Center, Covington, LA, United States

Sudesh K. Srivastav
Department of Biostatistics and Bioinformatics, Tulane University, New Orleans, LA, United States

Arpita Das
Division of Microbiology, Tulane National Primate Research Center, Covington, LA, United States

Clementine Wallet, Marco De Rovere, Jeanne Van Assche, Fadoua Daouad, Olivier Rohr and Christian Schwartz
Université de Strasbourg, EA7292, FMTS, IUT Louis Pasteur, Schiltigheim, France

Stéphane De Wit
Division of Infectious Diseases, Saint-Pierre University Hospital, Université Libre de Bruxelles (ULB), Brussels, Belgium

Christine Bourgeois, Delphine Desjardins, Roger Le Grand and Abderaouf Damouche
Center for Immunology of Viral Infections and Autoimmune Diseases, IDMIT Department, IBFJ, CEA, Université Paris Sud, INSERM U1184, Fontenay-aux-Roses, France

Jennifer Gorwood, Claire Lagathu, Jacqueline Capeau and Véronique Béréziat
INSERM UMR_S 938, Centre de Recherche Saint-Antoine, Institut Hospitalo-Universitaire de Cardio-Métabolisme et Nutrition (ICAN), Sorbonne Université, Paris, France

Aurélie Barrail-Tran and Olivier Lambotte
AP-HP, Service de Médecine Interne et Immunologie Clinique, Hôpital Bicêtre, Groupe Hospitalier Universitaire Paris Sud, Le Kremlin-Bicêtre, France

Jana L. Jacobs, Elias K. Halvas, Melissa A. Tosiano and John W. Mellors
Division of Infectious Diseases, Department of Medicine, University of Pittsburgh School of Medicine, Pittsburgh, PA, United States

Ziv Sevilya
Internal Medicine Department A, Assuta Ashdod Medical Center, Ashdod, Israel
Crusaid Kobler AIDS center, Tel-Aviv Sourasky Medical Center, Tel-Aviv, Israel

Ehud Chorin
Crusaid Kobler AIDS center, Tel-Aviv Sourasky Medical Center, Tel-Aviv, Israel
Sackler Faculty of Medicine, Tel-Aviv University, Tel-Aviv, Israel

Orit Gal-Garber and Einat Zelinger
Interdepartmental Equipment Facility, Robert H. Smith Faculty of Agriculture, Food and Environment, the Hebrew University, Rehovot, Israel

Gideon Berke
Department of Immunology, Weizmann Institute of Science, Rehovot, Israel

Dan Turner and Boaz Avidor
Crusaid Kobler AIDS center, Tel-Aviv Sourasky Medical Center, Tel-Aviv, Israel
Sackler Faculty of Medicine, Tel-Aviv University, Tel-Aviv, Israel

David Hassin
Internal Medicine Department A, Assuta Ashdod Medical Center, Ashdod, Israel
Crusaid Kobler AIDS center, Tel-Aviv Sourasky Medical Center, Tel-Aviv, Israel
Sackler Faculty of Medicine, Tel-Aviv University, Tel-Aviv, Israel
Faculty of Health Sciences, Ben Gurion University of the Negev, Beer-Sheva, Israel

Dinesh Devadoss, Marko Manevski and Hitendra S. Chand
Department of Immunology and Nano-Medicine, Herbert Wertheim College of Medicine, Florida International University, Miami, FL, United States

Shashi P. Singh, Neerad Mishra and Mohan Sopori
Respiratory Immunology Division, Lovelace Respiratory Research Institute, Albuquerque, NM, United States

Arpan Acharya, Palsamy Periyasamy, Siddappa N. Byrareddy and Shilpa Buch
Department of Pharmacology & Experimental Neuroscience, University of Nebraska Medical Center, Omaha, NE, United States

Kieu Chinh Do, Carmen S. Tellez and Steven A. Belinsky
Lung Cancer Program, Lovelace Respiratory Research Institute, Albuquerque, NM, United States

Sundaram Ramakrishnan
Department of Surgery, University of Miami Miller School of Medicine, Miami, FL, United States

Romina Cabrera-Rodríguez, Silvia Pérez-Yanes, Judith Estévez-Herrera, Daniel Márquez-Arce and Agustín Valenzuela-Fernández
Laboratorio de Inmunología Celular y Viral, Unidad de Farmacología, Sección de Medicina, Facultad de Ciencias de la Salud, e IUETSPC de la Universidad de La Laguna, Campus de Ofra s/n, Tenerife, Spain

Cecilia Cabrera
AIDS Research Institute IrsiCaixa, Institut de Recerca en Ciències de la Salut Germans Trias i Pujol (IGTP), Barcelona, Spain

Lucile Espert
Institut de Recherche en Infectiologie de Montpellier, Université de Montpellier, CNRS, Montpellier, France

Julià Blanco
AIDS Research Institute IrsiCaixa, Institut de Recerca en Ciències de la Salut Germans Trias i Pujol (IGTP), Barcelona, Spain
Universitat de Vic-Central de Catalunya (UVIC-UCC), Catalonia, Spain

Index

www.ingramcontent.com/pod-product-compliance
Lightning Source LLC
LaVergne TN
LVHW080928210926
848485LV00004B/751